D1587567

# Molecular Pathology

## A Practical Guide for the Surgical Pathologist and Cytopathologist

# Molecular Pathology

A Practical Guide for the Surgical Pathologist
and Cytopathologist

Edited by

**John M. S. Bartlett**
Ontario Institute for Cancer Research, Toronto, Ontario, Canada

**Abeer Shaaban**
Queen Elizabeth Hospital, Birmingham, UK, and Tanta University Hospital, Tanta, Egypt

**Fernando Schmitt**
The Laboratoire National de Santé, Dudelange, Luxembourg

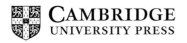

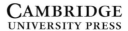

## CAMBRIDGE
### UNIVERSITY PRESS

University Printing House, Cambridge CB2 8BS, United Kingdom

Cambridge University Press is part of the University of Cambridge.

It furthers the University's mission by disseminating knowledge in the pursuit of education, learning and research at the highest international levels of excellence.

www.cambridge.org
Information on this title: www.cambridge.org/9781107443464

© Cambridge University Press 2015

First published 2015

Printed in the United Kingdom by Bell and Bain Ltd

*A catalogue record for this publication is available from the British Library*

*Library of Congress Cataloguing in Publication data*
Molecular pathology (2015)
Molecular pathology : a practical guide for the surgical pathologist and cytopathologist / edited by John M. S. Bartlett, Abeer Shaaban, Fernando Schmitt.
    p. ; cm.
Includes bibliographical references and index.
ISBN 978-1-107-08298-4 (Hardback) – ISBN 978-1-107-44346-4 (Mixed Media) – ISBN 978-1-316-01470-7 (ebook)
I. Bartlett, John M. S., editor.    II. Shaaban, Abeer, editor.
III. Schmitt, Fernando, editor.    IV. Title.
[DNLM: 1. Pathology, Molecular–methods.    2. Molecular Diagnostic Techniques–methods.  QZ 50]
RB113
616.07–dc23    2015022902

ISBN 978-1-107-44346-4 Mixed Media
ISBN 978-1-107-08298-4 Hardback
ISBN 978-1-316-01470-7 Cambridge Books Online

# Contents

# Contributors

**Sylvia L. Asa, MD, PhD**
Department of Pathology, University Health
Network, and the Department of Laboratory
Medicine and Pathobiology, University of Toronto,
Ontario, Canada

**John M. S. Bartlett, BSc (Hons), PhD, FRCPath**
Director of Transformative Pathology and Improved
Management of Early Cancer at the Ontario Institute
for Cancer Research, Toronto, Ontario, Canada

**Jane Bayani, PhD**
Ontario Institute for Cancer Research, Toronto,
Ontario, Canada

**Philippe L. Bedard**
Princess Margaret Cancer Centre, University Health
Network, Toronto, Ontario, Canada, and the
Department of Medicine, University of Toronto,
Toronto, Ontario, Canada

**Claudio Bellevicine, MD**
Pathology Division, Department of Public Health,
University of Naples, Federico II, Naples, Italy

**Hal K. Berman**
Princess Margaret Cancer Centre, University Health
Network, Toronto, Ontario, Canada, and the
Department of Laboratory Medicine and
Pathobiology, University of Toronto, Ontario, Canada

**Martha Bishop Pitman, MD**
Director of Cytopathology, Massachusetts General
Hospital, Boston, Massachusetts, USA, and Associate
Professor of Pathology, Harvard Medical School,
Boston, Massachusetts, USA

**Marsela Braunstein, PhD**
Ontario Institute for Cancer Research, Toronto,
Ontario, Canada, and Department of Immunology,
University of Toronto, Ontario, Canada

**Andrew M. K. Brown, PhD**
Ontario Institute for Cancer Research, Toronto,
Ontario, Canada

**Lukas Bubendorf, MD**
Institute of Pathology, University Hospital Basel,
Basel, Switzerland

**Sarah E. Coupland**
Professor and George Holt Chair in Pathology,
Deputy Head of Department of Molecular
and Clinical Cancer Medicine, Honorary
Consultant in Pathology, and Director of the
NWCR Centre, Department of Molecular and
Clinical Cancer Medicine, University of Liverpool,
Liverpool, UK

**Ben Davidson, MD, PhD**
Department of Pathology, Oslo University Hospital,
Norwegian Radium Hospital, and University of Oslo,
Faculty of Medicine, Institute of Clinical Medicine,
Oslo, Norway

**Paul J. van Diest, MD, PhD**
Professor and Head, Department of Pathology,
University Medical Centre Utrecht, Utrecht, the
Netherlands

**Pedro Farinha**
Pathology, Department of Molecular and Clinical
Cancer Medicine, University of Liverpool,
Liverpool, UK

**Maria Sofia Fernandes**
Institute of Molecular Pathology and Immunology
of the University of Porto (IPATIMUP), Porto,
Portugal

**Petra van der Groep, PhD**
Department of Pathology, University Medical Centre
Utrecht, Utrecht, the Netherlands

**Aaron R. Hansen**
Princess Margaret Cancer Centre, University Health Network, Toronto, Ontario, Canada, and the Department of Medicine, University of Toronto, Toronto, Ontario, Canada

**Carlo V. Hojilla, MD, PhD**
Department of Laboratory Medicine and Pathobiology, University of Toronto, Ontario, Canada

**Angela B. Y. Hui, PhD**
Ontario Cancer Institute, University Health Network, Ontario, Canada

**Suzanne Kamel-Reid**
Princess Margaret Cancer Centre, University Health Network, Toronto, Ontario, Canada, and Princess Margaret Cancer Centre, Ontario Cancer Institute, Toronto, Ontario, Canada

**Jerzy Klijanienko, MD, PhD, MIAC**
Associate Professor, Institut Curie, Paris, France

**Robert Kornegoor MD, PhD**
Department of Pathology, Gelre Hospital, Apeldoorn, the Netherlands

**Paul M. Krzyzanowski, PhD**
Ontario Institute for Cancer Research, Toronto, Ontario, Canada

**Sigurd F. Lax, MD, PhD**
Professor and Head at the Department of Pathology, General Hospital Graz West, and the Academic Teaching Hospital of the Medical University Graz, Graz, Austria

**Adhemar Longatto Filho, MSc, PhD, PMIAC**
Laboratory of Medical Investigation (LIM) 14, Faculty of Medicine University São Paulo, São Paulo, and the Molecular Oncology Research Center, Barretos Cancer Hospital, Pio XII Foundation, Barretos, Brazil; Life and Health Sciences Research Institute (ICVS), School of Health Sciences, University of Minho, Braga, Portugal; ICVS/3B's – PT Government Associate Laboratory, Braga/Guimarães, Portugal

**Umberto Malapelle, PhD**
Pathology Division, Department of Public Health, University of Naples, Federico II, Naples, Italy

**Kirsten D. Mertz, MD, PhD**
Institute of Pathology Liestal, Cantonal Hospital Baselland, Liestal, Switzerland

**Ozgur Mete, MD**
Department of Pathology, University Health Network, and the Department of Laboratory Medicine and Pathobiology, University of Toronto, Ontario, Canada

**Cathy B. Moelans, PhD**
Department of Pathology, University Medical Centre Utrecht, Utrecht, the Netherlands

**Susan Picton, BMedSci, BM BS, FRCPCH**
Consultant in Paediatric and Adolescent Oncology, Department of Paediatric Oncology, LTHT Leeds, UK

**Paul Roberts, FRCPath, BSc**
Consultant Cytogeneticist, Cytogenetics Department, LTHT Leeds, UK

**Manuel Salto-Tellez, MD, FRCPath, FRCPCH**
Northern Ireland – Molecular Pathology Laboratory, Centre for Cancer Research and Cell Biology, Queen's University, Belfast, UK

**Fernando Schmitt, MD, PhD, FIAC**
Director of the Department of Medicine and Pathology at the Laboratoire National de Santé, Dudelange, Luxembourg

**Raquel Seruca**
Institute of Molecular Pathology and Immunology of the University of Porto (IPATIMUP), Porto, Portugal, and the Faculty of Medicine, University of Porto, Porto, Portugal

**Abeer Shaaban, PhD, FRCPath, Diploma Health Research**
Consultant Pathologist, Clinical Academic Lead, Queen Elizabeth Hospital, Birmingham, and Honorary Senior Lecturer, University of Birmingham, UK, and Lecturer at the Department of Pathology, Tanta University Hospital, Tanta, Egypt

**Jens Stahlschmidt, MD, FRCPath**
Consultant Paediatric-Perinatal Histopathologist, Department of Cellular Pathology, LTHT Leeds, UK

**Mahadeo A. Sukhai**
Princess Margaret Cancer Centre, University Health Network, Toronto, Ontario, Canada and Princess Margaret Cancer Centre, Ontario Cancer Institute, Toronto, Ontario, Canada

**Stamatios Theocharis, MD, PhD**
Associate Professor of Pathology, Medical School, University of Athens, Athens, Greece

**Luigi Tornillo, MD, PhD**
Associate Professor of Pathology, University of Basel Department of Pathology, University Hospital of Basel, Basel, Switzerland

**Giancarlo Troncone, MD, PhD**
Pathology Division, Department of Public Health, University of Naples, Federico II, Naples, Italy

**Sérgia Velho**
Institute of Molecular Pathology and Immunology of the University of Porto (IPATIMUP), Porto, Portugal

**Elena Vigliar, MD**
Pathology Division, Department of Public Health, University of Naples, Federico II, Naples, Italy

**Jelle Wesseling, MD, PhD**
Department of Pathology, The Netherlands Cancer Institute, Amsterdam, the Netherlands

**Annette D. Wong, BSc**
Ontario Cancer Institute, University Health Network, Ontario, Canada

**Roseann I. Wu, MD, MPH**
Assistant Professor of Clinical Pathology & Laboratory Medicine, University of Pennsylvania Health System, Philadelphia, Pennsylvania, USA

**Benedict Yan, MD**
Department of Pathology and Laboratory Medicine, KK Women's and Children's Hospital Singapore, Singapore

**Bin Yang, MD, PhD**
Medical Director of Molecular Cytopathology, and Director of International Affairs of CCL at the Robert J. Tomsich Pathology and Laboratory Medicine Institute, Cleveland, Ohio, USA

**Philipe C. Zuzarte, PhD**
Ontario Institute for Cancer Research, Toronto, Ontario, Canada

# Preface

The practice of pathology has undergone significant evolution over the last few years. Molecular pathology has been instrumental in driving refined classifications of tumors and providing prognostic and predictive information based on the molecular phenotype of those tumors. As the wealth of targeted therapies in development is applied to the treatment of tumors, the demand for molecular diagnostic testing in pathology will inevitably increase.

Molecular pathology has therefore become an integral part of the daily diagnostic practice of pathologists. As defined by the Medical Research Council (MRC), molecular pathology is a discipline that seeks to describe and understand the origins and mechanisms of disease at the level of macromolecules (for example, DNA, RNA and protein) largely using patient samples. Pathologists are often asked to provide a large amount of diagnostic and prognostic information derived from molecular testing of tissue samples or cytological preparations. Moreover, through identifying the shared molecular characteristics in groups/strata of patients (stratified medicine), better diagnostic tools and effective therapeutic measures could be developed with significant health and economic benefits.

This book is aimed towards general and specialist practising and trainee pathologists to serve as an everyday manual for the practising pathologist. It contains the essential molecular pathology information in a format relevant to the reporting pathologist. It provides an overall view of current molecular pathology techniques followed by separate chapters detailing their clinical applications in various tissues covering both histopathology and cytopathology. We believe this book will aid pathologists in their daily practice of providing essential information for better diagnosis and management of patients.

# Glossary

**Accuracy:** In terms of biomarker measurements, accuracy is defined as how close the measurement of any particular analyte approaches its true value (see ASCO-CAP guidelines on HER2 2007). Such a definition presupposes the existence of a "gold standard" for the measurement of any particular analyte, which can represent a significant challenge to the demonstration of analytical accuracy in biomarker studies.

**Adjuvant therapy:** In the context of cancer therapy, adjuvant therapy is treatment, usually chemotherapy or radiotherapy, given to patients where the primary cancer has been eradicated (by surgery), but where there remains a statistical probability that undetected or undetectable disease persists elsewhere. It represents a clinical area where treatment is based not on evidence of disease, but on risk of disease.

**AFIP:** Armed Forces Institute of Pathology – US government institution, founded in 1862, which provides diagnostic consultation, education and research in pathology.

**Allele:** One of two or more variant DNA sequences occurring at a particular gene locus. Typically one allele is more common, and other alleles ("variants") are rare. Allelic variation may impact on gene function.

**Allele-specific oligonucleotide (ASO):** ASO is a short piece of synthetic DNA complementary to the sequence of a variable target DNA. It acts as a probe for the presence of the target in a Southern blot assay or, more commonly, in the simpler Dot blot assay.

**Amplification refractory mutation system (ARMS):** ARMS is a simple method for detecting any mutation involving single base changes or small deletions. ARMS is based on the use of sequence-specific PCR primers that allow amplification of test DNA only when the target allele is contained within the sample. Following an ARMS reaction, the presence or absence of a PCR product is diagnostic for the presence or absence of the target allele.

**Amplification:** An increase in the number of copies of a gene or DNA fragment usually as a result of a chromosomal alteration during tumor pathogenesis.

**Amsterdam Criteria (see also Bethesda guidelines):** The Amsterdam Criteria were developed following a consensus which arose out of the 1990 meeting of the International Collaborative Group on Hereditary Non-Polyposis Colorectal Cancer (ICG-HPNCC) or Lynch syndrome in order to assist clinicians in the identification of individuals or families who were likely to suffer from this condition.

**Aneusomy:** This describes the condition where there exists greater than two copies of a whole chromosome or chromosomal region in comparison to the normally expected two copies per cell in the human genome.

**Annealing temperature:** The temperature that allows for the formation of hydrogen bonds between complementary bases in a sequence and hence allows for hybridization.

**Annealing:** The process wherein complementary bases (e.g. dATP↔dTTP and dCTP↔dGTP) within a nucleic acid sequence align following formation of hydrogen bonds to create a double-stranded molecule.

**ASCO guidelines:** Guidelines developed under the auspices of the American Society of Clinical Oncology.

**ASCO-CAP guidelines:** Guidelines, usually with regard to diagnostic procedures developed by groups of experts under the auspices of the American Society of Clinical Oncology and the College of American Pathologists.

**Automated Childhood Cancer Information System (ACCIS):** An authoritative source of European data on cancer incidence and survival of children and adolescents.

**Autosomal dominant:** A disease trait where an inherited allele from only one parent is sufficient to confer risk of disease or disease itself. In this case, the second parental allele is recessive.

**Autosomal:** Pertaining to any of the paired (i.e. non-sex) chromosomes within a cell.

**Bacterial Artificial Chromosome (BAC):** BAC describes the use of a construct where a fragment of the desired DNA (between 150 and 300 kb) can be inserted into the F-plasmid and transformed into *Escherichia coli* (*E.coli*). Transformed *E.coli* are cultured and the DNA extracted to be used for molecular analyses.

**Base pair:** Two DNA nucleotides paired together in double-stranded DNA. When used as a quantity (e.g. 8 base pairs, or 8 bp), this term refers to the length of a nucleotide sequence.

**Bethesda guidelines (see also Amsterdam Criteria):** The Bethesda guidelines were developed by the American National Cancer Institute (NCI) as a means of screening for individuals who should be counseled to undergo testing for HNPCC or Lynch syndrome related tumors.

**Biliary intraepithelial neoplasia (BilIN):** BilIN is a precursor lesion of hilar/perihilar and extrahepatic cholangiocarcinoma. BilIN represents the process of multistep cholangiocarcinogenesis and is the biliary counterpart of pancreatic intraepithelial neoplasia (PanIN).

**Biochips, Chips or Microarray:** This describes the use of a solid substrate, such as glass or polystyrene plastics, as a matrix for binding test materials, typically DNA or RNA probes, such that several (hundred or thousand) tests can be performed at one time in a high-throughput manner.

**Bioinformatics:** This is a discipline of computer science applying the use of computer programming to develop strategies for the analysis and management of high-level biological data.

**Biomarker:** Any substance, structure or process that can be measured in the body or its products which may influence or predict the presence, type or outcome of disease, the effect of treatments, interventions and even unintended environmental exposure, such as to chemicals or nutrients. NIH definition – "a characteristic that is objectively measured and evaluated as an indicator of normal biologic processes, pathogenic processes, or pharmacologic responses to a therapeutic intervention."

**Blastema:** An aggregate of histologically undifferentiated, typically "small round blue cells." Blastema can differentiate into different cell types/tissues.

**Bouin fixative:** This is a compound fixative used in histology, composed of picric acid, acetic acid and formaldehyde in an aqueous solution.

**BRAF:** BRAF is a member of the Raf kinase family of growth signal transduction protein kinases. The protein plays a role in regulating the MAP kinase/ERK's signaling pathway, which affects cell division, differentiation and secretion. Mutated BRAF, especially of the V600E BRAF, is seen in melanomas and also benign naevi. Drugs that inhibit mutated BRAF have been approved for treating late-stage melanoma.

**Break-apart FISH probes:** Dual colour DNA probes with a 3' and 5' component mapping either side of the breakpoint of specific genetic rearrangement, which appear as a fusion signal on a normal chromosome. Genomic rearrangement within tumor cells separates the probes, allowing visualization of the two component parts as distinct entities and distinctly separate colors.

**Brightfield microscopy:** Microscopy using transmitted white light.

**CAP/IASLC/AMP lung biomarker guidelines:** The College of American Pathologists (CAP), the International Association for the Study of Lung Cancer (IASLC) and the Association for Molecular Pathology (AMP) set out to create standardized international guidelines for lung cancer biomarker testing.

**CAP:** The College of American Pathologists.

**Catalogue of somatic mutations in cancer (COSMIC):** a website (http://cancer.sanger.ac.uk/cancergenome/ projects/cosmic/) designed to store and display somatic mutation information and related details of human cancers. The mutation data and associated information are extracted from the primary literature and entered into the COSMIC database. Data from The Cancer Genome Atlas and the International Cancer Genome Consortium portals are also uploaded into COSMIC.

**CDK4 gene:** Cyclin-dependent kinase 4 gene, also known as cell division protein kinase 4, is an enzyme that is encoded by the CDK4 gene. CDK4 is a member of the cyclin-dependent kinase family.

**Cell-block:** A paraffin block, suitable for sectioning, staining and microscopic study, prepared from any suspension of cells in fluid (i.e. aspirates or washings); cells are concentrated by centrifugation or filtering, and the resulting aggregation is processed as if it were a solid specimen of tissue.

**Centromere:** This is described as the part of the chromosome where sister chromatids are most closely attached, and visualized as a constricted region. Centromeres are composed of DNA with unique repetitive DNA sequences called satellite repeats. Each chromosome contains one centromere and these are often targets for enumeration assays.

**Chimaeric fusion proteins:** Novel oncogenic proteins, often tumor-specific, formed from the rearrangement and fusion of two genes, most usually by a chromosome translocation.

**Chromatin immuopreciptiation (ChIP):** This describes a type of immunoprecipitation experimental technique used to investigate the interaction between proteins and DNA. The DNA-protein complex is precipitated using antibodies mobilized to a substrate. The protein is then unlinked from the DNA, and the subsequent DNA is extracted and analyzed.

**Chromogenic *in situ* hybridization (CISH):** This describes the detection of DNA or RNA in tissues or cells using specific probes that are visualized by bright-field microscopy.

**Chromosomal rearrangement:** This describes the disruption of the chromosome that results in the gain, loss or physical translocation/rearrangement of chromosomal material.The rearrangement may occur within the same chromosome (intrachromosomal), or between chromosomes (extrachromosomal, or chromosomal translocation). Rearrangements may be relatively simple or complex and involve several chromosomes.

**Chromosomal translocation:** This is a chromosome abnormality caused by rearrangement of varying-sized parts between non-homologous chromosomes. A gene fusion may be created when the translocation joins two otherwise separated genes: this is commonly observed in cancer, particularly NHL. Chromosomal translocations are detected on cytogenetics (e.g. by using fluorescence *in situ* hybridization, FISH) or a karyotype of the affected cells. Translocations can be **balanced** (in an even exchange of material with no genetic information extra or missing, and ideally full functionality) or **unbalanced** (where the exchange of chromosome material is unequal, resulting in extra or missing genes).

**Chromosome instability (CIN):** This is a phenotype where increased mis-segregation of chromosomes at mitosis leads to increasingly variable chromosome numbers within tumor cells. The phenotype is frequently a result of deregulation of key cell cycle checkpoints, especially those at G2/M. CIN is associated with increased sensitivity to DNA-damaging agents.

**Circulating tumor cells:** As cancerous cells within a tumor proliferate, they do not all stay in a neighborhood. Some tumor cells shed into the vasculature from a primary tumor and circulate in the bloodstream. These circulating tumor cells (CTCs) can remain loose in circulation, cluster together as they travel, or lodge themselves in new tissues. CTCs thus constitute seeds for metastasis in distant organs, a mechanism that is responsible for the vast majority of cancer-related deaths. The common origin of CTCs means that they hold information about the primary tumor. Detection of CTCs in peripheral blood can serve as a "liquid biopsy" approach, which can be used for diagnosis and disease monitoring.

**Class switch recombination:** A biological mechanism that changes a B lymphocyte's production of immunoglobulin (i.e. antibodies) from one class to another, such as from the isotype IgM to the isotype IgG. During this process, the constant-region portion of the immunoglobulin heavy chain is changed, but the variable region of the heavy chain stays the same (the terms "variable" and "constant" refer to changes or lack thereof between antibodies that target different epitopes). Since the variable region does not change, class switching does not affect antigen specificity. Instead, the antibody retains affinity for the same antigens, but can interact with different and additional effector molecules.

**Clone:** An identical copy of a DNA sequence or entire gene; one or more cells derived from and identical to a single ancestor cell OR to isolate a gene or specific sequence of DNA.

**Comparative Genomic Hybridization (CGH):** This describes a method of comparing two differentially labeled DNA for the changes in copy-number between them. A typical experiment compares equal amounts of the test DNA (i.e. tumor) to a reference (i.e. normal) DNA by ascertaining the differences at a particular genomic location. This is normally achieved by the changes in the ratio of the emitted fluorescence by the test DNA vs. the reference DNA.

**Copy-number Variation (CNV):** CNV refers to the genetic trait involving the number of copies of a particular gene present in the genome of an individual. Genetic variants, including insertions, deletions and duplications of segments of DNA, are also collectively referred to as CNVs. CNVs account for a significant proportion of the genetic variation between individuals. Also called copy-number variant or copy-number aberration (CNA).

**Core needle biopsy (CNB):** CNB is a diagnostic procedure that uses a larger, hollow needle to withdraw small cylinders (or cores) of tissues, maintaining the architectural structure.

**Coverage:** The proportion of a target sequence (a single gene, a whole genome, etc.) sequenced. Coverage is sometimes used interchangeably with depth, when referring to "average coverage."

**CpG island methylator phenotype (CIMP):** CIMP is a phenomenon where multiple CpG islands are hypermethylated in cancer (first described in colorectal cancer), leading to the putative deregulation of key genes.

**Cryoarrays:** Tissue microarrays of snap-frozen tissues in OCT. They allow performing studies that are very difficult on FFPE tissues (e.g. proteomic studies, RNA hybridization studies).

**DCIS:** Ductal Carcinoma *in situ* of the breast.

**Deletion:** A genetic alteration that occurs when a segment of DNA is absent. The size of the segment can range from a single base to multiple genes.

**Denaturation:** The process of applying heat to break bonds between complementary bases, which unwinds DNA and leads to the separation of a double strand into two single-stranded molecules.

**Depth:** The average number of times base pairs in a region are sequenced. Depth can also refer to the number of times a single position was sequenced. Sometimes used interchangeably with coverage.

**DFSP (dermatofibrosarcoma protuberans):** An uncommon skin tumor arising in the deeper layer of the skin (the dermis). It grows slowly and has a tendency to recur after excision, but rarely metastasizes.

**Diagnostic biomarker:** This biomarker gives an indication if a disease exists or not.

**DNA methylation:** An epigenetic mechanism for negatively regulating gene expression through methylation of CpG islands within gene promoters; tumor cells often have hypermethylation of tumor suppressor genes and hypomethylation of oncogenes.

**Double minute chromosome (DMs or dims):** DMs are small fragments of extrachromosomal DNA that have the ability to replicate and are a means by which DNA may become amplified. These are seen as multiple extrachromosomal paired structures. Frequently, double minute chromosomes harbor oncogenes.

**Down's syndrome:** Human genetic syndrome associated with an additional copy of chromosome 21.

**Driver gene:** Any gene key to the development or progression of cancer.

**Driver mutation:** A mutation in a driver gene that results in a deleterious effect on the protein and confers the cell with a survival advantage.

**EGFR tyrosine kinase inhibitors (TKIs):** These drugs occupy the TK adenosine triphosphate (ATP) binding site, thereby preventing EGFR activation and downstream signaling effects.

**Endobronchial ultrasound-guided fine-needle aspiration (EBUS-FNA):** This is a safe and minimally invasive bronchoscopic technique that allows both visualization and cytologic sampling with a high diagnostic yield in a patient with mediastinal lymphadenopathy. Besides the most common indication of staging for a patient with a primary lung carcinoma, EBUS-FNA can be used to identify benign infectious and non-infectious processes, as well as lymphoma and malignancy of unknown primary.

**Enzyme-linked Immunosorbant Assay (ELISA):** ELISA describes the detection of a protein typically in a liquid sample such as urine, serum or blood, using the antibody-antigen interaction. Standard ELISA entails the mobilization of the capture antibody to a substrate such as a plastic multi-welled plate. The sample to be tested is added to the well, allowing any antigens in the sample to be captured by the mobilized antibody. The captured antigen is then detected using an antibody conjugated to a detection system, such as a chromogen or fluorescent molecule.

**Epidermal growth factor receptor (EGFR) mutation analysis:** Part of the current standard of care in advanced non-small cell lung cancer (NSCLC).

**Epigenetics:** This describes the study of gene expression changes that are not due to modifications to the DNA sequence. Most commonly, epigenetics refers to the level of methylation experienced at cytosine residues.

**Exon:** The sequence of DNA present in mature messenger RNA, some of which encodes the amino acids of a protein. Most genes have multiple exons, with introns between them.

**Extension:** The addition of nucleic acid bases during nucleic acid replication.

**Fallopian tube tumors:** Neoplastic tissue originates from Fallopian tubes. Benign tumors (adenomatoid tumors) are originated from the subserosal area. Tubal adenocarcinomas are rare and are often associated to the BRCA germline mutation. Fallopian tube cells are also involved in ovarian carcinoma origin.

**Familial adenomatous polyposis:** An inherited condition in which numerous polyps (growths that protrude from mucous membranes) form on the inside walls of the colon and rectum. It increases the risk of colorectal cancer. Also called familial polyposis and FAP.

**Familial colorectal cancer type X syndrome (FCC-XS):** This term is often used to describe apparently familial or Lynch syndrome colorectal cancers where no underlying mismatch repair gene mutation or defect can be identified. To fall within this grouping, cancers must satisfy the "Amsterdam criteria," but have no evidence of mismatch repair defects.

**Fine-needle aspiration (FNA):** FNA biopsy (FNAB) or FNA cytology (FNAC) is a diagnostic procedure used to investigate superficial lumps or deep masses. In this technique, a thin needle is inserted into the lesion for sampling of cells that, after being stained, will be examined under a microscope.

**Flow cytometry:** This is a laser-based, biophysical technology employed in cell counting, cell sorting, biomarker detection and protein engineering, by suspending cells in a stream of fluid and passing them by an electronic detection apparatus. It allows simultaneous multiparametric analysis of the physical and chemical characteristics of up to thousands of particles per second. This technique is used in the diagnosis of several diseases, especially lymphoproliferative diseases, but has many other applications in basic research and clinical practice.

**Fluorescence *in situ* hybridization (FISH):** FISH describes the detection of DNA or RNA in tissues or cells using specific probes that are visualized by fluorescence microscopy. The genomics or cellular location of these labeled probes to their targets is achieved by complementary base pairing. It is important for visualizing and mapping of chromosomal abnormalities and rearrangements. FISH can also be used to determine how many chromosomes of a certain type are present in a cell. For FISH, small DNA strands called probes that have a fluorescent label attached and that are complementary to specific parts of a chromosome are used to look at specific areas of a chromosome. FISH does not need to be performed on cells that are actively dividing, which makes it a very versatile procedure that can be performed on formalin-fixed and paraffin-embedded tissues.

**Fluorescence microscopy:** Fluorescence microscopy uses fluorescence to generate the image. It makes use of filters to excite the fluorescent molecule at a particular wavelength, enabling it to emit a signal within the visual or non-visual range.

**Food and Drug Administration (FDA):** The US Food and Drug Administration is responsible for the regulatory oversight and licensing of new diagnostic tests and therapeutics (among other roles) in the United States.

**Formalin-fixed paraffin-embedded (FFPE):** A method of tissue preservation and storage wherein tissues are fixed using a formaldehyde-based medium (formalin) and embedded in a wax matrix (paraffin) that permits tissue sectioning.

**Fusion probes:** This describes the use of differentially labeled probes from two different chromosomal regions for the detection of a translocation event between them. When the two probes are co-localized, the fusion event has occurred. When the two probes are separate, the fusion event has not occurred.

**Gardner syndrome:** This is an autosomal dominant form of polyposis characterized by the presence of multiple polyps in the colon, together with tumors outside the colon. The extracolonic tumors may include osteomas of the skull, thyroid cancer, epidermoid cysts and fibromas, as well as the occurrence of desmoid tumors in approximately 15 percent of affected individuals.

**Gastrointestinal stromal tumor (GIST):** GIST is a neoplasm that arises in the smooth muscle pacemaker cells of Cajal. It is pathologically identified by a tyrosine kinase membrane receptor, c-kit protein (CD 177 antigen). Most occur in the stomach, and gastric GISTs have a lower malignant potential than tumors found elsewhere in the GI tract.

**GCP:** Good Clinical Practice is a system of quality management governing the performance of clinical research, including clinical trials, involving human subjects. The principles of GCP encompass ethical practices, documentation, privacy and all associated aspects of clinical research involving human subjects. Increasingly, where translational laboratory research is allied to clinical trials, this is linked to Good Laboratory Practice in a combined system of Good Clinical and Laboratory Practice.

**Gene expression profiling:** This is the measurement of the activity (the expression) of thousands of genes at once, to create a global picture of cellular function. These profiles can, for example, distinguish between cells that are actively dividing, or show how the cells react to a particular treatment. Many experiments of this sort measure an entire genome simultaneously, that is, every gene present in a particular cell.

**Germline mutation:** A gene change in a body's reproductive cell (egg or sperm) that becomes incorporated into the DNA of every cell in the body of the offspring. Germline mutations are passed on from parents to offspring and are present in every cell. They are also called hereditary mutation.

**GLP:** Good Laboratory Practice is a system of quality management and assessment of quality through quality controls implemented in research organizations and other bodies carrying out laboratory research. Implicit in this process is the assumption that: (a) quality management is an essential component of both pre-clinical and clinical research; and (b) all diagnostic procedures, which are regulated by other bodies in addition, will nonetheless adhere to GLP.

**Hamartomatous polyposis syndromes:** These are a heterogeneous group of disorders that share an autosomal-dominant pattern of inheritance and are characterized by hamartomatous polyps of the gastrointestinal tract. These syndromes include juvenile polyposis syndrome, Peutz-Jeghers syndrome and the PTEN hamartoma tumor syndrome. The frequency and location of the polyps vary considerably among syndromes, as does the affected patient's predisposition to the development of gastrointestinal and other malignancies.

**Hereditary non-polyposis colorectal cancer (HNPCC):** See also Lynch syndrome. HNPCC is an autosomal dominant genetic condition that has a high risk of colon cancer as well as other cancers, including endometrial cancer (second most common), ovary, stomach, small intestine, hepatobiliary tract, upper urinary tract, brain and skin. The increased risk for these cancers is due to inherited mutations that impair DNA mismatch repair.

**High-resolution melting analysis (HRMA):** HRMA is a post-PCR analysis method used to identify variations in nucleic acid sequences. The method is based on detecting small differences in PCR melting (dissociation) curves. It is enabled by improved dsDNA-binding dyes used in conjunction with real-time PCR instrumentation that has precise temperature ramp control and advanced data capture capabilities. Data are analyzed and manipulated using software designed specifically for HRM analysis.

**Hodgkin's lymphoma (HL):** HL was first described by Thomas Hodgkin in 1832 and later classified by Robert Luke in 1963. There are four particular subtypes of classic HL (excluding nodular lymphocyte predominant HL), based on the Reed-Sternberg cell morphology and accompanying reactive cell infiltrate and degree of sclerosis. HL tend to be more radiation sensitive than NHL.

**Homebox genes:** A large family of genes directly involved with human embryonic development. They can also regulate the activity of other genes, acting as transcription factors, and tumor suppressors. Deregulated activity or mutations of these genes are associated to the malignancies development.

**HPV (Human papillomavirus):** More than 150 types of this virus are currently identified which generally correlate with the three clinical categories applied to HPV infection: anogenital or mucosal, non-genital cutaneous, epidermodysplasia verruciformis. HPV is common: most people have the virus at some time in their lives. In most cases, the virus causes no symptoms and goes away on its own. Some types of HPV can cause changes in the cells of the cervix or the lining of the mouth and throat. They are known as high-risk HPVs. The changed cells have an increased risk of becoming malignant. Other types of HPV can cause warts, but do not usually cause cell changes that develop into cancer. They are therefore called low-risk HPVs.

**HPV testing:** Use of molecular identification of high-risk HPV for screening proposals in order to enhance the sensitivity of cervical lesions detection generally underestimated by conventional Pap test. The specificity is supposed to also be improved with cytology reflex test for cases tested positive for HPV.

**ICGC:** The International Cancer Genome Consortium is a collaborative network of cancer genome projects, including the TCGA (see TCGA). The goal of the ICGC (see ICGC.org) is "to obtain a comprehensive description of genomic, transcriptomic and epigenomic changes in 50 different tumor types and or subtypes which are of clinical and societal importance across the globe."

**Immunohistochemistry (IHC):** An immunostaining technique to detect protein expression in tissue sections by the use of antibodies that bind specifically to antigens in tissues and are visualized by a marker such as fluorescent dye, enzyme or colloidal gold. Immunohistochemistry is widely used in the diagnosis of malignant cells, to study the localization of biomarkers and differentially expressed proteins in different tissues.

***In situ* hybridization (ISH):** A method detecting mRNA or DNA *in situ* in tissue or cell block sections using chromogenic or fluorescent probes, allowing signal localization to specific cell populations.

**Indels:** Mutations that result in the insertion and/or deletion of nucleotides.

**Interphase cells:** This describes the state of nuclei within tissues that are not undergoing mitosis.

**Intraductal papillary mucinous neoplasia (IPMN):** Intraductal grossly visible (1 cm or more) epithelial neoplasm of mucin-producing cells, arising in main pancreatic duct or its branches; neoplastic epithelium is usually papillary; variable mucin secretion, duct dilatation (cyst formation) and dysplasia; classify based on the highest degree of cytoarchitectural atypia and invasiveness as IPMN with low- to intermediate-grade dysplasia, IPMN with high-grade dysplasia and IPMN with associated invasive carcinoma.

**Intrinsic subtypes:** molecular subtypes of breast cancer based on microarray gene expression patterns that improve prognostication and prediction of response to therapy compared with categories defined by classical clinicopathological characteristics.

**Karyotyping:** The classical method for identifying chromosome rearrangements in tumors. Almost all specific translocations known in soft tissue tumors have been detected using this method.

**Ki-67:** This is a cellular marker strictly associated with cell proliferation. During interphase, the Ki-67 antigen can be exclusively detected within the cell nucleus, whereas in mitosis most of the protein is relocated to the surface of the chromosomes. Ki-67 protein is present during all active phases of the cell cycle ($G_1$, S, $G_2$ and mitosis), but is absent from resting cells ($G_0$).

**Kleinfelter syndrome:** Human genetic syndrome affecting males where there is an extra chromosome X, in addition to the normal X and Y chromosome per cell.

**Laser capture micro-dissection (LCM):** The use of a laser to precisely dissect tissues under a microscope.

**Liquid-based cytology:** This is a method of preparing samples for examination in cytopathology. The sample is collected, by a small brush or needle, in the same way as for a conventional smear test, but rather than the smear being transferred directly to a microscope slide, the sample is deposited into a small bottle of preservative liquid.

**Ligation:** The enzymatic process of joining two DNA sequences by creating new phosphodiester bonds.

**Loss of heterozygosity (LOH):** This describes the condition where there is the loss of a copy of a given locus, gene or chromosomal region.

**Lynch syndrome** (see HNPCC)

**Malignant fibrous histiocytoma (MFH):** A type of sarcoma arising in bone and/or soft tissue. Controversy exists as to its cell of origin. In 2002, the World Health Organization (WHO) declassified MFH as a formal diagnostic entity and renamed it as an undifferentiated pleomorphic sarcoma not otherwise specified (NOS).

**Massively parallel sequencing:** Another term for next generation sequencing.

**MDM2 gene:** Murine double minutes 2, a gene that is commonly amplified in well-differentiated liposarcoma.

**Melting temperature:** The temperature at which 50 percent of the oligonucleotide primers are bound to their complementary sequence and the other 50 percent are separated into single-stranded molecules.

**MEN (Multiple Endocrine Neoplasia):** Familial syndromes that are attributable to germline mutations in tumor suppressor genes. These syndromes are inherited as autosomal dominant tumor syndromes with variable penetrance.

**Metabolomics:** A method by which the levels of different metabolites (sugars, lipids, phosphate-containing substances and others) are quantitatively measured; often altered in tumor cells compared to normal cells, as well as following tumor-targeting therapy, such as radiation and chemotherapy.

**Metaphase spreads/cells:** This describes the preparation of cells that enables the chromosomes to be visualized at metaphase. Mitotically active cells are inhibited at metaphase and fixed in solution to maintain chromosomal architecture.

**Metastasis:** This is the spread of a cancer disease from one organ or body part to another not directly connected with it.

**Microarrays:** This is a multiplex lab-on-a-chip. It is a 2D array on a solid substrate (usually a glass slide or silicon thin-film cell) that assays large amounts of biological material using high-throughput screening miniaturized, multiplexed and parallel processing and detection methods. There are many types of microarrays, including DNA microarrays, protein microarrays and tissue microarrays.

**MicroRNA:** A small non-coding RNA molecule (containing about 22 nucleotides) found in plants, animals and some viruses, which regulates gene expression by binding to the 3'-untranslated regions (3'-UTR) of specific mRNAs.

**Microsatellite instability (MSI):** MSI is one genotypic consequence of impaired DNA mismatch repair. It is detected by the presence of multiple errors in short repetitive DNA sequences (either mononucleotide or dinucleotide repeats or microsatellites).

**Mismatch repair (MMR):** MMR is a form of DNA repair which corrects errors in DNA replication or which arise as a result of faulty recombination or DNA damage. During normal replication, the daughter strand may contain errors and this form of DNA repair uses the parental strand as a template to correct mismatches in DNA sequence which result from such errors.

**Missense mutation:** A mutation that results in a different amino acid sequence.

**Monoclonal cells:** These are defined as a group of cells produced from a single ancestral cell by repeated cellular replication. Hence, they are suggested to form a single clone. Monoclonality testing using IgH-PCR or TCR-PCR is one way of providing additional evidence to morphology and immunohistological studies to define a lymphoproliferative lesion as being malignant (or not).

**Mononucleotide repeat:** These comprise multiple repeats of a single nucleotide in DNA and are frequently used in assays to diagnose mismatch repair syndromes. Due to the nature of long mononucleotide repeat sequences, they are prone to extension or deletion during DNA synthesis and a failure to detect and repair such errors is indicative of mismatch repair syndrome.

**Monosomy:** This describes the condition where there exists one copy of a whole chromosome or chromosomal region in comparison to the normally expected two copies per cell.

**Mucinous cystic neoplasias (MCN):** Benign or potentially low-grade malignant cystic epithelial neoplasm composed of cells which contain intracytoplasmic mucin (WHO). MCN is one of the three precursor lesions of pancreatic adenocarcinoma (see also PanIN, IPMN).

**Multi-colored FISH (MFISH):** MFISH describes the detection of more than two differentially fluorescently detected/labeled DNAs or RNAs in tissues or cells, by fluorescence microscopy.

**MYH-associated polyposis:** This is a condition predisposing to colorectal cancer, caused by germline mutations in the base excision repair (BER) gene

MUTYH (MYH). The phenotype is often undistinguishable from that of autosomal dominant familial adenomatous polyposis (FAP). The number of adenomas is often lower and affected patients are often sporadic cases. Biallelic MUTYH mutations have also been detected in patients affected with early-onset colorectal cancer (CRC) without polyps. Cancers are more frequently located in the proximal side of the colon compared to APC-related FAP. Generally, mean age at diagnosis of MAP is 48 to 56 years, later than in APC-related FAP.

**NATA:** National Association of Testing Authorities (Australia) is one of a number of national bodies responsible for overseeing adherence by members (in this case diagnostic laboratories) to both national and international standards.

**NET (neuroendocrine tumor):** NETs are a heterogenous group of neoplasms arising from neuroendocrine cells of the diffuse endocrine system. They can be seen in a variety of anatomic locations and although their morphologic features and hormonal activities can be similar, their pathogenesis appears to vary with the site.

**Next generation sequencing (NGS):** Also known as high-throughput sequencing, NGS is the "catch-all" term used to describe a number of different modern sequencing technologies, which allow us to sequence DNA and RNA in a massively parallel fashion (vs. single or a few DNA fragments) and more cheaply than the previously used capillary electrophoresis Sanger sequencing. As such, NGS has revolutionized the study of genomics and molecular biology.

**Non-Hodgkin's lymphoma (NHL):** A group of over 80 diverse malignancies that arise from lymphocytes, a type of white blood cell, normally found within the blood and tissues. The NHLs vary in their morphology, immunophenotype, genetic alterations and in the degree of clinical severity. They are distinct from Hodgkin's lymphoma.

**Nonsense mutation:** A mutation that results in a stop codon, which may produce a truncated protein.

**NSCLC subtyping:** The subtyping of NSCLC into adenocarcinoma and squamous cell carcinoma is crucial and may require beyond microscopy the use of specific immunostainings.

**Oligonucleotides:** Described as short, single-stranded DNA or RNA molecules that are synthesized for various molecular applications.

**Oncogene:** A gene involved in promoting cell growth or proliferation, which if altered can promote cancer.

**Ovarian cancer:** Ovarian epithelial carcinomas count for the majority of ovarian cancer and are divided into serous, endometrioid, mucinous or clear-cell carcinoma types. Other less frequently seen ovarian cancers include germ cell tumor, dysgerminoma, yolk sac tumor, teratoma and sex cord-stromal tumor.

**Pancreatic intraepithelial neoplasia (PanIn):** PanIn are the most common precursor lesions of pancreatic ductal adenocarcinoma; they are microscopic papillary or flat, non-invasive epithelial neoplasms that are usually <5 mm and confined to pancreatic ducts; they are composed of columnar to cuboidal cells with variable mucin, and are divided into three grades according to the degree of cytological and architectural atypia.

**Passenger mutation:** A mutation that does not result in a deleterious effect and does not confer the cell with a survival advantage.

**PBS (phosphate buffer saline):** PBS is a water-based salt solution containing sodium phosphate, sodium chloride and, in some formulations, potassium chloride and potassium phosphate. The osmolarity and ion concentrations of the solutions match those of the human body (isotonic).

**Philadelphia chromosome (Ph):** The name of a specific chromosomal translocation associated with chronic myelogenous leukemia (CML) resulting in the translocation between the ABL gene (9q32) and the BCR gene (22q11).

**PDFGRA:** Alpha-type platelet-derived growth factor receptor is a protein that is encoded by the PDGFRA gene. The gene is mutated in a subset of gastro intestinal stromal tumors (GISTS).

**Photolithography:** This describes a micromanufacturing process that is directed by light.

**Phred score:** A quality score (denoted "Q") related to the probability of an observation being an error. Phred scores are commonly used to describe the qualities of base calling and sequence mapping.

**Polymerase Chain Reaction (PCR):** A procedure that produces millions of copies of a short segment of DNA through repeated cycles of: (1) denaturation; (2) annealing; and (3) elongation. PCR is a very common procedure in molecular genetic testing and may be used to generate a sufficient quantity of DNA to perform a test (e.g. allele-specific amplification, trinucleotide repeat quantification).

**Polymerase:** An enzyme class that allows for the creation of DNA or RNA polynucleotides.

**Predictive assay/biomarker:** This identifies subpopulations of patients who are most likely to respond to a given therapy.

**Predictive biomarker:** Measurable indicator of a biological state which identifies patients who will benefit from a specific treatment.

**Primer:** A defined segment of DNA or RNA used to initiate replication of a sequence by DNA polymerase.

**Probe:** This refers to a known fragment of DNA or RNA (i.e. specific gene, locus) that is labeled and detectable by fluorescent or chromogenic means.

**Prognosis (see also residual risk):** The prognosis of a patient following a diagnosis of cancer is widely understood, correctly, to be a forecast of the likely course of the disease and its outcome. However, in its strictest context, prognosis relates to outcome *in the absence of treatment or intervention*. Almost no cancer patient is simply observed, all receive either treatment (be it surgery or chemo-/radiotherapy) or surveillance (for early prostate cancer). Frequently, therefore, when discussing *prognosis*, clinicians are in fact discussing "residual risk," i.e. the risk remaining after treatment of an adverse outcome. This is particularly important in an era of "residual risk assessment" using nonograms or diagnostic assays which may only apply in the context of the management of patients at the time they were developed.

**Prognostic assay/biomarker:** This indicates the likely course of the disease in an untreated individual.

**Prognostic biomarker:** Characteristics that can estimate the chance of survival or disease recurrence in the context of either no treatment or a previously performed treatment.

**Promotor hypermethylation:** Hypermethylation of cytosine residues within CpG islands located within or in proximity to promoters of regulating gene expression is one mechanism which is now understood to be important in the development of cancers. Hypermethylation of promoter regions of tumor suppressor genes can lead to "gene silencing" or loss of gene expression which may result, phenotypically, in a loss of gene expression similar to that seen following genetic loss through deletion.

**Pyrosequencing:** This is a method of DNA sequencing based on the "sequencing by synthesis" principle. It differs from Sanger sequencing, in that it relies on the detection of pyrophosphate release on nucleotide incorporation, rather than chain termination with dideoxynucleotides.

**Real-time PCR:** A PCR strategy that allows for the quantification of products as they are produced.

**Receptor tyrosine kinases (RTKs):** Surface molecules which induce cell survival and proliferation; often altered (mutated or amplified) in cancer, thereby extensively investigated for relevance in targeted therapy (e.g. EGFR, HER2, KIT).

**Recombinant DNA:** This describes the manipulation of DNA using the laboratory methods.

**Reflex testing:** A testing policy that does not require a separate clinician order for biomarker testing of lung tumors at diagnosis from patients presenting with stage I, II or III disease.

**Residual risk (see also prognosis):** Frequently confused with prognosis, residual risk is the risk of patients experiencing an adverse event (e.g. recurrence or death) after conventional treatments have been completed. While prognosis is an estimate of projected outcomes in the absence of treatments, "residual risk" implies the presence of a program of active interventions in the disease process including, but not limited to, surgery, radiotherapy and chemotherapy. Most "prognostic" algorithms or nonograms are in fact estimates of residual risk following conventional therapy.

**Residual risk assay or nonogram:** For many cancers, nonograms or residual risk assays (molecular diagnostic assays) may be of value in determining the risk/benefit of treatment interventions for certain groups of patients. Particularly in breast cancer, where multiple treatment options exist, such approaches are widely used to inform patients of the potential risks/benefits of different treatment options. Increasingly, molecular diagnostic approaches are being developed which claim to support such decisions.

**Restriction fragment length polymorphism (RFLP):** RFLP is a technique that exploits variations in homologous DNA sequences. It refers to a difference between samples of homologous DNA molecules that come from differing locations of restriction enzyme sites, and to a related laboratory technique by which these segments can be illustrated. In RFLP analysis, the DNA sample is broken into pieces (digested) by restriction enzymes and the resulting restriction fragments are separated according to their lengths by gel electrophoresis.

**Ring chromosome:** This describes a specialized chromosomal structure where the chromosome is in the shape of a ring and frequently contains several copies of a given DNA fragment.

**ROSE:** To enhance the adequacy rate of cytological samples for microscopic and molecular analysis, rapid on-site evaluation (ROSE) is performed at the time of sampling by a dedicated cytopathologist.

**RPMI:** This is a culture media containing a bicarbonate buffering system with variable amounts of amino acids and vitamins. It was developed at Roswell Park Memorial Institute, hence the acronym RPMI.

**Sanger sequencing:** The common name for capillary electrophoresis-based sequencing. Also called chain-termination sequencing, or first generation sequencing.

**Segmental chromosome aberrations (SCA):** Large-scale genomic dosage changes, often with loss or gain of whole chromosome arms.

**Sensitivity (of a biomarker):** The sensitivity of a biomarker test is a measure of how well the assay performs in picking up a disease or event (response to therapy, relapse, etc.) when the test is positive. Sensitivity can be calculated by dividing the number of true positives (test is positive and event occurs) by the sum of true positives and false negatives (where the test is negative but the event occurs).

**Serous effusions:** Accumulations of fluid within the peritoneal, pleural or pericardial space; associated with malignancy, as well as infectious, inflammatory and various other conditions.

**Silent mutation:** A mutation that results in no change in the translated amino acid sequence.

**Silver *in situ* hybridization (SISH):** SISH describes the detection of DNA or RNA in tissues or cells using silver particles that are visualized by bright-field microscopy.

**Single Nucleotide Polymorphism (SNP):** DNA variations that occur in over 1 percent of the population and do not cause disease. Each SNP represents a difference in one of the nucleotides adenine (A), thymine (T), cytosine (C) or guanine (G) in the genome and can differ between members of a species or paired chromosomes in an individual. Most SNPs have no effect on health or development. However, some SNPs are associated with certain diseases. These associations allow the evaluation of an individual's genetic predisposition to develop a disease.

**Somatic hypermutation (SHM):** SHM is a critical process used by B-cells to generate antibodies. The human immune system is highly adapted to generate an enormous diversity of antibodies against foreign pathogens using a limited set of genes within the genome. SHM has been highly conserved through mammalian biology and is the key process responsible for generating antibody diversity within B-cells.

**Somatic mutation:** A DNA alteration that occurs after conception. Somatic mutations can occur in any of the cells of the body except the germ cells (sperm and egg) and therefore are not passed on to children. These alterations can, but do not always, cause cancer or other diseases.

**Specificity (of a biomarker):** The specificity of a biomarker test is a measure of how well the assay performs in giving a true result for the population lacking disease or event (response to therapy, relapse, etc.) when the test is negative. Specificity can be calculated by dividing the number of true negatives (test is negative and event is absent) by the sum of true negatives and false positives (test is positive in the absence of event).

**Substitution mutation:** Also referred to as a point mutation, this is a genetic alteration where one nucleotide is exchanged for a different nucleotide. Depending on the effect on the translated protein, a substitution may be categorized as a silent, missense or nonsense mutation.

**Targeted therapy:** Type of treatment that acts by interfering with essential biochemical pathways or mutant proteins or tissue environment that contributes to cancer growth and survival.

**Telomere:** This describes the ends of sister chromatids where a specific DNA sequence exists to ensure protection of the chromosome ends during replication.

**The Cancer Genome Atlas (TCGA, see also ICGC):** A coordinated effort (http://cancergenome.nih.gov/) to accelerate our understanding of the molecular basis of cancer through the application of genome-wide analysis technologies, including large-scale genome sequencing. The TCGA Research Network has catalogued aberrations in the DNA (mutations, SNPs and methylation), mRNA and microRNA of thousands of tumors relative to matched normal genomes.

**Thymidylate synthase (TS):** TS is a key enzyme in the synthesis of 2'-deoxythymidine-5'-monophosphate, an essential precursor for DNA biosynthesis. For this reason, this enzyme is a critical target in cancer chemotherapy. As the first TS inhibitor in clinical use, 5-fluorouracil (5-FU) remains widely used for the treatment of several types of cancers.

**Tissue microarray (TMA):** Tissue microarrays are an ingenious means of collecting large numbers of samples from tumor specimens into a miniaturized tumor biobank. Usually, small punch core biopsies are taken from donor tissue blocks and assembled into a new recipient pathology block in an ordered and precise pattern. In this way, many hundreds or indeed thousands of tumor samples may be represented on a single tissue block to facilitate research. Increasingly, mini TMAs are used to assemble quality controls for conventional diagnostic approaches into a single strip which can, in some instances, be placed adjacent to the test sample,

allowing "in slide" controls for comparison of staining or ISH.

**TMPRSS2-ERG gene fusions:** TMPRSS2-ERG is a fusion of pieces of DNA from two different genes, TMPRSS2 and ERG. TMPRSS2-ERG gene fusion causes the ERG gene that contributes to cancer cell growth, survival and movement to become abnormally activated by hormones (e.g. testosterone) in the prostate.

**TMPRSS2-ETS gene fusions:** Fusions between the promoter of the androgen-regulated transmembrane protease serine 2 gene (TMPRSS2) and erythroblastosis virus E 26 (ETS) transcription factors in prostate cancer. These gene fusions result in androgen-dependent transcription of ETS factors in prostate cancer cells. The most common fusion is with ERG (ETS-related gene), a member of the ETS family, resulting in the TMPRSS2-ERG gene fusion in approximately 50 percent of prostate cancer cases. TMPRSS2 has also been identified in fusions with the ETS family members ETV1, ETV4 and ETV5 in prostate cancer.

**TNM staging:** The TNM staging system is a consensus staging approach to multiple cancers coordinated and maintained by the UICC (Union for International Cancer Control) and also adopted by the AJCC (American Joint Committee on Cancer). TNM staging includes: (1) a measure of primary tumor size, including notation of spread beyond the site of origin; (2) measurement of spread to local lymph nodes; and (3) measurement of distant metastases which combined make up the tumor nodes metastasis or TNM classification of tumors.

**Touton giant cell:** A type of multinucleated histiocytic giant cell with nuclei arranged in a ring-like fashion that surround central homogenous eosinophilic or amphophilic cytoplasm.

**Translocation:** A chromosomal abnormality in which a chromosome breaks and a portion of it reattaches to a different chromosomal location.

**Tumor cell enrichment:** To avoid mutant allele dilution into wild-type DNA, cytological and histological samples undergo microdissection to select for the testing the most pure neoplastic cell population.

**Tumor suppressor gene:** A gene that normally suppresses cell growth, which if inactivated or deleted can promote cancer.

**Tumor cellularity:** The proportion of a tumor made up of tumor cells.

**Tumor infiltrating lymphocytes (TILs):** Lymphocytes which infiltrate into the tumor area are increasingly thought to reflect differential aspects of the "host response" to tumors. This aspect of tumor biology is attracting increasing research and clinical interest as the presence of TILs of different subtypes (e.g. T-helper or T-suppressor cells) is linked to treatment response and disease outcome.

**Turcot syndrome:** This is a genetic disease characterized by polyps in the colon (large intestine) in addition to tumors in the brain. Skin abnormalities can also occur. Turcot syndrome is inherited in an autosomal recessive manner and can result from mutations in either the adenomatous polyposis coli (APC) gene or the mismatch repair genes underlying the syndrome of hereditary nonpolyposis colon cancer (HNPCC).

**Turner syndrome:** Also known as gonadal dysgenesis, this human genetic disorder affects females and is associated with the absence of one of two copies of the X chromosome per cell.

**Type I endometrial carcinoma:** Endometrial carcinoma (endometrioid and mucinous adenocarcinoma) that arise from the hyperplastic endometrium tissue are associated to estrogen activity, and show a favorable clinical outcome.

**Type II endometrial carcinoma:** Endometrial carcinomas (serous and clear cell carcinoma) arise from atrophic endometrium tissue, without estrogen association, and show an unfavorable clinical outcome.

**Urothelial carcinoma:** Urothelial carcinoma, also known as transitional cell carcinoma, is a malignant neoplasm derived from transitional epithelium, occurring mainly in the urinary bladder, ureters and kidney (renal pelvis). The cells lining these organs are called "transitional" because they can stretch and change shape without breaking. Urothelial carcinoma is the most common type of bladder cancer. Outside of the bladder, this is an uncommon cancer. It accounts for approximately 7 percent of kidney cancers. Urothelial carcinoma is the most common tumor of the renal pelvis.

**Vogelstein model:** A linear model of progression of colorectal cancer first proposed by Bert Vogelstein to explain the sequential development of mutations during the course of development and progression of colorectal cancer. Such linear models (applied to many cancers) are frequently referred to as "Vogelstein models." Like many models, this linear approach has been developed and expanded, including developments by Vogelstein himself, to include branched and other more complete model systems.

**Whole-exome sequencing:** A laboratory process that is used to determine the nucleotide sequence primarily of the exonic (or protein-coding) regions of an individual's genome and related sequences, representing approximately 1 percent of the complete DNA sequence.

**Whole-genome sequencing:** A laboratory process that is used to determine the sequence of nuclear DNA without enrichment for regions of interest. The human genome consists of approximately 3 billion nucleotides.

**World Health Organization (WHO):** An agency of the United Nations concerned with international health priorities across a broad spectrum of diseases, including cancer.

**Xenograft:** Tissue or organs from an individual of one species transplanted into or grafted onto an organism of another species, genus or family.

# An introduction to molecular pathology

John M. S. Bartlett

## Molecular pathology: time for a transformation?

Discoveries in both basic and applied science over the past five years are revolutionizing our understanding of cancer. Pivotal discovery projects, including the ICGC/TCGA consortia, are rapidly providing information on the broad mutational landscape of cancer, revealing ever-increasing levels of complexity [1–8]. Multiple mutational events (between 50 and 200) are identified in early cancers [1–8], highlighting a far greater degree of molecular diversity within cancers than previously thought. Recent reports, based on copy-number variation (CNV) data alone, suggest the existence of at least 10 molecular subtypes of early breast cancer [9, 10]. Each of these subtypes may respond differently to different chemotherapy approaches and this could explain to a large degree the relatively slow progress over recent years in improving outcomes for patients with early breast cancer. Linked research has identified a greater degree of polyclonality within cancers than previously appreciated [3, 4, 6]. There are increasing numbers of reports which document the existence of multiple subclones within patients which may be identified contemporaneously (for example, by single cell analysis [11–13]) or by sampling patients at different times or tumor sites [4, 6, 11]. We now recognize, perhaps as never before, the true molecular complexity, diversity and heterogeneity of even "common" cancers such as breast, colorectal, lung and prostate.

In response to such discoveries, clinical researchers and pharmaceutical companies have been adapting, albeit slowly, their strategies for the development of novel therapeutic agents. The past 10 to 15 years have seen the implementation of targeted therapeutics, specifically directed against molecular events which are pivotal drivers in subsets of cancers. This has led to implementation of an increasing number of molecular diagnostic approaches to predict therapeutic response and target molecular therapies [14–21]. However, the success of molecularly targeted therapies such as Herceptin, Gleevec, Iressa, etc. [22, 23] has, paradoxically, highlighted the growing gap between clinical validation of therapeutic agents and validation of diagnostic tests. Over 30 years after the introduction of tamoxifen as an ER-targeted therapy and over 10 years after the introduction of Herceptin as a HER2-targeted therapy, debate as to the optimal methods for diagnostic testing, the accuracy and interpretation of "personalized diagnostics" remains an area of continuing controversy [24–28]. For neither therapeutic approach was the predictive diagnostic test, currently used in diagnostic pathology laboratories, *prospectively* validated. Many, indeed the majority of, current molecular diagnostic tests were retrospectively, and some argue poorly, validated prior to implementation. Nonetheless, "targeted" or personalized therapy is rightly viewed as an essential component of future improvements in treatments for individual patients. The rapidly expanding portfolio of targeted therapies, either in pre-clinical development or undergoing testing through clinical trials, represents the potential for an extremely rapid extension of the spectrum and number of diagnostic molecular pathology tests which may be required to implement targeted therapies in the future. For these advances in knowledge to impact on patient management in the clinic, they must be translated into novel diagnostic approaches which match clinical needs, improve patient outcomes and impact on healthcare in a cost-effective manner.

*Molecular Pathology: A Practical Guide for the Surgical Pathologist and Cytopathologist*, ed. John M. S. Bartlett, Abeer Shaaban and Fernando Schmitt. Published by Cambridge University Press. © Cambridge University Press, 2016.

## Personalized medicine requires personalized diagnostics

*Personalized medicine* is the buzz word of patients, clinical managers, diagnosticians and healthcare professionals at all levels. As pathologists and diagnosticians, we recognize that future progress in personalized or targeted medicine depends entirely upon and requires significant and rapid progress in "personalized diagnostics." Major advances in diagnostic anatomical pathology are essential if we are to deliver new diagnostic approaches to support targeted treatment for cancer patients. Such advances will, nonetheless, require to be fully validated before being implemented into modern healthcare practices. Fundamentally, what was true at the turn of the twentieth century remains true today – *accurate and appropriate diagnosis is fundamental to the successful treatment of disease* – "As is your pathology, so is your medicine" (William Osler, 1849–1919). What has changed dramatically over the past 100 years is our understanding of the scope of the challenge and of the diversity of cancer as a group of diseases, and our ability to address these challenges through a rapid acceleration in technology which puts us in a unique position to provide the molecular diagnostic tools for the twenty-first century which will accelerate improvements in healthcare for the coming generations of cancer sufferers.

It is our conviction that to achieve these goals diagnostic pathologists will need to focus on the delivery of novel "fit for purpose" multiparametric, functional molecular diagnostic assays and, in parallel, deliver established tests to a consistently high standard and continue the process of developing future diagnostic assays. This requires a revolution in anatomical molecular pathology analogous to the rapid development of clinical biochemistry in the 1980s and 1990s. Anatomic pathologists are uniquely placed to facilitate and drive this transformation in diagnostic molecular pathology through a multidisciplinary approach to the development, validation and implementation of complex molecular diagnostic methods. However, the challenge ahead will require both a multidisciplinary collaboration between pathologists, scientist and ancillary laboratory staff and a readiness to innovate and improve existing diagnostic pathology approaches. Failure to rapidly grasp these challenges may lead to further erosion of the pivotal role of anatomical pathology in the management of disease, both within and beyond the scope of cancer diagnostics.

## Diagnostic molecular pathology: the challenge ahead

As will be clear from the review of molecular cell regulation (Chapter 2), the scope for both targeted therapeutics and targeted diagnostics is extensive. Even with existing targeted and conventional therapies, the range of candidate predictive and prognostic markers expands on a month-by-month basis. Validation of even a fraction of such markers will require further development of complex molecular diagnostic assays. Given the molecular complexity and heterogeneity of tumors, it is not unrealistic to propose that, within the next 5 to 10 years, diagnostic reporting of 10s to 100s of different molecular variants will be essential to provide relevant information to facilitate appropriate treatment decisions to be made.

Already significant numbers of "molecular diagnostic pathology" assays of varying utility and cost are being offered in different jurisdictions worldwide. These range from *in situ* based analysis of protein expression, gene copy-number/amplification, to mutational analysis, expression arrays of 10s to 100s of genes, etc. As outlined in the following chapters, the clinical challenge addressed ranges from prediction of response to specific therapies (mostly single gene/mutation assays at present), through prediction of residual risk or prognosis following treatment (increasingly multigene assays) to improved molecular classification (diagnosis) of tumors. As assays increase in complexity, we are experiencing a rapid switch from *in situ* manually or visually assessed approaches to multiplex analyses of mRNA, CNA and mutations. As the number of targeted therapies increase, so will the complexity and diversity of molecular diagnostic assays required to provide appropriate diagnostic information for personalized or targeted medicine approaches. In many cancers there is already a requirement for anatomical, expression, mutational and CNA data to be reported on the same tumor sample.

## Through a glass darkly – microscopy is *not* the future of molecular pathology?

As a result, from a personal overview of molecular diagnostic pathology, I have reached the conclusion that we are experiencing a critical transition point in our discipline – away from "slide-based" visual assessment of molecular markers towards high throughput and quantitative assessment of tumor markers in "liquid phase" assays such as multiplex polymerase chain reaction (PCR), targeted or whole genome sequencing and microarray platforms. The majority of chapters in this volume relating to molecular techniques represent this progressive switch. As molecular diagnostic assays are being developed, we do not conceptualize *in situ* approaches to mutation detection or methylation and increasingly expression and gene deletion or amplification (copy-number changes) are being addressed using moderate to high throughput liquid phase technologies (see Chapters 6 to 11). Currently, only protein (immunohistochemistry) and DNA/RNA hybridization technologies (see Chapter 5) continue to rely on *in situ* methodologies. However, these *in situ* methods represent some of the most challenging aspects of quality control among current molecular diagnostic assessments in clinical laboratories (see Chapter 4).

Since the advent of the light microscope almost 400 years ago, anatomical pathology has been built around the expertise of its practitioners in recognizing morphological patterns to discriminate tumor anatomical type, grade, local invasion, etc. With the advent of immunohistochemistry in the 1980s and *in situ* hybridization (ISH) in the 1990s, this expertise extended to assessment of protein expression (increasingly on a quantitative level) and gene alterations (deletions, fusions, amplifications). For many tumor types, pathological grade, type, protein expression (either qualitative or quantitative) or gene alterations by ISH are a pivotal part of the decision-making process in determining treatment. The challenge faced in performing subjective, visual assessments of the intensity of immunohistochemical staining, the degree of nuclear pleomorphisms or even the percentage of positive cells (either mitoses or MIB1/Ki67 stained) leads to significant inter-observer variation in each of these areas which can undermine, at least in part, the clinical utility of key pathological variables. Tumor grading, in almost all areas of pathology, is recognized as one of the most significant challenges facing diagnostic pathologists, resulting in considerable inter-observer variability (for example, [29, 30]). Indeed, a comprehensive review of breast cancer grading recognized that "despite the objective improvements that have been made to breast cancer grading

methods, any assessment of morphological characteristics inevitably retains a subjective element" [29]. Equally challenging has been the standardization of molecular *in situ* assessments of protein expression, again particularly when such measures are used to direct treatment (for example, estrogen receptor in breast cancer or Ki67 as a marker of proliferation). Recent ASCO-CAP and expert panel guidelines [24, 27, 31] recognize the significant challenges in reducing to practice quantitative or even qualitative assessment of molecular markers where inter-observer variation and subjective interpretation of results is a critical component of the assay. This is further reflected and emphasized by the review of quality assurance practices for molecular *in situ* assays (Chapter 4). These challenges by no means undermine the pivotal role of the expert pathologist in providing critical prognostic and predictive information through visual evaluation of tumor biopsies; they do, however, emphasize the critical need to adapt processes, even where improvements may simply increase the accuracy and reproducibility of current procedures and to re-evaluate procedures based on robust scientific evidence-based approaches to the diagnostic challenges ahead.

A second observation, outlined in brief above, is that the breadth of molecular assessments required will rapidly expand to exceed the capacity and capability of existing pathology laboratories if we remain focused on *in situ* approaches. Already, it can be challenging to examine multiple molecular markers on limited tissue samples available through diagnostic core biopsies. With a static or even shrinking budget, pathologists are called upon to deliver even more diagnostic results. Even with improvement in image-guided biopsy, microtomy and rapid processing of *in situ* assays, it is impossible to envisage a workflow which would allow high throughput analysis of 10s to 100s of markers per case which is reliant upon *in situ* approaches and manual or visual assessment by pathologists. This in parallel with the rapid expansion of mutational assays which cannot currently be assessed by *in situ* methods argues strongly against the continued development of slide-based assays for future molecular pathology.

Does this mean that the age of the microscope is past? Nearly 400 years after van Leeuwenhoek, is it time to abandon morphological assessment of tumor pathology? Will novel molecular approaches completely replace or supplant anatomical pathology?

I would strongly argue that this is not the case, and that while the future of pathology is increasingly bound up with molecular diagnostic approaches which require quantitative, accurate and reproducible assessment of multiple molecular components of tumors, these approaches will both develop alongside and require a firm foundation in anatomical pathology. As will be apparent in multiple examples from Chapters 12 to 22, molecular diagnostic approaches augment and supplement anatomical pathology assessments and are frequently, if not uniformly, dependent upon them. Detection of HER2 amplification in early breast cancer is essential to direct use of anti-HER2 therapies, but HER2 amplification in pre-invasive ductal carcinomas (DCIS) is more frequent than in invasive cancers [32, 33]. Similarly, assessment of HER2 expression in gastric cancers requires close linkage to the anatomical pathology context of disease. Discrimination between tumor subtypes in ovarian, breast, lung and other organs may ultimately drive the selection of appropriate treatments and molecular diagnostic assays. Furthermore, expression and mutation of key genes can be rapidly and quantitatively assessed by PCR and other methodologies, but normal tissues also express many of the key driver genes and indiscriminate homogenization of cancer biopsies can compromise molecular diagnostic approaches by dilution of the invasive tumor component with normal tissue (stroma, lymphocytes, etc.). Finally, tumor heterogeneity where subclones of invasive tumors may be molecularly distinct presents a clear challenge to novel diagnostic approaches.

The challenge ahead, therefore, is not to forget the past, but to build upon it. It is to develop a cooperative multidisciplinary approach to anatomical and molecular diagnostic pathology which incorporates the highest standards of care for the patient. Novel diagnostic assays must be accurate, reproducible, portable and rapidly scalable if we are to address coming challenges in molecularly targeted therapeutics [34–37]. Existing anatomical pathology approaches will survive only if they match these criteria as well as or to a greater extent than candidate molecular assays. Novel molecular approaches will only be viable to the degree that they *extend* our ability to manage patients beyond the significant information derived by "conventional" morphological and pathological assessments. To address the increasing complexity of cancer, to improve risk stratification and to accelerate delivery of personalized medicine will require a refocusing and repurposing of diagnostic anatomic and molecular pathology as a discipline at the center, rather than the periphery of modern healthcare. We expect, over the next three to five years, to see an acceleration of delivery of both single gene and pathway or panel-based multiparametric tests which are focused on delivery of personalized medicine. Within or beyond five years, it seems possible, even likely, that multiparametric molecular profiling of cancers will be the norm rather than the exception. The future of anatomical pathology is increasingly linked to development of molecular diagnostic assays which will deliver accurate information to direct clinical decisions by both the patients and their physicians.

## Personalized pathology for personalized medicine

As we witness an ever-expanding repertoire of molecular diagnostic tests, it appears that the days of "simple" diagnostic pathology are far behind us. Simply expanding the taxonomy of cancer to include molecular features has significant potential, but unless this expanded classification is linked to treatment decisions it will, ultimately, fail to impact on targeted treatment. In addition to addressing the conventional question, "what kind of cancer is it?" – diagnostic medicine must address two further questions: 1. How should I treat it? and 2. which drugs are likely to be the most effective?

## Prognostic, residual risk and predictive diagnostic assays

These, apparently simple, questions encompass a wide range of diagnostic challenges, firstly to determine the elements of tumor pathology and biology which impact on the natural course of disease, to determine the extent of treatment including surgery, local treatment and systemic treatment with cytotoxic and increasingly targeted agents. Patients with low-grade, organ-confined cancer are frequently low risk and can avoid some of the toxic sequelae of adjuvant chemotherapy. Conversely, patients with high-grade disease frequently benefit from aggressive treatment options. The use of conventional histopathological approaches to assess disease *prognosis*, or risk of recurrence following surgery and local therapy, has been a mainstay of treatment decision making for decades. Increasingly, molecular diagnostic assays, including multiplex assays, are impacting in this area. In breast cancer, where endocrine treatment is associated with relatively minor side effects, such assays increasingly inform patients of the "residual risk" of recurrence following local resection, radiotherapy and adjuvant endocrine therapy to aid in decisions relating to additional therapeutic options.

However, increasingly, with the advent of molecularly targeted therapies, *predictive* diagnostic assays, which discriminate between patients likely to benefit from treatments and those who require alternative treatment approaches, are required. These may be those developed in the context of specific molecularly targeted therapies, or possibly in the context of so-called "conventional" chemotherapies. The goal there is not risk assessment in the context of disease progression or prognosis, but specifically aiding treatment selection based on the molecular make up of particular tumors and the existence of molecularly targeted therapies.

Clearly, the individual diagnostic context will differ between tumor types; however, the key challenges of prognosis, residual risk and predicting response to therapeutic agents cross tumor boundaries. To design appropriate diagnostic assays, it will be critical to relate these to the appropriate disease context based on a clear understanding of the objective for which the test is being developed.

## Prognosis or residual risk

Almost all patients who receive a diagnosis of cancer have one major question in common with their physician. How likely is it that this cancer will kill me? Some "cancers," including superficial transitional cell carcinomas of the urinary bladder and non-melanoma skin cancers, rarely result in death, even if treated conservatively. Others, including pancreatic, ovarian and lung tumors are frequently diagnosed late in the disease course and are associated with high mortality. However, many patients, probably the majority, are faced with the dilemma of balancing their risk of succumbing to their disease against the potential costs and benefits of treatment. For most situations, surgical resection is a starting point, with progressively more aggressive local (radiotherapy) and systemic (chemotherapy)

treatments given the greater the risk of disease recurrence following surgery.

Strictly speaking, prognosis relates to the study of the natural history of a disease in the absence of intervention. Even the most basic form of intervention, surgery, changes the disease pattern. The result is that in almost every context cancer diagnosis, both conventional and molecular, is used to assess the residual risk of relapse following treatment. If that residual risk is low following surgery or local treatment, then additional adjuvant chemotherapy may be more harmful than beneficial.

Treatment of cancer in the "adjuvant" setting aims to eradicate residual tumor cells at sites distant from the primary tumor, *if present*, which are not detected and are not removed by conventional surgical approaches. By definition, therefore, adjuvant chemotherapy treats *risk* of disease – not its actual presence. For every patient for whom treatment is necessary may experience harmful side effects for no personal benefit. A significant minority of patients exposed to adjuvant chemotherapy are not destined for the cancer to recur even if untreated and molecular profiles are increasingly used to propose stratification of cancers and treatment selection [15, 38–42]. Even for patients who benefit from polychemotherapy, therapeutic choices are largely based on risk and average benefit across populations. Lacking a clear understanding of the mechanisms by which drugs act, and therefore the molecular features of tumors which markers prospectively select for response, reduces the ability to rationally develop predictive diagnostic assays. Pathology remains, as ever, rooted in both the understanding of disease mechanisms and the subsequent development of rational diagnostic approaches to disease [21].

Multiple strategies have been applied, particularly in early breast cancer, to develop tools to assess "residual recurrence risk" after surgery, radiotherapy and endocrine therapy to inform the choice between endocrine therapy and/or chemotherapy. These range from algorithms based on historical clinicopathological features (stage, grade, etc.) and patient factors (age, co-morbidities), such as "Adjuvant Online!" [43], through studies exploring the impact of *in situ* biomarkers on risk of relapse [44, 45], to complex multiparameter diagnostic assays such as Oncotype DX [46]. As this area of research evolves, the proliferation of multiple competing, and modestly selective, risk stratifiers [47] presents a twofold challenge to molecular pathologists: firstly, to contribute to research which optimizes risk stratification for individual patients; and, secondly, to offer robust molecular diagnostics in a cost-effective manner to inform clinicians and patients as to the optimal treatment strategy, *including* the potential for avoiding adjuvant chemotherapy. There exists clear potential for extension of this strategy into other tumors (prostate, transitional cell carcinoma of the bladder, etc.) where aggressive treatment is not beneficial for every patient and also into pre-invasive conditions such as DCIS.

In parallel with an increasing awareness that adjuvant therapy could be "personalized" by the exclusion of patients at either minimal or low risk of recurrence is the recognition that progressive small gains from stepwise advances in chemotherapy (CMF vs. CAF, CAF vs. TAC) [38, 48] may also mask the potential for personalized approaches to the selection of modern chemotherapies. Extensive research has, to date, failed to yield robust clinically viable diagnostic tests for personalized medicine choices [49–52], but this challenge remains one of the key deliverables identified by an international consultation for translational research in early breast cancer [53].

## Molecular pathology – the coming transformation

The developments highlighted above have, over the past decade or more, begun to impact on the delivery of molecular pathology services. Increasingly, anatomical pathology laboratories are adopting molecular pathology tests and implementing them into their routine workflow. However, increasingly complex, multiparametric assays are being offered by central, commercial laboratories as a solution to the perceived and actual challenges of disseminated molecular testing. More critically, when the "conventional" challenges outlined above (risk stratification, more accurate prediction/selection of both conventional and targeted therapeutics) are aligned with recent advances delineating the molecular landscape and the extent of molecular heterogeneity within common cancers, the scope of the challenge facing molecular pathology both in the clinic and at the research/validation phase becomes daunting.

The goal for the future delivery of molecular pathology is to focus research, both technical and applied, towards the development of clinically applicable and accurate diagnostics for a highly complex disease. Future diagnostic approaches will have to recognize the broad spectrum of molecular events which drive cancers (mutations, CNVs, transcriptional and proteomic changes), to address the increasing fragmentation/subtyping of so-called "common cancers" and to match a rapidly expanding pharmacopeia of conventional and targeted drugs to support the expected advent of personalized medicine.

## Summary

Personalized medicine requires personalized diagnostics which in turn requires robust, validated diagnostic tests which can be applied in routine diagnostic pathology laboratories. This is critical to the delivery of personalized medicine in cancer where novel diagnostics will drive improvements in therapeutic targeting by: improved assessment of risk (to exclude patients from unnecessary or harmful treatments); validation of predictive diagnostic assays to better personalize current therapeutic options; and development of theranostics, pairing diagnostics with drugs to accelerate delivery of targeted therapies.

Anatomical pathology is central to the future delivery of accurate diagnostic approaches to disease, particularly for cancer. This will require a rapid adoption of novel approaches to diagnostic medicine throughout the profession, from training to quality assurance programs. Anatomical pathologists are, as always, central to the appropriate treatment of disease because they deliver critical diagnostic information to inform treatment choice. Development of future approaches to personalized medicine cannot be delivered without rapid development and investment in anatomical molecular pathology. While progress has been slow in the past, there is now a wealth of opportunity to address the key challenges facing molecular anatomical pathology.

## Acknowledgement of research support

This study was conducted with the support of the Ontario Institute for Cancer Research through funding provided by the Ontario Ministry of Research and Innovation. The TEAM trial is a multinational study supported by an unrestricted research grant by Pfizer Inc., and funding from Cancer Research UK.

# References

1. Banerji, S., Cibulskis, K., Rangel-Escareno, C., Brown, K. K., Carter, S. L., Frederick, A. M. *et al.* Sequence analysis of mutations and translocations across breast cancer subtypes. *Nature* 2012; 486 (7403): 405–9.

2. Grasso, C. S., Wu, Y. M., Robinson, D. R., Cao, X., Dhanasekaran, S. M., Khan, A. P. *et al.* The mutational landscape of lethal castration-resistant prostate cancer. *Nature* 2012; 487(7406): 239–43.

3. Nik-Zainal, S., Alexandrov, L. B., Wedge, D. C., Van, L. P., Greenman, C. D., Raine, K. *et al.* Mutational processes molding the genomes of 21 breast cancers. *Cell* 2012; 149(5): 979–93.

4. Nik-Zainal, S., Van, L. P., Wedge, D. C., Alexandrov, L. B., Greenman, C. D., Lau, K. W. *et al.* The life history of 21 breast cancers. *Cell* 2012; 149(5): 994–1007.

5. Stephens, P. J., Tarpey, P. S., Davies, H., Van, L. P., Greenman, C., Wedge, D. C. *et al.* The landscape of cancer genes and mutational processes in breast cancer. *Nature* 2012; 486(7403): 400–4.

6. Swanton, C. Intratumor heterogeneity: evolution through space and time. *Cancer Res* 2012; 72(19): 4875–82.

7. Hudson, T. J., Anderson, W., Artez, A., Barker, A. D., Bell, C., Bernabe, R. R. *et al.* International network of cancer genome projects. *Nature* 2010; 464(7291): 993–8.

8. Pleasance, E. D. A comprehensive catalogue of somatic mutations from a human cancer genome. *Nature* 2010; 463(7278): 184–90.

9. Cheang, M. C. U., Voduc, D., Bajdik, C., Leung, S., McKinney, S., Chia, S. K. *et al.* Basal-like breast cancer defined by five biomarkers has superior prognostic value than triple-negative phenotype. *Clin Cancer Res* 2008; 14(5): 1368–76.

10. Curtis, C., Shah, S. P., Chin, S. F., Turashvili, G., Rueda, O. M., Dunning, M. J. *et al.* The genomic and transcriptomic architecture of 2,000 breast tumours reveals novel subgroups. *Nature* 2012; 486 (7403): 346–52.

11. Gerlinger, M., Rowan, A. J., Horswell, S., Larkin, J., Endesfelder, D., Gronroos, E. *et al.* Intratumor heterogeneity and branched evolution revealed by multiregion sequencing. *New Engl J Med* 2012; 366(10): 883–92.

12. Borresen-Dale, A. L., Hicks, J., Navin, N. and Russnes, H. G. Insight into the heterogeneity of breast cancer through next-generation sequencing. *J Clin Invest* 2011; 121(10): 3810–18.

13. Navin, N., Kendall, J., Troge, J., Andrews, P., Rodgers, L., McIndoo, J. *et al.* Tumour evolution inferred by single-cell sequencing. *Nature* 2011; 472 (7341): 90–4.

14. Alayev, A. and Holz, M. K. mTOR signaling for biological control and cancer. *J Cell Physiol* 2013; 228(8): 1658–64.

15. Banerjee, S. and Kaye, S. B. New strategies in the treatment of ovarian cancer: current clinical perspectives and future potential. *Clin Cancer Res* 2013; 19(5): 961–8.

16. Rexer, B. N. and Arteaga, C. L. Optimal targeting of HER2-PI3K signaling in breast cancer: mechanistic insights and clinical implications. *Cancer Res* 2013; 73 (13): 3817–20.

17. Chen, K. G. and Sikic, B. I. Molecular pathways: regulation and therapeutic implications of multidrug resistance. *Clin Cancer Res* 2012; 18(7): 1863–9.

18. Dancey, J. E., Bedard, P. L., Onetto, N. and Hudson, T. J. The genetic basis for cancer treatment decisions. *Cell* 2012; 148(3): 409–20.

19. Flaherty, K. T., Hodi, F. S. and Fisher, D. E. From genes to drugs: targeted strategies for melanoma. *Nat Rev Cancer* 2012; 12(5): 349–61.

20. Kurtz, J. E. and Ray-Coquard, I. PI3 kinase inhibitors in the clinic: an update. *Anticancer Res* 2012; 32 (7): 2463–70.

21. Wright, N. A. and Poulsom, R. Omnis cellula e cellula revisited: cell biology as the foundation of pathology. *J Pathol* 2012; 226(2): 145–7.

22. Hirsch, F. R., Varella-Garcia, M., Bunn, P. A., Jr., Franklin, W. A., Dziadziuszko, R., Thatcher, N. *et al.* Molecular predictors of outcome with gefitinib in a phase III placebo-controlled study in advanced non-small-cell lung cancer. *J Clin Oncol* 2006; 24(31): 5034–42.

23. Bell, R. What can we learn from Herceptin (R) trials in metastatic breast cancer? *Oncology* 2002; 63: 39–46.

24. Hammond, M. E. H., Hayes, D. F., Dowsett, M., Allred, D. C., Hagerty, K. L., Badve, S. *et al.* American Society of Clinical Oncology/College of American Pathologists guideline recommendations for immunohistochemical testing of estrogen and progesterone receptors in breast cancer (unabridged version). *Archives of Pathology & Laboratory Medicine* 2010; 134(7): E48–E72.

25. Bartlett, J. M. S., Ibrahim, M., Jasani, B., Morgan, J. M., Ellis, I., Kay, E. *et al.* External quality assurance of HER2 FISH and ISH testing three years of the UK National External Quality Assurance Scheme. *American J Clin Pathol* 2009; 131(1): 106–11.

26. Miller, K. D., Ibrahim, M., Barnett, S. and Jasani, B. Technical aspects of predictive and prognostic markers in breast

**7**

cancer: What UK NEQAS data shows. *Curr Diagn Pathol* 2007; 13 (2): 135–49.

27. Wolff, A. C., Hammond, M. E., Schwartz, J. N., Hagerty, K. L., Allred, D. C., Cote, R. J. *et al.* American Society of Clinical Oncology/College of American Pathologists guideline recommendations for human epidermal growth factor receptor 2 testing in breast cancer. *J Clin Oncol* 2007; 25(1): 118–45.

28. Miller, K., Rhodes, A. and Jasani, B. Variation in rates of oestrogen receptor positivity in breast cancer again. *BMJ* 2002; 324(7332): 298–9.

29. Rakha, E., Reis-Filho, J., Baehner, F., Dabbs, D., Decker, T., Eusebi, V. *et al.* Breast cancer prognostic classification in the molecular era: the role of histological grade. *Breast Cancer Res* 2010; 12(4): 207.

30. Engers, R. Reproducibility and reliability of tumor grading in urological neoplasms. *World J Urol* 2007; 25(6): 595–605.

31. Dowsett, M., Nielsen, T. O., A'Hern, R., Bartlett, J., Coombes, R. C., Cuzick, J. *et al.* Assessment of Ki67 in breast cancer: recommendations from the international Ki67 in breast cancer working group. *J Natl Cancer Inst* 2011; 103(22): 1656–64.

32. Han, K., Nofech-Mozes, S., Narod, S., Hanna, W., Vesprini, D., Saskin, R. *et al.* Expression of HER2neu in ductal carcinoma in situ is associated with local recurrence. *Clin Oncol (R Coll Radiol)* 2012; 24(3): 183–9.

33. Sauter, G., Lee, J., Bartlett, J. M., Slamon, D. J. and Press, M. F. Guidelines for human epidermal growth factor receptor 2 testing: biologic and methodologic considerations. *J Clin Oncol* 2009; 27(8): 1323–33.

34. Dancey, J. E., Dobbin, K. K., Groshen, S., Jessup, J. M.,

Hruszkewycz, A. H., Koehler, M. *et al.* Guidelines for the development and incorporation of biomarker studies in early clinical trials of novel agents. *Clin Cancer Res* 2010; 16(6): 1745–55.

35. Simon, R. M., Paik, S. and Hayes, D. F. Use of archived specimens in evaluation of prognostic and predictive biomarkers. *J Natl Cancer Inst* 2009; 101(21): 1446–52.

36. Taube, S. E., Clark, G. M., Dancey, J. E., McShane, L. M., Sigman, C. C. and Gutman, S. I. A perspective on challenges and issues in biomarker development and drug and biomarker codevelopment. *J Natl Cancer Inst* 2009; 101(21): 1453–63.

37. McShane, L. M., Altman, D. G., Sauerbrei, W., Taube, S. E., Gion, M. and Clark, G. M. Reporting recommendations for tumour MARKer prognostic studies (REMARK). *Br J Cancer* 2005; 93 (4): 387–91.

38. Abe, O., Abe, R., Enomoto, K., Kikuchi, K., Koyama, H., Masuda, H. *et al.* Effects of chemotherapy and hormonal therapy for early breast cancer on recurrence and 15-year survival: an overview of the randomised trials. *Lancet* 2005; 365(9472): 1687–717.

39. Abe, O., Abe, R., Enomoto, K., Kikuchi, K., Koyama, H., Nomura, Y. *et al.* Polychemotherapy for early breast cancer: an overview of the randomised trials. *Lancet* 1998; 352(9132): 930–42.

40. Oxnard, G. R. and Jänne, P. A. Power in numbers: meta-analysis to identify inhibitor-sensitive tumor genotypes. *Clin Cancer Res* 2013; 19(7): 1634–6.

41. Schoenborn, J. R., Nelson, P. and Fang, M. Genomic profiling defines subtypes of prostate cancer with the potential for therapeutic stratification. *Clin Cancer Res* 2013; 19(15): 4058–66.

42. Costello, E., Greenhalf, W. and Neoptolemos, J. P. New

biomarkers and targets in pancreatic cancer and their application to treatment. *Nat Rev Gastroenterol Hepatol* 2012; 9(8): 435–44.

43. Ravdin, P. M. Adjuvant! version 5. Underlying data and assumptions. *Breast Cancer Res Treat* 2003; 82: 321.

44. Bartlett, J. M. S., Brookes, C. L., Robson, T., van de Velde, C. J. H., Billingham, L. J., Campbell, F. M. *et al.* Estrogen receptor and progesterone receptor as predictive biomarkers of response to endocrine therapy: a prospectively powered pathology study in the tamoxifen and exemestane adjuvant multinational trial. *J Clin Oncol* 2011; 29(12): 1531–8.

45. Cuzick, J., Dowsett, M., Pineda, S., Wale, C., Salter, J., Quinn, E. *et al.* Prognostic value of a combined estrogen receptor, progesterone receptor, Ki-67, and human epidermal growth factor receptor 2 immunohistochemical score and comparison with the genomic health recurrence score in early breast cancer. *J Clin Oncol* 2011; 29(32): 4273–8.

46. Paik, S., Shak, S., Tang, G., Kim, C., Baker, J., Cronin, M. *et al.* A multigene assay to predict recurrence of tamoxifen-treated, node-negative breast cancer. *New Engl J Med* 2004; 351(27): 2817–26.

47. Hornberger, J., Alvarado, M. D., Rebecca, C., Gutierrez, H. R., Yu, T. M. and Gradishar, W. J. Clinical validity/utility, change in practice patterns, and economic implications of risk stratifiers to predict outcomes for early-stage breast cancer: a systematic review. *J Natl Cancer Inst* 2012; 104(14): 1068–79.

48. Peto, R., Davies, C., Godwin, J., Gray, R., Pan, H. C., Clarke, M. *et al.* Comparisons between different polychemotherapy regimens for early breast cancer: meta-analyses of long-term

outcome among 100,000 women in 123 randomised trials. *Lancet* 2012; 379(9814): 432–44.

49. Hertel, P. B., Tu, D., Ejlertsen, B., Jensen, M. B., Balslev, E., Jiang, S. *et al.* TIMP-1 in combination with HER2 and TOP2A for prediction of benefit from adjuvant anthracyclines in high-risk breast cancer patients. *Breast Cancer Res Treat* 2012; 132(1): 225–34.

50. Pritchard, K., Munro, A., O'Malley, F., Tu, D., Li, X., Levine, M. *et al.* Chromosome

17 centromere (CEP17) duplication as a predictor of anthracycline response: evidence from the NCIC Clinical Trials Group (NCIC CTG) MA.5 Trial. *Breast Cancer Res Treat* 2012; 131(2): 541–51.

51. Di Leo, A., Isola, J., Piette, F., Ejlertsen, B., Pritchard, K. I., Bartlett, J. M. S. *et al.* A meta-analysis of phase III trials evaluating the predictive value of HER2 and topoisomerase II alpha in early breast cancer patients treated with CMF or anthracycline-based

adjuvant therapy. *Cancer Res* 2009; 69(2): 99S.

52. Hayes, D. F., Thor, A. D., Dressler, L. G., Weaver, D., Edgerton, S., Cowan, D. *et al.* HER2 and response to paclitaxel in node-positive breast cancer. *New Engl J Med* 2007; 357(15): 1496–506.

53. Dowsett, M., Goldhirsch, A., Hayes, D. F., Senn, H. J., Wood, W. and Viale, G. International web-based consultation on priorities for translational breast cancer research. *Breast Cancer Res* 2007; 9(6): R81.

# Molecular regulation of cellular function

Marsela Braunstein and John M. S. Bartlett

## Overview

Within the human body exists a diversity of cells that perform specialized functions yet contain the same genetic material as all other cells. How, then, does a liver cell "know" how to function as a liver cell and a skin cell, with the same genetic blueprint, function in an entirely different manner? Cellular function is controlled by a highly complex and interconnected network of intracellular signaling pathways. Since all cells, apart from differentiated B-cells and enucleated red blood cells, contain the same DNA "codeset" to direct cellular function, it is clear that for different cellular functions to be manifest some signaling pathways must be activated and others deactivated. Activation of critical pathways, such as metabolic pathways, is common to all cells in the body; however, within cells, specific functional pathways may be "imprinted" during embryological development and differentiation, or modified by specific environmental or developmental cues. The process of silencing some pathways and activating others is fundamental to the development of specific tissue types. The resulting cell is functionally organized, which is a defining feature of a multicellular organism. Despite developmental commitment, however, it is becoming increasingly evident that even terminally differentiated cells retain a degree of developmental plasticity. In normal tissues, for example, monocytes may differentiate into either dendritic cells or macrophages depending on the cytokines produced by infected tissues. In response to extracellular stimuli, metastatic cancer cells may undergo epithelial-to-mesenchymal transition to detach from the tumor and migrate to distant tissues.

Cancer is a disease of deregulation of cellular control pathways and, therefore, to understand cancer it is essential that we understand the regulation of normal cellular function and its broad diversity. This chapter will provide an overview of molecular pathways, regulatory mechanisms and signaling networks that control normal cell function, and outline the challenges to development of therapeutic agents targeting deregulation of key pathways in pathological conditions such as cancer. We will begin by describing the concept of receptor signaling and a simple, linear signal transduction pathway. Additionally, we will discuss more complex pathways, how they engage in signaling networks during cross talk and describe regulatory inputs that control the effects of signaling events. To finish, we will discuss how complex molecular changes within an organism contribute to the continuing "evolution" of adaptive mechanisms in pathological conditions such as cancer.

## Signaling pathways

### Receptor signaling turns on a switch

Signaling pathways convey information from the extracellular environment to the interior of the cell that leads to a particular cellular response. Most signaling pathways involve a physical interaction between two components: a ligand and a receptor. Ligands, which may be secreted or membrane bound, bind to receptors on another or the same cell. A receptor molecule is usually a transmembrane protein that not only binds a ligand, but also acts to transmit the signal. In many cases, the intermediate molecules are protein or lipid kinases, which phosphorylate a target molecule to activate it. Signals are propagated like waves, which induce reversible changes to signaling intermediates: one activated kinase phosphorylates the next, which in turn phosphorylates another, triggering a chain reaction in a

*Molecular Pathology: A Practical Guide for the Surgical Pathologist and Cytopathologist*, ed. John M. S. Bartlett, Abeer Shaaban and Fernando Schmitt. Published by Cambridge University Press. © Cambridge University Press, 2016.

switch-like manner. The activated kinases are rapidly dephosphorylated by phosphatases, which return kinases into an inactive state until another extracellular stimulus arrives. The signaling pathway culminates in either activation or inhibition of a protein that participates in a cellular response, such as transcriptional activity, cellular motility, proliferation, growth or apoptosis.

# Major signaling pathways in animals: a view from linear to complex signal transduction cascade

Cell-fate decisions during development and later in the life of an animal are controlled by multiple signaling pathways (1). Of these, seven pathways are used repeatedly throughout development to activate different suits of target genes. These pathways include: Wnt (Wingless related), TGFβ (transforming growth factor β), Hedgehog, JAK/STAT (Janus kinase/Signal Transducer and Activator of Transcription), RTKs (receptor tyrosine kinases) superfamily, Notch and nuclear hormone receptor (2) (Table 2.1). The remaining ten pathways are used during organogenesis and throughout adult life, and include: toll-like receptors (TLR), apoptotic pathways, adhesion molecule signaling pathways (cadherin, integrin and gap junctions), ligand-gated ion channels, receptor phosphotyrosine phosphatase, receptor guanylate cyclise, nitric oxide receptor, as well as G-protein-coupled receptor superfamily (1).

With the exception of nuclear hormone and nitric oxide receptors, which are intracellular receptors binding hydrophobic ligands that diffuse across the cell membrane, the majority of signaling pathways involve ligand binding to a membrane-bound receptor. Of those, perhaps the simplest is the JAK/STAT pathway, which involves a linear activation of signaling intermediates and three signaling steps: 1. dimerization of cytokine/chemokine receptor subunits that induces cross-phosphorylation of JAKs; 2. subsequent phosphorylation and dimerization of two STAT molecules; and 3. nuclear translocation of STATs and activation of target gene expression (Figure 2.1). The pathway is negatively regulated by SOCS (suppressors of cytokine signaling) proteins that bind directly to JAK molecules and act as pseudosubstrates to inhibit JAK activity (5). The TGFβ pathway is conceptually similar to the JAK/STAT pathway as it involves phosphorylation and dimerization of SMAD transcription factors, but multiple protein modifications and extracellular regulators add additional levels of complexity to this pathway (6). The remaining pathways, Wnt, Notch, Hedgehog and RTKs, however, do not involve a linear activation of merely two signaling intermediates.

A good example of a complex signal transduction pathway is HER receptor signaling, a member of the RTK signaling pathway superfamily. The complexity initiates at the top of the signaling cascade: four HER receptors homo- and heterodimerize to generate 10 receptor combinations. When this receptor diversity is coupled to the existence of 30 different ligands, one can begin to appreciate the intricacy of the HER receptor signaling pathway that generates complex, yet distinct, signaling outcomes. In addition, activated HER receptor signaling utilizes multiple adaptor proteins and secondary messengers, which may branch into any one of the four major signaling cascades:

**Table 2.1** Seven signaling pathways used repeatedly during animal development and life (1, 3, 34)

| Pathway | Signaling molecule | Receptors | Ligands |
| --- | --- | --- | --- |
| Wnt | Wnt | 12 | 19 |
| TGFβ | TGFβ | 12 | 33 |
| Hedgehog | Hedgehog | 1 | 3 |
| Receptor tyrosine kinase superfamily (with 20 subfamilies) | RTK | 54 | 48 |
| Notch-Delta | Notch | 4 | 5 |
| Cytokine receptor superfamily | JAK/STAT | >70 | 7 |
| Nuclear hormone receptor superfamily | Nuclear hormone | 59 | Various lipophilic molecules |

**11**

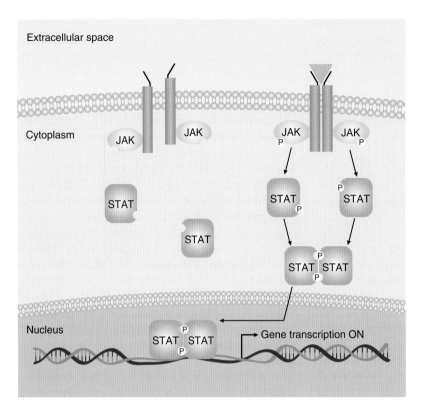

Extracellular space

Cytoplasm

Nucleus

Gene transcription ON

**Figure 2.1** JAK/STAT signaling pathway. © The Ontario Institute for Cancer Research (OICR).

1. MAPK (mitogen-activated protein kinase)/Erk pathway; 2. PI3K (phosphatidylinositide 3-kinase)/Akt/mTOR pathway; 3. STAT1/3 signaling pathway; and 4. PLCγ/IP3/DAG/PKC (phospholipase Cγ/inositol 1,4,5-triphosphate/diacylglycerol/proteink inase C) pathway (7)(Figure 2.2). Finally, this complex pathway is negatively regulated by dephosphorylation, ubiquitination and receptor endocytosis (7).

Since the complexity in signaling pathways arises from multiple ligand-receptor combinations (Table 2.1), it raises a question of how the specificity in cellular responses is achieved. For HER signaling, distinct activation of one signaling cascade but not others is largely determined by a combination of factors: the concentration of ligands, the composition of receptor and the rate of ligand-receptor dissociation (8, 9). In addition, at least five other mechanisms have been proposed to generate signaling specificity of receptors (10). Firstly, lipid-enriched microenvironments called lipid rafts are concentrated in protein kinases, adaptor molecules, scaffolds and other molecules involved in signaling pathways. As such, they can include and exclude proteins involved in signaling cascades, controling the specificity of

protein-protein interaction downstream of ligand-receptor engagement (11). Secondly, the same receptor may bind ligands with different affinities, which will lead to a distinct cellular response. For example, during HER signaling high-affinity receptor-ligand interactions activate canonical Ras/MAPK and PI3K/Akt pathways leading to cellular proliferation; in contrast, low-affinity interactions activate STAT factors, which inhibit proliferation and enhance cellular adhesion (12). Thirdly, multiple pathways may need to work cooperatively to stimulate gene expression. For example, Notch and Wnt signaling pathways stimulate hematopoietic stem cells to develop into T lymphocytes. Functional inactivation of key regulatory transcription factors downstream of either one of these pathways arrests thymocyte development or redirects differentiation into alternative blood lineages (13–17). Fourthly, the same receptor may activate different signaling cascades in different cells (10). Fifthly, the cells express tissue-specific transcriptional regulators that determine whether a cell responds to the activated pathway, a concept that we will elaborate on in the section entitled "Transcription factors are the effectors of signaling pathways."

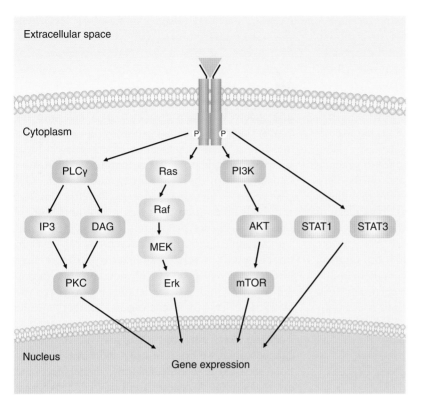

Extracellular space

Cytoplasm

Nucleus

Gene expression

**Figure 2.2** RTK pathway branches into distinct signaling cascades. © The Ontario Institute for Cancer Research (OICR).

# Receptors are grouped into families

The availability of the whole genome sequences of yeast, worm, fly, fish and human has made it possible to obtain a greater understanding of the signaling components in a given animal compared to a gene-by-gene approach utilized in the pre-genome era. Based on their conserved structure or function, receptors are grouped into distinct families. Frizzled receptors, which bind to Wnt ligands, belong to a family of receptors with a recruiting ability (18). Unlike RTKs, Frizzled has no catalytic activity; instead, ligand binding initiates accumulation of stabilized β-catenin in the cytoplasm, which translocates into the nucleus to activate target gene expression. RTKs and TGFβ receptors possess structural domains that phosphorylate the receptor itself as well as downstream signaling molecules, forming a family of receptors with intrinsic enzymatic activity. On the other hand, the Hedgehog receptor called Patched antagonizes Smoothened (SMO) activation in the absence of its ligands; however, once Hedgehog binds to Patched, the whole complex becomes internalized, which allows SMO to activate Gli transcription factors (19). Because of this translocation property, Hedgehog receptors belong to a family of transporter-like receptors (18). In fact, this is a superfamily consisting of five families, numerous subfamilies and nearly 800 genes in humans encoding for G-protein-coupled receptors (GPCR) (20). Although not structurally conserved, all GPCRs share a seven-transmembrane topology and undergo a conformational change upon ligand-receptor interaction. Next, Notch receptor signaling involves the activity of four Notch (Notch 1–4) receptors and five membrane-anchored ligands in humans: Delta-like (Dl)-1, Dl-3, Dl-4, Jagged-1 and Jagged-2 (21). Upon Notch-Dl interaction, γ-secretase cleaves the intracellular portion of Notch (ICN) for nuclear translocation. ICN is an active form of Notch that displaces a repressor and acts as a transcriptional activator. Thus, Notch receptors are unique in that they possess an intrinsic transcriptional activity. Nuclear receptors are similar to ICN in a sense that the receptor is classified as a transcription factor; however, while Notch receptors are membrane-bound, nuclear receptors are generally intracellular and typically located in the cytosol. Once a steroid hormone diffuses across the plasma membrane, it binds to the nuclear receptor; it is only in this form that the receptor is capable of executing a function of a transcription factor. Lastly, adaptive immune receptors expressed by T-cells (T-cell receptor; TCR) and B-cells (B-cell receptor; BCR) represent a unique class of rearranging receptors. The genes encoding for these two receptors are composed of multiple gene segments, called variable (V), diversity (D) and joining (J) segments, which are "cut and pasted" by RAG (recombination-activating gene) enzymes to generate an enormous repertoire of TCRs and BCRs. This enables the adaptive immune cells to bind to millions of different ligands, called antigens, regardless of whether they are used in self-recognition or activation of immune response upon non-self recognition. Unlike any other cellular receptor, BCR can improve its affinity for antigens by inserting random mutations into the ligand-binding component of BCR. This process, called affinity maturation, is a unique feature of BCRs that generates highly specific, secreted forms of BCR called antibodies.

## Signaling pathways form signaling networks

During animal development and later in life, signaling pathways are rarely activated in isolation; instead, the pathways engage in a cross-talk, which creates a sophisticated response to external stimuli (19). Some of these signaling networks are specific to stem cells, while other networks, or just components of signaling networks, are activated in differentiating tissues (19). Although the signal transduction components remain unchanged, the responses generated through these sophisticated networks may become unpredictable due to the variety of ligands and their receptors (Table 2.1), as well as the increasing number of their target genes. The following example illustrates the cross-talk interactions among RTK, Notch, Hedgehog and Wnt pathways (Figure 2.3A). Signaling through Notch and RTK activates PI3K/Akt, which in turn activates mTOR. Inhibitor of mTOR down-regulates not only mTOR but ICN as well, suggesting that mTOR positively regulates Notch signaling (22). Conversely, Notch1 siRNA (short interfering RNA) down-regulates Akt and mTOR, indicating that mTOR is also activated by Notch signaling (23). Cross-talk between Notch and Hedgehog pathways occurs through the activity of ICN, which up-regulates Sonic Hedgehog (24), a ligand for Patched

receptor. Conversely, signaling through SMO activates Gli1 transcription factors that induce expression of Jagged-2, a ligand for Notch receptors (19) (Figure 2.3A) and completes the positive feedback loop that exists between Notch and Hedgehog signaling pathways. In addition, Gli1 transcription factors up-regulate Wnt, engaging in a cross-talk with the Wnt/β-catenin signaling pathway. Depending on the context, Wnt signaling could be negatively regulated by Hedgehog, which is found to inhibit Wnt signaling through the activity of SFRP-1 (25) (Figure 2.3A). Signaling pathways, therefore, interact with each other as parts of larger, multidimensional signaling networks that cannot be fully appreciated with a simple illustration. However, one can envision this complex network resembling a constellation map when 17 major signaling pathways converge during development and differentiation (Figure 2.4). The interactions contain numerous nodes that may be partially or fully activated, or inhibited, upon receptor signaling. Yet, even this road map is "subject to change" when we begin to layer additional information, such as developmental time, tissue space and external stimuli. A systems approach will help generate more comprehensive receptor signaling networks and gene regulatory circuits, which will still have to be qualified based on the spatial, temporal and environmental contexts.

## Transcription factors are the effectors of signaling pathways

### Molecular regulation of gene expression

The actions and properties of cells are determined by the differential gene expression, which refers to an entire process whereby the information encoded by genes is decoded into proteins in response to external stimuli or particular developmental cues. Gene expression is initiated by RNA polymerase complex, which transcribes genes into mRNA; processed and spliced mRNA translocates to the cytoplasm where translation occurs. Regulatory mechanisms exist at each step of gene expression; however, the most important mechanisms in eukaryotes center on the transcriptional initiation. This process is controlled by transcription factors, which are executers of signaling pathways. They bind to the regulatory DNA sequences that consist of promoters, which position RNA polymerase close to the transcription-initiation

A

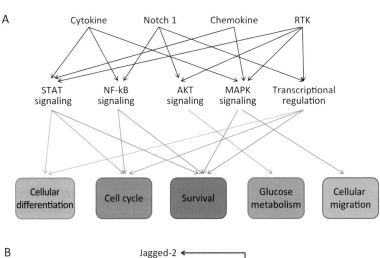

**Figure 2.3** Cross-talk among signaling pathways creates a signaling network.

B

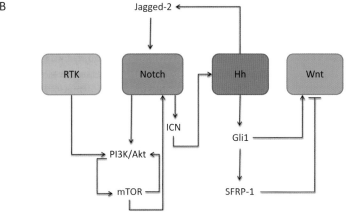

**Figure 2.4** A network resembling a constellation map when all 17 signaling pathways converge during development and differentiation.

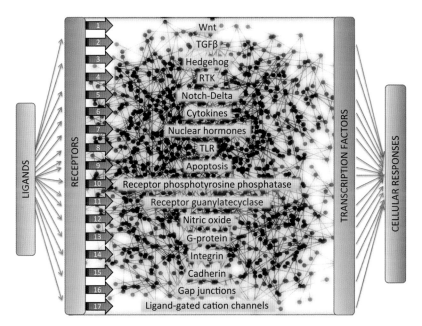

site, and enhancers, which stimulate transcription from a promoter in a tissue-specific manner. Transcription factors are proteins that bind to promoter and enhancer regulatory elements and function as activators or repressors of protein-coding genes.

The control of gene expression can be visualized as involving five levels: three-dimensional (3D), epigenetic, transcriptional, translational and posttranslational (Figure 2.5). The development of modern chromosome visualizing techniques, such as 3C (chromosome conformation capture) technology, has allowed the analysis of physical interactions among chromosomes. In particular, it has become evident that widely spaced chromosomal regions can loop and interact with each other to connect genes and regulatory regions separated by thousands of kilobases into so-called transcription factories (26) (Figure 2.5, part 1). The transcriptional activity of the interacting regions will depend on the state of the chromatin structure, which is determined by epigenetic modifications (Figure 2.5, part 2). DNA that is tightly bound by histones is closed, thus inhibiting unwanted gene transcription. When histones are modified by changing the acetylation and methylation patterns, the chromatin is in an open state allowing transcription factors to access DNA regulatory

elements (Figure 2.5, part 3). Activators interact with other proteins in the complex and bind to DNA to turn on transcription from a nearby promoter. Repressors, on the other hand, inhibit the activity of the transcription factors in the complex, thereby turning off the expression of the nearby gene (Figure 2.5, part 3). Even if the gene is successfully transcribed, mRNA stability may be compromised in response to a change in environmental conditions. Numerous mechanisms exist to ensure that there is a balance between protein translation and mRNA-decay. One mechanism involves nucleases, which are enzymes that bind to mRNA and initiate RNA-decay. Another mechanism, called RNA interference (27), involves the activity of microRNA (miRNA; Figure 2.5, part 4), which are 20 to 30 basepair short, non-coding RNA molecules that are complementary to mRNA. Upon binding, they prevent translation and cause mRNA degradation. Lastly, posttranslational modifications ensure that newly synthesized peptides are stable and functional. Most common protein-stabilizing modifications involve protein phosphorylation (Figure 2.5, part 5), glycosylation and acetylation; in contrast, misfolded proteins are subjected to poly-ubiquitination and subsequent degradation by proteasomes (Figure 2.5, part 5).

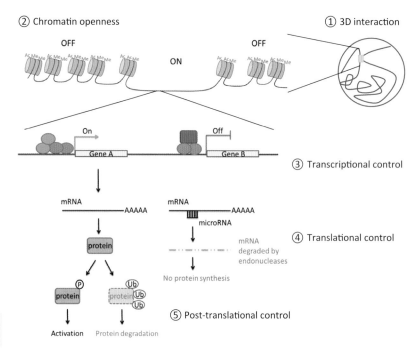

Figure 2.5 Molecular regulation of gene expression.

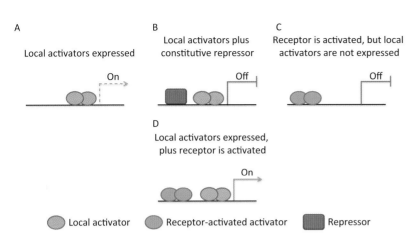

A

Local activators expressed

B

Local activators plus
constitutive repressor

C

Receptor is activated, but local
activators are not expressed

D

Local activators expressed,
plus receptor is activated

⬤ Local activator    ⬤ Receptor-activated activator    ▮ Repressor

**Figure 2.6** Receptor signaling alone is insufficient to activate gene expression.

## Signaling pathways alone are insufficient to activate gene expression

Signaling through a receptor activates a pathway; however, not all cells respond equally, or at all, to the same environmental cue. This is an important feature contributing not only to normal cellular development and function, but also to cancer. Three fundamental mechanisms of gene regulation are shared by most signaling pathways: activator insufficiency, default repression and cooperative activation (2). Whether a cell responds to receptor signaling is ultimately determined by the presence of local activators. Activator insufficiency refers to a scenario where a receptor-activated transcription factor alone cannot activate gene expression due to the absence of local activators (Figure 2.6C). These are usually tissue-specific factors, which ensure gene activation only within correct temporal and spatial contexts. In Notch-Delta pathway for instance, combinatorial and synergistic interaction among Notch-target genes and tissue-specific factors, such as GATA factors and bHLH proteins, provides differential signaling outcomes by the mechanisms that are not yet well understood (28). Default repression, on the other hand, ensures that local activators are not weakly and constitutively active (Figure 2.6A) and that genes are kept off until appropriate receptor signaling switches it on (Figure 2.6B). Importantly, by having fully occupied DNA regulatory sites, receptor signaling can trigger rapid gene transcription and initiate an appropriate cellular response. Default repression is by far the most common regulatory mechanism of gene expression: of the seven major signaling pathways (Table 2.1), the JAK/STAT pathway is the only one without a

known default repressor. Lastly, cooperative activation refers to a combinatorial action of local activators and receptor-regulated transcription factors (Figure 2.6D), which allows robust and highly specific activation of target genes. Robust cooperative activation may be due to additive effects of signaling inputs, or due to enhanced physical interaction of activators, co-activators and basal transcription factors at the gene regulatory sequences (2). Overall, these regulatory mechanisms explain why some cells respond with precision to receptor signaling, while other neighboring cells remain unresponsive. Furthermore, it also suggests that mutations in regulatory regions would be insufficient to drive ectopic gene expression.

## Challenges in pathological conditions

Building a network with all participating pathways and being able to predict a cellular response is currently an area of intense research. Although we may not be able to piece together all cross-talk interactions in this complex network in the next 5 to 10 years, we are certainly getting closer to identifying the participating players in the context of normal and pathological cell development and differentiation. Figure 2.3B illustrates an example of a "simple" network showing inputs that a single T lymphocyte receives upon activation of cytokine, chemokine, RTK and Notch receptors. Ligands activate a number of effector molecules, such as Akt, MAPK, NF-κB, STAT or various other transcriptional regulators, which engage in a cross-talk to activate cellular responses such as differentiation, proliferation, survival, migration or metabolic changes (Figure 2.3B).

One can envision how convoluted a regulatory network becomes once all 17 signaling pathways are activated in a cell (Figure 2.4). In a pathological condition such as cancer, a particular cellular response may be changed with an alteration as simple as a DNA mutation. For instance, p53 gene loss-of-wild-type function mutations produce a protein that exerts a dominant-negative function over wildtype p53 and often functions in a wildtype p53-independent manner, allowing cancer cells to grow uncontrollably (29, 30). Conversely, gain-of-function mutations in Notch1 gene constitutively activate Notch/Delta signaling pathway and downstream target genes that contribute to the development of T-cell leukemia (31). Alternatively, gene amplification and over-expression of HER2 in certain breast cancers represents yet another alteration that modifies a gene regulatory network. Other mechanisms include gene deletions as well as epigenetic changes, including methylation and acetylation patterns. Thus, the "road map" to a particular cellular response in cancer may change considerably, rendering the signaling networks established for normal cells somewhat redundant.

To add to this complexity, cancers are composed of heterogeneous populations (32) where some cells fully activate a particular pathway and other cells do not. Furthermore, cancers are not only heterogeneous within, but between different patients, making it extremely difficult to devise a specific, yet universal treatment option. This begs a question as to how cancer cells remain functional despite numerous environmental and therapeutic insults. The increased complexity of signaling networks is a reflection of cancer evolution due to selection pressures that include environmentally derived genotoxicity, cancer therapeutics and niche availability (33). After a selection pressure is applied, some clones become distinct, while others survive and expand into a newly available microenvironment. For example, an increased hypoxic condition within the tumor mass represents an environmental selection pressure that limits which cancer cells are fit to survive. Tumor evolution involves up-regulation of VEGF (vascular epithelial growth factors) that stimulate development of new blood vessels, increasing nutrient and oxygen supply to the growing tumor mass (34). Later, the evolution may involve a selection of clones with mutations in molecular targets against which a particular pharmaceutical agent is used. Ultimately, what drives tumor evolution is a combination of existing and acquired molecular changes. This continuous selection and adaptation of cancer cells makes it difficult to predict what effects pharmaceutical agents will have on a target pathway for an extended period of time; consequently, as cancer adapts, so must the treatment.

Let us consider a specific example, such as targeting Hedgehog signaling pathway in the cancer cells (Figure 2.7). Blocking antibodies, which prevent formation of Hedgehog-Patched complex, are among the most important negative regulators of Hedgehog pathway (35) (Figure 2.7A). In basal cell cancer, the adaptation involves inactivating mutations in Patched receptor and activating mutations in SMO, which bypass the requirement for Hedgehog ligand and, therefore, constitutively activate Gli factors (Figure 2.7B). As a result, pharmaceutical companies have focused on developing small-molecule inhibitors against SMO. The most common inhibitors range from naturally derived cyclopamine that is already commercially available, to potent small-molecule SMO inhibitor GDC-0449 (Figure 2.7C), which is in stage II clinical trials (19). The effects of the SMO inhibitors are eventually surpassed as the cells acquire resistance to drugs. The most common mechanism involves the up-regulation of efflux pumps, which actively transport drugs across the plasma membrane into the extracellular environment, hence decreasing the intracellular concentration of inhibitors. In addition, frequent mutations in suppressor of fused homolog (SUFU), which keeps Gli factors in an inactive form, liberates Gli factors that positively regulate cell cycle progression in cancer cells (36) (Figure 2.7D). Emerging therapies in pre-clinical development include silencing Gli factors by siRNA (Figure 2.7E). However, even if many of these approaches successfully down-regulate Hedgehog pathway signaling, the problem of cross-talk still remains. In the case of Hedgehog signaling pathway, it is the epidermal growth factor receptor (EGFR) pathway that up-regulates cell cycle progression via Akt and MAPK signaling intermediates (35) (Figure 2.7F). Thus, it is the integration of cell signaling networks and diverse regulatory mechanisms in both normal and pathological conditions that will determine the biological effect in response to the exogenous stimuli.

Increasing our understanding of these sophisticated cellular functions will determine how well prepared we are to tackle complex pathological

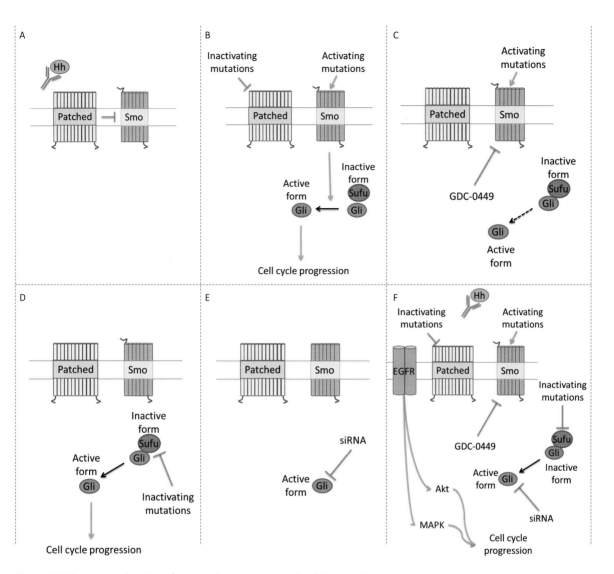

**Figure 2.7** Continuous adaptation of cancer cells to environmental and therapeutic changes.

conditions such as cancer. The advances in molecular technologies and the establishment of centralized data portals, The Cancer Genome Atlas (TCGA) and The Cancer Genome Consortium, have enabled researchers not only to generate a wealth of genomic data, but also to easily access, share and systemically analyze thousands of tumors. For example, the TCGA Pan-

Cancer project identified 127 mutated genes across 12 tumor types; surprisingly, the average number of driver mutations is low, ranging from two to six mutations per gene (37). Such efforts hold promise in delivering specific therapies on a per-patient basis, bringing us closer to the aspirations of personalized medicine.

# References

1. Gerhart, J. Warkany lecture: signaling pathways in development. *Teratology* 1998; 60(4): 226–39.

2. Barolo, S. and Posakony, J. W. Three habits of highly effective signaling pathways: principles of transcriptional control by developmental cell signaling. *Genes Dev* 2002; 16(10): 1167–81.

3. Robinson, D. R., Wu, Y.-M. and Lin, S.-F. The protein tyrosine

kinase family of the human genome. *Oncogene* 2000; 19(49): 5548–57.

4. Moustakas, A. and Heldin, C.-H. The regulation of TGFbeta signal transduction. *Development* 2009; 136(22): 3699–714.

5. Yoshimura, A., Naka, T. and Kubo, M. SOCS proteins, cytokine signalling and immune regulation. *Nat Rev Immunol* 2007; 7(6): 454–65.

6. Massague, J. TGFbeta signalling in context. *Nat Rev Mol Cell Biol* 2012; 13(10): 616–30.

7. Lemmon, M. A. and Schlessinger, J. Cell signaling by receptor tyrosine kinases. *Cell* 2010; 141(7): 1117–34.

8. Pinkas-Kramarski, R., Soussan, L., Waterman, H., Levkowitz, G., Alroy, I., Klapper, L. et al. Diversification of Neu differentiation factor and epidermal growth factor signaling by combinatorial receptor interactions. *EMBO J* 1996; 15(10): 2452–67.

9. Zaczek, A., Brandt, B. and Bielawski, K. P. The diverse signaling network of EGFR, HER2, HER3 and HER4 tyrosine kinase receptors and the consequences for therapeutic approaches. *Histol Histopathol* 2005; 20(3): 1005–15.

10. Pires-daSilva, A. and Sommer, R. J. The evolution of signalling pathways in animal development. *Nat Rev Genet* 2003; 4(1): 39–49.

11. Simons, K. and Toomre, D. Lipid rafts and signal transduction. *Nat Rev Mol Cell Biol* 2000; 1(1): 31–9.

12. Krall, J. A., Beyer, E. M. and MacBeath, G. High- and low-affinity epidermal growth factor receptor-ligand interactions activate distinct signaling pathways. *PLoS ONE* 2011; 6(1): e15945.

13. Li, L., Leid, M. and Rothenberg, E. V. An early T cell lineage commitment checkpoint

dependent on the transcription factor Bcl11b. *Science* 2010; 329 (5987): 89–93.

14. Li, P., Burke, S., Wang, J., Chen, X., Ortiz, M., Lee, S. C. et al. Reprogramming of T cells to natural killer-like cells upon Bcl11b deletion. *Science* 2010; 329(5987): 85–9.

15. van de Wetering, M., de Lau, W. and Clevers, H. WNT signaling and lymphocyte development. *Cell* 2002; 109(Suppl.): S13–S19.

16. Ikawa, T., Hirose, S., Masuda, K., Kakugawa, K., Satoh, R., Shibano-Satoh, A. et al. An essential developmental checkpoint for production of the T cell lineage. *Science* 2010; 329(5987): 93–6.

17. Braunstein, M. and Anderson, M. K. HEB-deficient T-cell precursors lose T-cell potential and adopt an alternative pathway of differentiation. *Mol Cell Biol* 2011; 31(5): 971–82.

18. Ben-Shlomo, I., Yu, H. S., Rauch, R., Kowalski, H. W. and Hsueh, A. J. Signaling receptome: a genomic and evolutionary perspective of plasma membrane receptors involved in signal transduction. *Sci STKE* 2003; 2003(187): RE9.

19. Takebe, N., Harris, P. J., Warren, R. Q. and Ivy, S. P. Targeting cancer stem cells by inhibiting Wnt, Notch, and Hedgehog pathways. *Nat Rev Clin Oncol* 2011; 8(2): 97–106.

20. Katritch, V., Cherezov, V. and Stevens, R. C. Structure-function of the G protein-coupled receptor superfamily. *Annu Rev Pharmacol Toxicol* 2013; 53: 531–56.

21. Radtke, F., Wilson, A. and MacDonald, H. R. Notch signaling in T- and B-cell development. *Curr Opin Immunol* 2004; 16(2): 174–9.

22. Ma, J., Meng, Y., Kwiatkowski, D. J., Chen, X., Peng, H., Sun, Q. et al. Mammalian target of rapamycin regulates murine and human cell differentiation

through STAT3/p63/Jagged/Notch cascade. *J Clin Invest* 2010; 120(1): 103–14.

23. Wang, Z., Li, Y., Banerjee, S., Kong, D., Ahmad, A., Nogueira, V. et al. Down-regulation of Notch-1 and Jagged-1 inhibits prostate cancer cell growth, migration and invasion, and induces apoptosis via inactivation of Akt, mTOR, and NF-kappaB signaling pathways. *J Cell Biochem* 2010; 109(4): 726–36.

24. Androutsellis-Theotokis, A., Leker, R. R., Soldner, F., Hoeppner, D. J., Ravin, R., Poser, S. W. et al.Notch signalling regulates stem cell numbers in vitro and in vivo. *Nature* 2006; 442(7104): 823–6.

25. Borday, C., Cabochette, P., Parain, K., Mazurier, N., Janssens, S., Tran, H. T. et al.Antagonistic cross-regulation between Wnt and Hedgehog signalling pathways controls post-embryonic retinal proliferation. *Development* 2012; 139(19): 3499–509.

26. Gibcus, J. H. and Dekker, J. The hierarchy of the 3D genome. *Mol Cell* 2013; 49(5): 773–82.

27. Wilson, R. C. and Doudna, J. A. Molecular mechanisms of RNA interference. *Annu Rev Biophys* 2013; 42: 217–39.

28. Bray, S. and Bernard, F. Notch targets and their regulation. *Curr Top Dev Biol* 2010; 92: 253–75.

29. Petitjean, A., Mathe, E., Kato, S., Ishioka, C., Tavtigian, S. V., Hainaut, P. et al.Impact of mutant p53 functional properties on TP53 mutation patterns and tumor phenotype: lessons from recent developments in the IARC TP53 database. *Hum Mutat* 2007; 28(6): 622–9.

30. Muller, P. A. and Vousden, K. H. p53 mutations in cancer. *Nat Cell Biol* 2013; 15(1): 2–8.

31. Aster, J. C., Blacklow, S. C. and Pear, W. S. Notch signalling in T-cell lymphoblastic

leukaemia/lymphoma and other haematological malignancies. *J Pathol* 2011; 223 (2): 262–73.

32. De Sousa E. Melo, F., Vermeulen, L., Fessler, E. and Medema, J. P. Cancer heterogeneity – a multifaceted view. *EMBO Rep* 2013; 14(8): 686–95.

33. Greaves, M. and Maley, C. C. Clonal evolution in cancer. *Nature* 2012; 481(7381): 306–13.

34. Carmeliet, P. VEGF as a key mediator of angiogenesis in cancer. *Oncology* 2005; 69(Suppl. 3): 4–10.

35. Mimeault, M. and Batra, S. K. Frequent deregulations in the hedgehog signaling network and cross-talks with the epidermal growth factor receptor pathway involved in cancer progression and targeted therapies. *Pharmacol Rev* 2010; 62(3): 497–524.

36. Taylor, M. D., Liu, L., Raffel, C., Hui, C. C., Mainprize, T. G., Zhang, X. *et al.* Mutations in SUFU predispose to medulloblastoma. *Nat Genet* 2002; 31(3): 306–10.

37. Kandoth, C., McLellan, M. D., Vandin, F., Ye, K., Niu, B., Lu, C. *et al.* Mutational landscape and significance across 12 major cancer types. *Nature* 2013; 502 (7471): 333–9.

# Chapter 3

# Practical application of molecular techniques in diagnostic histopathology and cytopathology and clinical management

Abeer Shaaban and Fernando Schmitt

## Introduction

The application of molecular techniques has changed the practice of histopathology and cytopathology. Currently, the use of these techniques is widely accepted as an adjuvant to morphological diagnosis. Moreover, the study of diagnostic markers of therapeutic response has been helpful in several types of neoplasms. While most of these techniques have been applied to formalin-fixed paraffin-embedded (FFPE) material, there are advantages to the use of cytological material to perform molecular studies, including ease of obtaining fresh material, ability to check the quality of the material immediately after harvest and better preservation of DNA and RNA [1–3]. The possibility of performing genomic and proteomic studies in small amounts of material obtained, for example, by core needle biopsy or fine-needle aspiration (FNA), can minimize invasive procedures and allow the monitoring of cancer. Techniques such as *in situ* polymerase chain reaction (PCR), microarrays, proteomics and sequencing (including next generation sequencing) are now being validated in some centers, but are still not disseminated in routine clinical practice [4–6]. PCR methods are ideal for cytology material and some applications such as detection of viral sequences, gross chromosomal alterations as deletions and translocations or even point mutations in individual genes. PCR applications are centered in diagnosis of solid tumor detecting gene mutations or detecting clone gene rearrangement in lymphoproliferative disorders. *In situ* hybridization (ISH) can also be applied to both cytology and histological material, permitting, with either fluorescent or chromogenic markers, detection of numerical or structural chromosomal or gene level aberrations. This technique is used to detect deletions, insertions or translocations and is used to detect gene amplifications like HER2 in breast carcinoma or MYCN in neuroblastomas [2–4].

## Technical aspects

Validated protocols for fixation/processing of tissue and/or cytological material must be followed to ensure good quality of the test sample. The main challenges for the application of molecular techniques to pathology are to select the proper test for a limited sample quantity and quality, and to use appropriate controls for diagnostic tests and materials [7]. Validation is an essential step for any molecular diagnostic and rigorous standards must be applied to meet the need for technical accuracy, reproducibility and clinical utility. Evaluation of Genomic Applications in Practice and Prevention (EGAPP) [1, 2], an initiative with a public health focus, was established by the National Office of Public Health Genomics at the Centers for Disease Control and Prevention in the United States. EGAPP supports the development and implementation of a rigorous, evidence-based process for evaluating genetic tests and others that impact on clinical and public health practice. One of the major components of the evaluation is the analytical validity, which includes test sensitivity, specificity, reliability (for example, repeatability of test results) and assay robustness (for example, resistance to minor changes in pre-analytical and analytical factors) [8, 9]. Laboratories should follow the EGAPP criteria for genetic/molecular testing, where available [10].

## Specimens

Proper specimen processing is of utmost importance for any diagnostic technique. While molecular testing can be performed on a variety of specimens ranging from fresh or snap frozen tissue, most current molecular diagnostic procedures have been adapted to the workflow of the diagnostic pathology laboratory and are applied to FFPE or cytology samples. It is worth noting here that other fixatives, in particular Bouin's fixative, which gained favor some 30 to 40 years ago due to the enhanced morphology provided in such samples, may adversely affect the ability to perform modern molecular analyses. The acidic environment in Bouin's fixative, for example, is a major cause for DNA degradation and makes extraction from Bouin's fixed samples very difficult. Some attempts, however, have been made to extract DNA and RNA from those Bouin's fixed samples with limited success [11, 12].

Several molecular techniques can be applied to a variety of histological samples, including core biopsies, punches, standard and large blocks from excision specimens and tissue microarrays. Advances in DNA and RNA extraction techniques have enabled the use of archival FFPE material to provide DNA and RNA for molecular testing. In contrast to DNA, high-quality mRNA is more difficult to extract as mRNA is more sensitive to the effect of fixation, rapidly degraded by ubiquitous RNases and requires stringent RNase free conditions during specimen handling and preparation.

To overcome the issue of tumor heterogeneity, extracting DNA from selected tissue compartment down to a single cell of interest can be done by microdissection. Laser capture microdissection (LCM) allows dissection of area(s) of interest within a histological section and can be applied to various cytological and histological preparations, including FFPE sections [13]. The technique uses a low energy infrared laser pulse to target a visually selected area of tissue section into a thermoplastic membrane. Loss of heterozygosity (LOH) and other DNA-based studies were applied successfully to LCM samples. In combination with whole genome amplification, comparative genomic hybridization (CGH) was used on microdissected samples. In heterogeneous tissue, LCM has also been used to obtain good quality mRNA from FFPE samples by reverse transcription PCR (RT-PCR).

Cytology laboratories process different types of material such as fine-needle aspirates (FNAs), cell suspensions and various types of exfoliative collections. The most commonly used preparations are direct smears, cytospin centrifugations, cell blocks and liquid-based cytology (LBC) preparations. Direct smears are prepared from FNA material, brushings or sediment fresh effusions. Direct smear can be used for molecular studies. After removing the coverslip with xylene or substitute, it is possible to scrap the cells previously stained to an Eppendorf tube, to perform lysis and extract DNA of good quality for PCR or DNA sequencing [14]. Removing the glass coverslips for retrieving DNA from archival slides can be time-consuming and, traditionally, xylene or substitute has been used as the solvent for glass coverslip removal, which can take several days and thereby impose delays in molecular assays. Recently, a method that applies "freezing" to old stained slides has been described to overcome this problem, shortening the time required for getting the slides ready for DNA extraction [15]. According to the "freezer method," the slide should be placed flat in the freezer as the initial step. The slides can rest in the freezer (at a temperature of –20°C) for 1 to 2 minutes. Following that, the coverslip can be removed using the tip of a scalpel blade while the slide is still frozen. Cytospin preparations are prepared from cell suspensions in non-fixative solutions such as PBS, RPMI, etc., of FNA material or effusions. Air-dried cytospin slides can be stored for many years at –70°C with excellent DNA preservation. LBC preparation systems are today available in most cytology laboratories. Several slides can be produced from LBC material and these slides, post-fixed in 95% ethanol, can be stored for months at –70°C. LBC preparations are suitable for preserving cell samples and DNA with sufficient quality to be used in several molecular analyses such as PCR, RFLP and even sequencing [3, 16]. PCR analysis can be performed directly with fresh collected material from FNA, in LBC samples or even with cells scraped from slides. In the first condition, the needle should be washed up in ethanol, methanol or culture mediums like RPMI. The amount and quality of DNA obtained by FNA for PCR assay does not seem to be a problem and 50 to 100 cells are adequate to obtain good PCR results. Monolayer smears are ideal for ISH techniques and slides with ethanol or air-dried fixed preparations are equally suitable. Cell blocks can be prepared from all types of cytological specimens, except preparations with low cellularity such as cerebrospinal fluids. There are several techniques to produce cell blocks, such as cytocentrifugation, either with direct formalin fixation or fixation after addition of plasma-tromboplastin. In addition, there are commercially available systems which offer a standardized technique with a high reproducibility [17].

The choice of whether to use cytological preparations or histological sections for testing depends on the clinical setting and also on technical issues. Cytological samples are easier and quicker to obtain and may be the only material obtainable in certain settings (for example, metastatic tumors, patients who cannot tolerate biopsy). Moreover, molecular techniques that have been standardized for FFPE material can be applied to cell blocks of cytological samples.

On the other hand, tissue sample is superior in confirming the morphological diagnosis (for example, *in situ* versus invasive malignancy), which cannot be achieved using cytological smears. In primary breast carcinoma, testing of hormone receptor and HER2 is recommended on tissue samples (core biopsy or excision) since this is the only type of sample that can distinguish between *in situ* and invasive malignancy. Tissue stained sections are of superior quality, provide wider sampling and allow architectural correlation and scoring within the tumor areas of interest for treatment purposes.

## Controls

The basis of a good and valid technique is a correct choice of positive and negative controls verifying the sensitivity and specificity of the technique.

A range of materials can be used as positive controls, including tumor tissue samples and cell lines with known validated genomic characteristics. On setting up new tests (for example, next generation sequencing for somatic mutations), it is important to include positive control samples, previously validated by other techniques such as qPCR assays. In certain experiments, a range of positive controls should be included. If no clinical samples are readily available for use as controls, as in cases of rare mutations, commercially available cell lines with known mutation status can be used as controls.

Negative controls to ensure procedural success should also be included with each run.

Laboratories that are involved in diagnostic molecular testing should follow all the accreditation requirements required by the relevant accreditation authorities such as the College of American Pathologists (CAP) in the United States, Clinical Pathology

Accreditation (CPA) in the United Kingdom or equivalent. They should use validated assays (for example, those approved by the US Food and Drug Administration (FDA)). The UK NEQAS provides a comprehensive external quality assessment service for laboratories to ensure reliability and reproducibility of laboratory tests, including in clinical and molecular genetics, and provides advice on the appropriate controls for each diagnostic test (www.ukneqas.org.uk). Similarly, NordiQC is an independent scientific organization that promotes quality of immunohistochemistry and molecular testing by providing validated protocols and recommendations for improvements (www.nordiqc.org).

## Procedures

There is a wide range of molecular techniques such as ISH, PCR, RT-PCR, microarrays and sequencing that can be used to study DNA and mRNA alterations in tissue and cytological specimens. These techniques will be discussed in detail in the following chapters of this book. The introduction of these molecular techniques raises an important point: how to preserve good quality material maintaining cellular morphology and DNA/RNA integrity. As stated previously, LBC material is suitable for the preservation of cell samples and DNA with sufficient quality to be used in several molecular techniques. DNA/RNA is stable for a period of up to three years in this type of media [7, 16]. However, the horizons for the use of molecular techniques on cytological specimens have been expanded, with studies showing the applicability of these techniques to archival FNA samples, which are extremely useful in situations in which the diagnostic material may be limited to certain slides. The application of protocols that test the quality and quantity of storage DNA is a rule of good practice [7, 21]. Annaratone *et al.* showed that the leftover, residual material from the smearing procedures of FNA samples contains an important source of fresh cells, suitable for banking and appropriate for molecular analysis of breast lesions [6]. The results demonstrate that RNA can be successfully extracted from the FNA leftovers for gene expression profiling using oligonucleotide microarrays. Clusters generated by global expression profiles partitioned samples in well-distinguished subgroups that overlapped with clusters obtained using "biologic scores" (cytohistologic variables) and differed from clusters based on "technical scores" (RNA/complementary RNA/ microarray quality). Microarray profiling used to measure the grade of differentiation and ER and HER2 status reflected the results obtained by histology and immunohistochemistry. Given that proliferative status in the FNA material is not always assessable, a multiprobe genomic signature for proliferation genes was designed and strongly correlated with the Ki67 index examined on histologic material. These findings show that cells residual to cytological smears of FNA are suitable for obtaining high-quality RNA for high-throughput analysis even when taken from small breast lesions. High-quality, fresh-frozen human neoplastic and normal tissues may be stored in tumor banks through validated procedures for collection, storage, retrieval, shipping and tracking of samples. We demonstrated that cells obtained from fine-needle sampling of breast cancer surgical specimens are an effective tissue-sparing method for cell collection and banking with the preservation of high-quality RNA [10]. This methodology is a useful alternative for keeping material for molecular studies from small tumors in which we need to include all the material for histological evaluation. Recently, a commercially available gene expression classifier has been used for the preoperative identification of benign thyroid nodules whose cytology is indeterminate [19, 20]. The cytological material is collected in a liquid-media and morphological control runs in parallel. Morphological control may be one of the most crucial issues in the application of molecular techniques to cytology. Pang *et al.* [21] have shown the value of the enrichment of tumor cells in microdissection and how this should maintain the analytical sensitivity of the test, which, in their case, was 10% of malignant cells in a background of 90% of non-neoplastic cells. The role of the pathologist is mandatory in the collection and selection of cells [13]. For sequencing, in our laboratory we set at 20% of tumor cells present in the sample with the method sensitivity. We observed that the global rate detection of mutations increase from 26% to 40% when we consider only specimens with more than 20% of tumor cells. ISH is one of the techniques where the interpretation of the molecular changes is simultaneous with the morphological control. Chromosomal translocations are one of the most common genetic alterations studied in pathology. Several methods exist to evaluate them, including conventional cytogenetics, RT-PCR and ISH. ISH offers several advantages over

conventional cytogenetics. Its main advantage is that non-dividing (interphase) nuclei can be evaluated, making it unnecessary to evaluate the neoplastic cells in culture. ISH is especially advantageous in small samples, in which it may not be possible to submit tissue for cytogenetics. ISH also offers several benefits over RT-PCR. For a given translocation with multiple breakpoints, multiple primers are necessary to evaluate all possible fusion transcripts; whereas with fluorescence *in situ* hybridization (FISH), this can be achieved by using break-apart probes (with split signals reflecting the presence of gene fusion) or dual-fusion translocation probes (with fusion of signals indicating the presence of gene fusion). Therefore, one set of FISH probes can identify essentially all known breakpoints of a given translocation, resulting in increased sensitivity. In addition to the advantages of evaluating multiple breakpoints, FISH is also helpful in situations in which one translocation partner is constant, but the second translocation partner changes. This event occurs in Ewing's sarcoma/ primitive neuroectodermal tumor (ES/PNET), in which the ES receptor 1 gene (EWSR1) translocates with different partners, and in myxoid/round cell liposarcoma, in which the DNA-damage-inducible transcript 3 (DDIT3) gene in chromosome 12 translocates with chromosome 16, and the chromosome 22 translocation t(12,16), and the t(12,22). When analyzing FISH results, the examiner must be aware that the same gene is often involved in translocations present in different soft tissue neoplasms. Therefore, the same set of probes can also be used for a gene rearranged in multiple diagnostic entities: EWSR1 is rearranged in ES/PNET, in desmoplastic round cell tumor, in extraskeletal myxoid chondrosarcoma in some myxoid/round cell sarcomas, and in clear cell sarcoma. Translocations of ALK gene is detailed further in the lung section. Rapid advances in sequencing technologies have brought the cost of sequencing DNA down. Traditional sequencing technologies rely on a labor- and resource-intensive process of cloning fragments of sample DNA into bacteria, selecting and growing the clones, and then sequencing purified copies of a single fragment. Each traditional sequencing reaction yields approximately 1 kb (1,000 bp) of DNA sequence; typically about 100 reactions are run in parallel. In contrast, next generation sequencing technologies take advantage of miniaturization and automation to sequence hundreds of thousands to millions of DNA fragments in parallel using

25

extremely small amounts of chemical reagents per reaction. A single sequencing run with next generation technologies can yield more than 100 gb (100 billion bp) of DNA sequence in a matter of hours or days, depending on the particular technology used. On the horizon are "$1,000 genome" technologies that further refine sequencing by allowing direct sequencing of individual DNA molecules. Such refinements have the potential to eliminate the need for sample amplification, further reduce the use of chemical reagents, and produce highly accurate sequence data more rapidly. Next generation DNA sequencing is revolutionizing cancer genomics [5]. Whole genome resequencing of tumors is within our reach. High-quality reference genome sequences provide us with the prospect to study genetic variation on an unprecedented scale. Genes, genomic regions and whole genomes can be resequenced, aligned to appropriate references, and genetic peculiarity between individuals can be detected. There are many applications of this high-throughput method. The possibility to detect many genetic alterations in one "shot" opens avenues to study a panel of mutation, many of them that can be "druggable" targets. The demonstration that during lung cancer evolution there are several genotypic and phenotypical changes that can imply in acquisition a drug resistance and in some cases later loss of this mutation and development of drug response is an opportunity to apply this technology in cytology to follow these patients [22]. Actually, our group is performing next generation sequencing (NGS) technologies in cytological material obtained from metastatic sites in an attempt to compare the profiling of mutations with the primary tumors [23]. A summary of the technical aspects of molecular studies in pathology and cytology is shown in Table 3.1.

## Main applications

There are many possible applications of the use of molecular techniques in different organs using histological and cytological material. Molecular techniques currently play a pivotal role in diagnostic pathology, providing unique signatures that cannot be obtained via other techniques to allow a specific diagnosis to be made. Molecular pathology also provides prognostic information and predicts the likelihood of response to particular therapies. Increasingly, molecular profiling of tumor samples is used to randomize patients into clinical trials and to optimize patient treatment in the primary and metastatic settings. These applications will be described in detail among the different chapters of this book. Here, we briefly mention possible applications in metastatic cancer.

## Metastatic cancer

An important example to use molecular assessment in metastatic cancer is metastatic breast cancer (MBC). MBC is usually diagnosed by a combination of clinical and imaging findings. Once diagnosed, the choice of systemic therapy is based on the ER, PR and HER2 status from the patient's primary tumor. Biopsy of suspected metastatic lesions can be done where clinically indicated. However, tumor characteristics can change and discrepancies between primary and metastasis are described with variations until 30% for the hormonal receptors and 5 to 10% in HER2 [17]. Wilking *et al.* [24], using FISH for HER2 in FNA samples from metastatic sites of breast cancer, showed an intra-patient agreement in HER2 status of 76% and a disagreement of 10%. The multivariable Cox analysis showed a significantly increased risk of dying in the patient group with changed HER2 status. The unstable status for

**Table 3.1** A summary of the technical aspects of molecular studies in pathology

| Target | Pre-analytical issues | Fixation | Techniques | Applications |
|---|---|---|---|---|
| DNA | Very stable | Any kind, including air-dried | PCR, ISH, sequencing | Detection of mutations, translocations |
| RNA | Very unstable | Dedicate sampling for adequate preservative | Microarrays, RT-PCR | Gene expression profiling |
| Protein | Variable | Alcohol-fixed, formalin-fixed, LBC preservatives | IHC, flow cytometry | Expression of proteins (markers) |

HER2 in breast cancer is clinically significant and should motivate more frequent testing of recurrences. In our own experience, we observed 15% of disagreement between HER2 assessment in primary and respective metastases of breast cancer, using FISH on FNA material [25]. For metastatic treatment, KRAS and BRAF gene mutations in patients with metastatic colorectal cancer are molecular markers that predict the sensitivity of tumors to anti-EGFR therapeutics. Patients with tumors that harbor KRAS mutations have a lower drug response rate; however, a significant percentage of patients with KRAS-WT tumors also do not respond to anti-EGFR drugs [26]. One of the many possible reasons for this is the discrepancy between KRAS status in the primary tumor and in metastasis. Moreover, it is estimated that 20% of the target patient population will present with metastatic disease and there will not be access to archive material from the primary tumor. In both situations, FNA material obtained from metastatic sites is a good, safe and cheap alternative for determining KRAS status in metastatic colon cancer [21]. Another example in the management of metastatic disease is metastatic melanoma, for which FNA is frequently used to diagnose it at a metastatic site. Fifty percent of melanoma cases harbor mutation of the BRAF gene and recently inhibitors of BRAF were described and tested with success [27]. It is thus now imperative that all metastatic melanomas be tested for BRAF mutations, and FNA biopsies have proven to be suitable for such tests. Hookim *et al.* [28] showed that the use of cytologic direct smears proved to be a robust and reliable methodology for molecular testing. In this study, mutation testing was successfully performed using cellular material microdissected from archived, Diff-Quick-stained smears. From these given examples, it is clear that cytology coupled with modern molecular techniques has a definitive role in helping to tackle many of the challenges presented by tumor heterogeneity and metastatic disease. NGS is the ideal method for "multiple" genomic alterations assessments in one single test, thus limiting the amount of biological material needed and therefore making it a promising method to couple with FNA sampling.

In the near future, we expect that biopsy of metastatic sites will help to clarify many mechanisms of tumor evolution. For this, re-biopsying of metastases may increasingly become a part of standard of care clinical practice. We expect that the knowledge generated by biopsies of metastatic tissue will contribute to a better understanding of the development of treatment resistance and will help to uncover therapeutic choices that will prolong the survival and enhance the quality of life of patients with metastatic cancer. As such, we believe that cytopathology can become a discipline with a central role in state-of-the-art diagnoses and treatment of metastatic disease [23].

## Learning points

- Collection of good and well-preserved material
- Validation in large-scale molecular studies on cytological and histological material
- Controlling the cases morphologically

## References

1. Schmitt, F. C., Longatto-Filho, A., Valent, A. and Vielh, P. Molecular techniques in cytopathology practice. *J Clin Pathol* 2008; 61(3): 258–67.

2. Schmitt, F. C. and Barroca, H. Possible use and role of molecular techniques in fine needle aspiration. *Diagn Histopathol* 2011; 17(7): 286–92.

3. Schmitt, F. C. and Vielh, P. Molecular biology and cytopathology. Principles and applications. *Ann Pathol* 2012; 32(6): e57–63.

4. Schmitt, F. and Barroca, H. Role of ancillary studies in fine-needle aspiration from selected tumors. *Cancer Cytopathol* 2012; 120(3): 145–60.

5. Di Lorito, A. and Schmitt, F. C. Cytopathology and sequencing: next (or last) generation? *Diagn Cytopathol* 2012; 40(5): 459–61.

6. Annaratone, L., Marchio, C., Renzulli, T., Castellano, I., Cantarella, D., Isella, C. *et al.* High-throughput molecular analysis from leftover of fine needle aspiration cytology of mammographically detected breast cancer. *Translational Oncology* 2012; 5(3): 180–9.

7. Schmitt, F. C. Molecular cytopathology and flow cytometry: pre-analytical procedures matter. *Cytopathology* 2011; 22(6): 355–7.

8. Teutsch, S. M., Bradley, L. A., Palomaki, G. E., Haddow, J. E., Piper, M., Calonge, N. *et al.* The Evaluation of Genomic Applications in Practice and Prevention (EGAPP) initiative: methods of the EGAPP Working Group. *Genet Med* 2009; 11(1): 3–14.

9. Berg, A. O. The CDC's EGAPP initiative: evaluating the clinical evidence for genetic tests. *Am Fam Physician* 2009; 80(11): 1218.

10. Evaluation of Genomic Applications in Practice and Prevention (EGAPP) Working Group. Recommendations from the EGAPP Working Group: testing for cytochrome P450 polymorphisms in adults with nonpsychotic depression treated with selective serotonin reuptake inhibitors. *Genet Med* 2007; 9(12): 819–25.

11. Longy, M., Duboue, B., Soubeyran, P. and Moynet, D. Method for the purification of tissue DNA suitable for PCR after fixation with Bouin's fluid. Uses and limitations in microsatellite typing. *Diagn Mol Pathol* 1997; 6(3): 167–73.

12. Bonin, S., Petrera, F., Rosai, J. and Stanta, G. DNA and RNA obtained from Bouin's fixed tissues. *J Clin Pathol* 2005; 58(3): 313–16.

13. Fend, F. and Raffeld, M. Laser capture microdissection in pathology. *J Clin Pathol* 2000; 53(9): 666–72.

14. Arcila, M. E. Simple protocol for DNA extraction from archival stained FNA smears, cytospins, and thin preparations. *Acta Cytol* 2012; 56(6): 632–5.

15. Santos, G. C., Schroder, M., Zhu, J. B., Saieg, M., Geddie, W., Boerner, S. *et al.* Minimizing delays in DNA retrieval: the "freezer method" for glass coverslip removal. *Cancer Cytopathol* 2013; 121(9): 533.

16. Longatto-Filho, A., Gonçalves, A. E., Martinho, O., Schmitt, F. C. and Reis, R. M. Liquid-based cytology in DNA-based molecular research. *Anal Quant Cytol Histol* 2009; 31(6): 395–400.

17. Gorman, B. K., Kosarac, O., Chakraborty, S., Schwartz, M. R. and Mody, D. Comparison of breast carcinoma prognostic/predictive biomarkers on cell blocks obtained by various methods: cellient, formalin and thrombin. *Acta Cytol* 2012; 56(3): 289–96.

18. Eloy, C., Amendoeira, I. and Schmitt, F. C. Fine-needle aspiration as an alternative method for frozen tissue banking of breast cancer. *Diagn Cytopathol* 2009; 37(1): 76–7.

19. Duick, D., Klopper, J., Diggans, J., Friedman, L., Kennedy, G., Lanman, R. *et al.* The impact of benign gene expression classifier test results on the endocrinologist–patient decision to operate on patients with thyroid nodules with indeterminate fine-needle aspiration cytopathology. *Thyroid* 2012; 22(10): 996–1001.

20. Alexander, E., Kennedy, G., Baloch, Z., Cibas, E., Chudova, D., Diggans, J. *et al.* Preoperative diagnosis of benign thyroid nodules with indeterminate cytology. *New Engl J Med* 2012; 367(8): 705–15.

21. Pang, N. K. B., Nga, M. E., Chin, S. Y., Ismail, T. M., Lim, G. L., Soong, R. *et al.* KRAS and BRAF mutation analysis can be reliably performed on aspirated cytological specimens of metastatic colorectal carcinoma. *Cytopathology* 2011; 22(6): 358–64.

22. Sequist, L. V., Waltman, B. A., Dias-Santagata, D., Digumarthy, S., Turke, A. B., Fidias, P. *et al.* Genotypic and histological evolution of lung cancers acquiring resistance to EGFR. *Sci Transl Med* 2011; 3(75): 75ra26.

23. Beca, F. and Schmitt, F. Growing indication for FNA to study and analyze tumor heterogeneity at metastatic sites. *Cancer Cytopathol* 2014; 122(7): 504–11.

24. Wilking, U., Karlsson, E., Skoog, L., Hatschek, T., Lidbrink, E., Elmberger, G. *et al.* HER2 status in a population-derived breast cancer cohort: discordances during tumor progression. *Breast Cancer Res Treat* 2011; 125(2): 553–61.

25. Niikura, N., Odisio, B. C., Tokuda, Y., Symmans, F. W., Hortobagyi, G. N. and Ueno, N. T. Latest biopsy approach for suspected metastases in patients with breast cancer. *Nat Rev Clin Oncol* 2013; 10(12): 711–19.

26. Lievre, A., Bachet, J., Boige, V., Cayre, A., Le Corre, D., Buc, E. *et al.* KRAS mutations as an independent prognostic factor in patients with advanced colorectal cancer treated with cetuximab. *J Clin Oncol* 2008; 26(3): 374–9.

27. Flaherty, K. T., Infante, J. R., Daud, A., Gonzalez, R., Kefford, R. F., Sosman, J. *et al.* Combined BRAF and MEK inhibition in melanoma with BRAF V600 mutations. *New Engl J Med* 2012; 367(18): 1694–703.

28. Hookim, K., Roh, M. H., Willman, J., Placido, J., Weigelin, H. C., Fields, K. L. *et al.* Application of immunocytochemistry and BRAF mutational analysis to direct smears of metastatic melanoma. *Cancer Cytopathol* 2012; 120(1): 52–61.

# Fluorescent and non-fluorescent *in situ* hybridization

Jane Bayani and John M. S. Bartlett

## Introduction

The number of tools contained within pathologists' molecular "toolboxes" has expanded rapidly over the past three decades. Recent technological advances in molecular biology have transformed the traditional discipline of pathology, giving rise to the sub-specialty of "molecular pathology." While the architecture and associated features of diseased tissues remain essential for accurate diagnosis, the inclusion of molecular markers, whether DNA, RNA or protein, has greatly enhanced our ability to further characterize disease – and directly impact patient care. The value of immunohistological markers has been well established and continues to be the mainstay of routine clinical testing in pathology laboratories; however, the use of DNA markers is now critical for appropriate diagnosis and treatment of cancer and the use of DNA and RNA markers is expanding rapidly.

Since Theodore Boveri's observations in the early 1900s (1), scientists have recognized the contribution of aberrant chromosomes/DNA to cancer and congenital abnormalities (reviewed by (2) and (3)). The refinement of cytogenetic fixation procedures set the stage for studies linking genotypes to phenotypes; which were later improved by the ability to distinguish and decipher the banding patterns that characterized each chromosome. Improved staining and microscopy techniques led scientists to identify abnormalities at the whole or sub-chromosomal level, exemplified by the identification of trisomy 21 as the cause of Down's syndrome 1959; followed by Turner syndrome (OX) and Kleinfelter syndrome (XXY) (2). In 1960, the first translocation event, the Philadelphia (Ph) chromosome was identified (4), but it required over 10 years before this was confirmed as a translocation between the ABL gene (9q32) and the BCR

gene (22q11) (5). Rapidly thereafter, more subtle recurrent chromosomal abnormalities, such as deletions and other translocations, were observed. Studies of solid tumors and hematological malignancies rapidly revealed variable levels of both numerical and structural karyotypic complexity; but studies were limited to the resolution afforded by cytogenetic preparations and banding patterns. Also during this time, unique chromosomal structures such as double minute (DMs) chromosomes, homogeneously staining regions (HSRs) and ring chromosomes were documented and confirmed by other molecular techniques as contributing to genomic amplification. This growing understanding of the complexity of DNA underpinned a need to increase the resolution of existing techniques, such that information regarding copy-number or structural/rearrangement status could be specifically ascertained at the level of the genomic locus or single gene. The ability to stably clone DNA fragments and label them for molecular analyses played a significant role in developing *in situ* hybridization techniques. Gall and Pardue (6), reported the first *in situ* hybridization experiments in 1969, utilizing radioactively labeled nucleotides. Whilst of pivotal importance for research applications, radiolabeled *in situ* hybridization (ISH) probes were insufficiently rapid (requiring weeks or days of exposure to develop) for diagnostic pathology applications. It required development of indirect- and directly labeled fluorescent-probes in the early 1980s (7) to set the scene for diagnostic applications of ISH; and it would take another five years to optimize fluorescence *in situ* hybridization (FISH) to human chromosomes, resulting in the first gene mapping experiment using non-radioactive probes of the thyroglobulin gene (8). Mapping the chromosomal, and indeed

*Molecular Pathology: A Practical Guide for the Surgical Pathologist and Cytopathologist*, ed. John M. S. Bartlett, Abeer Shaaban and Fernando Schmitt. Published by Cambridge University Press. © Cambridge University Press, 2016.

sub-chromosomal, location of genes, and (due to cross-hybridization) sometimes their high-homology family members, could now be performed rapidly and reliably; but more importantly, the status of key genes within a cancer genome could now be examined. FISH enabled the verification of rearrangement events between specific genes such as the Ph chromosome, but despite the significant improvement in resolution over classical cytogenetics, locus-specific FISH was still limited in the information that it could provide. During the early 1990s, the use of labeled ISH probes led to the development of comparative genomic hybridization (CGH) which subsequently was replaced by array-based CGH (aCGH) (9), and with it, other multi-color, multi-locus FISH assays (reviewed by Bayani and Squire (10)). What resulted were whole genome analyses, identifying recurrent DNA copy-number aberrations characterizing cancers. However, the bulk-extracted DNAs used for these whole genome surveys only provided the net copy-number changes within a potentially heterogeneous tumor. It was unclear as to whether these changes were clonally derived, or represented a subset of cells. Furthermore, there was no way to determine whether all the copy-number changes seen were present in all cells, or whether there were certain combinations of copy-number alterations. Among the greatest of recent advances in molecular pathology is the ability to evaluate the DNA copy-number or rearrangements *in situ*. Diagnostic formalin-fixed paraffin-embedded (FFPE) tissues provide a wealth of information by maintaining the cellular and tissue architecture. *In situ*-based detection of nucleic acids has the advantage of providing information in the context of tissue anatomy. With an extensive base of genomic information built on traditional chromosomal studies, together with data from FISH-based, locus-specific and whole-genome studies, we are now able to apply those specific and clinically relevant research techniques to routinely derived patient material. Currently, there are two major ways of assessing DNA copy-number/rearrangement status *in situ* – fluorescence-based methods – FISH; and bright-field-based methods – chromogenic *in situ* hybridization (CISH). Both FISH and CISH utilize the complementary base-pairing properties of DNA and/or RNA (11) with the ability to detect a labeled DNA probe (12). This chapter will review the advantages and disadvantages of these methods and,

briefly, their current and future applications in clinical and research settings.

# FISH, D-FISH, M-FISH, CISH, DDISH, SISH, GOLDFISH: what's in a name?

Particularly in the field of breast cancer HER2 detection, the proliferation of chromogenic assays based on silver, 3',3' diaminobenzidine (DAB) or other colored substrates has led to a confusing proliferation of names for chromogenic *in situ* hybridization. For the remainder of this chapter, we will use the term CISH for chromogenic *in situ* hybridization, recognizing that whether silver *in situ* hybridization (SISH), gold-facilitated *in situ* hybridization (GOLD-FISH) (13), dual *in situ* hybridization (DDISH) (Table 4.1) or variants thereof are discussed, the goal is to use a chromogen to visualize nucleic acids *in situ*. While, in the strictest sense, fluorochromes could be included in this definition, we have retained the distinction between CISH and FISH (for fluorescence *in situ* hybridization) for two pivotal reasons: firstly, because the use of fluorochromes provides the distinct advantage of allowing *direct* labeling of probes and the avoidance of signal amplification steps which can pose significant challenges (see below); and, secondly, because the use of fluorochromes is linked to the use of fluorescent microscopy with the linked requirement to work in reduced light conditions. We recognize that FISH may be performed using secondary antibodies followed by a fluorochrome-conjugated antibody, but such FISH methods are not utilized in diagnostic laboratories, remaining almost exclusively in the research domain. Indeed, as already mentioned, directly labeled fluorescence probes avoid the additional treatment of specimens, while decreasing assay time. As with CISH, the term FISH is generically used to include dual-colored assays (D-FISH), multicolored probe configurations (M-FISH) and specialty FISH assays to be discussed later (Table 4.1).

## Principles of *in situ* hybridization (ISH)

*In situ* hybridization can be used to describe the detection of DNA or RNA in their cellular context. The basic principles of ISH are simple: (1) the use of a specific probe that is detectable; and (2) hybridization of that probe to its target as either fixed cells or tissues. Similarly, the detection of nucleic acids;

**Table 4.1** Alternative names for CISH and FISH

| Name | Description |
|------|-------------|
| | **CISH** |
| DISH | Double *in situ* hybridization<br>Dual *in situ* hybridization |
| SISH | Silver *in situ* hybridization |
| GOLD-FISH | Gold-facilitated *in situ* hybridization |
| | **FISH** |
| D-FISH | Double color fluorescence *in situ* hybridization<br>Dual-color fluorescence *in situ* hybridization |
| M-FISH | Multicolored fluorescence *in situ* hybridization |
| | **Specialty FISH assays** |
| SKY | Spectral karyotyping |
| Mband | Multicolor banding |
| COBRA-FISH | Combined binary ratio labeling fluorescence *in situ* hybridization |
| mCGH | Metaphase comparative genomic hybridization |
| | **Other** |
| RNA-ISH | RNA-*in situ* hybridization |

whether DNA or RNA, relies on complementary base pairing between the probe and target sequences. Finally, visualization of the protein or nucleic acid of interest can be achieved by either bright-field or fluorescence microscopy (Figure 4.1). In this chapter, we will focus on the detection of DNA.

We have previously discussed that both assays had their beginnings as extensions of the first *in situ* hybridization experiments using radioactively labeled isotopes (6). The disadvantages associated with the use of radioactive isotopes, together with technological improvements for biological reagents, quickly drove the development of non-radioisotopic methods. The most commonly used reporter molecules for indirect-labeling of nucleic acids are biotin and digoxigenin; however, the vast majority of commercial sources for FISH probes are in ready-to-use, fluorochrome-directly-labeled formats. The standard DNA-based *in situ* protocol requires a labeled DNA probe, target pre-treatment, denaturation, hybridization and probe detection (Figure 4.1).

# Probes

For the clinical laboratory, commercially prepared probes eliminate the need for in-house labeling of cloned DNA, assuring a quality controlled reagent. Probes may be derived from a number of sources, such as customed-labeled oligonucleotides, Bacterial Artificial Chromosomes (BACs), Yeast Artificial Chromosomes (YACs), Plasmid Artificial Chromosomes (PACs) or cosmids. Nick translation is the traditional method of labeling, which utilizes the action of DNAse I to nick double-stranded DNA, then incorporates the labeled nucleotide ("X"-dUPT) in the master mix via DNA polymerase I (14). The DNA fragment to be used as the probe may be labeled "directly" with a fluorochrome; or "indirectly" with a reporter molecule such as biotin or digoxigenin. The latter format requires subsequent incubations with primary and secondary antibodies for subsequent probe detection. The DNA can also be labeled by PCR-based methods such as random-primed labeling, or degenerate oligonucleotide-primed PCR (DOP-PCR). Peptide Nucleic Acid (PNA) probes (15) are probes derived from an analog of DNA with a pseudopeptide backbone, instead of a normal sugar, which is conjugated to a fluorochrome. The advantage of PNA probes lies in their ability to bind with greater affinity to the complementary nucleic acid strand, resulting in higher specificity and greater stability. Generally, high probe/target specificity increases the sensitivity of the assay. Thus, the ideal probe should possess a limited number of repeat elements, to prevent cross-hybridization, and cover a large area of the target region, which will produce a larger signal. The resolution and specificity of probes used for FISH has improved significantly. Investigators are no longer limited to large genomic fragments on the order of hundreds of kilobases (kb) to reliably detect their region of interest. As more efficient labeling strategies emerged, together with improved stability of fluorochromes and/or detection systems, probes between 1 kb and 10 kb became more easily detectable. The suppression of repeat elements, contributing to cross-hybridization, is facilitated by the use of COT-1 DNA. However, this can also be minimized through the removal of repeat elements from the cloned DNA or by specific primer design. Probe design depends largely on the type of information that is sought from the test. Finally, probes can be classified as a locus-specific or painting probe

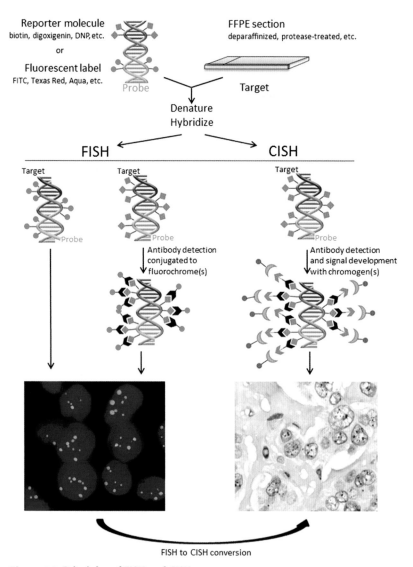

**Figure 4.1 Principles of FISH and CISH**
Shown is a comparison between the basic FISH and CISH protocols. The DNA probe may be labeled "directly" with a fluorochrome, shown in green; or "indirectly" with a reporter molecule, shown in grey diamonds. The use of directly or indirectly labeled probes will influence the length of the protocol. If multiple genes/loci will be assessed using indirectly labeled probes, the appropriate antibodies must be used and in the correct sequence. The target DNA comes from the sample to be tested such as a FFPE section. For both FISH and CISH, the probe and slides are processed, denatured and allowed to hybridize with each other. Directly labeled probes need no further processing, and following hybridization can be washed and mounted in DAPI and antifade and visualized by fluorescence microscopy. Indirectly labeled probes for FISH must be detected with antibodies and intervening blocking and washing steps, with the final antibody conjugated to a fluorochrome, shown in green. CISH probes must similarly be detected using antibodies, with the final signal detection using a chromogen such as DAB. Additional reagents have now become available, permitting the conversion of FISH signals (green-fluorescing FITC and red-fluorescing Texas Red) to CISH signals. Shown below are examples of FISH detecting copy-number changes in breast cancers using HER2 (red) and centromere 17 (green); as well as the comparable CISH assay with HER2 shown as black/blue signals and centromere 17 as red signals. Images courtesy of John M. S. Bartlett.

(Figure 4.2). Locus-specific probes may correspond to a specific gene or a portion of that gene; or span a few hundred contiguous kb, encompassing several genes. Special classes of locus-specific probes include centromere probes and telomere probes. Such probes may be specific to a particular chromosome, requiring the labeling of the sequences unique to that chromosome within the telomeric/centromric

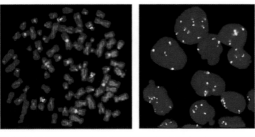

**Figure 4.2 Metaphase and interphase analyses**
Shown are the fundamental similarities and differences between metaphase and interphase analyses when using different classes of DNA probes. Metaphase analysis restricted to the use of metaphase spreads is prepared by cytogenetic methods. Interphase analyses can be accomplished through the use of different tissue sources. Metaphase analysis is amenable to the use of both locus-specific probes as well as painting probes; whereas interphase analysis is restricted to the use of locus-specific probes within the clinical setting. Ideograms within the table illustrate the different classes of probes described in the text. Unpublished images courtesy of Jane Bayani.

| | Metaphase analyses | Interphase analyses |
|---|---|---|
| **Target** | • Metaphase preparation | • Metaphase preparation<br>• Cytological smears<br>• Touch-preparations<br>• Formalin-fixed paraffin-embedded tissues |
| **Locus-specific probes** | **Metaphase analyses** | **Interphase analyses** |
| • gene/locus-specific probes<br>• centromere-specific probes (chromosome specific)<br>• telomere-specific (chromosome specific) | Amplification, gain, deletion, rearrangement, translocation | |
| • all centromere probe<br>• all telomere probe | Ploidy assessment, multi-centric chromosomes, telomere fusion, telomere shortening (research) | Ploidy assessment, telomere shortening (research) |
| **Painting probes** | **Metaphase analyses** | **Interphase analyses** |
| • whole-chromosome(s) or whole-chromosome arm(s)<br>• 24-color whole chromosome<br>• multi-color, band specific | Copy-number, translocation, rearrangements | Chromosome domain studies (research) |

regions; or may be non-chromosome specific, such that all telomeric/centromeric sequences can be detected. Painting probes, as their name suggests, are composed of labeled DNA that hybridize to large chromosomal regions, such as the entire chromosome or chromosomal arms, or to specific chromosomal bands (Figure 4.2 and Figure 4.4).

## Target DNA and pre-treatment

The second stage of the assay involves exposing the target DNA, which may be in the form of FFPE tissues, fixed cytological smears/touch preps, or cytogenetically prepared cells. Traditional cytogenetic analyses relied on short-termed culturing of mitotically active cells, arresting them at metaphase then fixing the cells and applying them to microscope slides. This yields not only metaphase spreads for analyses, but also interphase nuclei. The advantage of metaphase analyses is in the ability to directly visualize the chromosomes involved and the context for which the copy-number changes or structural changes are manifested in the karyotype. Unfortunately, this can only be inferred by interphase analyses (Figure 4.2). However, short-term culturing of solid tumors is laborious, can promote the outgrowth of normal cells and can yield poor mitotic indices. Moreover, the required disaggregation of these solid tissues destroys the tissue architecture, essentially mixing tumor and normal cells into a bulk cellular suspension. It is for this reason, as well as others, that the use of FFPE is desired. The quality of the original tissue and the method of fixation will significantly influence the quality of *in situ* results. Some fixatives, including Bouin's fixative, should be avoided at all costs. Each type of cellular fixation requires different pre-treatment protocols that enable the maximal access of the labeled DNA probes to the target DNA (for the purposes of this chapter, we will focus primarily on FFPE tissues). For FFPE tissues, the fixation and embeding procedures serve to maintain tissue architecture and ensure ease of sectioning. To account for the range of fixation and embeding methods, a number of convenient commercial kits are available for the pre-treatment of the target specimen, which is particularly useful in the clinical laboratory where assay consistency is desirable. In general terms, the removal of paraffin is facilitated by treatment with xylenes followed by rehydration steps in graded alcohols. A mild acid treatment helps to deproteinize tissues, enabling probe access; which is followed by treatment with proteases such as pepsin or proteinase K. The length of time and concentration of protease treatment is critical, since over-digestion will lead to poor tissue morphology and degradation of the DNA; while under-digestion will prevent access of the probe to the target DNA (16). The use of DAPI staining, before probe hybridization, to assess digestion can be of significant benefit during the optimization of ISH protocols (16).

## Hybridization and probe detection

The DNA probe and target DNA are denatured to generate single-stranded DNA, then allowed to hybridize together such that the probe and target anneal according to complementary base pairing. Hybridization is facilitated by the use of a hybridization solution containing varying concentrations of salts and formamide (50–65%), which helps to maintain the single-stranded state of the probe at lower temperatures, only allowing the annealing of the probe to the target that has the greatest complementarity. Hybridization times can vary from as little as 2 hours to overnight. Generally, one can modulate the stringency of probe hybridization by altering the salt

and formamide concentration. Thus, increasing the temperature and formamide concentration in the wash solutions permits only those probes with high complementarity to remain bound to the target. This can similarly be achieved by decreasing the salt concentration in the wash buffers. Directly labeled fluorescent probes require no further detection steps, and the slides can be counterstained, typically with blue-fluorescing 4',6-diamidino-2-phenylindole (DAPI) mounted in an antifade medium to prevent photobleaching of the signal. For CISH, the probe is similarly processed by incubations with the appropriate antibodies and detergent washes, then typically developed with 3, 3'-diaminobenzidine (DAB) as the chromogen (12). Counterstaining with hematoxylin, additional washes and fixation completes the experiment, and the slides can be mounted in standard mounting medium and ready for analysis. Both FISH and CISH have the capability of being performed with more than one probe. For such multi-locus experiments, one is only limited by the number of ways in which the DNA probes can be differentially labeled and subsequently detected. Until recently, CISH has been performed using one probe, posing a limitation for its use and implications for accurate copy-number assessment (to be discussed below). However, dual probe CISH (DISH) assays have now become commercially available to overcome this limitation and are currently undergoing validation (17–23). The detection of probe by precipitated silver molecules, termed SISH, utilizes 2,4-Di-Nitrophenyl (DNP) as the label for DNA and is visualized as black signals. The use of a DNP-labeled probe means that a probe cocktail could be generated in combination with hapten-labeled probes, provided there are sufficient secondary antibodies and chromogens to distinguish the differentially labeled probes. Although the visualization of black/brown or red signals are commonly seen by CISH, there are now other color options, such as blue or green chromogens conjugated to horseradish peroxidase or alkaline phosphatase, that can improve visualization. Also, reagents that can convert the fluorescence signals (i.e. red-fluorescing Texas Red and/or green-fluorescing FITC) into bright-field CISH signals (DAKO DuoCISH™) have been developed, affording the flexibility of utilizing the greater variety and availability of FISH probes in a CISH setting. In this case, FITC/Texas Red become the reporter molecules. While two probes appear to be the current limit to the number of probes that can be detected by CISH, FISH can be performed in up to 24 different colors (24); however, within a standard clinical laboratory setting, up to five different probes can be comfortably assayed.

## Quality control of diagnostic DNA *in situ* assays

Without a doubt, the success of these diagnostic tests, whether FISH or CISH, lie both with proper execution of the assay and interpretation of the results (25–30). For this reason, all laboratories, whether diagnostic or research, should always implement best practices; including the use of a clear and comprehensive protocol for each assay being performed and the use of proper controls. Indeed, those performing and interpreting the results of the test must understand the nature of the test being utilized (i.e. amplification, deletion, translocation, rearrangement, etc.), as there will be different criteria for detecting these abnormalities. Moreover, variations in protocols will also be influenced by the type of specimens being interrogated (i.e. FFPE, cytological smears, cytogenetically fixed cells).

Before one can detect an abnormality with certainty, one must recognize how the probe(s) appears in normal cells. Assuming optimum probe hybridization, signal detection and low-leveled background, accurate results from both metaphase-based and interphase-based analyses can be easily achieved. For cytogenetically prepared cells, metaphase and interphase cells do not suffer from the effects of cellular truncation as do (interphase) cells derived from FFPE. In the context of interphase analyses in FFPE, normal cells for a given chromosomal locus will typically yield copy-numbers from 1.4 to 1.7 copies per cell, rather than 2. This range of copy-number in normal tissues reflects the effects of cellular truncation, due to sectioning, as well as technical aspects related to the assays themselves. Therefore, for each probe/probe set used, it is strongly recommended that comprehensive assessment of the "normal" range of copy-number be established. Manufacturers of the probe will often provide guidelines for signal interpretation, and the laboratory must integrate these guidelines, as well as those provided by other governing bodies such as the American Society of Clinical Oncology (ASCO), College of American Pathologists (CAP) and United Kingdom National External Quality Assessment Service

(UK-NEQAS), among others. It is also imperative that those charged with interpreting the results do so with consistency. Intra- and inter-observer variation can impact the results of the test, with typical variation between observers as high as 10%. To minimize this variation, dual-observer scoring can be an important quality control measure that reduces scoring bias and aids in identification of probe inefficiencies. Finally, the accuracy of a laboratory in performing a test should be assessed internally as well as externally. A set of control tissues, comprising normal tissues and abnormal tissues confirmed to carry the abnormality, should be used for such internal assessments as well as the (ongoing) training of technical staff. These tissue controls become invaluable particularly if the performance of reagents comes into question. Similarly, participation in external testing supports the credibility of the laboratory and, as for all diagnostic tests, assures external validation of and quality control of results reported to patients.

## Current diagnostic utility of DNA ISH

The increasing use of CISH over the past 10 years was preceded at least 15 years ago by the already well-established use of FISH both in the research and clinical setting. Unquestionably, the ability to clone, label and detect specific regions of a gene or locus has improved our ability to diagnose disease, and offers better predictions for outcome and response to therapies. The largest impact to date of this technology has been in the field of directing targeted therapy against the HER2 oncogene, originally in breast cancer (31–34) and more recently in gastric cancer (35). Together with new information generated by large cancer genome consortiums, the repertoire of clinically relevant DNA biomarkers will continue to increase, leading to improved personalized care. Currently, the most common uses for FISH or CISH has been used to assess the status of a gene(s) or chromosomes in the patient specimen, and for many tests, this is restricted primarily to copy-number or rearrangement status (Table 4.2). While the vast majority of studies to date utilize FISH due to its significant lead time in use, there are increasingly growing numbers of comparable CISH studies. The technical advances and experiences from molecular cytogenetics and genomics, coupled with important diagnostic and prognostic findings from these and other molecular studies, helped to pave the way for

Table 4.2 Partial compendium of common diagnostic or companion tests performed by FISH or CISH

| Aberration | Neoplasm | Genes or locus | Aberration type | Probe type(s) |
|---|---|---|---|---|
| *Hematological malignancies* | | | | |
| t(8;14)(q24;q32) | Burkitt's lymphoma Diffuse large B-cell | MYC/IGH | Translocation/ rearrangement | Break apart dual color (MYC) Break apart dual color (IGH) Tri-color fusion (MYC/IGH/CEP8) |
| t(8;22)(q24;q11.2) | Burkitt's lymphoma | MYC/IGL | Translocation/ rearrangement | Break apart dual color (MYC) |
| t(11;14)(q13;q32) | Mantle cell lymphoma | CCND1-XT/IGH | Translocation/ rearrangement | Break apart dual color (CCND1) |
| t(14;18)(q32;q21) | Follicular lymphoma | IGH/BCL2 | Translocation/ rearrangement | Break apart dual color (IGH) Break apart dual color (BCL2) Dual color fusion (IGH/BCL2) |
| t(3;var)(q27;var) | Follicular lymphoma | BCL6 | Translocation/ rearrangement | Break apart dual color (BCL6) |
| t(8;22)(q24;q11.2) | Burkitt's lymphoma Diffuse large B-cell lymphoma | MYC/IGL | Translocation/ rearrangement | Break apart dual color (MYC) Break apart dual color (IGH) Tri-color fusion (MYC/IGH/CEP8) |
| t(11;18)(q21;q21) | Marginal zone of MALT type lymphoma | BIRC3/MALT1 | Translocation/ rearrangement | Dual color fusion (BIRC3/MALT1) |
| t(14;18)(q32;q21) | Marginal zone of MALT type lymphoma | IGH/MALT1 | Translocation/ rearrangement | Break apart dual color (IGH) |
| t(9;22)(q34;q11.2) | CLL B-Cell ALL AML | BCR/ABL Imatinib benefit | Translocation/ rearrangement | Dual color dual fusion (BCR/ABL) Dual color single fusion (BCR/ ABL) |
| t(8;21)(q22;q23) | AML | RUNX1T1/ RUNX1 | Translocation/ rearrangement | Dual color dual fusion (RUNX1T1/ RUNX1) |
| t(12;21)(p13;q22) | B-Cell ALL | ETV6/RUNX1 | Translocation/ rearrangement | Break apart dual color (ETV6) |
| 11q23 | B-Cell ALL T-Cell ALL MDS B-Cell lymphoma T-Cell lymphoma | MLL | Translocation/ rearrangement | Break apart dual color (MLL) |
| 5q31 | AML | EGR1 | Deletion | Dual probe set (EGR1 and 5p15.2) |
| 11q22.3 | CLL | ATM | Deletion | Locus-specific single probe (ATM) Dual-color probe set (ATM and CEP 11) |
| +8 | MDS AML CML | Centromere 8 | Trisomy 8 | Single probe CEP8 |

Table 4.2 (*cont.*)

| Aberration | Neoplasm | Genes or locus | Aberration type | Probe type(s) |
|---|---|---|---|---|
| | | | *Solid tumors* | |
| 1p36/19q | Oligodendroglioma | | Deletion | Dual color probe set |
| 13q14 | Alveolar rhabdomyosarcoma | FOXO1 | Translocation/ rearrangement | Break apart dual color (FOXO1) |
| 22q12 | Ewing sarcoma | EWSR1 | Translocation/ rearrangement | Break apart dual color (EWSR1) |
| 2p24 | Neuroblastoma | MYCN | Amplification | Locus-specific single probe (MYCN) Dual color probe set (MYCN and CEP2) |
| 17q12 | Breast cancer Gastrointestinal cancers | HER2 Trastuzumab benefit | Amplification | Locus-specific single probe (HER2) Dual color (HER2 and CEP17) |
| 2p23 | Lung cancer | ALK Crizotinib benefit | Translocation/ rearrangement | Break apart dual color (ALK) |
| 18q11.2 | Synovial sarcoma | SS18 | Translocation/ rearrangement | Break apart dual color (SS18) |
| 12q13 | Myxoid/round cell liposarcoma | DDIT3 | Translocation/ rearrangement | Break apart dual color (DDIT3) |
| Centromere 3, 7, 17, 9p12 UroVision (Abbott Molecular) | Bladder cancer | | Polysomy centromere 3, 7, 17; deletion 9p12 | Four-color probe set |
| 10q23 | Glioma | PTEN | Deletion | Dual color probe (PTEN and CEP10) |

Probe configurations based on probe sets available by Abbott Molecular.

a practical utilization of CISH as a viable option in diagnostic laboratories. In the following sections, we will discuss some of the current diagnostic and clinical uses of FISH and CISH, as well as some of the current research and future applications of these technologies.

# Copy-number assessment

## Amplification

With the exception of the genes located on the Y chromosome, all other genes in the human genome are normally presented in two copies per cell. For many cancers, malignant transformation is associated with a change in DNA copy-number. There are now a number of commercially available tests used to determine the copy-number status of genes or loci across different cancers, as well as genetic syndromes. Many pathology or molecular cytogenetic laboratories may perform these companion tests to complement standard diagnostic testing. Amplification of oncogenes such as the MYC family of genes, MYC (8q24) or MYCN (2p24), are often predictors of poor prognosis among neuroblastomas, medulloblastomas and prostate cancer (reviewed by Vita and Henriksson (36)). Recommendations by the International Collaboration on Cancer Reporting (ICCR) (www.cap.org) suggest the assessment of MYCN copy-number in neuroblastoma (currently by FISH), using dual-color probe set for MYCN and centromere 2 as standard testing.

Interestingly, recent studies in breast cancer have shown that those patients with altered copy-number of MYC predicts an added benefit to Trastuzumab (37), thus breast cancer patients may benefit from MYC assessment. The amplification of the Epidermal Growth Factor Receptor (EGFR), at 7p11.2, has treatment implications for lung (38) and colorectal cancer (CRC) (39). Specifically, both EGFR gene amplification and/or high polysomy are associated with clinical benefit in patients with non-small cell lung carcinoma (NSCLC), who are treated with tyrosine kinase inhibitors (TKI), such as Gefitinib and Erlotinib (38). However, recent CAP guidelines suggest EGFR status by FISH, or CISH, should not be used as a selection criteria of patients for EGFR TKI therapy (40), since the mutational status of EGFR showed greater correlation to TKI benefit. Nonetheless, gene amplification testing for many cancers continues to be performed to support diagnostic findings and treatment options. Interestingly, however, Ji *et al.* (41) utilized PCR-generated FISH probes for exons 2 to 7 for the detection of the EGFR vIII deletion in a small survey of lung cancers, suggesting that there is the possibility of utilizing *in situ*-based assays for identifying those patients who may benefit from TKIs. Patents for a probe set designed to detect the vIII EGFR mutant have been recently filed by Abbott Molecular Inc., thus offering the possibility of a commercial product. EGFR amplification is also frequently seen among glioblastoma (GBM) patients and is associated with poor prognosis (42). For example, in an ongoing clinical trial (NCT01112527), patients with recurrent GBM and EGFR amplification, as assessed by FISH, will be treated with a potent irreversible EGFR inhibitor (Dacomitinib), which can cross the blood-brain barrier, unlike other TKIs. The results of the trial may help to ascertain the benefit of routine EGFR copy-number assessment among GBM patients, identifying those who may benefit from Dacomitinib, which could be enhanced if a commercial probe set for the EGFR vIII mutant comes quickly to market. Amplification of EGFR has also been seen in breast cancer, although the prognostic implications of amplification are not as clear as for HER2 (to be discussed in detail below). Although the amplification of topoisomerase II-a (TOP2A), which maps telomeric to HER2 at 17q21, has been investigated, its value as a predictive marker remains unclear (43, 44). Indeed, the assessment of HER2, TOP2A and centromere 17 may have predictive significance, underlining the

importance of ascertaining the copy-number status of these two genes in the same tumor cell. This approach was recently utilized by Fountzilas *et al.* (45), where a multicolor FISH probe set comprising HER2/TOP2A and centromere 17 was used in a series of breast cancers testing their prognostic significances.

## Deletion

While gene amplification is an important mechanism driving tumorigenesis and disease progression, gene deletions contribute an equally important role in cancer biology. Classical cytogenetics and whole genome profiling have identified regions of recurrent genomic loss, suggesting the presence of important genes with tumor suppressive qualities. The assessment of genomic deletion *in situ* is technically more challenging than ascertaining gains/amplification; due primarily to the effects of cell truncation during the histological preparation of the sections. For this reason, it is critical to have reliable controls and cut-off values for determining the deletions. However, the information from deletion studies is invaluable, since deletion data derived from bulk-extracted molecular methods suffer from the normalization effects of normal cell contamination or genomic heterogeneity. *In situ* analyses permit the selective scoring of only tumor cells. Deletions occur frequently among congenital syndromes, for which a large compendium of probe sets for FISH is available and typically applied to metaphase or interphase preparations derived from chorionic villus, amniotic specimens or blood. For solid tumors, numerous FISH studies have evaluated the deletion status of many important genes, including tumor suppressor genes RB1 (13q14), TP53 (17p13), p16 (9p21) and PTEN (10q23), among others. However, currently there are no comprehensive studies utilizing CISH for routine diagnostic assessment of gene deletion, although a small number of research-based investigations have utilized the non-fluorescent CISH technique, primarily as single probes, including PTEN (10q23)(46), BMI1 (10p13)(47) and NF2 (22q12) (48, 49).

## Aneusomy and ploidy

The detection of specific whole chromosome aneusomies or overall changes in ploidy has implications for pre-natal diagnostics and oncology. FISH lends itself well in this respect as multiple probes can be used in one experiment, thereby capturing a more comprehensive picture of the genetic information in these cells. For high-risk pregnancies and those resulting from *in vitro* technologies, FISH using the commercial Vysis AneuVysion Multicolour (Abbott Molecular) probe kit may be ordered. This five-probe FISH cocktail includes the RB1 gene (13q14), a locus at 21q22.13, centromeres 18, X and Y; with other pre-natal/pre-implantation probe sets available. Similarly, the Food and Drug Administration (FDA)-approved multicolor probe set for bladder cancer (UroVysion Bladder Cancer Kit, Abbott Molecular) is utilized for detecting cancer and monitoring recurrence from cells derived from urine. This multicolor probe set allows the detection of chromosomes 3, 7, 17 poly-somy as well as the presence of deletion at 9p12 which has been shown to characterize higher grade tumors. The selection of 3, 7 and 17 alpha-centromeric alpha satellites in the probe set reflects the frequent finding of copy-number gains of these chromosomes during recurrence of, and potentially as predictive markers for progression of, superficial transitional cell carci-momas of the urinary bladder (50–59). The deletion of 9p12 appears to be a characteristic of early and non-invasive tumors (50–52,57–59).

## Gene rearrangement or translocation status

Since the identification of the Ph chromosome in 1960 (4), and its confirmation as a translocation between the ABL gene (9q32) and the BCR gene (22q11) (5), scientists have continued to search for recurrent translocation events, resulting in an exten-sive list of recurrent translocations in both hemato-logical malignancies as well as solid tumors (http://cgap.nci.nih.gov/Chromosomes/Mitelman). In the case of the BCR-ABL translocation, the resultant fusion gene produces a constitutively active and oncogenic ABL tyrosine kinase, and is the target for Imatinib (Novartis Pharmaceutical Corp.) in the treatment of chronic myelogenous leukemia (CML). Originally, identification of rearrangement events were determined by the preparation of metaphase spreads, a laborious process, which requires the col-lection of viable tissue for diagnostic specimens, and in this context can be challenging for samples with low mitotic rates. The advent of labeled DNA probes permitted the interrogation of interphase nuclei to derive the rearrangement status of a gene without the requirement of visualizing the chromosomes.

Because the majority of translocation and rearrange-ment probes have been manufactured and optimized for FISH, the majority of the discussion will be based on these probe sets. However, comprehensive CISH evaluation studies have now been conducted for translocation status, and will be discussed further below.

The detection of gene fragmentation can be visu-alized by differential labeling of the gene on either side of the breakpoint – typically referred to as a "break-apart" probe (Figure 4.3). For example, the 3' side of the breakpoint may be detected by a red-(fluorescing) signal, while the 5' side of the breakpoint may be detected by a green-(fluorescing) signal. When the gene is intact, signals will be co-localized and produce a yellow signal, indicative of the fusion of the two probe signals. When the gene is involved in a rearrangement, the red and green signal will be separated. Utilization of the break-apart probe is of value when it is sufficient to know that the gene of interest has been disrupted, and the identity of the gene partner is not necessary. In contrast, when the identity of the specific translocation partners are required to be confirmed, a "fusion" probe set may be used (Figure 4.3). In this case, each of the genes involved in the translocation event are differentially labeled. Using the BCR-ABL translocation as an example, the entire BCR gene may be identified with a red-(fluorescing) signal and the entire ABL gene with a green-(fluorescing) signal. In a normal cell, two separate signals for each color (gene) would be identified, yielding a total of four separate signals. However, in a Ph+ positive CML, the translocation event would produce two yellow fusion signals – one representing the BCR-ABL translocation, and one representing the reciprocal ABL-BCR translocation – hence the term "double fusion" probe set (Figure 4.3). Also present in the Ph+ cell would be a single green and red signal, indicative of the normal, and non-rearranged, copy of BCR and ABL. Alternatively, in a "single fusion" probe set, the region 3' to the breakpoint on the ABL gene would be labeled in red, while the region 5' on the BCR gene would be labeled in green, resulting in one fused yellow signal when the translocation event is present, and with one single signal each on the unaffected chromosomes (Figure 4.3). Many mainstream DNA probe manufac-turers provide such dual-color probe sets for the identification of the common structural aberrations. In fact, because of the number of variant

## Break-apart probe

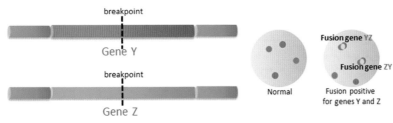

## Double fusion probe

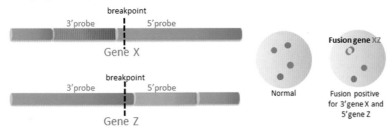

## Single fusion probe

**Figure 4.3 Probe configuration for rearrangement/translocation events**
Commercially available probe sets may utilize different probe configurations to determine whether a gene has undergone a rearrangement event, or whether a specific translocation event between two genes has occurred. "Break-apart" probes comprise differentially labeled probes representing either side of the breakpoint in the gene of interest, shown in red for the 3′ side of the breakpoint, and green for the 5′ side of the breakpoint in gene X. In normal cells, the colocalization of the signals are shown as green and red signals juxtaposed to each other, or sometimes seen as yellow signals, due to their colocalization. In a cell positive for the rearrangement, the two signals will be separated. "Double fusion" probes comprise differentially labeled probes that span each gene across their breakpoints, shown as red for gene Y and green for gene Z. In a normal cell, two separate signals for each gene can be seen. When the translocation is present, two fusion signals will be seen; each representing the translocation (i.e. oncogenic fusion) and reciprocal translocation, in addition to the unaffected chromosomes. In this case, the oncogenic fusion cannot be distinguished from the non-oncogenic fusion. "Single fusion" probes comprise differentially labeled probes specific for the translocation of interest (i.e. the oncogenic fusion), and not the reciprocal translocation. In this example, the 3′ side of the breakpoint of gene X is labeled in red, while the 5′ side of the breakpoint of gene Z is labeled in green. As in double fusion probes, a normal cell will possess two signals for each probe. In a translocation positive cell, specifically that the 3′ end of gene X is expected to translocate to the 5′ end of gene Z, one fusion signal will be seen.

translocations and the elucidation of microdeletions associated with some of the translocation events, multicolor probe sets (presently for FISH only) have been generated to provide this additional information. Moreover, the addition of other chromosomal abnormalities associated with the translocations, such as whole chromosomal gains, can be included such that several aberrations can be assayed in the same cell at the same time. It is worth noting that, since the

break-apart and fusion gene sets rely on the detection of a fused yellow signal where the red and green signals from the probes are interacting to produce a yellow signal, this application is currently unable to be used for chromogenic *in situ* assays.

The identification of a number of recurrent translocation and gene rearrangement events in leukemias and lymphomas has permitted rapid detection, enhanced monitoring of disease recurrence, and provided putative targets for therapeutic intervention. Several sarcomas also possess recurrent translocations (http://cgap.nci.nih.gov/Chromosomes/Mitelman); however, high-frequency recurrent translocations do not appear to be as common among other solid carcinomas. Nevertheless, there have been a handful of recurrent rearrangements that have become of clinical significance. The ALK gene (2p23) is a receptor tyrosine kinase, whose oncogenic activity can be mediated by mutation, copy-number or by an oncogenic gene fusion. In lung cancer, the presence of the oncogenic EML4-ALK fusion occurs in 2–7% of pulmonary adenocarcinomas, with other ALK partners such as KIF5B (10p11) and TFG (3q12) comprising a minority of the rearrangements (40). The recent approval by the FDA for the use of the ALK inhibitor, Crizotinib (Pfzier Inc.), in treating pulmonary adenocarcinomas requires diagnostic ISH assays to identify those patients who may benefit from the drug. The EML4-ALK fusion results from a pericentric inversion, inv (2)(2p21p23), such that the amino-terminal end of EML4 becomes fused with the intracellular region of ALK, eliminating the normal 13 mb gap between them. CAP recommendations for ALK testing suggest the use the FDA-approved companion diagnostic dual-labeled break-apart FISH probe by Abbott Molecular, for selecting patients for ALK TKI therapy. Indeed, recommendations also indicate the use of FISH over RT-PCR (40). The expected FISH pattern for a rearrangement positive cell would be the presence of split green and red signals, since the probe configuration comprises an orange probe corresponding to the 3' end of ALK, and green probe mapping on the 5' end. Since the partners for ALK are not required for selecting patients eligible for ALK TKI therapy, this probe configuration is sufficient.

## Research applications of DNA ISH and related technologies

## Identification of whole chromosome or whole genome copy-number imbalances and structural rearrangements

Dual-color FISH enables investigators to perform simple gene mapping and copy-number experiments (reviewed by Bayani and Squire (60)). FISH is now commonly applied to FFPE samples or chromatin fibers (60). The routine use of two-colored FISH to

chromosomes provided the foundation for whole genome profiling. In 1992, the Pinkel group (9) published a seminal paper in *Science* describing Comparative Genomic Hybridization (CGH). The precursor to today's array-based CGH and comparative expression assays, this two-color FISH experiment entailed the hybridization of equal amounts of differentially labeled tumor and normal reference DNA to denatured normal metaphase spreads. Each metaphase spread was digitally imaged and the individual chromosomes paired so that the average green:red (tumor:normal) ratio change in fluorescence for each chromosome, and across several metaphase spreads, could be determined. Despite the fact that the lower level of resolution was limited to the size of a chromosomal band (approximately 10 mb), researchers could now better identify regions of recurrent copy-number change and subsequently verify those findings by FISH, using locus-specific probes. Today, rather than the comparatively lower-resolution metaphase chromosomes, such whole genome profiling now occurs at the level of the gene. The contribution of CGH – whether metaphase-, array-, sequencing- or bead-based – to our understanding of cancer genomes is evident, as there are numerous online repositories for both public and controlled access. Through these studies, investigators have identified many potential drivers for cancer initiation and progression and providing putative biomarkers for translation to the clinic (61).

As fluorescence microscopy and digital imaging improved for the growing discipline of molecular cytogenetics, other metaphase FISH-based technologies were born, including Spectral Karyotyping (SKY), Multi-Color FISH (MFISH) and Combined Binary Ratio labeling-FISH (COBRA-FISH). Using combinatorial labeling of both directly and indirectly labeled DNA, a whole genome cocktail composed of 24 whole chromosome painting probes could be used in one experiment. SKY (62), Multi-colour FISH (63) and COBRA-FISH (64) are 24-color whole chromosome painting assays able to detect numerical and structural aberrations at the resolution of the metaphase chromosome (Figure 4.4). However, their differences lie in the way in which the fluorochromes are detected. SKY acquires the FISH image in two stages: one for the DAPI counterstain, and one for all the chromosomes. Unique spectral signatures are associated with each chromosome, which are based on the combinatorial labeling using five different fluorochromes. The spectral signatures across the length of a given chromosomal structure are compared with the combinatorial library, enabling the identification of the origins of the chromosomal segments in question. In contrast, MFISH utilizes the presence or absence of signal upon image acquisition under different filters. Thus, a typical MFISH acquisition cycle would include the DAPI counterstaining image, with additional acquisition under five different filters (Figure 4.4). Like SKY, the combinatorial labeling of each chromosome would serve as the reference and the analysis software identifies the chromosome. COBRA-FISH is less commonly used, but similarly exploits sequential imaging with specific filters, but employs both combinatorial and ratio labeling to generate the chromosome library. Using these whole genome FISH techniques, structural aberrations were exquisitely identified, illustrating the previously unimaginable karyotypic complexity of these cancer genomes. In this way, investigators could integrate the findings from both CGH and SKY/MFISH and validating such changes by locus-specific FISH assays (63, 65–67). A variation of MFISH, MBand (Multi-colour Banding), was also introduced and utilized the combinatorial labeling strategy of SKY and MFISH, but applied it to specific chromosomal bands, such that one chromosome could be differentially labeled from the p-arm to the q-arm in large segments (Figure 4.4) (68). The strength of MBand lies in its ability to better localize breakpoints and in determining the presence of intrachromosomal rearrangements, such as deletions, inversions and duplications, not always revealed by SKY/MFISH or traditional banding analyses (Figure 4.4). The weakness of these techniques is the need to generate metaphase chromosomes for hybridization and intense image analysis, which has led to the development of sequencing and array-based techniques.

## Detection of aberrant biological mechanisms

The use of centromere or telomere probes, either chromosome specific or common to all chromosomes, reveals important information regarding DNA recombination events and errors in mitotic segregation. The use of chromosome-specific centromere probes has already been discussed in the context of determining copy-number; however, applying centromere probes to metaphase spreads aids detection of abnormal chromosomal structures such as multi-centric chromosomes, indicating errors in

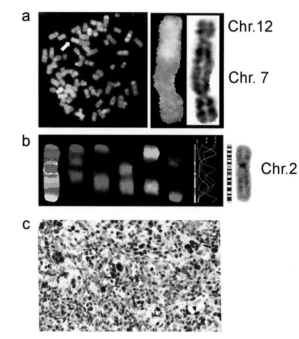

**Figure 4.4 Applications of ISH**
**(a) Spectral karyotyping (SKY).** Shown is a representative metaphase spread from the breast cancer cell line MCF-7 hybridized with the SKY probe set (Applied Spectral Imaging). Changes in fluorochrome color along the length of a given chromosome represent the presence of a different chromosome. A dicentric chromosome composed of chromosomes 12 and 7 (arrow) is shown to the right, with chromosome 12 material appearing as yellow/ orange fluorescence and chromosome 7 appearing as yellow/green fluorescence. Numerous chromosomal translocations involving multiple chromosomes can be seen in the metaphase spread. **(b) Normal chromosome 2 Mband.** Shown from left to right are the pseudocolored chromosome 2 banding pattern resulting from the combinatorial labeling and detection of various bands along the length of chromosome 2. In this probe set, five different fluorochromes are used in a combinatorial fashion to delineate different chromosomal bands. The presence or absence of signal along the length of the chromosome, as detected through specific filters, is compared to the combinatorial reference for that chromosome. **(c) *In situ* detection of the small non-coding nuclear RNA U6.** Shown is a representative image of a FFPE section from a serous ovarian cancer hybridized with a digoxigenin-labeled locked nucleic acid (LNA) probe for the small non-coding nuclear RNA U6 (Exiqon) and detected as dark purple/blue by the enzymatic reaction between alkaline phosphatase and nitro-blue tetrazolium and 5-bromo-4-chloro-3′-indolyphosphate (NBT-BCIP).
Unpublished images courtesy of Jane Bayani.

DNA repair and recombination (reviewed by Bayani *et al.* (69)). Moreover, application of centromere probes can determine ploidy changes and the presence of segregation errors, particularly when positive signals are present in micronuclei. However, care must be taken in extrapolation of changes in pericentromeric alpha and beta satellite repeats, which are the actual target of these "centromere enumeration probes" (CEPs), to changes in whole chromosomes. Alterations to specific arms, or even smaller sub-chromosomal regions, can appear to reflect "aneusomy" in interphase nuclei when in fact only the region containing the CEP has been altered (70, 71). Similarly, chromosome-specific telomeric probes to both metaphase and interphase cells have been used to identify the presence of isochromosomes, which characterize some cancer genomes, such as the i17(q) in CML and in medulloblastomas (http://cgap.nci.nih.gov/Chromosomes/Mitelman). Like centromere probes, telomere probes can identify errors in DNA repair through the detection of telomeric fusions between different chromosomes, often yielding multicentric chromosomes. Telomeres, which are located at the ends of chromosomes, are characterized by a unique sequence of repetitive DNA, whose length shortens after each cycle of replication. When the cell has reached its critically shortest length, the cell is triggered to undergo senescence and eventual apoptosis. In cancers, telomerase becomes activated, and telomere length is maintained. As such, scientists have investigated the relationship between telomere length and tumorigenesis (reviewed by Aubert *et al.* (72)). Additionally, radiosensitivity studies have been conducted using centromeric and/or telomeric probes to determine the severity of DNA damage upon ionizing radiation, allowing for genotype-phenotype analyses.

## RNA ISH applications

ISH is not limited to DNA. In fact, ISH has been routinely used to examine RNA expression both in a fluorescence and bright-field context for several decades (Figure 4.4). Labeling of a complementary segment of nucleic acid for RNA detection is performed in a similar fashion to DNA detection. Since the RNA species to be detected is the mature, single-stranded RNA, no denaturation of the target is required, eliminating the potential for the probe to hybridize with their DNA counterpart in the nucleus. *In situ* RNA detection is challenged by the fact that RNA is more susceptible to degradation and different mRNAs possess variable half-lives. Live cells, grown *in situ*, then fixed, produce the best results. Frozen tissue sections can also yield acceptable results provided proper fixation and probe access is facilitated. Results from FFPEs can be variable due to fixation

procedures; however, in general, reliable results can be obtained. The applicability of RNA ISH to the diagnostic laboratory has been tested using HER2, most predominantly in the bright-field context (73). Moreover, recent studies have applied the integration of standard HER2 immunohistochemistry (IHC) together with single locus HER2 copy-number evaluation (74) within the same section. In general, the quantification of RNA by ISH in these studies was largely concordant with results obtained by IHC, FISH or CISH. The possibility of utilizing RNA as an alternative test requires more rigorous evaluation and guidance; however, this suggests that a simultaneous approach for assessing DNA, RNA and protein (or combinations thereof) can be achieved, ideally in a multicolored approach using fluorescence microscopy; providing additional information to improve diagnosis or resolve problematic cases.

RNA ISH is not limited to the detection of mature mRNA; indeed, in recent years, FFPE has been an optimal source for examining microRNA (miRNA) expression *in situ*. Comprising a class of non-coding RNAs, miRNAs are involved in the post-transcriptional regulation of gene expression. As the importance of miRNA expression is becoming more apparent, in time miRNA expression will no doubt be included in diagnostic molecular panels and used as an *in situ* biomarker in the clinic (75).

## To CISH or FISH … that is the question …

It is apparent from the review of the basic methods for both bright-field- and fluorescent-based *in situ* assays that there are a number of advantages and disadvantages to each technique (Table 4.3). By virtue of being the first mainstream assay used for diagnostic molecular cytogenetics, FISH has already been well optimized and routinely performed. However, these experiences have been easily translated into CISH platforms for selected applications, only requiring simple steps for validation and acceptance as a viable alternative to FISH.

## Technical expertise, reagents, equipment and cost

In general, the technical expertise required for performing either CISH or FISH is similar; however, performance of the assay and in particular reporting

Table 4.3 Comparison of techniques/advantages/disadvantages

|  | CISH | FISH |
| --- | --- | --- |
| Target specimens | FFPE, cytological smears, touch preparations<br>Metaphase chromosomes<br>Chromatin fibers | FFPE, cytological smears, touch preparations, metaphase chromosomes, chromatin fibers |
| Probe<br>labeling<br>Number of probes | Indirectly labeled: requires antibody detection steps, can contribute to background<br>1–2<br>Dependent on availability of reporter molecules and ability to differentially detect labels | Directly and indirectly labeled: more common use of directly labeled probes minimizes issues related to background<br>1–24<br>Combined use of directly fluorescently labeled probes and indirectly labeled probes provides greater ability to generate multi-probe cocktails |
| Overall reagent costs | High | High |
| FDA-approved reagents | Yes | Yes |
| Bench time and analysis | 2–3 days | 2–3 days |
| Amenable to automation<br>Performing of assay<br>Image acquisition<br>Image analysis | <br>Yes<br>Yes<br>Yes | <br>Yes<br>Yes<br>Yes |
| Technical expertise for analysis | High | High |
| Microscope<br>magnification | Light microscope<br>20–40X<br>Dry objectives | Fluorescent microscope + appropriate filters<br>60–100X<br>Oil objectives |
| Cellular morphology | Variable | Variable |
| Ability to distinguish signals from background | High | High |
| Multi-gene/locus analysis ability | Restricted | High |
| Signal stability | High<br>Slides archivable | Low<br>Signals fade over time |

the diagnostic analysis appears to vary from institution to institution/country to country. Bench time for both assays remains essentially the same, although newer generation CISH assays and some FISH protocols are performed on automated platforms and can be performed within a day, as compared to the standard overnight FISH protocol; which has significant implications for how quickly a sample could be analyzed and reported. A number of commercial sources provide reagents in a ready-to-use fashion, reducing batch-to-batch variability and QA issues of in-house probe generation. Furthermore, the ability to process slides using automated histological stainers, which are commonly found in routine pathology laboratories,

serves as another benefit of performing CISH and FISH. Indeed, since the same reagents for routine IHC are used for CISH, and reagent modules can be easily exchanged for specific CISH reagents, CISH can be easily adopted with an existing pathology laboratory workflow. In terms of short-term and long-term storage, CISH slides have the convenience of being stored at room temperature with minimal or insignificant loss of signal over time following microscopy. FISH slides, however, suffer from the loss of signal intensity following exposure to microscopic analysis, requiring storage at –20°C to prevent signal deterioration. Ultimately, there is an eventual loss of fluorescence, making the possibility of successful long-term archiving unlikely. Although it has been previously believed that fluorescent-based assays bear a higher reagent cost, this was likely the case over a decade ago; however, the increasing popularity of CISH has made a dent in the FISH monopoly, driving reagent costs to near equivalency.

## Signal visualization and cellular architecture

The similarity of CISH staining to routine histo-pathology slides also provides the comfort of familiarity in visualizing cell morphology and architecture that is sometimes unclear under the fluorescent setting. However, insufficient development of the signal, high non-specific background, the inability to distinguish between similar or saturated chromogens, or debris in the bright-field context can result in ambiguous scoring and inconclusive results. In fact, the use of directly labeled, fluorescent probes minimizes the potential for non-specific background, which can plague experiments that require several antibody treatment steps. The inability to discriminate between the chromogens when signals are overlapping also poses a concern when determining presence or absence of a signal as well as enumerating signal numbers. By the same token, FISH may also be confounded by autofluorescence of surrounding tissues. Certainly, the primary advantage of CISH is the use of a standard light microscope for visualization, rather than a more costly fluorescent microscope with appropriate filters. However, the gap in cost, for a medium to high-end light microscope and associated digital hardware, with a fluorescent microscope, is reducing as the popularity of CISH increases. The ability to switch between different filters under fluorescence microscopy provides the advantage of better visualization of overlapping signals; not afforded by light microscopy.

## Multi-color analyses

Perhaps the greatest advantage FISH has over CISH is the ability to hybridize more than two probes in one experiment, and the access to a wider variety of commercially available probe sets. Furthermore, the use of probes directly labeled with the fluorochrome endows FISH with a significant advantage over CISH, which requires additional antibody incubations and final signal detection steps. Combinatorial labeling with multiple fluorochromes or in combination with reporter molecules by FISH permits the evaluation of multiple DNA loci in one experiment; resulting in the use of less patient material and generating more data for a given cell. This can minimize the concerns that arise with interpreting genetic data from serial sections. In particular, break-apart and fusion ISH based assays are, to date, limited to FISH systems. However, Hoff *et al.* (76) recently described the use of reagents for the conversion of FISH probes to dual-color CISH. The authors reported a 100% concordance between the FISH and CISH results following the subsequent conversion to CISH, using HER2/CEP17, EGFR/CEP7 and TOP2A/CEP17. As this is the only published study of its kind to date, it remains to be seen in a larger sample size and across different laboratories whether the concordance remains high. Conversion of FISH to CISH would certainly incur significant additional costs and lengthening of the procedure; however, it permits access to well-established commercial probe sets. Despite the ability to convert dual-color FISH probes (presumably at this time only FITC and Texas Red) to a bright-field environment, bright-field analysis is still essentially limited to two probes/color. Therefore, the potential to perform multi-probe analyses by fluorescence still translates into the ability to generate more genomic information within the same cell, and using less precious patient material.

## Microscopy and digital image acquisition

Another aspect that should be considered when deciding whether to CISH or FISH is the reporting, analysis and archiving of data. In an ever-increasing digital age, and recognizing that samples may need to be revisited or re-analyzed, together with the increasing number of molecular pathology tests available to patients today, there is a strong drive towards rigorous data archiving, reporting and analysis. We have previously mentioned that the use of standard light microscopy for CISH can reduce the start-up and ongoing costs as compared to fluorescence microscopy. However, it is rare that microscopes today are not associated with image acquisition equipment and software. For the purposes of basic documentation, many of the mainstream microscope manufacturers possess fundamental acquisition software and hardware; composed essentially of a camera connected to a

**45**

generic desktop computer with simple report templates. Admittedly, fluorescence imaging tends to incur higher initial and ongoing costs than bright-field. However, most often, the ability to image in bright-field already comes integrated with the higher-priced fluorescence modules. The difference in cost may come when choosing the module for which image analysis will be conducted. For FISH, image capture requires the acquisition of separate images using the appropriate filter and using the appropriate light source, typically a mercury or xenon lamp, although LED options are increasingly popular. Thus, for a standard two-color FISH experiment using green- and red-fluorescing signals, three images would be taken: one under the DAPI filter; one using a filter appropriate for the green-fluorescing signal; and one for the red-fluorescing signal. Taken as grey-scale images, the individual images are assigned the appropriate color and merged together to create the final color image. The same process is carried out for multicolor probe sets, unless the SKY method of image acquisition and analyses is utilized. Because of this, the time required to acquire the FISH images is generally longer, and requires more computing power and memory. Moreover, the slide is subjected to increased exposure time, contributing to eventual photobleaching, jeopardizing the possibility of successful long-term storage. In bright-field imaging, which uses transmitted light, a color digital camera acquires a color image. This poses a limitation for bright-field imaging and analysis since the camera will only be able to take images from the visible range, unlike fluorescence, for which signals emitted from the visible and non-visible range can be acquired. Comparatively, bright-field images can be acquired much quicker. Since only one image is taken, the file sizes are relatively smaller, unless taken at high resolution. Despite these limitations, image analysis for bright-field microscopy has advanced significantly, allowing for different chromogens to be distinguished by separating the color image into its basic red, green and blue (RGB) layer components and analyzing the relative intensities across each layer.

## Manual and automated analyses and quality control

Traditionally, the scoring of CISH or FISH signals has been performed by direct visualization and manual analysis; and the vast majority of laboratories continue to perform analysis in this fashion. However, direct visualization and manual scoring is labor intensive and, despite efforts to maintain best laboratory practices, manual scoring can still be subject to scoring bias and scoring variability. To accommodate the trends in remote access, analysis, documentation and to reduce scoring bias, image analysis modules capable of automatically scoring acquired cells have been developed. While there is no requirement for a specific light or fluorescent microscope for scoring, scanning or imaging, other than possessing the appropriate filters, light sources and objectives, there has been the move in the clinical setting to have FDA-approved imaging systems in place. To date, the FDA has approved the BioView™ Duet System for automated FISH scanning and Applied Spectral Imaging's GenASIs for automated scanning. Both offer the ability to image and analyze FISH signals using automated cell segmentation and signal enumeration algorithms to generate signal ratios. Other mainstream microscope manufacturers or digital pathology companies such as Applied Imaging, Leica Biosystems, Metasystems, Carl Zeiss, Aperio and others also provide comparable automated image capture and analysis software. In most cases, additional modules can accommodate the imaging of CISH slides. It should be cautioned that the results of "fully automated" analysis require some manual quality control and scoring to ensure that automated scoring algorithms are robust. Nevertheless, in some problematic cases, whether FISH or CISH, automated imaging and/or analysis may not be feasible, requiring manual scoring.

Irrespective of the assay chosen, it is critical that sufficient training and internal QA standards are maintained. We have already discussed the importance of both internal and external laboratory assessment, as well as adherence to guidelines for scoring set forth by recognized organizations such as ASCO and CAP (77). Standard reporting elements should include: the protocol and reagents used; positive and negative controls; scoring criteria; number of independent observers and the variation between those observers; and validation of scoring methods (i.e. manual and/or automated). Ultimately, the decision to use CISH or FISH becomes one of preference; therefore, laboratories must comply with all the necessary quality control measures and additional validation to achieve the greatest level of sensitivity and specificity.

## Analysis of copy-number *in situ*: the challenge of truncation and accurate signal enumeration

Unlike interphase analyses from cytogenetic suspensions or direct cytological smears, copy-number analysis of interphase cells *in situ* possesses challenges, with significant implications in a diagnostic setting. Copy-number analyses of intact nuclei from cytogenetic preparations or cytological smears are considerably easier and more reliable, subject only to the phase of the cell cycle and, more importantly, inefficiencies of hybridization and background. Thus, enumeration of a given locus in a normal cell can yield the expected two copies in over 98% of cells (78). Unfortunately, this is not the case for FFPE tissues, which is a challenge for both CISH and FISH. As we have previously discussed, the effects of nuclear truncation will alter the observed copy-number for a given locus. Indeed, the range of gene copy in normal breast tissues analyzed in paraffin section is 1.6 ± 0.8 (mean ± SD) for chromosome centromere 17 (79), generating a range of 1.3 to 1.85. Based on this rationale, values less than 1.35 reflect monosomy, while values greater than 1.85 indicate polysomy. Controversies as to the value of single locus enumeration without the benefit of a reference locus, such as the corresponding centromere, continue. Single probe guidelines for HER2 suggest that copy-numbers greater than 6.0 are amplified; while less than 4.0 copies are not considered amplified; and 4.0 to 6.0 copies require validation with a parallel section with centromere 17. This strategy fails to account for the possibilities in changes of chromosome 17. However, we have previously demonstrated the value of performing dual locus copy-number studies in the context of HER2 (70). Consider the situation where a mean HER2 copy-number of 3 from single locus evaluation would render this case non-amplified. However, if analyzed with the chromosome 17 centromere possessing a ratio of 1.4, the current guidelines would consider this as HER2 amplified. In fact, the consideration of these "low copy" cases provided the impetus for our study demonstrating the value of performing dual-color analyses on the outset to improve the accuracy of diagnosis for HER2 (70). Clearly, dual-color FISH or CISH provides valuable additional information, and as we have discussed above, is greatly enhanced by the ability to discriminate the signals, particularly when they are overlapping. Indeed, the instances of centromere amplification can confound analysis and interpretation, thus the assay that can best discriminate between signals is desirable.

## HER2 assessment: a tale of two assays

To illustrate the advantages and limitations between FISH and CISH, the assessment of HER2 (17q12) copy-number for breast cancer will used as a model, since the vast majority of studies comparing FISH and CISH are based on this important predictive marker. The over-expression of HER2 occurs in approximately 18–20% of breast cancers and is associated with tumor aggressiveness and poor prognosis (77, 80). However, HER2 amplification identifies patients who would benefit from treatment with Trastuzumab (Herceptin®) (Genentech Inc.), the humanized monoclonal antibody against HER2 (77, 80), Lapatinib and other HER2-directed therapies. Therefore, accurate identification of HER2 positivity is critical, as therapeutic benefit from treatment with Trastuzumab is only seen in patients with HER2-positive disease (77). The standard clinical algorithm for HER2 testing typically begins with immunohistochemical analyses. Patients exhibiting equivocal HER2 protein expression (2+) are then subjected to reflex assays for validation, typically by FISH, and more recently by CISH (77). The importance of establishing HER2 positivity has resulted in the rapid generation of clinical assays for reflex testing and their cross-validation (17–23). Because single-probe CISH was initially available, CISH testing comprised the enumeration of only HER2. In this case, high amplification was defined as a cell with 10 or more copies or present in clusters in more than 50% of cancer cells; low-leveled amplification defined as 6 to 10 copies, or present as multiple copies, and small clusters in more than 50% of cancer cells; and non-amplified when HER2 was present in five or fewer copies, in more than 50% of cells. However, in cases where HER2 was present in fewer than six copies, it was unclear as to whether these cases were truly (non-)amplified, resulting in the recommendation that centromere 17 CISH should also be assessed to account for chromosome 17 aneusomy in a serial section (70). More recently, dual-color CISH has enabled the enumeration of both HER2 and centromere 17 on the same tissue section to generate the HER2/centromere 17 ratio; and which distinguishes between true gene amplification, chromosome

17 polysomy or variability copy-number due to truncation and differences in replication timing. Thus, most laboratories assess HER2 copy-number by enumerating the number of HER2 and centromere 17 signals per cell, in 60 intact and non-overlapping cells, to generate the HER2/centromere 17 ratio. Using the HER2/centromere 17 ratio, HER2-amplified cells are described as possessing a ratio greater than 2.2; non-amplified when possessing a ratio of less than 1.8. In those equivocal cases which generate ratios between 1.8 and 2.2, it is recommended to score an additional 30 cells per technologist. There is, of course, continuing controversy regarding the usefulness of a single HER2 probe for detecting amplification, as a cancer may be deemed as amplified using the single probe assay, but non-amplified using the dual probe/ratio classification (70).

In a multicenter evaluation of 45 (17) and 30 (22) breast cancers studied by our group, comparing the use of the FDA-approved HER2 PathVision FISH test (Abbott Molecular) to Ventana's FDA-approved INFORM HER2 ISH assay (Ventana Medical Systems Inc.), and under the guidelines of the UK National External Quality Assessment Scheme (UK NEQAS), it was demonstrated that both tests resulted in equivalent results. Briefly, the PathVision probe set comprises two differentially labeled fluorescent probes: a directly labeled HER2-Spectrum Orange and directly labeled-centromere 17/CEP17-Spectrum Green. In contrast, the first generation of the INFORM SISH assay (17) required the staining of separate slides for HER2 and centromere 17; however, the second generation of INFORM (22) comprises two differentially labeled probes – a DNP-labeled HER2 and digoxigenin-labeled centromere 17 – chromogenically detected as black and red signals respectively. Indeed, the results showed an impressive overall success rate of 94.8% in determining HER2 status across several laboratories, using the same tissue microarray (TMA), with the INFORM SISH assay (17). This was comparable to the success rate of 86.7% of cases for HER2 determination using the standard FISH method in the reference laboratory. In a direct comparison between INFORM-SISH and PathVision, a 94.8% concordance was found, which just exceeds the ASCO/CAP guidelines (greater than 90% concordance) to validate a novel FISH or immunohistochemical procedure (77). The results for the INFORM HER2 Dual ISH (22) showed similar findings, with a 93.3% overall success rate with the PathVision FISH-derived results.

These findings are consistent with others (18, 23) and have been reviewed extensively by Rosa *et al.* (81), showing high concordance between FISH and dual-color CISH.

However, the situation appears to be more difficult for those cases where patterns of copy-number change are ambiguous. Recently, Mansfield *et al.* (82) compared CISH (INFORM HER2 Dual ISH) to FISH (PathVision) in 251 samples enriched for common and difficult-to-assess HER2 status, originally assessed by FISH and IHC. In addition to cases with straightforward genomic patterns, the anomalous categories included cases with high-level HER2 amplification; cases with chromosome 17 aneusomy; cases with HER2 deletion or duplication; as well as cases with equivocal results. While the initial FISH failure rate was 8.5%, retesting by FISH was successful, in contrast to the CISH failure rate of 11%, with 2.8% failing repeated testing. The concordance between FISH and CISH, based on the categorized anomaly, was 64%. The comparison between FISH and CISH was 83% when categorized according to the ASCO/CAP guidelines of amplified, equivocal or non-amplified. In general, these findings demonstrated that CISH generated lower HER2/centromere 17 ratios than FISH, with agreement between FISH and CISH appearing worse at higher ratios. Thus, relative to FISH results (which continues to be the gold standard), this study demonstrated that 28% of tumors that would have been considered HER2 amplified with FISH would have been classified as normal by CISH. This has a significant impact on patient care regarding these women, as CISH results would have resulted in them not being offered HER2-targeted therapy. Moreover, CISH could not reliably detect HER2 amplification against a background of centromere 17 co-amplification, leading the authors to suggest that the advantages of CISH are outweighed by the higher false-negative rates in these anomalous cases.

Thus, it appears that the majority of studies have concluded that CISH for HER2 assessment is comparable to assessment by FISH, opening the door for CISH to be used in place of FISH. Although the CAP guidelines suggest FISH be used for the detection of the ALK rearrangement, it does not restrict the use of in-house or other commercial probes, or CISH, provided it attains or exceeds the performance of the Abbott probe set. With this in mind, Schildhaus *et al.* (83) reported their findings of the direct comparison between the Abbott probe set with a break-apart dual-color ALK CISH probe set by ZytoVision (Germany) in 100 lung adenocarcinomas. The digoxigenin- and DNP-labeled probes were detected by horseradish peroxidase, visualized with a green chromogen, and alkaline phosphatase, visualized with a red chromogen, respectively. Blinded to the FISH results, CISH identified 16 of 16 ALK rearranged tumors, with no false positives. The authors reported 100% sensitivity and specificity by CISH for correct classification of ALK positive or negative. Seven percent of ALK-negative cases represented a subgroup of diagnostically difficult cases by FISH, in contrast to 3.5% of cases by CISH. Moreover, in a comprehensive evaluation by van Rijk *et al.* (84), the consistency between CISH and FISH was assessed, using split-signal probes in 540 of 11 lymphoma entities and reactive, benign lymphoid tissues, collected from eight different pathology laboratories, arrayed on 15 FISH pre-stained TMAs, which were double stained for the chromogenic hybridization for the following genes: BCL10 (1p22); IGK (2p11); ALK (2p23); BCL6 (3q27); TCRG (7p14); TCRB (7q34); MYC (8q24); PAX5 (9p13); CCND1 (11q13); TCRAD (14q11); TCL1 (14q32); IGH (14q32); MALT1 (18q21); BCL2 (18q21); BCL3 (19q13); and IGL (22q11); all in the context of two-color experiments. For each core, morphology and actual signal were compared to the original fluorescence hybridization results. The authors reported an impressive 97% concordance, arguing for CISH as a viable tool for diagnostic samples. Similarly, Lass and colleagues (85) assessed CISH as an alternative to FISH for the diagnostic assessment of the 1p/19q deletion status that characterizes the oligodendroglioma subtype of gliomas. Their findings across 42 consecutive gliomas showed reproducibility between FISH and CISH findings of 93% (n = 39/42). Those non-concordant cases were re-evaluated by FISH and microsatellite analysis for loss of heterozygosity (LOH), confirming the initial CISH results. Other CISH to FISH comparative studies have been performed to assess aneusomies for various solid tumors such as ependymomas (86) and chondromas (87).

## Concluding remarks

There seems to be ongoing debate with molecular laboratories as to whether ISH-based testing will still have a future, as array-based and sequencing costs begin to decline and the speed at which these analyses can be performed increases. However, this brings us back to the point that ISH-based analysis has its strength of assessing copy-number or rearrangement status on a cell-by-cell basis and within the cellular context of the tissue, which cannot be accounted for through the bulk extraction of nucleic acids. A recent publication by Gerdes *et al.* (88) described a multiplex assay for quantitative single-cell analysis and subcellular characterization of multiple analytes as well as FISH in FFPE, using fluorescence microscopy and in-house generated imaging algorithms. While this application currently remains in the research domain, the move to a diagnostic application will most definitely come, as most laboratories already have the foundations for such technology. The decision for a laboratory to FISH or CISH is not a trivial one. Cost and efficient turnover of testing is important to the operation of a clinical laboratory, but one must not forget that at the end of each specimen is a patient for which the results of the test have life-changing implications. When performed to the highest technical standards, FISH and CISH can produce equivalent results. However, as we have discussed, each assay carries with it both strengths and weaknesses that must be weighted according to both the current and future needs of the laboratory. Perhaps the benefits of CISH include the fact that many of the reagents used to perform the assay are already in use in the laboratory. Coupled with the fact that the results of CISH appear similar to routine histological slides, and contribute to the ease of analysis, the greatest advantage of using CISH technology would be for a laboratory that does not already have a FISH program in place. The recent availability of different chromogens to visualize the signals has improved the ability to discriminate signals and utilize two-color strategies. Moreover, the ability to access the variety of existing FISH probes and convert them to CISH signals no longer limits the type tests that can be performed. However, the FISH to CISH conversion comes at a cost – an increase in reagent cost and time at the bench. Moreover, CISH is still limited primarily to two colors. In contrast, FISH has been implemented in many laboratories, with commercial probe sets and reagents already well optimized. The robustness of probes directly labeled with fluorochromes eliminates the need to perform detection steps using antibody incubations, which can contribute to background. In fact there are a variety of fluorochromes both within the visual and non-visual range of detection that can be utilized to create multi-probe cocktails. The detection of each fluorochome through its specific filter affords the ability to distinguish signals even when overlapping, which is not always the case in bright-field microscopy. FISH provides the flexibility to provide more genomic information in one experiment, reducing the number of individual tests and the amount of patient material. No matter which assay is used, strict quality control measures must always be implemented so that the assay can perform to its highest standard, bearing in mind that the results of the test directly impact the future of that patient.

ISH is a powerful tool that can provide valuable insights into the mechanisms of disease; and the

assessment of DNA imbalances will continue to be an important element of diagnostic and prognostic testing.

## Learning points

- *In situ*-based DNA analyses provide important copy-number information at a by-cell level, offering additional information that is lost through bulk extraction of nucleic acids
- CISH and FISH are robust assays capable of providing copy-number and rearrangement status information
- FISH offers greater assay flexibility than CISH, since more than two fluorochromes can be easily visualized

## References

1.  Boveri, T. Concerning the origin of malignant tumours by Theodor Boveri. Translated and annotated by H. Harris. *J Cell Sci* 2008; 121(Suppl. 1): 1–84.

2.  Trask, B. J. Human cytogenetics: 46 chromosomes, 46 years and counting. *Nat Rev Genet* 2002; 3(10): 769–78.

3.  Speicher, M. R. and Carter, N. P. The new cytogenetics: blurring the boundaries with molecular biology. *Nat Rev Genet* 2005; 6(10): 782–92.

4.  Nowell, P.C. and Hungerford, D. A. Chromosome studies on normal and leukemic human leukocytes. *J Natl Cancer Inst* 1960; 25(1): 85–109.

5.  Rowley, J. D. Letter: a new consistent chromosomal abnormality in chronic myelogenous leukaemia identified by quinacrine fluorescence and Giemsa staining. *Nature* 1973; 243(5405): 290–3.

6.  Gall, J. G. and Pardue, M. L. Formation and detection of RNA-DNA hybrid molecules in cytological preparations. *Proc Natl Acad Sci USA* 1969; 63(2): 378–83.

7.  Bauman, J. G., Wiegant, J., Borst, P. and van Duijn, P. A new method for fluorescence microscopical localization of specific DNA sequences by in situ hybridization of fluorochromelabelled RNA. *Exp Cell Res* 1980; 128(2): 485–90.

8.  Landegent, J. E., Jansen in de Wal, N., van Ommen, G. J., Baas, F., de Vijlder, J. J., van, D. P. *et al.* Chromosomal localization of a unique gene by non-autoradiographic in situ hybridization. *Nature* 1985; 317(6033): 175–7.

9.  Kallioniemi, A., Kallioniemi, O. P., Sudar, D., Rutovitz, D., Gray, J. W., Waldman, F. *et al.* Comparative genomic hybridization for molecular cytogenetic analysis of solid tumors. *Science* 1992; 258(5083): 818–21.

10. Bayani, J. and Squire, J. A. Application and interpretation of FISH in biomarker studies. *Cancer Lett* 2007; 249(1): 97–109.

11. Alba, J., Gutierrez, J., Coupe, V. M., Fernandez, B., Vazquez-Boquete, A., Alba, J. *et al.* HER2 status determination using RNA-ISH – a rapid and simple technique showing high correlation with FISH and IHC in

141 cases of breast cancer. *Histol Histopathol* 2012; 27(8): 1021–7.

12. Summersgill, B., Clark, J. and Shipley, J. Fluorescence and chromogenic in situ hybridization to detect genetic aberrations in formalin-fixed paraffin embedded material, including tissue microarrays. *Nat Protoc* 2008; 3(2): 220–34.

13. Tubbs, R., Pettay, J., Skacel, M., Powell, R., Stoler, M., Roche, P. *et al.* Gold-facilitated in situ hybridization: a bright-field autometallographic alternative to fluorescence in situ hybridization for detection of Her-2/neu gene amplification. *Am J Pathol* 2002; 160(5): 1589–95.

14. Bayani, J. and Squire, J. A. Fluorescence in situ hybridization (FISH). *Curr Protoc Cell Biol* 2004; Chapter 22: Unit 22.4.

15. Egholm, M., Buchardt, O., Christensen, L., Behrens, C., Freier, S. M. and Driver, D. A. *et al.* PNA hybridizes to complementary oligonucleotides obeying the Watson-Crick hydrogen-bonding rules. *Nature* 1993; 365(6446): 566–8.

16. Watters, A. D. and Bartlett, J. M. S. Fluorescence in situ hybridization in paraffin tissue sections – pretreatment protocol.

*Mol Biotechnol* 2002; 21(3): 217–20.

17. Bartlett, J. M., Campbell, F. M., Ibrahim, M., Wencyk, P., Ellis, I., Kay, E. *et al.* Chromogenic in situ hybridization: a multicenter study comparing silver in situ hybridization with FISH. *Am J Clin Pathol* 2009; 132(4): 514–20.

18. Brugmann, A., Lelkaitis, G., Nielsen, S., Jensen, K. G. and Jensen, V. Testing HER2 in breast cancer: a comparative study on BRISH, FISH, and IHC. *Appl Immunohistochem Mol Morphol* 2011; 19(3): 203–11.

19. Mollerup, J., Henriksen, U., Muller, S. and Schonau, A. Dual color chromogenic in situ hybridization for determination of HER2 status in breast cancer: a large comparative study to current state of the art fluorescence in situ hybridization. *BMC Clin Pathol* 2012; 12: 3.

20. Penault-Llorca, F., Bilous, M., Dowsett, M., Hanna, W., Osamura, R. Y., Ruschoff, J. *et al.* Emerging technologies for assessing HER2 amplification. *Am J Clin Pathol* 2009; 132(4): 539–48.

21. Arnould, L., Roger, P., Macgrogan, G., Chenard, M. P., Balaton, A., Beauclair, S. *et al.* Accuracy of HER2 status determination on breast core-needle biopsies (immunohistochemistry, FISH, CISH and SISH vs FISH). *Mod Pathol* 2012; 25(5): 675–82.

22. Bartlett, J. M., Campbell, F. M., Ibrahim, M., O'Grady, A., Kay, E., Faulkes, C. *et al.* A UK NEQAS ISH multicenter ring study using the Ventana HER2 dual-color ISH assay. *Am J Clin Pathol* 2011; 135(1): 157–62.

23. Garcia-Caballero, T., Grabau, D., Green, A. R., Gregory, J., Schad, A., Kohlwes, E. *et al.* Determination of HER2 amplification in primary breast cancer using dual-colour chromogenic in situ hybridization

is comparable to fluorescence in situ hybridization: a European multicentre study involving 168 specimens. *Histopathol* 2010; 56(4): 472–80.

24. Bayani, J. and Squire, J. Multi-color FISH techniques. *Curr Protoc Cell Biol* 2004; Chapter 22: Unit 22.5.

25. Bartlett, J. M. S., Going, J. J., Mallon, E. A., Watters, A. D., Reeves, J. R., Stanton, P. *et al.* Evaluating HER2 amplification and overexpression in breast cancer. *J Pathol* 2001; 195(4): 422–8.

26. Bartlett, J., Mallon, E. and Cooke, T. The clinical evaluation of HER-2 status: which test to use? *J Pathol* 2003; 199(4):411–7.

27. Bartlett, J. M. S., Mallon, E. A. and Cooke, T. G. Molecular diagnostics for determination of HER2 status. *Curr Diagn Pathol* 2003; 9(1): 48–55.

28. Dowsett, M., Bartlett, J., Ellis, I. O., Salter, J., Hills, M., Mallon, E. *et al.* Correlation between immunohistochemistry (HercepTest) and fluorescence in situ hybridization (FISH) for HER-2 in 426 breast carcinomas from 37 centres. *J Pathol* 2003; 199(4): 418–23.

29. Ellis, I. O., Bartlett, J., Dowsett, M., Humphreys, S., Jasani, B., Miller, K. *et al.* Updated recommendations for HER2 testing in the UK. *J Clin Pathol* 2004; 57(3): 233–7.

30. Bartlett, J. M. S., Ibrahim, M., Jasani, B., Morgan, J. M., Ellis, I., Kay, E. *et al.* External quality assurance of HER2 fluorescence in situ hybridisation testing: results of a UK NEQAS pilot scheme. *J Clin Pathol* 2007; 60(7): 816–19.

31. Piccart, M., Lohrisch, C., Di Leo, A. and Larsimont, D. The predictive value of HER2 in breast cancer. *Oncology* 2001; 61(Suppl. 2): 73–82.

32. Perez, E. A., Roche, P. C., Jenkins, R. B., Reynolds, C. A., Halling, K. C., Ingle, J. N. *et al.* HER2 testing in patients with breast cancer: poor correlation between weak positivity by immunohistochemistry and gene amplification by fluorescence in situ hybridization. *Mayo Clinic Proceedings* 2002; 77(2): 148–54.

33. Romond, E. H., Perez, E. A., Bryant, J., Suman, V. J., Geyer, C. E., Davidson, N. E. *et al.* Trastuzumab plus adjuvant chemotherapy for operable HER2-positive breast cancer. *New Engl J Med* 2005; 353(16): 1673–84.

34. Wolff, A. C., Hammond, M. E., Schwartz, J. N., Hagerty, K. L., Allred, D. C., Cote, R. J. *et al.* American Society of Clinical Oncology/College of American Pathologists guideline recommendations for human epidermal growth factor receptor 2 testing in breast cancer. *J Clin Oncol* 2007; 25(1): 118–45.

35. Bartlett, J. M. S., Starczynski, J., Atkey, N., Kay, E., O'Grady, A., Gandy, M. *et al.* HER2 testing in the UK: recommendations for breast and gastric in-situ hybridisation methods. *J Clin Pathol* 2011; 64(8): 649–53.

36. Vita, M. and Henriksson, M. The Myc oncoprotein as a therapeutic target for human cancer. *Semin Cancer Biol* 2006; 16(4): 318–30.

37. Perez, E. A., Jenkins, R. B., Dueck, A. C., Wiktor, A. E., Bedroske, P. P., Anderson, S. K. *et al.* C-MYC alterations and association with patient outcome in early-stage HER2-positive breast cancer from the north central cancer treatment group N9831 adjuvant trastuzumab trial. *J Clin Oncol* 2011; 29(6): 651–9.

38. Peled, N., Yoshida, K., Wynes, M. W. and Hirsch, F. R. Predictive and prognostic markers for epidermal growth factor receptor inhibitor therapy in non-small cell

lung cancer. *Ther Adv Med Oncol* 2009; 1(3): 137–44.

39. Di, F. F., Sesboue, R., Michel, P., Sabourin, J. C. and Frebourg, T. Molecular determinants of anti-EGFR sensitivity and resistance in metastatic colorectal cancer. *Br J Cancer* 2010; 103(12): 1765–72.

40. Lindeman, N. I., Cagle, P. T., Beasley, M. B., Chitale, D. A., Dacic, S., Giaccone, G. et al. Molecular testing guideline for selection of lung cancer patients for EGFR and ALK tyrosine kinase inhibitors: guideline from the College of American Pathologists, International Association for the Study of Lung Cancer, and Association for Molecular Pathology. *J Thorac Oncol* 2013; 8(7): 823–59.

41. Ji, H., Zhao, X., Yuza, Y., Shimamura, T., Li, D., Protopopov, A. et al. Epidermal growth factor receptor variant III mutations in lung tumorigenesis and sensitivity to tyrosine kinase inhibitors. *Proc Natl Acad Sci USA* 2006; 103(20): 7817–22.

42. Taylor, T. E., Furnari, F. B. and Cavenee, W. K. Targeting EGFR for treatment of glioblastoma: molecular basis to overcome resistance. *Curr Cancer Drug Targets* 2012; 12(3): 197–209.

43. Press, M. F., Sauter, G., Buyse, M., Bernstein, L., Guzman, R., Santiago, A. et al. Alteration of topoisomerase II-alpha gene in human breast cancer: association with responsiveness to anthracycline-based chemotherapy. *J Clin Oncol* 2011; 29(7): 859–67.

44. Bartlett, J. M., Munro, A., Cameron, D. A., Thomas, J., Prescott, R., Twelves and C. J. Type 1 receptor tyrosine kinase profiles identify patients with enhanced benefit from anthracyclines in the BR9601 adjuvant breast cancer chemotherapy trial. *J Clin Oncol* 2008; 26(31): 5027–35.

45. Fountzilas, G., Dafni, U., Bobos, M., Kotoula, V., Batistatou, A., Xanthakis, I. et al. Evaluation of the prognostic role of centromere 17 gain and HER2/topoisomerase II alpha gene status and protein expression in patients with breast cancer treated with anthracycline-containing adjuvant chemotherapy: pooled analysis of two Hellenic Cooperative Oncology Group (HeCOG) phase III trials. *BMC Cancer* 2013; 13: 163.

46. Huttner, A. J., Kieran, M. W., Yao, X., Cruz, L., Ladner, J., Quayle, K. et al. Clinicopathologic study of glioblastoma in children with neurofibromatosis type 1. *Pediatr Blood Cancer* 2010; 54(7): 890–6.

47. Hayry, V., Tanner, M., Blom, T., Tynninen, O., Roselli, A., Ollikainen, M. et al. Copy number alterations of the polycomb gene BMI1 in gliomas. *Acta Neuropathol* 2008; 116(1): 97–102.

48. Begnami, M. D., Rushing, E. J., Santi, M. and Quezado, M. Evaluation of NF2 gene deletion in pediatric meningiomas using chromogenic in situ hybridization. *Int J Surg Pathol* 2007; 15(2): 110–15.

49. Begnami, M. D., Palau, M., Rushing, E. J., Santi, M. and Quezado, M. Evaluation of NF2 gene deletion in sporadic schwannomas, meningiomas, and ependymomas by chromogenic in situ hybridization. *Hum Pathol* 2007; 38(9): 1345–50.

50. Hopman, A. H., Moesker, O., Smeets, A. W., Pauwels, R. P., Vooijs, G. P. and Ramaekers, F. C. Numerical chromosome 1, 7, 9, and 11 aberrations in bladder cancer detected by in situ hybridization. *Cancer Res* 1991; 51(2): 644–51.

51. Bartlett, J. M. S., Watters, A. D., Ballantyne, S. A., Going, J. J., Grigor, K. M. and Cooke, T. G. Is chromosome 9 loss a marker of disease recurrence in transitional cell carcinoma of the urinary bladder? *Br J Cancer* 1998; 77(12): 2193–8.

52. Edwards, J., Duncan, P., Going, J. J., Watters, A. D. and Bartlett, J. M. S. Loss of heterozygosity on chromosome 9 as a potential marker of recurrence and progression in bladder cancer. *Br J Cancer* 2000; 83(12): 190.

53. Edwards, J., Duncan, P., Going, J. J., Grigor, K. M., Watters, A. D. and Bartlett, J. M. S. Loss of heterozygosity on chromosomes 11 and 17 are markers of recurrence in TCC of the bladder. *Br J Cancer* 2001; 85(12): 1894–9.

54. Edwards, J., Duncan, P., Going, J. J., Watters, A. D. and Bartlett, J. M. S. Loss of heterozygosity on chromosome 11 is a marker of recurrence in TCC of the bladder cancer. *Br J Cancer* 2001; 85(12): 74.

55. Watters, A. D., Stacey, M. W., Going, J. J., GRIGOR, K. M., Cooke, T. G., Sim, E. et al. Genetic aberrations of NAT2 and chromosome 8: their association with progression in transitional cell carcinoma of the urinary bladder. *Urol Int* 2001; 67(3): 235–9.

56. Latif, Z., Watters, A., Dunn, I., Grigor, K., Underwood, M. and Bartlett, J. HER2 abnormalities in transitional cell carcinomas of the bladder with detrusor muscle invasion at presentation compared with carcinomas progressing to detrusor muscle invasion. *J Urol* 2002; 167(4): 110.

57. Watters, A. D., Latif, Z., Forsyth, A., Dunn, I., Underwood, M. A., Grigor, K. M. et al. Genetic aberrations of c-myc and CCND1 in the development of invasive bladder cancer. *Br J Cancer* 2002; 87(6): 654–8.

58. Watters, A. D., Going, J. J., Grigor, K. M. and Bartlett, J. M. S. Progression to detrusor-muscle invasion in bladder carcinoma is associated with polysomy of

chromosomes 1 and 8 in recurrent pTa/pT1 tumours. *Eur J Cancer* 2002; 38(12): 1593–9.

59. Watters, A. D., Ballantyne, S. A., Going, J. J., Grigor, K. M. and Bartlett, J. Aneusomy of chromosomes 7 and 17 predicts the recurrence of transitional cell carcinoma of the urinary bladder. *BJU Int* 2004; 85(1): 42–7.

60. Bayani, J. M. and Squire, J. A. Applications of SKY in cancer cytogenetics. *Cancer Invest* 2002; 20(3): 373–86.

61. Chin, L. and Gray, J. W. Translating insights from the cancer genome into clinical practice. *Nature* 2008; 452(7187): 553–63.

62. Schrock, E., du Manoir, S., Veldman, T., Schoell, B., Wienberg, J., Ferguson-Smith, M. A. *et al.* Multicolor spectral karyotyping of human chromosomes. *Science* 1996; 273(5274): 494–7.

63. Speicher, M. R., Gwyn, B. S. and Ward, D. C. Karyotyping human chromosomes by combinatorial multi-fluor FISH. *Nat Genet* 1996; 12(4): 368–75.

64. Tanke, H. J., Wiegant, J., van Gijlswijk, R. P., Bezrookove, V., Pattenier, H., Heetebrij, R. J. *et al.* New strategy for multi-colour fluorescence in situ hybridisation: COBRA: COmbined Binary RAtio labelling. *Eur J Hum Genet* 1999; 7(1): 2–11.

65. Bayani, J., Brenton, J. D., Macgregor, P. F., Beheshti, B., Albert, M., Nallainathan, D. *et al.* Parallel analysis of sporadic primary ovarian carcinomas by spectral karyotyping, comparative genomic hybridization, and expression microarrays. *Cancer Res* 2002; 62(12): 3466–76.

66. Bayani, J., Marrano, P., Graham, C., Zheng, Y., Li, L., Katsaros, D. *et al.* Genomic instability and copy-number heterogeneity of chromosome 19q, including the kallikrein locus, in ovarian

carcinomas. *Mol Oncol* 2011; 5(1): 48–60.

67. Pandita, A., Bayani, J., Paderova, J., Marrano, P., Graham, C., Barrett, M. *et al.* Integrated cytogenetic and high-resolution array CGH analysis of genomic alterations associated with MYCN amplification. *Cytogenet Genome Res* 2011; 134(1): 27–39.

68. Chudoba, I., Hickmann, G., Friedrich, T., Jauch, A., Kozlowski, P. and Senger, G. mBAND: a high resolution multicolor banding technique for the detection of complex intrachromosomal aberrations. *Cytogenet Genome Res* 2004; 104(1–4): 390–3.

69. Bayani, J., Selvarajah, S., Maire, G., Vukovic, B., Al-Romaih, K., Zielenska, M. *et al.* Genomic mechanisms and measurement of structural and numerical instability in cancer cells. *Semin Cancer Biol* 2007; 17(1): 5–18.

70. Bartlett, J. M., Campbell, F. M. and Mallon, E. A. Determination of HER2 amplification by in situ hybridization: when should chromosome 17 also be determined? *Am J Clin Pathol* 2008; 130(6): 920–6.

71. Bartlett, J. M., Munro, A. F., Dunn, J. A., McConkey, C., Jordan, S., Twelves, C. J. *et al.* Predictive markers of anthracycline benefit: a prospectively planned analysis of the UK National Epirubicin Adjuvant Trial (NEAT/BR9601). *Lancet Oncol* 2010; 11(3): 266–74.

72. Aubert, G., Hills, M. and Lansdorp, P. M. Telomere length measurement-caveats and a critical assessment of the available technologies and tools. *Mutat Res* 2012; 730(1–2): 59–67.

73. Wang, Z., Portier, B. P., Gruver, A. M., Bui, S., Wang, H., Su, N. *et al.* Automated quantitative RNA in situ hybridization for resolution of equivocal and heterogeneous ERBB2 (HER2)

status in invasive breast carcinoma. *J Mol Diagn* 2013; 15(2): 210–19.

74. Reisenbichler, E. S., Horton, D., Rasco, M., Andea, A. and Hameed, O. Evaluation of dual immunohistochemistry and chromogenic in situ hybridization for HER2 on a single section. *Am J Clin Pathol* 2012; 137(1): 102–10.

75. Sachs, R. K., Chen, A. M. and Brenner, D. J. Review: proximity effects in the production of chromosome aberrations by ionizing radiation. *Int J Radiat Biol* 1997; 71(1): 1–19.

76. Hoff, K., Jorgensen, J. T., Muller, S., Rongaard, E., Rasmussen, O. and Schonau, A. Visualization of FISH probes by dual-color chromogenic in situ hybridization. *Am J Clin Pathol* 2010; 133(2): 205–11.

77. Wolff, A. C., Hammond, M. E., Schwartz, J. N., Hagerty, K. L., Allred, D. C., Cote, R. J. *et al.* American Society of Clinical Oncology/College of American Pathologists guideline recommendations for human epidermal growth factor receptor 2 testing in breast cancer. *Arch Pathol Lab Med* 2007; 131(1): 18–43.

78. Bayani, J., Paderova, J., Murphy, J., Rosen, B., Zielenska, M. and Squire, J. A. Distinct patterns of structural and numerical chromosomal instability characterize sporadic ovarian cancer. *Neoplasia* 2008; 10(10): 1057–65.

79. Watters, A. D., Going, J. J., Cooke, T. G. and Bartlett, J. M. Chromosome 17 aneusomy is associated with poor prognostic factors in invasive breast carcinoma. *Breast Cancer Res Treat* 2003; 77(2): 109–14.

80. Bartlett, J. M. Pharmacodiagnostic testing in breast cancer: focus on HER2 and trastuzumab therapy. *Am J Pharmacogenomics* 2005; 5(5): 303–15.

**53**

81. Rosa, F. E., Santos, R. M., Rogatto, S. R. and Domingues, M. A. Chromogenic in situ hybridization compared with other approaches to evaluate HER2/neu status in breast carcinomas. *Braz J Med Biol Res* 2013; 46(3): 207–16.

82. Mansfield, A. S., Sukov, W. R., Eckel-Passow, J. E., Sakai, Y., Walsh, F. J., Lonzo, M. *et al.* Comparison of fluorescence in situ hybridization (FISH) and dual-ISH (DISH) in the determination of HER2 status in breast cancer. *Am J Clin Pathol* 2013; 139(2): 144–50.

83. Schildhaus, H. U., Deml, K. F., Schmitz, K., Meiboom, M., Binot, E., Hauke, S. *et al.* Chromogenic in situ hybridization is a reliable assay for detection of ALK rearrangements in adenocarcinomas of the lung. *Mod Pathol* 2013; 26(1): 1468–77.

84. van Rijk, A., Svenstroup-Poulsen, T., Jones, M., Cabecadas, J., Cigudosa, J. C., Leoncini, L. *et al.* Double-staining chromogenic in situ hybridization as a useful alternative to split-signal fluorescence in situ hybridization in lymphoma diagnostics. *Haematologica* 2010; 95(2): 247–52.

85. Lass, U., Hartmann, C., Capper, D., Herold-Mende, C., von Deimling, A., Meiboom, M. *et al.* Chromogenic in situ hybridization is a reliable alternative to fluorescence in situ hybridization for diagnostic testing of 1p and 19q loss in paraffin-embedded gliomas. *Brain Pathol* 2013; 23(3): 311–18.

86. Santi, M., Quezado, M., Ronchetti, R. and Rushing, E. J. Analysis of chromosome 7 in adult and pediatric ependymomas using chromogenic in situ hybridization. *J Neurooncol* 2005; 72(1): 25–8.

87. Walter, B. A., Begnami, M., Valera, V. A., Santi, M., Rushing, E. J. and Quezado, M. Gain of chromosome 7 by chromogenic in situ hybridization (CISH) in chordomas is correlated to c-MET expression. *J Neurooncol* 2011; 101(2): 199–206.

88. Gerdes, M. J., Sevinsky, C. J., Sood, A., Adak, S., Bello, M. O., Bordwell, A. *et al.* Highly multiplexed single-cell analysis of formalin-fixed, paraffin-embedded cancer tissue. *Proc Natl Acad Sci USA* 2013; 110(29): 11982–7.

# Chapter 5

# Clinical applications of the polymerase chain reaction for molecular pathology

Angela B. Y. Hui, Annette D. Wong and Carlo V. Hojilla

## Introduction

A relatively simple yet ground-breaking method of amplifying nucleic acids was introduced in the Nobel Prize award-winning discovery by Mullis and colleagues (1). Since then, the polymerase chain reaction (PCR) has proven to be a very versatile and highly adaptable method that advanced the fields of microbiology, genetics, oncology and anatomic pathology (2, 3). PCR continues to evolve and remains an indispensable tool for research and clinical diagnostics.

Core to the principle of PCR is the amplification of a DNA region of interest (4, 5). In this chapter, we will discuss the technical details of PCR as well as optimization and troubleshooting aspects of the reaction. We will also elaborate on the variations and types of PCR. Finally, several current and prospective clinical applications of PCR will be discussed.

## Basic steps and principles of PCR

The basic PCR consists of a target deoxyribonucleic acid (DNA) template, site-specific primers, enzyme buffer and a heat-stable polymerase. The standard PCR protocol is extensively reported (2, 6–8) and often well established in research and clinical labs. PCR is divided into three basic steps, namely: thermal-induced denaturing of target DNA; annealing of synthetic oligonucleotide primers to the target sequence; and extension of the annealed primer-target sequence by a DNA polymerase (Figure 5.1). These steps are repeated in 25 to 40 cycles. PCR products are then analyzed by a variety of methods.

## Step 1: the denaturing step

Double-stranded DNA (dsDNA) is denatured into single-stranded DNA (ssDNA) to allow the hybridization of ssDNA primers. The main factor that determines the denaturation of dsDNA is its melting temperature. The melting temperature is determined by the nucleotide composition, and in particular its guanine-to-cytosine content ("GC content"), because these pair-bonds require higher energy to break than adenosine-to-thymidine bonds. As such, this step is often the limiting step in the reaction. Initial denaturation of target DNA is typically set at 94°C for 6 to 8 minutes, as most dsDNA initially are those of the target DNA (commonly genomic DNA). As replicated or product DNA increases in subsequent cycles, the denaturation temperature can be theoretically lowered due to lower melting temperatures of the amplicon. Practically, however, the temperature is maintained at 94°C to ensure complete denaturation of both target and product DNA. The denaturation step length is commonly reduced to 1 to 2 minutes as the PCR progresses.

## Step 2: the annealing step

Similar to the denaturation step, the primer annealing step is largely determined by the nucleotide composition of the primer and its melting temperature. The ideal annealing temperature is eventually determined empirically and runs for 1 to 2 minutes. Having primers in molar excess concentration promotes target-to-primer hybridization over target ssDNA re-annealing.

## Step 3: the extension step

The primer extension step is primarily determined by two factors: temperature and length. The extension temperature is a functional property of the DNA polymerase, while the extension length is determined

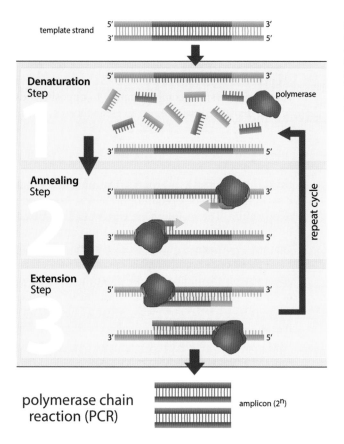

template strand

**Denaturation Step**

polymerase

**Annealing Step**

**Extension Step**

repeat cycle

**polymerase chain reaction (PCR)**

amplicon $(2^n)$

**Figure 5.1** **A simplified schematic of the basic steps of a polymerase chain reaction**
A typical PCR cycle consists of three steps: (1) a denaturation step to separate the double-stranded DNA template into two single stands; (2) an annealing step where the primers anneal to the template; and (3) an extension step where a complementary copy is made by the polymerase enzyme (Pol) (blue arrow = forward primer; green arrow = reverse primer).

by both the polymerase and the length of the target. For the commonly used DNA polymerases, the typical extension temperature is 72°C, with an extension time of 1 minute per kilobase (kb) of product DNA. Extension time specific for each reaction is optimized empirically.

## Repeat steps 1 to 3 – optimizing the cycle number

Given that target DNA is doubled for every PCR cycle, the theoretical exponential PCR production can be calculated by the formula $2^x$, where x is the number of cycles. However, as the reaction progresses past 25 cycles, the production begins to plateau due to the reaction components (most often deoxyribonucleotide triphospahates (dNTPs)) being consumed by the reaction. There is also a steady decline in efficiency of the DNA polymerase due to thermal denaturation. This concept is known as cycle plateauing and is an important factor for quantitative applications of PCR.

In practice, the optimal cycle repeat number is determined empirically. The number of cycles required is inversely dependent on the starting copy-number of the target DNA. As a starting point, for example, $10^5$ template molecules requires 25 cycles for an ethidium bromide-visible signal on gel electrophoresis. Lower copy-numbers of target DNA require longer cycles of amplification. A typical PCR cycle number of 25 to 30 cycles will yield a detectable product for a target DNA of <6 kb in size.

## Final extension, termination and storage

At the end of the 25 to 30 cycles, consumable reagents are depleted, a detectable amount of replicated dsDNA is produced and the PCR is essentially complete. However, most PCR recipes include a final extension and termination step which is a function of the DNA polymerase used. Typically, this step runs at 72°C for 5 to 10 minutes. Theoretically, this allows for the DNA polymerase to continue extending incompletely replicated ssDNA and increase product yield. Practically, however, this step can take advantage of the inherent terminal deoxynucleotidyltransferase (TdT) activity of DNA polymerases, which adds non-template-directed nucleotides to the 3' ends of PCR amplified products. For example, the TdT activity of Taq polymerase tends to add adenosine bases to the ends of PCR products, which can be useful for cloning procedures into specialized cloning vectors. If, however, blunt-ended PCR products are essential, recombinant DNA polymerases lacking TdT activity can be substituted.

The absolute final step of the PCR program often involves an incubation step of 4°C for an indefinite amount of time. This minimizes any enzymatic activity while storing DNA products in a stable buffered solution until further analysis.

# Starting reagents of PCR

## DNA template

The nucleic acid source can be cloned DNA, genomic DNA, mitochondrial DNA or even ribonucleic acid (RNA) that is reverse transcribed into complementary DNA (cDNA). DNA can come from various anatomic sources such as peripheral blood, tissues (fine-needle aspirates, biopsies, resections) or other material such as saliva, hair or nail samples (4). Tissues can be fresh or fixed, including frozen, air-dried, alcohol-fixed or formalin-fixed paraffin-embedded (FFPE). PCR is so remarkably robust that even fragmented DNA in nanogram quantities, which is often the case for archived material, can be sufficient for amplification (9).

Often, before PCR can proceed, obtaining a pure, good quality, template DNA is the main initial step. If cloned DNA is the source template, then retrieval is often not an issue. However, in clinical settings, the source is often tissue material. In general, proteinase K digestion of fresh tissue yields the highest and best quality DNA (10). However, this process is time-consuming and may involve exposure to organic solvents due to the use of multiple phenol-chloroform extraction steps. An alternative, more rapid extraction method, but one that produces a lower yield and quality, is achieved by boiling the fresh tissue in sterile water for 15 minutes. DNA can also be extracted successfully from archival samples, stained sections or cytological preparations using either approach described above.

## Allele-specific primers

In a basic PCR, two single-strand primers are used that flank the 5' and 3' ends of the desired dsDNA sequence. The primers (designated as the forward and reverse primers) are complementary to opposite ends of the denatured ssDNA of the sequence of choice (designated correspondingly, as the reverse or forward strands). In other variations of PCR, primer number and design can be complex and elaborate.

Primer design should incorporate three main concepts: inter- and intra-sequence specificity, primer concentration and annealing temperature. First, the primer sequence should be unique in the target DNA sequence to minimize the chance of non-specific amplification. Primers should have minimal intra- and inter-sequence complementarity to mitigate the formation of primer-dimer sequences, which can negatively impact the yield and specificity of the reaction. Complicated sequences such as palindromic sequences or having more than three or four of the same base should be avoided, primarily to avoid secondary structures such as hairpin loops that can interfere with the reaction. Secondly, primer concentration should be added in molar excess compared to the target DNA to promote primer-target hybridization, which becomes key as the PCR progresses and primers are consumed. Finally, annealing temperature (or primer melting temperature) is essential to specificity as non-specific binding occurs in lower annealing temperatures (4).

## DNA polymerase

The use of thermostable DNA polymerases from micro-organisms surviving in extreme temperatures was a key breakthrough for PCR. These polymerases are functional at temperatures required to denature dsDNA where most other proteins are denatured. Three commonly used DNA polymerases are Pfu (Pyrococcus furiosus), Vent or Tli (Thermococcus litoralis) and Taq polymerase (Thermus aquaticus), with the latter being the most common commercially available polymerase (4). The optimal working temperature for these enzymes is 70°C. Like other enzymes, Taq polymerase has a half-life of activity of $>2$ hours at 92.5°C, 40 minutes at 95°C and 5 minutes at 97.5°C. This temperature dependence explains the decline in fidelity and the plateau effect towards cycles greater than 25. Other PCR recipes call for a lower denaturation temperature, or a shorter denaturation step length, or even lower PCR cycle number in order to preserve as much polymerase fidelity for the course of the reaction. Overall, though, these polymerases are functionally quite robust in that they can amplify at a wide range of temperatures as long as a primer-template hybrid is present. Notably, Taq polymerase lacks a 3' to 5' proofreading exonuclease activity leading to an error rate of 1 in 9,000 bases (11). Additionally, Taq polymerase is sensitive to $Mg^{++}$ concentration. As mentioned above, most polymerases have a TdT activity that adds non-template-directed nucleotides to the 3' ends of PCR amplicons.

## PCR kits

Most commercially available PCR reagents come as proprietary "PCR kits" with common reagents such as deoxyribonucleotide triphosphate bases (dNTPs) and the reaction buffer included with the DNA polymerase. dATP, dTTP, dCTP, dGTP and dUTP bases are prepared for a final working concentration of 50 to 200 μM, which is sufficient to synthesize 6.5 to 25 μg of DNA (11). Tris reaction buffer at a concentration of 10mM and pH of 8.5 and 9.0 at 25°C is the buffer of choice. The pH of Tris is temperature-dependent such that a buffer made to pH 8.8 at 25°C will have a pH value of 7.4 at 72°C, which is the optimal working temperature and pH for Taq polymerase (11).

## PCR optimization

Discussed below are the most commonly optimized variables in a PCR protocol. Often, these are determined empirically when initially designing an amplification setup. Inherent in any PCR run is the use of a negative (for example, a "no DNA template" control) and a positive control (for example, a cloned dsDNA template containing the region of interest).

## Melting and annealing temperature

The melting temperature ($T_m$) serves as a starting point for choosing the annealing temperature for the primers and the template DNA in the PCR. It is the temperature at which 50% of the oligonucleotide primers are bound to their complementary sequence and the other 50% are separated into single-stranded molecules. The $T_m$ of the primer depends on both its length and its nucleotide sequence composition, specifically, the ratio of the

number of G:C bases to the number of A:T bases. Commonly, for primer sequences less than 14 nucleotides to be used under the standard PCR conditions of 50 nM of primer solution, 50 mM of $Na^+$, and pH 7.0, the formula is:

$$T_m = (wA + xT)^* 2 + (yG + zC)^* 4$$

where w, x, y and z are the number of the bases A, T, G and C in the sequence, respectively.

Melting temperatures can be calculated manually as above or are available through primer design tools online (especially useful for primer sequences >14 nucleotides or for multiple primers). The optimal annealing temperature for the PCR is usually determined by trial and error. Concomitant reactions are prepared that vary the annealing temperature by 0.5°C above and below the calculated melting temperature.

The concept of melting temperature is utilized as a powerful tool to analyze mutations in real-time PCR. Mutations as small as single-base pair changes can alter the $T_m$ and this change in $T_m$ is detectable. Thus, melting point analysis/melting curve analysis (discussed further below) can be used to characterize mutations or single nucleotide polymorphisms (12, 13).

## Magnesium ion concentration

Magnesium ions are essential co-factors to DNA polymerases, facilitating the association with DNA and dNTPs. Because of this, $[Mg^{++}]$ can affect the fidelity of the DNA polymerase and, consequently, the specificity of the PCR. As a rule of thumb, the magnesium concentration in the reaction mixture is generally 0.5 to 2.5 mM greater than the concentration of dNTPs. The optimal concentration, however, is specific and must be determined empirically per reaction.

## Thermal cyclers

Thermal cyclers allow for the cyclical, very rapid temperature ramping and cooling that is essential to PCR. Different commercial models are available and they all share common features such as a heating block with thermal uniformity, a heated cover, a cooling system and a programmable memory. Manufacturer-specific variations of thermal cyclers may include the type of reaction vessels used (plates vs. tubes vs. glass slides) and the capacity of reaction tubes. Some thermal cyclers have precise temperature control in specific sections of the heating block, allowing for multiple reactions to run simultaneously. This feature is especially useful when optimizing $Mg^{++}$ concentration or annealing temperatures per reaction. In real-time PCR, thermal cyclers are capable of exciting fluorophores and detecting emitted light wavelengths. Furthermore, they have post-amplification software to analyze fluorescence values that can be used to optimize the reaction, quantify PCR amplified products or perform melting curve analyses.

## Common PCR types and modifications

## Reverse transcriptase PCR (RT-PCR)

One of the most widely used applications of PCR is the study of gene expression by the ability to amplify RNA. This was made possible by the use of viral reverse transcriptase (RT) enzymes that can transcribe mRNA sequences into cDNA, which can then serve as the DNA template for the subsequent PCR (14, 15). Most RT enzymes used so far have been isolated from viruses, such as the avian myeloblastosis virus and the Moloney murine leukemia virus.

Several strategies for priming the reverse transcriptase reaction are available. First and most commonly used are oligo d(T) primers designed against the poly(A) tail of mRNA. Because of the non-specific nature, oligo d(T) primers suffer fidelity issues with long mRNA sequences or those with secondary RNA structures. A second similar strategy is the use of random hexamer primers which have the same disadvantage as oligo d(T) primers. Both random hexamer and oligo d(T) primer strategies readily create a cDNA template that can proceed to the remainder of the PCR amplification all within the same tube (i.e. a one-step reaction). The third strategy uses a downstream antisense PCR primer annealed to the RNA. This method allows for greater specificity of the reverse transcription, but limits the subsequent PCR to a single product and will necessitate the use of paired sense and antisense primers in a new reaction tube (i.e. a two-step reaction). Once cDNA is obtained, the remainder of the reaction proceeds similar to that described above.

## Real-time PCR or quantitative PCR

Real-time PCR is a modification that combines product amplification with simultaneous detection and analysis of PCR products (16, 17). Fluorescent probes as well as thermal cyclers that can excite and detect fluorescence are utilized so that PCR products can be measured with extremely high analytic sensitivity as they are synthesized in real time. Post-amplification software at the end of each cycle records the fluorescence intensity produced and plots it against the PCR cycle number. A fluorescence intensity threshold is initially set by the software early in the log-linear growth phase of the PCR amplification curve. The cycle number at which this threshold is reached is called the crossing threshold or cycle threshold ($C_t$) for the reaction. Since the $C_t$ corresponds to the starting amount of the template DNA, PCR products can be quantified as they are produced. Depending on the probe design and the post-amplification software used, real-time PCR is quite robust in its application. Commonly, real-time PCR can be used to quantify the gene expression levels of a target cDNA.

In general, two broad fluorescence-based detection strategies are used in real-time PCR (4). First, non-specific fluorescence makes use of an intercalating dye such as SYBR or ethidium bromide (EtBr), which binds to the minor groove of dsDNA. The advantage of this method is its cost-effectiveness, but it suffers from low specificity as other double-stranded sequences such as primer-dimers will be detected.

The second strategy makes use of specific oligonucleotide probes which are fluorescently labeled. The probes include a DNA primer coupled with a fluorophore (with or without a nearby quencher moiety) that is excitable and emits light at a detectable wavelength. Whatever the probe design strategy used, all produce a fluorescence signal that is proportional to the amount of amplicon generated. The most commonly employed probe designs include hybridization probes, hydrolysis or TaqMan® probes, minor groove binding (MGB) probes, and Molecular Beacon probes (Figure 5.2) (4).

The hybridization probe method uses two oligonucleotide probes, which are both fluorescently labeled. This method depends on fluorescence resonance energy transfer (FRET), wherein a donor fluorophore from the donor probe is excited by the thermal cycler light source and emits a specific wavelength in the absorption range of the second reporter fluorophore of the reporter probe. During the annealing step of the PCR, FRET occurs only when donor and reporter are in close proximity, with the

## **Hybridization**-based probe design

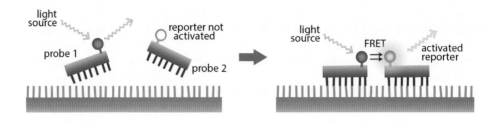

## **Hydrolysis**-based probe design

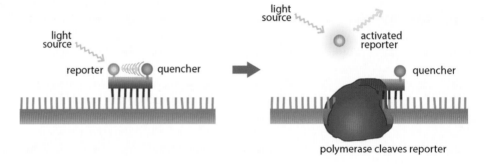

## **Molecular beacon**-based probe design

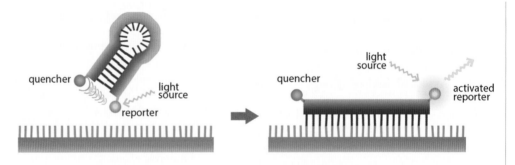

# methods of probe design

**Figure 5.2 Common real-time quantitative PCR probe design strategies**
A. hybridization-based; B. hydrolysis-based; and C. molecular beacon-based probes. FRET = fluorescence resonance energy transfer.

reporter absorbing the donor emission and fluorescing at a specific wavelength. Since the reporter probe is designed to be downstream of the donor probe along the template DNA sequence, occurrence of FRET ensures an added level of specificity. The amount of product generated per cycle is proportional to the FRET fluorescence generated. In practice, hybridization probes are useful for detection of

small deletion or insertion mutations. These can be detected after the PCR by performing melting curve analyses on the products, as the mutated sequence will have a different $T_m$.

The hydrolysis (commercially known as the *Taq*-Man) probe method requires two main components. Firstly, the probe is labeled with a reporter fluorophore at the 5'-end which is coupled to a fluorescence quencher at its 3'-end. At the beginning of the PCR, there is no fluorescence emitted due to the quencher. The second component of the hydrolysis method is a DNA polymerase with a 5'-exonuclease activity. During the extension step, exonuclease activity of the DNA polymerase cleaves and hydrolyzes the incorporated probe and releases the reporter dye from the effect of the quencher. The level of free fluorescence accumulates and is thus proportional to the amount of PCR product formed. Minor groove binding (MGB) probes work in a similar principle to the hydrolysis probe method in that it uses a dual-labeled probe and requires a 5'-hydrolysis activity. MGB, however, has a covalently linked molecule that binds to the minor groove of dsDNA (for example, dihydrocyclopyrroloindole tripeptide). This has a twofold advantage. Firstly, MGB probes are particularly useful for shorter probes due to the inherent stability of the minor groove-binding. Secondly, minor grove binding further stabilizes the annealing of the probe to target DNA and raises the $T_m$ of the reaction.

The molecular beacon probe method (Figure 5.2) shares a similar design to the hydrolysis probes, except that the 5' and 3' terminal sequences of the probe are complementary to one another, creating a hairpin loop secondary structure with a double-stranded terminal stem. As such, the fluorophore and quencher are brought to close proximity during the unbound state. During PCR, the stem is melted and the loop portion, which is complementary to the target DNA, is allowed to anneal. This permits separation of the fluorophore and quencher and allows for light emission. Unlike the hydrolysis probe, a 5'-exonuclease activity is not required and no free probe is generated. The probe is simply displaced, making it available for use in subsequent cycles.

A recent modification to this strategy was introduced as the Scorpion probe system (18). The main modification is the inclusion of the primer sequence to the hairpin loop fluorophore-quencher model, but separated with a 3'-end amplification blocker, usually hexethylene glycol monomers, which is non-amplifiable. This prevents read-through, which would lead to unfolding of the hairpin loop in the absence of a specific target. In the first cycle of PCR, extension occurs as usual with the primer. During the subsequent steps, the hairpin loop stem denatures and the probe sequence unfolds and binds to the specific target sequence downstream of the primer. This method is considered a unimolecular reaction as the

fluorescent probe is incorporated into the new strand, which contrasts with the bimolecular hydrolysis-based probe methods. The Scorpion method creates amplicons that are reportedly more thermodynamically stable than the original hairpin loop, which translates to a faster and more specific amplification, with amplicons that can be measured very accurately.

## Multiplex PCR

Multiplex PCR allows for more sophisticated amplification and analysis of multiple targets in one reaction using multiple, mutually exclusive primer sets. Many protocols are available for multiplex PCR (19). We briefly describe a commercial multiplex PCR platform, the multiplex ligation-dependent probe amplification (MLPA) system (20), that is unique in its methodology yet amenable to current clinical PCR protocols that employ fluorescence detection and capillary electrophoresis.

MLPA is a multiplex PCR-based method that can detect point mutations, changes in gene copy-number status and even DNA methylation status simultaneously (20). The unique methodology uses DNA hemi-probes with one set of common primers attached to each probe set, as well as stuffer sequences of specific size. For each target DNA sequence there are two DNA hemi-probe sets. The MLPA reaction is divided into two steps. The first step involves the denaturation of the target DNA sequence and hybridization with the DNA hemi-probes. Upon hybridization to the target DNA, the hemi-probes are in proximity of one another and are enzymatically ligated. In the second step, it is then the probes themselves that are amplified by PCR instead of the target DNA sequence, with only the use of one set of common primers. The amplicons/probes are then differentiated and analyzed according to their fragment size. Current applications can accommodate up to 50 MLPA probes for one reaction. Included in this probe complement are various reference probes for use in quantification as well as allowing for comparison between samples. MLPA amplifies probes that are 50 to 100 bp in length and hence is ideal for use even in fragmented DNA such as those from FFPE tissues.

One of the primary uses of MLPA is to assess gene copy-number status, particularly in tumor diagnostics. Changes in the copy-number (deletion or amplification) of a target probe is semi-quantitatively estimated by comparing the relative signal of this probe with the average relative signal of the same probe in a reference sample of normal DNA. Furthermore, the use of reference probes (distributed throughout different chromosomes) allows for the comparison of results between reactions and controls for possible heterogeneity in a sample.

## Digital PCR

Digital PCR was described and developed by Vogelstein and Kinzler (21) as a modification to traditional PCR in order to increase its sensitivity for detection and quantification of rare mutations. Basically, digital PCR is a single DNA molecule amplification. The reagents are similar to that of a conventional PCR. The reaction tube is then serially diluted and partitioned such that there are thousands of reactions per sample, with each PCR vessel containing one single DNA molecule. Amplification is detected via a fluorescence signal. Absolute quantification is achieved by counting the number of reactions with a positive amplification (22, 23).

The partitioning of the master PCR mix is the rate-limiting step and there are generally two commercial Digital PCR strategies available to achieve this: microdroplet and microfluidic platforms. The microdroplet platform generates microdroplets in an oil emulsion. In the Droplet Digital PCR platform, for example, a 20 μl PCR master mix is partitioned into approximately 20,000 microdroplets, with each containing a single DNA molecule. Analysis and quantification is via flow cytometry. Microdroplet strategies have a reported level of sensitivity of 0.0005% to 0.01% (22).

In the microfluidic platform, the master mix is added to a rectangular chamber with thousands of microfluidic chambers and separated via surface tension-based or valve-based technology. The target volume per PCR reaction is 1 pL, which equates to 1 million reactions per μL of PCR master mix. The chambers are analyzed by a microarray scanner. The reported sensitivity of this platform is 0.001% (22).

The advantages of Digital PCR are the ability to detect rare variants, accurately calculate allele frequency and discriminate low-fold copy-number variation. As each reaction contains one single molecule, post-amplification quantification is as simple as counting the number of positive reactions. Melting curve analyses are not required as amplicon level and signal detection occurs with a linear relationship.

From a practical standpoint, there is no pre-amplification or enrichment of template required due to the inherent sensitivity of the reaction. Furthermore, there is no need for internal normalization control and overall no need to optimize the PCR, since each reaction is being evaluated in a binary fashion. Finally, the various Digital PCR platforms are cross-platform compatible with emerging next generation sequencing technologies.

The main disadvantage of Digital PCR lies in the dilution of the PCR master mix and the uniformity of each partition volume. This is usually achieved by using statistics and assuming a Poisson distribution across the dilution to achieve a single DNA molecule per volume. As such, investing in this technology requires an investment into a commercial package with proprietary partitioning, amplification and quantification technologies. A second disadvantage is that because of Digital PCR's increased sensitivity, the reaction is very sensitive to contamination by DNA from extraneous sources. As it is currently marketed, the throughput is low, multiplexing is not yet feasible and clinical validation will be required.

## Post-PCR amplification analyses

The most common post-PCR analyses are quantification and identification of the product. Historically, the DNA product after PCR was identified by a combination of gel electrophoresis and Southern blotting. Briefly, PCR-generated products were identified by electrophoresis through EtBr-stained agarose gels that allow for separation according to size. Product size was visualized by ultraviolet (UV) light illumination and estimated via DNA size ladder markers. For definitive identification of the PCR product, Southern blotting was performed which required the hybridization of a radioactively labeled, complimentary ssDNA probe (for example, the template DNA sequence) against the generated PCR amplicon, which was fixed on a nitrocellulose membrane. Agarose gel electrophoresis remains a cost-effective and quick method of analyzing PCR products, but lacks specificity since identification is by fragment size only. Primer-dimers and other small products also appear as diffuse bands close to the leading edge of the gel and may further confound analyses (24). It also suffers from using hazardous substances such as EtBr and UV. Similarly, Southern blotting has fallen out of favor due to its laborious methodology and use of radioactivity.

Currently, PCR products are analyzed by using fluorescence-based methods of size estimation via capillary electrophoresis. Definitive identification is performed by fluorescence-based DNA sequencing. Discussed further below are the most common indirect (restriction fragment length polymorphism analysis) and direct (DNA sequencing) methods of identification.

## Restriction fragment length polymorphism analysis

Restriction enzymes are bacterial enzymes capable of cleaving specific DNA sequences. This ability is now used for various laboratory applications primarily as a way to identify DNA sequence alterations. Mutations may create a new restriction site or disrupt a known sequence. Wild-type can be differentiated from mutated DNA by the differential migration of fragments following the restriction enzyme digestion; a process known as restriction fragment length polymorphism (RFLP) analysis (10, 25).

RFLP analysis is an indirect method of identifying DNA PCR products that is quick and cost-effective. For some applications, RFLP analysis has sufficient sensitivity to detect low-level mutations. Careful selection of restriction sites should differentiate between wild-type and mutant sequences. New mutations with specific restriction sites can also be incorporated within the primer design, as an additional way of identifying PCR products or for DNA cloning strategies. The restriction digest reaction is usually performed in the same newly amplified PCR product tube, which streamlines the process, increases sample throughput and minimizes product loss. The digestion products are then analyzed by gel electrophoresis. In general, the obliteration of a restriction site generates a larger DNA sequence, whereas the introduction of a restriction site will produce at least two shorter DNA fragments via electrophoresis. The use of fluorescently labeled primers and capillary electrophoresis with fluorescence detectors allow for automated, more sophisticated size-based identification.

## DNA sequencing and next generation sequencing

The most direct way of identifying PCR products is by DNA sequencing. The most common method is the chain termination method or the Sanger sequencing method (26). This has been further elaborated on with the use of fluorescence and capillary electrophoresis. The demand for high throughput, low-cost sequencing methods have led to various "next generation sequencing" methods, which are different approaches that use massive, multiplex and parallel sequencing methods. Sanger-based and next generation sequencing are beyond the scope of this chapter and the readers are directed to the relevant chapters elsewhere in this book.

## PCR product quantification

Quantification of DNA product may be used for optimizing the PCR conditions or to estimate gene expression levels, especially in the setting of RT-PCR. Most quantification analyses are semi-quantitative, wherein levels are usually compared relative to an internal control. Methods discussed below include densitometry-based and fluorescence-based semi-quantitative analyses. Absolute level quantification will be more commonplace and accurate as newer, more sophisticated technologies such as Digital PCR become clinically validated.

The traditional and most cost-effective method of quantifying a PCR product is a densitometry-based analysis of the subsequent gel electrophoresis. This method is semi-quantitative as it compares the densitometry of product compared against that of a known housekeeping gene such as GAPDH, which is assumed to be present at constant levels. Currently, more accurate estimates of product amount are achieved by quantitative real-time PCR. As mentioned above, the quantification is based on the inverse relationship between the cycle threshold and the amount of starting DNA template. This relationship can be used for relative quantification of a target relative to an internal housekeeping gene control or for absolute quantification against a known set of standards by generating a standard curve (4,10).

## Clinical applications of PCR

Standard clinical protocols for PCR for tissue-based molecular analyses are now available in most academic and community anatomic pathology departments (2). The impetus is most often the role of PCR in molecular diagnostic pathology (27, 28). As the field matures, the role of PCR continues to expand and include detection of DNA changes that have prognostic and therapeutic implications. Essentially,

Table 5.1 A snapshot of the many clinical applications of PCR

| Clinical applications | Specific example and references |
|---|---|
| Forensic or kinship identification | • 10–15 short tandem repeat loci (29) |
| Mutation detection for diagnosis or prognostic and therapeutic stratification | • EGFR in lung cancer (30)<br>• BRAF in melanoma (30)<br>• KRAS in colorectal cancer (30) |
| miRNA expression | • In FFPE tissues (31) |
| Microsatellite instability testing | • MSI in Lynch syndrome (32) |
| Chromosomal rearrangements | • lymphoma/leukemia (33)<br>• 1p/19q deletion in oligodendroglial tumors (34)<br>• Various soft tissue sarcoma |
| Tumor clonality assessment | • Lymphoma (35) |
| Detection of carcinogenic infectious agents | • HPV in cervical lesions (36)<br>• EBV in Hodgkin's lymphoma, nasopharyngeal carcinoma and post-transplant lymphoproliferative disease (37) |
| Minimal residual disease detection | • BCR-Abl in CML (38) |
| Prenatal screening | • Trisomies 13, 18 and 21 and sex chromosome aneuploidies (39) |
| Detection of infectious agents | • HIV (40)<br>• M. tuberculosis and treatment-resistant M. tuberculosis (41) |
| Methylation analysis for imprinted genes | • Prader-Willi and Angelmann syndromes (42) |

the use of PCR methods is allowing for the full realization of the concept of personalized medicine. In addition, PCR is also implemented in clinical settings outside of oncology, such as microbiology (pathogen recognition), reproductive medicine (aneuploidy detection) and forensic medicine (identification).

The majority of current clinical laboratory applications of PCR are on single mutation detection. Table 5.1 provides a snapshot of some common, clinically utilized and validated PCR protocols for mutation detection for the purposes of diagnosis, prognosis or therapeutic selection. More comprehensive discussion of these common mutations, their pathobiology and their testing are well documented and outside the scope of this chapter. Instead, readers are directed to other sources for their background and detailed descriptions (43, 44). Briefly, however, we would like to highlight potential areas that we believe are viable substrates for the use of PCR in the rapidly evolving field of disease subtyping, whereby genomic alterations between normal and disease are analyzed in terms of global

patterns. In particular, we would like to discuss the role of multigene expression assays for prognosis, DNA methylation and epigenetic patterns, disease-associated single nucleotide polymorphisms and microRNA expression.

## Prognostic multigene classifiers

As the molecular underpinnings of tumorigenesis are unraveled at an exponential pace, so has the ability to detect said changes. While most molecular changes are clinically detected to aid in diagnosis, an ever-increasing number of specific changes are detected that aid in clinical prognostication; whether it be via the natural course of a tumor bearing that mutation or the therapeutic response of a tumor that harbors such molecular alterations (45). Furthermore, sophisticated informatics and analyses have allowed for the simultaneous analyses of multiple gene expression profiles, which can further stratify clinical outcome (45). For most of the available platforms, PCR and RT-PCR are central to these tests for reasons explained above. Most are still in the research and development phase, but more are achieving clinical validation and some are even successfully commercialized.

Breast cancer diagnostics leads the field in the adoption of multigene expression profiles as ancillary tests that accompany histopathologic diagnosis as well as hormone receptor status and HER2 scoring via immunohistochemistry (IHC) or *in situ* hybridization (ISH) methods (46, 47). Studies have shown that these are able to predict for overall prognosis and response to treatments. Most are commercialized and use either IHC, ISH, microarray or RT-PCR platforms. Of the RT-PCR-based platforms, Oncotype DX is perhaps the most widely used and one of the first to impact patient management.

Oncotype DX is a commercial RT-PCR based, clinically validated test that analyses 21 genes from FFPE tissues: five reference genes as well as 16 cancer-related genes (subgrouped as proliferation genes, invasion genes, HER2 genes, Estrogen genes and others) (46). This test is appropriate for stage I or II, node-negative, ER-positive breast cancers, and is generally used for detecting breast cancers with a low potential for recurrence (47). The test produces a tripartite recurrence score (RS; up to 17, low risk; between 18 and 30, intermediate risk; and greater than 30, high risk), which predicts for the 10-year risk of recurrence for those treated with tamoxifen. In addition, a high Oncotype DX recurrence score predicted for the added benefit of CMF chemotherapy (47).

Another RT-PCR-based test is the Predictor Analysis of Microarrays test that uses a 50-gene set (PAM50) which is designed to be a distributed test available in hospital laboratories (46, 48). This measures the expression of 50 classifier genes and five control genes on FFPE tissues to identify molecular subtypes of cancer. Thus, in addition to characterizing the biology of the tumor, PAM50 further provides quantitative data on predictive biomarkers. A recent comparison between PAM50 risk-of-recurrence and Oncotype DX recurrence score showed that PAM50 provided more prognostic information than Oncotype DX (48).

As the time of writing, there are already a multitude of multigene assays available and more yet to come. For example, there is now also an Oncotype DX score for colorectal cancer (49). One needs to be mindful that regardless of the testing platform, these are ancillary tests that accompany, and do not supersede, histopathologic diagnosis. Importantly, clinical validation is required for any test to ensure that it is applicable in clinical diagnostic practice (50).

## Methylation analysis

DNA methylation is a common epigenetic mechanism that cells use to control gene expression in cellular processes, such as embryonic development, genomic imprinting, X-chromosome inactivation and preservation of chromosome stability (51). DNA methylation occurs at CpG dinucleotides of eukaryotic DNA, with a methyl group added to cytosine forming 5-methyl-cytosine via DNA methyltransferase (DNMT) activity (52). In mammals, most CpG dinucleotides are distributed sparsely throughout the entire genome and are usually methylated. Unmethylated CpGs are often grouped into clusters called "CpG islands" which are associated with the 5' regulatory regions of promoters (52). Gene transcription is inhibited when promoter activity is suppressed by methylated promoter CpG islands (53).

Aberrant DNA methylation includes genome-wide hypomethylation, promoter hypermethylation or an increased DNMT expression (54). Genome-wide hypomethylation can lead to chromosome instability and increased mutation rates (54). Hypermethylation typically occurs at CpG islands in the promoter regions of tumor suppressor genes (TSG), leading to transcriptional silencing. Hence, detection of promoter hypermethylation of TSGs has been suggested as potential cancer biomarkers. However, since DNA methylation patterns are heterogeneous, careful selection of putative biomarkers must include DNA regions with differential methylation levels between normal and disease. Furthermore, analysis of CpG islands of the entire promoter region is required. The majority of the methylation detection methods start with bisulfate treatment of genomic DNA to convert unmethylated cytosine to uracil bases, while maintaining 5-methyl-cytosines. This is followed by a PCR amplification that replaces uracil with thymine and 5-methyl-cytosine with cytosine; hence, differentiating methylated from un-methylated sequences.

## Single nucleotide polymorphism

Single nucleotide polymorphisms (SNP) are the most common type of variation of DNA sequences in the human genome (55). It refers to the presence of an allele of a gene in more than 1% of the population. The human genome has about 10 million polymorphisms, which are located on coding, non-coding, as well as intragenic regions (55). Thus, the potential effects of SNPs are wide ranging, and can include gene splicing, transcription factor binding and messenger RNA degradation, among many others. Furthermore, gene variants can predispose individuals to diseases, but are usually not the major causative factor.

The International HapMap Project is an international collaboration with the goal to compare the genetic sequences of different individuals and identify chromosomal regions where genetic variants are shared (56). The database provides a complete catalogue of the common genetic variants to facilitate identification of disease-associated SNPs. With this SNP database, haplotypes (a set of SNPs on a chromosome) are being analyzed as possible indicators of disease susceptibility, and it is particularly amenable to genome-wide association studies. If a particular haplotype occurs more frequently in affected individuals, the disease-associated SNPs may be located within or near that haplotype. A SNP may indicate disease susceptibility if found to be significantly and frequently detected in the affected population compared to the control group (57). Disease-associated SNPs have been reported as potential genetic markers for many common diseases, such as cancers, diabetes, and autoimmune, cardiovascular and neurodegenerative diseases (57). SNPs can be analyzed by real-time PCR by using end-point plateau phase analysis or melting curve analysis.

## MicroRNAs

MicroRNAs (miRNA) are small (~22 nucleotides[nt]) endogenous non-coding RNA which regulate mRNA expression. As depicted in Figure 5.3, miRNA is originally transcribed by RNA polymerase II in the nucleus to form a long primary transcript (pri-miRNA) (58). They are processed by Drosha ribonuclease into ~70 nt hairpin precursors (pre-miRNA), which are transported to the cytoplasm. Within the cytoplasm, pre-miRNA duplex is further cleaved by the RNase Dicer into 22-nt mature miRNA duplex. One of the mature strands of the duplex will incorporate into RNA-induced silencing complex (RISC) for gene regulation. Usually, a "guide" strand will be retained in the RISC and the "passenger" strand will

be degraded. MicroRNAs can bind with either perfect complementarity to the open reading frame or 5' untranslated region (UTR) of target mRNA to cleave mRNAs, or with imperfect complementarity to the 3' UTR of mRNA to inhibit protein synthesis (59, 60). Thus, gene regulation results from mRNA cleavage or translational repression (59). The current miRDatabase (www.mirbase.org) has catalogued more than 1,400 human sequences. With their ability to target mRNA with imperfect complementarity, miRNA have been predicted to regulate the expression of around one-third of all human transcripts and are considered to be among the largest class of gene regulators.

MicroRNA profiling has been suggested to be a superior biomarker over mRNA profiling. MiRNAs are more stable in FFPE tissues than mRNAs since they are less affected by the fixation process and can be readily extracted from FFPE samples due to their small sizes (~22 nt in length) (61). Moreover, there is emerging interest in the investigation of miRNAs as non-invasive biomarkers in cancer. Aberrations of miRNAs have been associated with almost all cancer types, including both hematologic and solid malignancies (62). For example, miR-21 is one of the most commonly over-expressed miRNA in human malignancies which was first reported in glioblastoma, then described in epithelial cancers (63). Over-expression of miR-21 is usually associated with worse outcomes and has been shown to increase cell proliferation, migration, invasion and survival (64).

MiRNAs have also been detected in body fluids and are found to be shed into the extracellular environment via exosomes (65, 66). In a B-cell lymphoma study, higher levels of miR-155, miR-210 and miR-21 were found in patient serum samples, with miR-21 expression associated with relapse-free survival (67). Several studies have been conducted to measure circulating miRNAs in epithelial malignancies. For example, a 21-miRNA signature in plasma samples has been reported to aid in lung cancer patient diagnosis and prognosis (68). Both intact and functional miRNAs have been frequently reported in cancer-isolated exosomes, whereas peripheral blood-derived exosome miRNAs have been shown to correlate with tumor-derived miRNAs in ovarian and lung cancers (65, 68).

Since the discovery of miRNA, global miRNA profiling has been conducted in cancer samples using PCR-based molecular techniques. Despite the

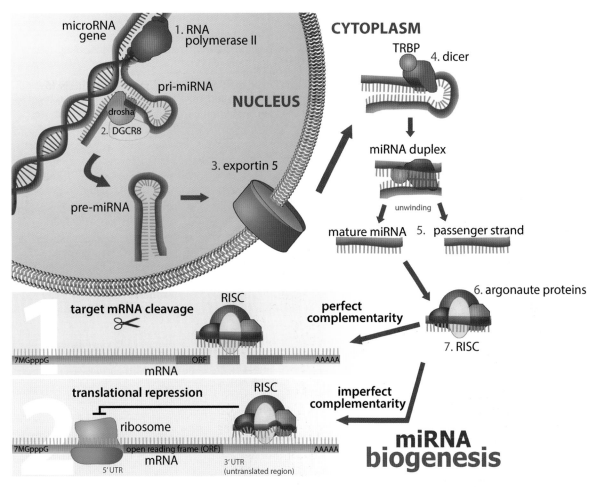

**Figure 5.3 Schematic illustration of miRNA biogenesis**
(1) Inside the nucleus, miRNA is transcribed by RNA polymerase II into pri-miRNA. (2) Drosha cleaves pri-miRNA to form pre-miRNA. (3) Pre-miRNA is transported to the cytoplasm via Exportin-5. (4) In the cytoplasm, Dicer cleaves pre-miRNA and removes the hairpin loop to form 22-nt mature miRNA duplex. (5) MiRNA duplex unwind, with the passenger strand usually degraded. (6) Argonaute binds to one of the mature strands to form RNA-induced silencing complex (RISC). (7) MicroRNAs can bind with perfect complementarity to the open reading frame or 5′ untranslated region (UTR) of target mRNA, or with imperfect complementarity to the 3′ UTR of mRNA to inhibit translation.

promising data supporting the potential application of miRNAs as cancer biomarkers, many challenges remain. Firstly, robust platforms, as well as appropriate statistical and bio-computational analyses, are essential to identify potential candidate prognostic miRNA signatures. Secondly, the selection of appropriate reference controls is extremely important for normalization of biological variation, as recent reports have shown that some commonly utilized reference miRNAs can in fact fluctuate (69). Hence, it is critical to determine the most stable miRNAs for each disease in evaluation of miRNA expression.

## Conclusions

From the basic PCR tenet as a method of DNA amplification, innovations in automation and miniaturization, as well as improvements in post-amplification analyses, have solidified the role of PCR within the clinical diagnostic domain. Increasingly, the genetic changes that are commonly assayed in academic and community labs are also being done for prognostic and therapeutic purposes. Soon, coupled with "next generation techniques" and multiplex platforms, PCR will be central for the production of complex genetic signatures that can identify disease, and subtype them accordingly, with the intent of working towards the true realization of personalized medicine.

## Learning points

- PCR is a simple, established molecular technique used in research and clinical laboratories.
- RT-PCR is a derivation of the PCR technique that is an indispensible tool for analyzing gene expression.
- The most common clinical application of PCR is as an ancillary test to aid or provide prognostic information in histopathologic diagnostics.
- Multigene classifiers, methylation profiling, SNP analyses and microRNA signatures are current and potential clinical tests that rely heavily on PCR.

## References

1. Mullis, K., Faloona, F., Scharf, S., Saiki, R., Horn, G. and Erlich, H. Specific enzymatic amplification of DNA in vitro: the polymerase chain reaction. *Cold Spring Harb Symp Quant Biol* 1986; 51(Pt 1): 263–73.

2. Hunt, J. L. Molecular pathology in anatomic pathology practice: a review of basic principles. *Arch Pathol Lab Med* 2008; 132(2): 248–60.

3. Gonzalez-Angulo, A. M., Hennessy, B. T. and Mills, G. B. Future of personalized medicine in oncology: a systems biology approach. *J Clin Oncol* 2010; 28(16): 2777–83.

4. Bossler, A. and van Deerlin, V. Conventional and real-time polymerase chain reaction, in Tubbs, R. R. and Stoler, M. H. (eds.), *Cell and Tissue Based Molecular Pathology* (Philadelphia, PA: Churchill Livingstone Elsevier Inc., 2009), pp. 33–49.

5. Rennert, H. and Leonard, D. G. B., Molecular methods in the diagnostic laboratory, in Leonard, D. G. B. (ed.), *Diagnostic Molecular Pathology* (Philadelphia, PA: Saunders, 2003), pp. 25–52.

6. Coleman, W. G. and Tsongalis, G. J. *Essential Concepts in Molecular Pathology* (San Diego, CA: Elsevier, 2010).

7. Lo, Y. M. and Chan, K. C. Setting up a polymerase chain reaction laboratory. *Methods Mol Biol* 2006; 336:11–18.

8. Remick, D. G., Kunkel, S. L., Holbrook, E. A. and Hanson, C. A. Theory and applications of the polymerase chain reaction. *Am J Clin Pathol* 1990; 93(4 Suppl. 1): S49–54.

9. Mies, C. Molecular biological analysis of paraffin-embedded tissues. *Hum Pathol* 1994; 25(6): 555–60.

10. Farkas, D. H. and Holland, C. A. Overview of molecular diagnostic techniques and instrumentation, in Tubbs, R. R. and Stoler, M. H. (eds.), *Cell and Tissue Based Molecular Pathology* (Philadelphia, PA: Churchill Livingstone Elsevier Inc, 2009), pp. 19–35.

11. Baumforth, K. R., Nelson, P. N., Digby, J. E., O'Neil, J. D. and Murray, P. G. Demystified . . . the polymerase chain reaction. *Mol Pathol* 1999; 52(1): 1–10.

12. Ririe, K. M., Rasmussen, R. P. and Wittwer, C. T. Product differentiation by analysis of DNA melting curves during the polymerase chain reaction. *Anal Biochem* 1997; 245(2): 154–60.

13. Wienken, C. J., Baaske, P., Duhr, S. and Braun, D. Thermophoretic melting curves quantify the conformation and stability of RNA and DNA. *Nucleic Acids Res* 2011; 39(8): e52.

14. Joyce, C. Quantitative RT-PCR. A review of current methodologies. *Methods Mol Biol* 2002; 193: 83–92.

15. Oliver, D. Polymerase chain reaction and reverse transcription-polymerase chain reaction, in Cagle, P. T. and Allen, T. C. (eds.), *Basic Concepts of Molecular Pathology* (New York: Springer, 2009), pp. 73–85.

16. Deepak, S., Kottapalli, K., Rakwal, R., Oros, G., Rangappa, K., Iwahashi, H. *et al.* Real-time PCR: revolutionizing detection and expression analysis of genes. *Curr Genomics* 2007; 8(4): 234–51.

17. Freeman, W. M., Walker, S. J. and Vrana, K. E. Quantitative RT-PCR: pitfalls and potential. *Biotechniques* 1999; 26(1): 112–22, 24–5.

18. Whitcombe, D., Theaker, J., Guy, S. P., Brown, T. and Little, S. Detection of PCR products using self-probing amplicons and fluorescence. *Nat Biotechnol* 1999; 17(8): 804–7.

19. Edwards, M. C. and Gibbs, R. A. Multiplex PCR: advantages, development, and applications. *PCR Methods Appl* 1994; 3(4): S65–75.

20. Homig-Holzel, C. and Savola, S. Multiplex ligation-dependent probe amplification (MLPA) in tumor diagnostics and prognostics. *Diagn Mol Pathol* 2012; 21(4): 189–206.

21. Vogelstein, B. and Kinzler, K. W. Digital PCR. *Proc Natl Acad Sci USA* 1999; 96(16): 9236–41.

22. Day, E., Dear, P. H. and McCaughan, F. Digital PCR strategies in the development and analysis of molecular biomarkers for personalized medicine. *Methods* 2013; 59(1): 101–7.

23. McCaughan, F. and Dear, P. H. Single-molecule genomics. *J Pathol* 2010; 220(2): 297–306.

24. Killeen, A. A. *Principles of Molecular Pathology* (Totowa, NJ: Humana Press, 2004).

25. Lo, Y. M. and Chan, K. C. Introduction to the polymerase chain reaction. *Methods Mol Biol* 2006; 336: 1–10.

26. Sanger, F., Nicklen, S. and Coulson, A. R. DNA sequencing with chain-terminating inhibitors. *Proc Natl Acad Sci USA* 1977; 74(12): 5463–7.

27. Bernard, P. S. and Wittwer, C. T. Real-time PCR technology for cancer diagnostics. *Clin Chem* 2002; 48(8): 1178–85.

28. Crocker, J. Demystified . . . molecular pathology in oncology. *Mol Pathol* 2002; 55(6): 337–47.

29. Thompson, R., Zoppis, S. and McCord, B. An overview of DNA typing methods for human identification: past, present, and future. *Methods Mol Biol* 2012; 830: 3–16.

30. McCourt, C. M., McArt, D. G., Mills, K., Catherwood, M. A., Maxwell, P., Waugh, D. J. *et al.* Validation of next generation sequencing technologies in comparison to current diagnostic gold standards for BRAF, EGFR and KRAS mutational analysis. *PLoS ONE* 2013; 8(7): e69604.

31. Goswami, R. S., Waldron, L., Machado, J., Cervigne, N. K., Xu, W., Reis, P. P. *et al.* Optimization and analysis of a quantitative real-time PCR-based technique to determine microRNA expression in formalin-fixed paraffin-embedded samples. *BMC Biotechnol* 2010; 10: 47.

32. Goel, A., Nagasaka, T., Hamelin, R. and Boland, C. R. An optimized pentaplex PCR for detecting DNA mismatch repair-deficient colorectal cancers. *PLoS ONE* 2010; 5(2): e9393.

33. Lin, M. T., Tseng, L. H., Rich, R. G., Hafez, M. J., Harada, S., Murphy, K. M. *et al.* Delta-PCR, a simple method to detect translocations and insertion/deletion mutations. *J Mol Diagn* 2011; 13(1): 85–92.

34. Chaturbedi, A., Yu, L., Linskey, M. E. and Zhou, Y. H. Detection of 1p19q deletion by real-time comparative quantitative PCR. *Biomark Insights* 2012; 7: 9–17.

35. Liu, H., Bench, A. J., Bacon, C. M., Payne, K., Huang, Y., Scott, M. A. *et al.* A practical strategy for the routine use of BIOMED-2 PCR assays for detection of B- and T-cell clonality in diagnostic haematopathology. *Br J Haematol* 2007; 138(1): 31–43.

36. Lindemann, M. L., Dominguez, M. J., de Antonio, J. C., Sandri, M. T., Tricca, A., Sideri, M. *et al.* Analytical comparison of the cobas HPV Test with Hybrid Capture 2 for the detection of high-risk HPV genotypes. *J Mol Diagn* 2012; 14(1): 65–70.

37. Thijsen, S. F. and Deege, M. P. Molecular diagnosis of Epstein-Barr virus infections. *Expert Opin Med Diagn* 2008; 2(1): 21–31.

38. van der Velden, V. H., Hochhaus, A., Cazzaniga, G., Szczepanski, T., Gabert, J. and van Dongen, J. J. Detection of minimal residual disease in hematologic malignancies by real-time quantitative PCR: principles, approaches, and laboratory aspects. *Leukemia* 2003; 17(6): 1013–34.

39. Onay, H., Ugurlu, T., Aykut, A., Pehlivan, S., Inal, M., Tinar, S. *et al.* Rapid prenatal diagnosis of common aneuploidies in amniotic fluid using quantitative fluorescent polymerase chain reaction. *Gynecol Obstet Invest* 2008; 66(2): 104–10.

40. Shan, L., Rabi, S. A., Laird, G. M., Eisele, E. E., Zhang, H., Margolick, J. B. *et al.* A novel PCR assay for quantification of HIV-1 RNA. *J Virol* 2013; 87(11): 6521–5.

41. Park, K. S., Kim, J. Y., Lee, J. W., Hwang, Y. Y., Jeon, K., Koh, W. J. *et al.* Comparison of the Xpert MTB/RIF and Cobas TaqMan MTB assays for detection of mycobacterium tuberculosis in respiratory specimens. *J Clin Microbiol* 2013; 51(10): 3225–7.

42. Procter, M., Chou, L. S., Tang, W., Jama, M. and Mao, R. Molecular diagnosis of Prader-Willi and Angelman syndromes by methylation-specific melting analysis and methylation-specific multiplex ligation-dependent probe amplification. *Clin Chem* 2006; 52(7): 1276–83.

43. Igbokwe, A. and Lopez-Terrada, D. H. Molecular testing of solid tumors. *Arch Pathol Lab Med* 2011; 135(1): 67–82.

44. Allen, T. C., Cagle, P. T. and Popper, H. H. Basic concepts of molecular pathology. *Arch Pathol Lab Med* 2008; 132(10): 1551–6.

45. Pickl, M., Ruge, E. and Venturi, M. Predictive markers in early research and companion diagnostic developments in oncology. *N Biotechnol* 2012; 29(6): 651–5.

46. Kittaneh, M., Montero, A. J. and Gluck, S. Molecular profiling for breast cancer: a comprehensive review. *Biomark Cancer* 2013; 5: 61–70.

47. Ross, J. S. Multigene classifiers, prognostic factors, and predictors of breast cancer clinical outcome. *Adv Anat Pathol* 2009; 16(4): 204–15.

48. Dowsett, M., Sestak, I., Lopez-Knowles, E., Sidhu, K., Dunbier, A. K., Cowens, J. W. *et al.* Comparison of PAM50 risk of recurrence score with oncotype DX and IHC4 for predicting risk of distant recurrence after endocrine therapy. *J Clin Oncol* 2013; 31(22): 2783–90.

49. Kelley, R. K. and Venook, A. P. Prognostic and predictive markers in stage II colon cancer: is there a role for gene expression profiling? *Clin Colorectal Cancer* 2011; 10(2): 73–80.

50. Halling, K. C., Schrijver, I. and Persons, D. L. Test verification and validation for molecular diagnostic assays. *Arch Pathol Lab Med* 2012; 136(1): 11–13.

51. Robertson, K. D. DNA methylation and human disease. *Nat Rev Genet* 2005; 6(8): 597–610.

52. Bird, A. P. CpG-rich islands and the function of DNA methylation. *Nature* 1986; 321(6067): 209–13.

53. Herman, J. G. and Baylin, S. B. Gene silencing in cancer in association with promoter hypermethylation. *New Engl J Med* 2003; 349(21): 2042–54.

54. Baylin, S. B., Herman, J. G., Graff, J. R., Vertino, P. M. and Issa, J. P. Alterations in DNA methylation: a fundamental aspect of neoplasia. *Adv Cancer Res* 1998; 72: 141–96.

55. Lander, E. S. The new genomics: global views of biology. *Science* 1996; 274(5287): 536–9.

56. International HapMap Consortium, A haplotype map of the human genome. *Nature* 2005; 437(7063): 1299–320.

57. Kruglyak, L. Prospects for whole-genome linkage disequilibrium mapping of common disease genes. *Nat Genet* 1999; 22(2): 139–44.

58. Lund, E., Guttinger, S., Calado, A., Dahlberg, J. E. and Kutay, U. Nuclear export of microRNA precursors. *Science* 2004; 303 (5654): 95–8.

59. Bartel, D. P. MicroRNAs: target recognition and regulatory functions. *Cell* 2009; 136(2): 215–33.

60. Bentwich, I., Avniel, A., Karov, Y., Aharonov, R., Gilad, S., Barad, O. *et al.* Identification of hundreds of conserved and nonconserved human microRNAs. *Nat Genet* 2005; 37(7): 766–70.

61. Nelson, P. T., Baldwin, D. A., Scearce, L. M., Oberholtzer, J. C., Tobias, J. W. and Mourelatos, Z. Microarray-based, high-throughput gene expression profiling of microRNAs. *Nat Methods* 2004; 1(2): 155–61.

62. Esquela-Kerscher, A. and Slack, F. J. Oncomirs – microRNAs with a role in cancer. *Nat Rev Cancer* 2006; 6(4): 259–69.

63. Volinia, S., Calin, G. A., Liu, C. G., Ambs, S., Cimmino, A., Petrocca, F. *et al.* A microRNA expression signature of human solid tumors defines cancer gene targets. *Proc Natl Acad Sci USA* 2006; 103(7): 2257–61.

64. Si, M. L., Zhu, S., Wu, H., Lu, Z., Wu, F. and Mo, Y. Y. miR-21-mediated tumor growth. *Oncogene* 2007; 26(19): 2799–803.

65. Taylor, D. D. and Gercel-Taylor, C. MicroRNA signatures of tumor-derived exosomes as diagnostic biomarkers of ovarian cancer. *Gynecol Oncol* 2008; 110(1): 13–21.

66. Valadi, H., Ekstrom, K., Bossios, A., Sjostrand, M., Lee, J. J. and Lotvall, J. O. Exosome-mediated transfer of mRNAs and microRNAs is a novel mechanism of genetic exchange between cells. *Nat Cell Biol* 2007; 9(6): 654–9.

67. Lawrie, C. H., Gal, S., Dunlop, H. M., Pushkaran, B., Liggins, A. P., Pulford, K. *et al.* Detection of elevated levels of tumour-associated microRNAs in serum of patients with diffuse large B-cell lymphoma. *Br J Haematol* 2008; 141(5): 672–5.

68. Boeri, M., Verri, C., Conte, D., Roz, L., Modena, P., Facchinetti, F. *et al.* MicroRNA signatures in tissues and plasma predict development and prognosis of computed tomography detected lung cancer. *Proc Natl Acad Sci USA* 2011; 108(9): 3713–18.

69. Gee, H. E., Buffa, F. M., Camps, C., Ramachandran, A., Leek, R., Taylor, M. *et al.* The small-nucleolar RNAs commonly used for microRNA normalisation correlate with tumour pathology and prognosis. *Br J Cancer* 2011; 104(7): 1168–77.

# Are microarrays ready for prime time?

Jane Bayani and John M. S. Bartlett

Microarray technology has significantly contributed to defining the "-omics" era, which has moved molecular research forward at an astounding pace. The routine use of microarrays in the research space has provided the framework for their use in the diagnostic space. Gene signatures of clinical relevance for cancer have been discovered and validated, but cannot move to the bedside until they satisfy comprehensive and rigorous evaluation with regard to clinical validity and utility. In this chapter we will review the evolution of microarrays, their uses and their role in clinical diagnostics.

## Introduction

It is an exciting and challenging time for clinical diagnostics. Compared to a decade ago, when the draft of the human genome was released and subsequently completed (1, 2), technological advances have made it possible to interrogate the human genome in a fraction of the time and cost. A catalogue of genes comprising the human genome, coupled to the ability to synthesize and immobilize biomolecules at high density, and to detect them with high specificity and sensitivity, has enabled microarrays to change the way in which we ask and answer both biological and clinical questions. As the technology and associated computational algorithms mature, the question is whether these techniques are ready for primetime in clinical diagnostic laboratories.

In research, microarrays focus on deciphering information generated by normal and diseased cells at the DNA, RNA or protein level (see Table 6.1). None of this would be possible without recent technological milestones in molecular biology: including cloning and recombinant DNA, sequencing, polymerase chain reaction (PCR); coupled to those of computer sciences and bioinformatics, yielding sequence alignment algorithms, databases and repositories; as well as advances in manufacturing to modify and adapt lessons learned in other industries to biomolecular materials. Glimpses of modern microarrays can be seen in the early use of recombinant libraries arrayed to filters used by researchers in the 1980s. Later, glass slides became the substrates of choice for the deposition of nucleic acids for array-based experiments. Photolithographic methods, such as those used by Affymetrix Inc. (3), produced biochips where oligonucleotides were chemically synthesized on glass slides. It was also around this time that Patrick Brown's laboratory at Stanford University performed the first expression microarray experiments that revolutionized the way in which molecular research could be conducted (4). Forty-five cDNAs from the *Arabi-*

**Table 6.1** Types of microarrays currently used in molecular pathology

| Target type | Aberration detected |
| --- | --- |
| DNA | Gene/locus copy-number (aCGH) |
| | Copy-number variations (CNVs) |
| | Gene rearrangements and structural aberrations |
| | Sequence mutations: |
| | Gene mutations |
| | Single nucleotide polymorphism (SNPs) |
| | Chromatin modification (ChIP on Chip) |
| | Methylation |
| RNA | Expression profiling |
| miRNA | Expression profiling |
| Protein | Protein expression profiling |
| | Enzymatic activity |

*Molecular Pathology: A Practical Guide for the Surgical Pathologist and Cytopathologist*, ed. John M. S. Bartlett, Abeer Shaaban and Fernando Schmitt. Published by Cambridge University Press. © Cambridge University Press, 2016.

*dopsis* genome were spotted onto a glass slide, to which equal amounts of differentially and fluorescently labeled RNAs from a transgenic and wild-type plant were hybridized to the deposited cDNAs. The difference in relative fluorescence reflected the differential gene expression between the transgenic and wild-type plant. Shortly after this, microarrays initially fabricated for the detection of expression changes would be refined for the detection of DNA copy-number changes, and give rise to other applications. In the decade since those initial reports, the amount of generated information is staggering; creating the greater need for biostatisticians, informaticians and computer language development. Indeed, international consortiums, such as the International Cancer Genome Consortium (ICGC) (http://icgc.org/) and The Cancer Genome Atlas (TCGA) (http://cancer genome.nih.gov/), were created based on the availability of next generation sequencing and microarray technology. However, the promises of molecular profiling efforts have not been translated into significant benefit for patients, and both geneticists and pathologists are limited in the ability to use genomic data when counseling patients. Nevertheless, microarrays have significantly impacted on all fields of molecular biology and molecular medicine. In this chapter, we will review the use of microarrays in molecular medicine both in the research and clinical

space, with a specific focus on the use of microarrays in the clinical setting.

## Applications of microarrays

There are now a number of uses for microarray-based technology, including the relative quantification of RNA, DNA or proteins. The utilization of microarrays has now expanded to identifying sequence polymorphisms, variant and fusion RNA transcripts, translocations and epigenetic modifications.

## Expression

Expression-based arrays have their origins in classic northern blotting techniques (5). Later, total RNAs were directly spotted onto membranes and probed with a labeled gene of interest to determine relative expression across the spotted RNAs. In fact, such arrays were applied to examining the relative expression of a given gene across RNAs extracted from different tissues (i.e. multiple organs, normal tissue vs. diseased, etc.). By the mid to late 1990s, companies like Clonetech Laboratories Inc. produced various filter-based expression array panels comprising over 500 different cDNAs and controls spotted in replicate, to which radioactively labeled or chemiluminescently labeled RNAs were hybridized to it and subsequently exposed to x-ray film (Figure 6.1). The earliest

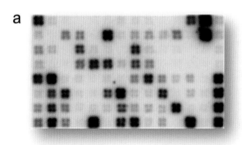

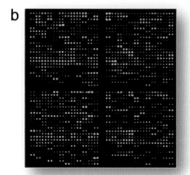

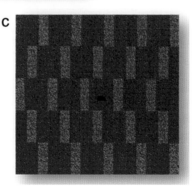

**Figure 6.1 Evolution of microarray technology**
(a) X-ray film developed following chemiluminescence detection of labeled RNAs hybridized to a spotted cDNA cancer array panel on a nitrocellulose array produced by Clonetech Laboratories Inc., showing differential gene expression of quadruplicate spots (image courtesy of J. Bayani). (b) Merged TIFF image of a two-color expression array experiment to the Agilent array platform, with yellow spots indicative of relative equal copy-numbers between normal and cancer-derived DNAs; red spots indicative of gene amplification; and green spots indicative of gene deletion (image courtesy of J. Bayani). (c) A TIFF image from the single channel Affymetrix gene chip showing the high density of oligonucleotides. Image courtesy of Affymetrix Inc.

microarray experiments examined differential gene expression using cDNAs (4); however, the vast majority of current commercially available expression microarrays are oligonucleotide-based, offering better sensitivity and specificity. This has enabled investigators to comprehensively compare gene expression differences using both *in vitro* and *in vivo* experimental models. Detecting changes in gene expression, particularly in the context of cancer, is not only limited to total or messenger RNA, but to the non-coding RNAs such as microRNAs (6); while efforts have also been made to create custom arrays to detect fusion gene products (7). The power of expression profiling has become evident in the translation of some gene expression signatures to the clinic, which will be discussed in greater detail later in this chapter.

## Copy-number

Shortly after the introduction of expression microarrays, researchers quickly adapted the principle to looking at changes in DNA copy-number. Recognizing the important information generated from metaphase-based comparative genomic hybridization (CGH) (8), but requiring greater resolution to narrow gains, losses and amplification to the gene level, investigators looked to the example of expression arrays and their growing utility. Since the cDNA platform was already available, these microarrays were first used to generate copy-number information (9). Later, copy-number microarrays utilized spotted bacterial artificial chromosome (BAC) clones (10) in tiling configurations to improve coverage, then moved to more stable and sequence-specific oligonucleotides (3). Current arrays are significantly higher in resolution and coverage; and have eliminated issues plaguing early generation microarrays, such as the presence of highly repetitive sequences, which commonly contributed to background and inconsistent results. In fact, due to the early microarray experiments, scientists were able to appreciate the extent of copy-number variations (CNVs) of these repeat elements among individuals (11).

## Sequence polymorphisms

The ability to identify copy-number imbalances at the level of the gene or sequence led to the development of microarrays that could detect polymorphisms which are exclusively oligonucleotide-based. Single nucleotide polymorphisms (SNPs) are defined as a variation in a single nucleic acid. The frequency and observed variation allows for sensitive genotyping and permits cataloguing for comprehensive genotype-phenotype studies. Moreover, the ability to detect and quantify these variations also allows investigators to obtain copy-number information. SNP-based arrays can detect other types of genomic alterations which have implications for clinical diagnosis of genomic disorders (12) such as germline mutations, microdeletions/duplications, loss of heterozygosity (LOH) or uniparental disomy (13).

## Epigenetic modifications

Epigenetics are largely associated with DNA methylation of cytosine residues at CpG dinucleotides and have a central role in normal human development and disease. Profiling of the methylome has been advanced significantly by microarrays or second-generation sequencing-based approaches, enabling quantitative analysis of DNA methylation at CpG loci throughout the genome. The use of microarray-based technology for methylation profiling was first reported by Gitan *et al.* (14), where targets were derived from PCR products of bisulfite-modified DNA, hybridized to oligonucleotide probes discriminating between converted (unmethylated cytosine) and unconverted (methylated cytosine) nucleotides. Similar to identifying methylation changes, interactions between proteins and DNA can also be assessed by microarray-based technology. Chromatin immunoprecipitation (ChIP) with microarray analysis (chip) has allowed the profiling of the cistrome – the transcription factor binding sites or histone modifications in a genome-wide fashion. The goals of ChIP-on-chip analyses are the identification of protein-binding sites that may help to identify functional elements in the genome. These analyses were first performed in budding yeast to reveal the distribution of cohesins along yeast chromosome III (15). ChIP-on-chip has now been successfully applied to all of the open reading frames (ORF) in the human genome (16).

## Protein

While the vast majority of effort in microarray technology has been relegated to DNA and RNA, the development of protein arrays has its roots in protein detection methods such as enzyme-linked immunosorbent assay (ELISA). Central to this technology is the ability of the antigen to be recognized by an antibody and detected through subsequent fluorescence or chromogenic methods. The first antibody matrices were introduced in the early 1980s (17), though saw little development until recently. Analytical protein microarrays function on a similar principle as their DNA and RNA cousins, with capture molecules arrayed on the solid surface. The array is probed with a complex protein solution such as a cell lysate, with subsequent analysis binding reactions detected, allowing for comparative analyses (18). In contrast, function protein arrays or target protein arrays are constructed by the immobilization of purified full-length functional protein or protein domains, and are used to identify protein-protein, protein-DNA, protein-RNA, protein-phospholipid and protein-small molecule interactions, to assay enzymatic activity and to detect antibodies and demonstrate their specificity (19). Reverse phase protein microarrays (RPPA) involve complex samples, such as tissue lysates, which are arrayed onto the support and probed with antibodies against the target protein (20).

## Principles of microarray technology

### Sequence recognition

The fundamental process that makes it possible to profile DNA or RNA is based on their basepair complementarity. Following the description of the DNA double helix, it was discovered that the strands could be separated by heat or with an alkali, but would then renature based on sequence complementarity. Hybridization microarrays exploit this complementarity. Typical microarray nomenclature designates the known sequence (i.e. cDNA, RNA, cloned DNA, etc.) as the "probe"; while the unknown mixture of nucleic acid to be hybridized to the array is termed the "target."

### Microarray probes, substrates and fabrication

The substrates on which the probes are mobilized have evolved. In the early days of recombinant DNA technology, cloned cDNAs were spotted onto charged membranes. Membranes had their advantages, as they provided a larger surface area for binding as well as allowing for larger volumes of material to be used. However, this method still relied on the use of

radioactivity or chemiluminescence and the development of the signal through (often repeated) exposure to x-ray film (Figure 6.1a). The use of glass slides, however, was already routinely used for fluorescence-based detection and microscopy in many disciplines, making it a sensible choice for the next iteration of the microarray (Figure 6.1b). Covalent modifications using epoxy-silane, amino-silane, lysine or polyacrylamide enhanced attachment of the probes to the glass substrate. More recently, silicon chips form the solid surface, and such microarrays are commonly referred to simply as "chips" or "biochips." However, some microarrays are no longer limited to the traditional platforms using silicon chips or glass slides, but have been extended to polystyrene microspheres, as in the case of the Ilumina platform (Ilumina Inc.) (21), or to hybrid technologies like NanoString (22).

The fabrication of current microarrays/biochips is carried out by photolithography (3) (Figure 6.1c) or by the direct mechanical deposition, spotting or printing of biomaterials to glass slides (23). For classical spotted arrays, probes were synthesized prior to their deposition to the solid surface. Probes included may be cDNAs or recombinant DNAs, such as BACs or Yeast Artificial Chromosomes (YACs), but most commonly oligonucleotides, due to their ease of synthesis and increased resolution. Photolithography permits the fabrication of probes *in situ* (3). Using a silica substrate, the biochips are created by repeated exposure to each nucleotide using light and light-sensitive masking agents to "build" sequences one nucleotide at a time across the entire array. Finally, platforms like Ilumina (21) utilize microspheres to which each bead is covered with hundreds of thousands of copies of a specific oligonucleotide "address" that acts as the capture sequence, in addition to the sequence of interest. The beads can then be arranged on a solid support and identified according to the specific oligonucleotide address and subsequently read and analyzed. In the case of NanoString, which is not a traditional microarray platform, the code sets utilize a pair of oligonucleotide probes per RNA of interest – a biotinylated capture probe and a uniquely fluorescently labeled reporter probe. Both capture probe and reporter bind the target RNA in a hybridization step similar to traditional microarrays; and following hybridization, unbound target and probe are removed and the hybrids are applied to a streptavidin-coated slide. Application of an electrical charge across the slides orients the hybrids so that the differentially labeled reporter probes can be quantified by a fluorescent scanner (22). Its categorization as a microarray platform is due to the scalability of the codeset to number in the several hundred.

## Target labeling and hybridization

The target for any microarray experiment may be DNA, RNA or derivatives of these molecules. Ideally, non-amplified targets are desired as this minimizes artifacts due to the amplification process. However, if amplification or modification of the original nucleic acid is necessary, minimal manipulation and rounds of amplifications are preferred. High-quality starting DNA or RNA contributes to the reliability of the results of the experiment. However, the ability to obtain sufficient amounts of DNA or RNA from fresh or frozen tissues or cells can be a challenge in both research and diagnostic laboratories; particularly when limited to small core needle biopsies. Furthermore, most diagnostic samples are formalin-fixed paraffin-embedded (FFPE), posing a challenge in obtaining sufficient diagnostic material for analyses. Extraction of nucleic acids from FFPE tissues often yields lower molecular-sized fragments, with sometimes significant proportions of these nucleic acids degraded to sizes that are not amenable to direct labeling or to amplification. Despite these challenges, extraction methods and labeling procedures have been improved and the use of nucleic acids extracted from FFPE samples is less of a hindrance for molecular studies. Labeling of nucleic acids is increasingly accomplished using sophisticated polymerase chain reaction strategies (PCR) to minimize the rounds of amplification as well as ensuring amplification is uniform across the entire genome (24). However, despite the ability to amplify nucleic acids, the question of bias remains. Therefore, it is desirable when choosing a diagnostic platform that technologies avoid amplification, or strive to minimize amplification and account for potential bias. As each platform has specific labeling protocols, generally, the target DNA or RNA is labeled with a detectable reporter – typically a fluorescent molecule. The labeled nucleic acids are precipitated from the labeling reaction reagents and re-suspended in a hybridization solution which helps to maintain the single-stranded state following denaturation and only permits annealing between sequences with the greatest homology. Hybridization typically occurs around 37°C, although specific protocols may suggest other temperatures suited to their platform. Like other hybridization-based assays, any unbound labeled target must be removed through a series of washes composed of different concentrations of salts and detergents before detection.

## Detection, image processing, transformation and normalization

Detection of the labeled target hybridized to the probes is once again platform-specific, but generally involves detection and quantification of the fluorescent signal. Typically, a fluorescent image of the array is acquired by laser-scanning confocal microscopy. The microarray scanner contains a set of lasers that produce light at the necessary wavelengths to excite fluorescent molecules. The intensity of the emitted light is quantified by a photomultiplier tube. A composite image is then created from the scans and the resulting quantified light intensities converted into ratios of relative expression. Microarray platforms are detected as single channel or two-channel (Figure 6.2). Single-channel analysis is primarily used in the context of microarrays created by photolithography (25), where quantification for each sample is generated on a different chip, with a single fluorescent tag, and the different images compared. In contrast, two-channel platforms differ in that a pair of samples is compared. Nucleic acid pairs are differentially labeled fluorescently, allowed to hybridize together on a single microarray, and scanned to generate a fluorescent image from the two channels (4). While both platforms can produce high-quality and reproducible results, the advantages of single channel detection lies in the fact that the results of a given experiment will not affect the data derived from another sample, since there is only one labeled DNA/RNA hybridizing to the microarray. In contrast, the poor quality of one sample could impinge on the results of the analysis of the other sample when performing two-channel assays. However, single channel analysis requires the use of more chips for analysis. Once the image has been captured, the relative intensity information must be converted into numerical information relating to gene expression. Commercial microarray providers such as Affymetrix, Agilent and others have integrated image-processing software tailored to their respective platforms, whereas in-house facilities must develop custom software suited for their particular needs.

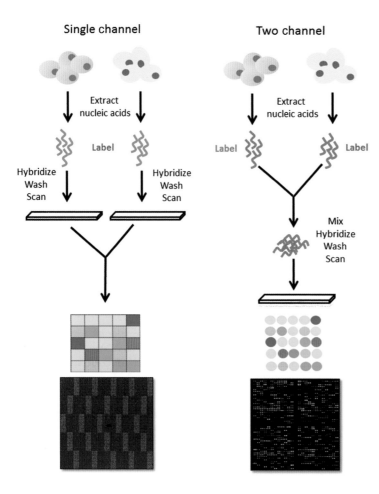

**Single channel**

Extract
nucleic acids

Label

Hybridize
Wash
Scan

**Two channel**

Extract
nucleic acids

Label

Label

Mix
Hybridize
Wash
Scan

**Figure 6.2 Single and two channel-based microarray assays**
In each case, nucleic acids from the test and/or reference samples are extracted and labeled; however, two-channel assays require differential labeling. Single channel methods, such as those used by Affymetrix Inc., hybridize, wash and scan each sample to its own chip. Relative analyses are then performed through the integration of the necessary chips in the study series. In contrast, two-channel assays require the mixing of the differentially labeled nucleic acids, which are then hybridized to the array. The relative fluorescence of each of the differentially labeled nucleic acids is then determined. Images courtesy of Affymetrix Inc. and J. Bayani.

Central to all microarray image analysis is the ability to identify the spot, properly separate the spot from other spots, quantify the signal intensity and perform quality assessments of the spot.

The raw intensity values are commonly converted into logarithmic intensities prior to proceeding with analysis. Transforming raw values to their logarithmic values serves to ensure that there is a reasonable distribution of intensities across the dataset, and that such intensities all fall within the expected bell-shaped distribution (26). To account for missing information, either due to poor hybridization between the target and probe, background or scratches to the array; pre-processing algorithms must consider the situation that a complete dataset may not always be possible. Various missing data estimation approaches

are available and form part of the pre-processing features of both commercially available and in-house generated software (27). Despite the fact that microarrays have been in common use for over a decade, there are still multiple and different methods for normalizing data (28). For more comprehensive description of normalization methods, the reader is directed to methods described by Quackenbush (28). Briefly, normalization of data refers to the removal of the effects of any source of variation that is not due to sample biology. These factors may include differential incorporation of fluorescent molecules into the target nucleic acid, the effects of fluorescence quenching of one dye when exposed to the excitation wavelength of another, or imperfections due to microarray fabrication (i.e. spot deposition, scratches, surface chemistry, etc). Integral to this point is the presence of proper experimental and technical controls that provide information on the sensitivity and reliability of the results by minimizing the number of both false-positive and false-negative features. Most commercially produced microarrays are integrated with such controls and replicates to ensure that the produced results are within acceptable parameters. There are three broad types of normalization: normalization that attempts to minimize the variances among the features within an array; normalization between multiple arrays, which reduces the variation between arrays; and normalization based on replicate experiments. Of these normalization procedures, global normalization methods and intensity-dependent normalization approaches are most commonly applied within the context of normalization within the array (28). Global normalization considers the total intensities of all the features on the array; while intensity-dependent normalization accounts for intensity variances between features particularly for those features at very low intensities as well as those at intensities that exceed the saturation level. When analysis of a given sample is covered over multiple arrays, then values need to be scaled to the same level for subsequent analysis. Finally, the robustness of microarray data can be assessed through replicate experiments, thus normalizations based on replicates can utilize the mean or median of each gene across the replicate experiments.

## Analysis

The analysis of microarray experiment continues to be the subject of controversy, debate and modification, and is dependent on the nature of the information that is being sought and whether such information is being collected in the context of research/discovery/validation or for clinical diagnostics. There is no shortage of methods for the analyses of microarray data and the reader should access these resources for more detailed explanations of the varying methods. In its basic form, microarray analysis serves to identify similarities or differences between samples (Figure 6.3a, b, c). For RNA, the convention has been to detect a twofold change in expression relative to the comparator (Figure 6.3a), while for DNA copy-number, the goal is to detect features that deviate from the expected normal of two copies per cell. The use of microarrays in the research space

focused largely on the discovery of expression or copy-number signatures between diseased and normal states or clinical parameters, as well as the elucidation molecular pathways and targets of therapeutic intervention. To identify such gene signatures or genes of significance, a number of analyses methods have been devised as reviewed by Butte (29) and will be briefly summarized here.

Supervised approaches are used to find genes with characteristics (i.e. expression, copy-number) that are different between groups of samples, as well as finding genes that can accurately predict a characteristic of that sample. Supervised analyses rely on an *a priori* knowledge or expectation of a particular pattern or outcome, for which the significance of the genes selected are evaluated by parametric and non-parametric tests, as well as analysis of variance (30). When conducting supervised analyses, four characteristics are generally considered: absolute expression level; subtractive degree of change between groups; fold change between groups; and reproducibility of the measurement (29). In contrast, unsupervised methods attempt to elucidate relationships in the dataset with no pre-existing expectation of the results (Figure 6.3b). There are several main forms of unsupervised classes: feature determination, such as principal-components analysis (PCA) (31); cluster determination, such as nearest neighbor clustering (32), self-organizing maps (33), k-means clustering and one- and two-dimensional hierarchical clustering (34); and network determination by Boolean (35) or Bayesian networks (36). The use of either method of analyses relies heavily on the nature of the hypothesis.

## From discovery to diagnostics

Microarray technology has been refined and developed over two decades and the key question is whether microarrays can be reliably used in the diagnostic setting. The use of microarray platforms in the diagnostic setting requires comprehensive quality control measures to ensure the fidelity of the results, as the tolerance for error in this setting is extremely low. Large discovery studies, most prominently in the context of breast cancer, have led to the development of expression microarrays of reduced gene sets for diagnostic purposes or to multiplex qRT-PCR assays suitable for clinical diagnostics (37–41). The availability of a number of these risk-prediction tests to breast cancer patients has increased pressure on healthcare

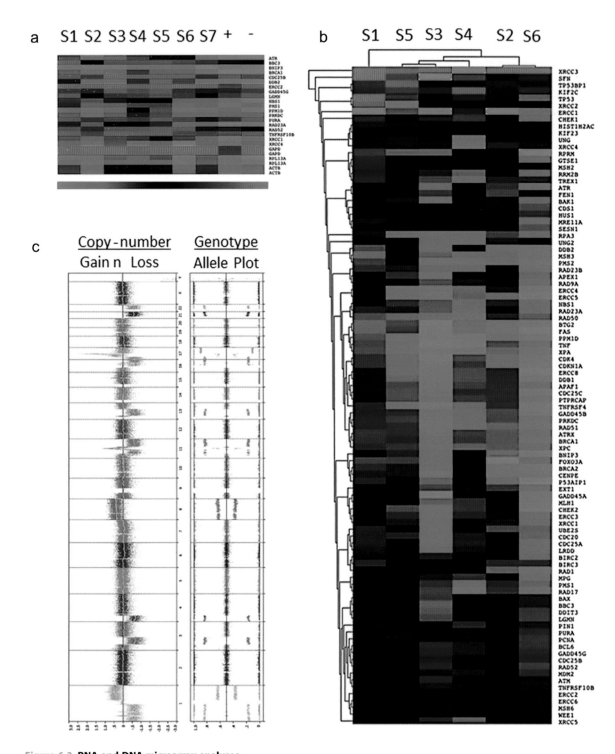

**Figure 6.3 RNA and DNA microarray analyses**

A. RNA expression plots of individual cancer RNAs in columns with gene annotations across the rows normalized against normal tissues, housekeeping genes and controls. Relative expression intensities are shown below, with red indicating relative over-expression and green indicating relative decreased expression in the cancer compared to the normal tissues (images courtesy of J. Bayani). B. Unsupervised clustering using the Eisen Clustering software (34) showing relationships between all samples based on their relative gene expression, and

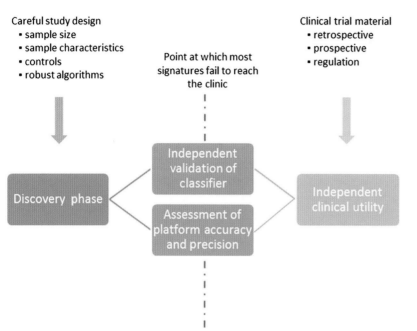

Careful study design
- sample size
- sample characteristics
- controls
- robust algorithms

Point at which most
signatures fail to reach
the clinic

Clinical trial material
- retrospective
- prospective
- regulation

**Figure 6.4** Steps to bringing a test to the clinic.

Discovery phase

Independent
validation of
classifier

Assessment of
platform accuracy
and precision

Independent
clinical utility

systems to evaluate their utility (to be discussed below). Furthermore, the information generated by high density of SNP arrays and alike have resulted in many of these technologies slowly replacing cytogenetic analyses such as G-banding analysis and FISH for pre-natal diagnostics and clinical genetics (42). Paralleled improvements in software and hardware now permit many of these diagnostic tests to be performed in hospital or clinic settings, rather than samples being delivered to reference laboratories. However, despite the vast amount of discovery data generated by microarrays, very few microarray gene signatures have made their way to the clinic, due to the challenges of signature validation and assay stability. A number of basic requirements must be met before microarrays can be used in a diagnostic setting (Figure 6.4).

## Accuracy and precision

Many microarray-based signatures fail to move towards the clinic due to an inability to perform independent validation. A major concern for clinical diagnostics is whether molecular markers can be accurately detected and whether the platforms upon which the markers will be assayed produce reproducible results. Accuracy is generally defined as how close a measurement is to the actual or true value; whereas precision is related to the reproducibility of the measurement under the same conditions. It can be argued, however, that it is uncertain whether accuracy can be truly assessed in the context of RNA, as it is still unclear as to how RNA molecules should be quantified. This should not, however, restrict the use of appropriate surrogates to determine accuracy.

To address these issues, the Microarray Quality Control (MAQC) project was initiated by the Food and Drug Administration (FDA) to assess reproducibility between different microarray platforms and laboratories, to provide a framework for quality control tools and to develop guidelines for microarray analyses. The MAQC project currently provides large reference datasets, together with accessible reference RNA samples (www.fda.gov/nctr/science/centers/toxi coinfomatics/maqc). Other consortiums such as the

---

Figure 6.3 (*cont.*) indicates sample 1 is less similar than all other samples. Additionally, samples 5 and 3, and samples 2 and 6, show more similarity to each other than between each other (images courtesy of J. Bayani). C. DNA copy-number and allele frequency analyses using the Affymetrix SNP array. Copy-number gains and losses are reflected to the left of the figure for each feature represented across each chromosome in the human genome. The plot to the right illustrates the allele frequency of each SNP represented on the array. A normal heterozygote call has a frequency of 0.5, with shifts in allele frequency due to loss of heterozygosity. Images courtesy of Affymetrix Inc. (22).

External RNA Control Consortium (ERCC) and Microarray Gene Expression Data (MGED) Society have been involved with developing consistency and reliability of microarray platforms. The first phase of the MAQC evaluated seven microarray platforms produced by Applied Biosystems, Affymetrix, Agilent Technologies, GE Healthcare, Illumina, Eppendorf and the National Cancer Institute (43). At least three independent test sites evaluated each platform, with five replicates of each platform on four different reference sample types, provided by MAQC. The four reference RNA samples comprised a mixture of a Universal Human Reference RNA (UHRR; Stratagene) and Human Brain Reference RNA (HBRR; Ambion), created in the following manner: 100% UHRR; 100% HBRR; 75% UHRR:25% HBRR and 25% UHRR:75% HBRR. Additionally, the RNA pools were tested on alternative platforms, including the TaqMan Gene Expression system (Applied Biosystems), StaRT-PCR (Gene Express) and QuantiGene (Panomics), as an independent method for accessing the relative accuracy of the microarray platforms being evaluated. Reassuringly, results were reproducible within the test sites, between test sites and comparable across the seven platforms. The median coefficient of variation for within-laboratory replicates ranged from 5% to 15%; with 10% to 20% variability between laboratory replicates, despite each platform differing in array fabrication, probe design, labeling and detection (44). Moreover, comparison of microarray results of several hundreds of genes by qRT-PCR showed correlation coefficients from 0.79 to 0.92. While encouraging, the detected variability could be challenging in the context of diagnostic medicine. Nevertheless, the results of phase I led to the publication of guidelines for the submission of genomic data to the FDA in the initial steps of bringing molecular markers to the clinical setting (www.fda.gov/downloads/Drugs/GuidanceComplianceRegulatoryInformation/Guidances/ucm079855.pdf). Our own studies have shown that variability between microarray platforms can be minimized through careful experimental design at the outset (45) and accounting for intra-experimental variation (46). The assessment of technical variation between replicate hybridizations of UHRR and individual or pooled breast-tumor RNAs between Affymetrix and Illumina platforms identified systemic noise in all datasets, which appeared to be the greatest at the sample preparation stage of the experimental workflow. Replicate extractions accounted for 40.6% of the

total variation, in contrast to 13.9% due to amplification and labeling; and 10.8% due to replicate hybridizations (45). These results have implications for both diagnostic medicine and the use of reference controls, as it was shown from this work that long periods of frozen storage and repeated freeze-thaw cycles contributed to less variability than re-extracting the same tissue, or even preparing a new cDNA source from the same RNA. Moreover, it calls into question the proper calibrator for reference samples, which is often dictated by the nature of the information being sought. Nevertheless, it suggests that such reference samples should be derived from a pooled source. As with the MAQC study (43), probe design can affect the observed expression findings; and results from our study showed that a significant trend was seen in favor of low-GC content in the core set of probes consistently affected by inter-run and inter-chip variation between sample duplicates (45). This is not entirely surprising, as hybridization conditions favor greater probe:target annealing at higher GC-content.

An additional requirement is the development of reproducible multivariate gene expression-based prediction models, also referred to as classifiers. Such models take gene expression data from a patient as input and, as an output, produce a prediction of a clinically relevant outcome for that patient. Therefore, the second phase of the MAQC project (MAQC-II) focused on the reproducibility of classifiers (47), studying how they are developed and evaluated. A number of factors affect the reliability of a classifier, as benchmarking studies may have been derived from datasets split at random with one part used for training, and the other for validation, as well as biases in sampling and quality of tissues within and across participating institutions during the months/years of accrual. The MAQC-II utilized six microarray datasets which were analyzed by 36 independent teams to generate predictive models with regard to 13 endpoints. Over 30,000 models were built, with model prediction performance being endpoint-dependent. Interestingly, both experienced and novice data analyses teams were prone to simple errors, strongly indicating that a mechanism must be implemented to ensure the reliability of the results being reported by microarray experiments. The MAQC-II project made the following recommendations for model building: (1) study design should include a sample set that is sufficiently powered to provide a good ratio between the sample size and classifier complexity; (2)

pilot study or internal validation can be accomplished by bootstrap or cross-validation methods. Samples from the pilot study are not replaced for the pivotal study, but are added to achieve the "appropriate" target size; (3) the pivotal or external validation sets should be completely separate, but there is value in swapping samples to test the reliability of the model; and (4) re-use of the independent validation set after modifications to an originally designed and validated data analysis algorithm continues to be of concern, and the MAQC strongly recommends against this approach.

## Validation for clinical use

The scientific literature contains many reports of promising gene signatures. However, few attain the level I evidence required (48) to enter clinical practice (see Table 6.3). The first step in bringing a gene signature, or any test, to the clinic is the ability to independently validate the biomarker. The Mamma-Print® 70-gene signature (Agendia), which is an array-based test commercially available to women with breast cancer, was initially developed in a series of untreated node negative patients from the Netherlands Cancer Institute diagnosed with primary breast cancer analyzed by the whole-genome-expression of 25,000 genes (49). Unsupervised clustering identified a number of significant genes that predicted a good prognosis (i.e. no distant metastasis >5 years) and poor prognosis signature (i.e. distant metastasis <5 years), which was refined to the final 70 genes associated with metastasis. However, prior to entering clinical use, subsequent signature validation studies had to be performed, including demonstration of accuracy and precision of the diagnostic array. With clinical validation of the 70-gene signature, the move towards a diagnostic test still required conversion from a 25,000 60-mer oligonucleotide microarray in the original study (49) to a diagnostic version of the 70-gene signature, MammaPrint®, and the evaluation of the platform's robustness for use in the clinical setting (50) as mini-arrays. The conversion to mini-arrays enabled an increase in precision. Comparison of the tumors hybridized to the mini-array as compared to the original study showed a Pearson correlation of 0.92 (p<0.0001). The overall accuracy was identified by calculating the odds ratio for the development of distant metastases within five years. The odds ratio of the mini-array

(OR = 13.95%, CI 3.9 to 44) was highly comparable to the original data (OR = 15%, CI 2.1 to 19). The authors recognized that while the technical reproducibility of the diagnostic assay was high, the chance of misclassification was higher among patients who were further away from the two prognosis thresholds. Based on the cases analyzed at the time of the evaluation (2006), this affected less than 1.1% of samples.

With the robustness of the platform assessed, clinical validation studies utilized a subset of patients (41), performed to evaluate the ability to estimate the risk of metastases. The probability of a patient remaining free of distant metastases, and overall survival according to the prognosis profile, between the original data and that generated by the diagnostic test was highly similar, with a Pearson correlation of 0.88 (p<0.0001).

## Do microarray-based signatures add clinical value?

While a commercial test may be available, the question remains as to whether it adds clinical value. The current challenges for women newly diagnosed with breast cancer include the ability to predict their prognosis, and to predict which additional systemic chemo- or endocrine-therapy is needed. Prognostic indices such as Adjuvant!Online (www.adjuvanton line.com/) and the Nottingham Prognostic Index (51) are meant to act as a guide for clinical management based on clinical and pathologic variables, but still lack prognostic power. In comparing Mamma-Print® to Adjuvant!Online, the 70-gene signature was found to be a better prognostic biomarker than Adjuvant!Online and provided an independent risk assessment, with a 28% to 35% discordance between the two, in low- and high-risk groups; suggesting that discordant patients had clinical outcomes that were more accurately predicted by the microarray assay (52, 53). Moreover, analyses showed that in patients who received either endocrine treatment or chemotherapy followed by endocrine treatment, the distant disease-free survival at five years was determined for MammaPrint® high- and low-risk groups. Those in the MammaPrint® low-risk group who received endocrine therapy alone had a distant disease-free survival (DDFS) of 93% compared with 99% for those patients who received chemotherapy plus endocrine therapy (HR = 0.26, 95% CI, 0.03– 2.02; p = 0.20). The high-risk patients who received endocrine therapy had a DDFS of 76%, compared to 88% among patients who received endocrine therapy plus chemotherapy (HR = 0.35, 95% CI, 0.17– 0.71; p > 0.01). Results were similar in multivariate analysis (54).

With a robust test available, the next question was the impact of such tests in treatment decision making. In this respect, clinical trials are required to answer these questions. In the prospective microaRAy-prognoSTics-in-breast-cancER (RASTER) study, 427 patients were evaluated and adjuvant systemic treatment decisions were based on the Dutch CBO 2004 guidelines, the 70-gene signature and doctors' and patients' preferences. The five-year distant-recurrence-free-interval (DRFI) probabilities confirmed the additional prognostic value of MammaPrint® to clinicopathological risk estimations such as Adjuvant! OnLine. In those patients who were deemed low risk by MammaPrint®, the omission of adjuvant chemotherapy appeared not to compromise outcome (55). These findings led to the evaluation of MammaPrint's® clinical value and impact on healthcare economics. The Microarray In Node-negative and 1 to 3 positive lymph node Disease may Avoid ChemoTherapy (MINDACT) trial was developed with the primary purpose of determining whether the gene array signature by MammaPrint® (genomic prognosis) was superior to conventional clinical pathology parameters (clinical prognosis) in determining which patients would benefit from chemotherapy. In addition, MINDACT also compared two different chemotherapy regimens and two different hormonal therapy regimens. The recent findings of the pilot phase of 800 patients showed that the potential reduction in adjuvant chemotherapy by using the genomic signature and compliance to treatment assignment were in accordance with the trial hypotheses (56). Similarly, recruitment of breast cancer patients has just begun for the United Kingdom Optimal Personalised Treatment of early breast cancer using Multiparameter Analysis (UK-OPTIMA) trial, which evaluates technologies, including microarray-based assays, that are available for improving patient selection for chemotherapy, and is the first to focus on the relative cost-effectiveness of alternate predictive assays and the impact test-guided treatment has on the patient (57). There are still no commercial microarray assays that predict those who may benefit from a particular treatment in contrast to those who would not benefit and could be spared the toxicities of treatment, although there are a number of proof-of-

principle studies that have attempted to identify patients sensitive and resistant to various chemotherapeutics (58).

Perhaps a crucial factor of whether a signature has clinical value lies in the answer to the question of what is "low" enough risk that will lead a patient to forgo systemic chemotherapy. Indeed, the categorization of "low" risk must consider not only the absolute risk of relapse, but the risks associated with treatment side effects, personal preferences of the patient and their ability to pay for treatment. The risk of adverse reactions may be deemed a necessary risk for the small gains in survival for some; while others are not willing to undergo the toxicities associated with these treatments for little or uncertain benefit.

## Regulation and guidelines

The Evaluation of Genomic Applications in Practice and Prevention (EGAPP) Working Group was established as an independent panel to develop a systematic process for evidence-based assessment, focused on genetic tests and other applications of genomic technology (59). Similarly, sub-committees of the National Cancer Institute and European Organisation for Research and Treatment of Cancer (NCI-EORTC) generated Reporting Recommendations for Tumor Marker Prognostic Studies (REMARK) (60), as have the National Association of Clinical Biochemists (NACB) (USA) (61). These working groups have helped to define the framework for validation of molecular markers. Common to all of these guidelines is the requirement for clinical utility and analytical and clinical validation (48) (Table 6.2). Within the FDA, the Office of *in vitro* Diagnostics (OIVD) within the Center for Devices and Radiological Health (CDRH) regulates clinical devices. FDA recommendations on *In Vitro* Diagnostic Multivariate Index Assays (IVDMIAs) continue to be developed in the context of all Laboratory Developed Tests (LDTs); and as these regulatory debates carry on, biotechnology companies continue to strive for level I evidence in validation studies, to satisfy clinicians, stakeholders and regulators.

## Status of microarrays in the clinic
## Diagnostic RNA profiling

A number of commercially available risk assessment tests for breast cancer initially derived by expression

**Table 6.2** NACB recommendations for use of microarrays in cancer diagnostics

**Recommendations**

Gene expression microarrays are new and promising devices used for cancer diagnosis, prognosis, prediction of therapeutic response, and monitoring and selection of therapy. The level of evidence from most published studies, according to Hayes (48), is level V [lowest category]. Consequently, microarrays should continue to be used as research devices, but not as tools for making clinical decisions.

Standardization and clinical validation of expression microarrays is warranted.

Quality control and quality assurance programs for expression microarrays need to be further developed.

Microarray automation is encouraged for improving reproducibility, throughput and robustness.

Tissue microarrays are devices suitable for high-throughput analysis of large numbers of samples and are recommended for use in clinical trials and retrospective studies for evaluating and validating new tumor markers by immunohistochemical analysis.

Use of microarrays for single nucleotide polymorphism analysis is recommended for establishing haplotypes and for correlating these haplotypes to disease predisposition.

Use of microarrays is recommended for high-throughput genotyping and mutation/sequence variation detection for cancer diagnostics and pharmacogenomics. More validation is necessary to ensure equivalent results between standard technologies (such as DNA sequencing) and microarray analysis.

Protein microarrays and other similar technologies are recommended as research tools for multiparametric analysis of large numbers of proteins. The level of evidence is not as yet high enough for clinical applications.

Standardized protocols should be developed for sample collection, handling and processing.

Adapted from the National Association of Clinical Biochemists (NABC) Laboratory Medicine Practice Guidelines (61).

**Table 6.3** Levels of evidence

| Level | Description |
|---|---|
| I | Evidence from a single, high-powered, prospective, controlled study that is specifically designed to test marker, or evidence from a meta-analysis, pooled analysis or overview of level II or III studies. |
| II | Evidence from a study in which marker data are determined in relationship to prospective therapeutic trial that is performed to test therapeutic hypothesis, but not specifically designed to test marker utility. |
| III | Evidence from large prospective studies. |
| IV | Evidence from small retrospective studies. |
| V | Evidence from small pilot studies. |

Based on Hayes (48).

microarray analysis include: the 50-gene intrinsic subtyping and risk assessment signature Prosigna (NanoString Technologies) (49, 52, 57); the risk assessment 21-gene test, Oncotype DX® (Genomic Health) (51, 64); and the 70-gene signature of risk, MammaPrint® Agendia (53, 64). TargetPrint® is a microarray-based gene expression assay that provides quantitative assessment ER, PR and HER2, while BluePrint® (62) is an 80-gene signature profile for the classification of breast cancer tumors into Basal-type, Luminal-type and ERBB2-type subclasses (40). Comparison between the three tests showed that use of the Agendia suite of tests performed as well as locally performed tests by IHC or FISH/ISH, while minimizing the lack of standardization for IHC markers like Ki67 (63). Of these RNA-based expression tests, only MammaPrint®, BluePrint® and TargetPrint® remain as traditional microarray-based tests.

However, another intrinsic subtyping and risk test, Prosigna, based on NanoString technology (34), has recently received FDA 510(k) approval for use. Like BluePrint®, the Prosigna 50-gene intrinsic-subtyping signature was developed around the study by Perou *et al.* (40), through the hierarchical clustering of cDNA results, grouping genes on the basis of similarity in the pattern of expression, and giving rise to the intrinsic subtypes Luminal A, Luminal B, ERBB2 Enriched, Basal-like and the Normal-like groups. Integration of subtype and tumor size, called the C-index, was a significant improvement on either the clinicopathologic model or subtype models alone. The intrinsic subtype model predicted neoadjuvant chemotherapy efficacy with a negative predictive value for pCR of 97%. These studies were validated

83

based on a qRT-PCR platform; however, the FDA-approved Prosigna test has been developed and validated on the NanoString platform (34). Recent data presented by Chia and colleagues indicate the benefit of the 50-gene signature for the prognosis and prediction of benefit from adjuvant tamoxifen (37).

Agendia has also made available a microarray-based gene expression profile for predicting the recurrence of stages II and III colon cancer patients called ColoPrint® (64). Using the same strategy as MammaPrint®, ColoPrint® was clinically validated on 135 patients who underwent curative resection (R0) for colon cancer stage II. The last member of the Agendia repertoire of microarray-based tests is the ThernaPrint® panel of 56 genes that have been identified as potential targets for prognosis and therapeutic response to a variety of therapies.

## Diagnostic DNA profiling

The transition of DNA profiling using microarrays into the clinic has been relatively more simple due to the routine use of cytogenetic techniques and sequencing. Chromosomal analyses have confirmed the relationship between chromosomal abnormalities and congenital syndromes as well as in cancer, and this has been discussed at length in Chapter 4. There is now an increasing movement in many molecular and clinical cytogenetic laboratories to adopt whole genome DNA analysis for the identification of mutations and copy-number aberrations associated with disease.

Considerable progress has been made in the implementation of microarrays for pre- and postnatal diagnostics; however, the situation for cancers is much different. To date, there are no diagnostic DNA assays for cancers. However, the findings in medulloblastomas are promising, with genomic profiling revealing patterns that segregated these childhood brain tumors into clinically distinct groups (65).

## The future of microarrays and summary

We have discussed the use of microarrays in a diagnostic setting provided the assays are robust and reproducible, that the intended results obtained for the tests have been validated and that they add clinical value. However, there is an argument that the reduction of large gene signatures to a handful of critical genes can be assayed by quantitative PCR methods, which have been already been standardized, validated and are scalable. Moreover, sequencing technologies are becoming less expensive and less prone to errors, suggesting that cancers may be sequenced diagnostically both at the DNA and RNA levels in the future.

## References

1. International Human Genome Sequencing Consortium. Finishing the euchromatic sequence of the human genome. *Nature* 2004; 431(7011): 931–45.

2. Lander, E. S., Linton, L. M., Birren, B., Nusbaum, C., Zody, M. C., Baldwin, J. *et al.* Initial sequencing and analysis of the human genome. *Nature* 2001; 409 (6822): 860–921.

3. Fodor, S. P., Read, J. L., Pirrung, M. C., Stryer, L., Lu, A. T. and Solas, D. Light-directed, spatially addressable parallel chemical synthesis. *Science* 1991; 251(4995): 767–73.

4. Schena, M., Shalon, D., Davis, R. W. and Brown, P. O. Quantitative monitoring of gene expression patterns with a complementary DNA microarray. *Science* 1995; 270(5235): 467–70.

5. Alwine, J. C., Kemp, D. J. and Stark, G. R. Method for detection of specific RNAs in agarose gels by transfer to diazobenzyloxymethyl-paper and hybridization with DNA probes. *Proc Natl Acad Sci USA* 1977; 74(12): 5350–4.

6. Di Leva, G. and Croce, C. M. miRNA profiling of cancer. *Curr Opin Genet Dev* 2013; 23(1): 3–11.

7. Lovf, M., Thomassen, G. O., Bakken, A. C., Celestino, R., Fioretos, T., Lind, G. E. *et al.* Fusion gene microarray reveals cancer type-specificity among fusion genes. *Gene Chromosome Canc* 2011; 50(5): 348–57.

8. Kallioniemi, A., Kallioniemi, O. P., Sudar, D., Rutovitz, D., Gray, J. W., Waldman, F. *et al.* Comparative genomic hybridization for molecular cytogenetic analysis of solid tumors. *Science* 1992; 258(5083): 818–21.

9. Pollack, J. R., Perou, C. M., Alizadeh, A. A., Eisen, M. B., Pergamenschikov, A., Williams, C. F. *et al.* Genome-wide analysis of DNA copy-number changes using cDNA microarrays. *Nat Genet* 1999; 23(1): 41–6.

10. Pinkel, D., Segraves, R., Sudar, D., Clark, S., Poole, I., Kowbel, D. *et al.* High resolution analysis of DNA copy number variation using comparative genomic hybridization to microarrays. *Nat Genet* 1998; 20(2): 207–11.

11. Carter, N. P. Methods and strategies for analyzing copy

number variation using DNA microarrays. *Nat Genet* 2007; 39(7 Suppl.): S16–S21.

12. Lupski, J. R. Genomic disorders: structural features of the genome can lead to DNA rearrangements and human disease traits. *Trends Genet* 1998; 14(10): 417–22.

13. Emanuel, B. S. and Saitta, S. C. From microscopes to microarrays: dissecting recurrent chromosomal rearrangements. *Nat Rev Genet* 2007; 8(11): 869–83.

14. Gitan, R. S., Shi, H., Chen, C. M., Yan, P. S. and Huang, T. H. Methylation-specific oligonucleotide microarray: a new potential for high-throughput methylation analysis. *Genome Res* 2002; 12(1): 158–64.

15. Blat, Y., Protacio, R. U., Hunter, N. and Kleckner, N. Physical and functional interactions among basic chromosome organizational features govern early steps of meiotic chiasma formation. *Cell* 2002; 111(6): 791–802.

16. Ren, B., Robert, F., Wyrick, J. J., Aparicio, O., Jennings, E. G., Simon, I. *et al.* Genome-wide location and function of DNA binding proteins. *Science* 2000; 290(5500): 2306–9.

17. Chang, T. W. Binding of cells to matrixes of distinct antibodies coated on solid surface. *J Immunol Methods* 1983; 65(1–2): 217–23.

18. Bertone, P. and Snyder, M. Advances in functional protein microarray technology. *FEBS J* 2005; 272(21): 5400–11.

19. Zhu, H., Bilgin, M., Bangham, R., Hall, D., Casamayor, A., Bertone, P. *et al.* Global analysis of protein activities using proteome chips. *Science* 2001; 293(5537): 2101–5.

20. Speer, R., Wulfkuhle, J. D., Liotta, L. A. and Petricoin, E. F., III. Reverse-phase protein microarrays for tissue-based analysis. *Curr Opin Mol Ther* 2005; 7(3): 240–5.

21. Oliphant, A., Barker, D. L., Stuelpnagel, J. R. and Chee, M. S. BeadArray technology: enabling an accurate, cost-effective approach to high-throughput genotyping. *Biotechniques* 2002; 56(8): 60–1.

22. Geiss, G. K., Bumgarner, R. E., Birditt, B., Dahl, T., Dowidar, N., Dunaway, D. L. *et al.* Direct multiplexed measurement of gene expression with color-coded probe pairs. *Nat Biotechnol* 2008; 26(3): 317–25.

23. Eisen, M. B. and Brown, P. O. DNA arrays for analysis of gene expression. *Methods Enzymol* 1999; 303: 179–205.

24. Richter, A., Schwager, C., Hentze, S., Ansorge, W., Hentze, M. W. and Muckenthaler, M. Comparison of fluorescent tag DNA labeling methods used for expression analysis by DNA microarrays. *Biotechniques* 2002; 33(3): 620–8, 630.

25. Lockhart, D. J., Dong, H., Byrne, M. C., Follettie, M. T., Gallo, M. V., Chee, M. S. *et al.* Expression monitoring by hybridization to high-density oligonucleotide arrays. *Nat Biotechnol* 1996; 14(13): 1675–80.

26. Thygesen, H. H. and Zwinderman, A. H. Comparing transformation methods for DNA microarray data. *BMC Bioinformatics* 2004; 5: 77.

27. Troyanskaya, O., Cantor, M., Sherlock, G., Brown, P., Hastie, T., Tibshirani, R. *et al.* Missing value estimation methods for DNA microarrays. *Bioinformatics* 2001; 17(6): 520–5.

28. Quackenbush, J. Microarray data normalization and transformation. *Nat Genet* 2002; 32(Suppl.): 496–501.

29. Butte, A. The use and analysis of microarray data. *Nat Rev Drug Discov* 2002; 1(12): 951–60.

30. Butte, A. J., Ye, J., Haring, H. U., Stumvoll, M., White, M. F. and Kohane, I. S. Determining significant fold differences in gene expression analysis. *Pac Symp Biocomput* 2001; 6: 6–17.

31. Raychaudhuri, S., Stuart, J. M. and Altman, R. B. Principal components analysis to summarize microarray experiments: application to sporulation time series. *Pac Symp Biocomput* 2000; 455–66.

32. Golub, T. R., Slonim, D. K., Tamayo, P., Huard, C., Gaasenbeek, M., Mesirov, J. P. *et al.* Molecular classification of cancer: class discovery and class prediction by gene expression monitoring. *Science* 1999; 286 (5439): 531–7.

33. Toronen, P., Kolehmainen, M., Wong, G. and Castren, E. Analysis of gene expression data using self-organizing maps. *FEBS Lett* 1999; 451(2): 142–6.

34. Eisen, M. B., Spellman, P. T., Brown, P. O. and Botstein, D. Cluster analysis and display of genome-wide expression patterns. *Proc Natl Acad Sci USA* 1998; 95(25): 14863–8.

35. Szallasi, Z. and Liang, S. Modeling the normal and neoplastic cell cycle with "realistic Boolean genetic networks": their application for understanding carcinogenesis and assessing therapeutic strategies. *Pac Symp Biocomput* 1998; 66–76.

36. Friedman, N., Linial, M., Nachman, I. and Pe'er, D. Using Bayesian networks to analyze expression data. *J Comput Biol* 2000; 7(3–4): 601–20.

37. Chia, S. K., Bramwell, V. H., Tu, D., Shepherd, L. E., Jiang, S., Vickery, T. *et al.* A 50-gene intrinsic subtype classifier for prognosis and prediction of benefit from adjuvant tamoxifen. *Clin Cancer Res* 2012; 18(16): 4465–72.

38. Nielsen, T. O., Parker, J. S., Leung, S., Voduc, D., Ebbert, M., Vickery, T. *et al.* A comparison of PAM50

intrinsic subtyping with immunohistochemistry and clinical prognostic factors in tamoxifen-treated estrogen receptor-positive breast cancer. *Clin Cancer Res* 2010; 16(21): 5222–32.

39. Paik, S., Tang, G., Shak, S., Kim, C., Baker, J., Kim, W. *et al.* Gene expression and benefit of chemotherapy in women with node-negative, estrogen receptor-positive breast cancer. *J Clin Oncol* 2006; 24(23): 3726–34.

40. Perou, C. M., Sorlie, T., Eisen, M. B., van de Rijn, M., Jeffrey, S. S., Rees, C. A. *et al.* Molecular portraits of human breast tumours. *Nature* 2000; 406(6797): 747–52.

41. van de Vijver, M. J., He, Y. D., van't Veer, L. J., Dai, H., Hart, A. A., Voskuil, D. W. *et al.* A gene-expression signature as a predictor of survival in breast cancer. *New Engl J Med* 2002; 347(25): 1999–2009.

42. Miller, D. T., Adam, M. P., Aradhya, S., Biesecker, L. G., Brothman, A. R., Carter, N. P. *et al.* Consensus statement: chromosomal microarray is a first-tier clinical diagnostic test for individuals with developmental disabilities or congenital anomalies. *Am J Hum Genet* 2010; 86(5): 749–64.

43. Shi, L., Reid, L. H., Jones, W. D., Shippy, R., Warrington, J. A., Baker, S. C. *et al.* The MicroArray Quality Control (MAQC) project shows inter- and intraplatform reproducibility of gene expression measurements. *Nat Biotechnol* 2006; 24(9): 1151–61.

44. Patterson, T. A., Lobenhofer, E. K., Fulmer-Smentek, S. B., Collins, P. J., Chu, T. M., Bao, W. *et al.* Performance comparison of one-color and two-color platforms within the MicroArray Quality Control (MAQC) project. *Nat Biotechnol* 2006; 24(9): 1140–50.

45. Kitchen, R. R., Sabine, V. S., Simen, A. A., Dixon, J. M., Bartlett, J. M. and Sims, A. H. Relative impact of key sources of systematic noise in Affymetrix and Illumina gene-expression microarray experiments. *BMC Genomics* 2011; 12: 589; doi: 10.1186/1471-2164-12-589.

46. Kitchen, R. R., Sabine, V. S., Sims, A. H., Macaskill, E. J., Renshaw, L., Thomas, J. S. *et al.* Correcting for intra-experiment variation in Illumina BeadChip data is necessary to generate robust gene-expression profiles. *BMC Genomics* 2010; 11: 134; doi:10.1186/1471-2164-11-134.

47. Shi, L., Campbell, G., Jones, W. D., Campagne, F., Wen, Z., Walker, S. J. *et al.* The MicroArray Quality Control (MAQC)-II study of common practices for the development and validation of microarray-based predictive models. *Nat Biotechnol* 2010; 28(8): 827–38.

48. Hayes, D. F. Prognostic and predictive factors for breast cancer: translating technology to oncology. *J Clin Oncol* 2005; 23(8): 1596–7.

49. van't Veer, L. J., Dai, H., van de Vijver, M. J., He, Y. D., Hart, A. A., Mao, M. *et al.* Gene expression profiling predicts clinical outcome of breast cancer. *Nature* 2002; 415(6871): 530–6.

50. Glas, A. M., Floore, A., Delahaye, L. J., Witteveen, A. T., Pover, R. C., Bakx, N. *et al.* Converting a breast cancer microarray signature into a high-throughput diagnostic test. *BMC Genomics* 2006; 7: 278.

51. Galea, M. H., Blamey, R. W., Elston, C. E. and Ellis, I. O. The Nottingham Prognostic Index in primary breast cancer. *Breast Cancer Res Treat* 1992; 22(3): 207–19.

52. Mook, S., Schmidt, M. K., Viale, G., Pruneri, G., Eekhout, I., Floore, A. *et al.* The 70-gene prognosis-signature predicts disease outcome in breast cancer patients with 1–3 positive lymph nodes in an independent validation study. *Breast Cancer Res Treat* 2009; 116(2): 295–302.

53. Mook, S., Schmidt, M. K., Weigelt, B., Kreike, B., Eekhout, I., van de Vijver, M. J. *et al.* The 70-gene prognosis signature predicts early metastasis in breast cancer patients between 55 and 70 years of age. *Ann Oncol* 2010; 21(4): 717–22.

54. Knauer, M., Mook, S., Rutgers, E. J., Bender, R. A., Hauptmann, M., van de Vijver, M. J. *et al.* The predictive value of the 70-gene signature for adjuvant chemotherapy in early breast cancer. *Breast Cancer Res Treat* 2010; 120(3): 655–61.

55. Drukker, C. A., Bueno-de-Mesquita, J. M., Retel, V. P., van Harten, W. H., van Tinteren, H., Wesseling, J. *et al.* A prospective evaluation of a breast cancer prognosis signature in the observational RASTER study. *Int J Cancer* 2013; 133(4): 929–36.

56. Cardoso, F., Van't Veer, L., Rutgers, E., Loi, S., Mook, S. and Piccart-Gebhart, M. J. Clinical application of the 70-gene profile: the MINDACT trial. *J Clin Oncol* 2008; 26(5): 729–35.

57. Bartlett, J., Canney, P., Campbell, A., Cameron, D., Donovan, J., Dunn, J. *et al.* Selecting breast cancer patients for chemotherapy: the opening of the UK OPTIMA trial. *Clin Oncol (R Coll Radiol)* 2013; 25(2): 109–16.

58. Mulligan, J. M., Hill, L. A., Deharo, S., Irwin, G., Boyle, D., Keating, K. E. *et al.* Identification and validation of an anthracycline/cyclophosphamide-based chemotherapy response assay in breast cancer. *J Natl Cancer Inst* 2014; 106(1): djt335.

59. Teutsch, S. M., Bradley, L. A., Palomaki, G. E., Haddow, J. E.,

Piper, M., Calonge, N. *et al.* The Evaluation of Genomic Applications in Practice and Prevention (EGAPP) Initiative: methods of the EGAPP Working Group. *Genet Med* 2009; 11(1): 3–14.

60. McShane, L. M., Altman, D. G., Sauerbrei, W., Taube, S. E., Gion, M. and Clark, G. M. REporting recommendations for tumour MARKer prognostic studies (REMARK). *Eur J Cancer* 2005; 41(12): 1690–6.

61. Sturgeon, C. M., Hoffman, B. R., Chan, D. W., Ch'ng, S. L., Hammond, E., Hayes, D. F. *et al.* National Academy of Clinical Biochemistry Laboratory Medicine Practice Guidelines for use of tumor markers in clinical practice: quality requirements. *Clin Chem* 2008; 54(8): e1–e10.

62. Krijgsman, O., Roepman, P., Zwart, W., Carroll, J. S., Tian, S., de Snoo, F. A. *et al.* A diagnostic gene profile for molecular subtyping of breast cancer associated with treatment response. *Breast Cancer Res Treat* 2012; 133(1): 37–47.

63. Nguyen, B., Cusumano, P. G., Deck, K., Kerlin, D., Garcia, A. A., Barone, J. L. *et al.* Comparison of molecular subtyping with BluePrint, MammaPrint, and TargetPrint to local clinical subtyping in breast cancer patients. *Ann Surg Oncol* 2012; 19(10): 3257–63.

64. Maak, M., Simon, I., Nitsche, U., Roepman, P., Snel, M., Glas, A. M. *et al.* Independent validation of a prognostic genomic signature (ColoPrint) for patients with stage II colon cancer. *Ann Surg* 2013; 257(6): 1053–8.

65. Northcott, P. A., Shih, D. J., Peacock, J., Garzia, L., Morrissy, A. S., Zichner, T. *et al.* Subgroup-specific structural variation across 1,000 medulloblastoma genomes. *Nature* 2012; 488(7409): 49–56.

# Tissue microarrays

**Chapter 7**

Luigi Tornillo

## Introduction

During the last three decades, the molecular machinery of the cancer cell has been deeply investigated, at different levels. High-throughput techniques (for example, cDNA microarrays, arrayCGH, protein array) led to the discovery of many candidate molecular biomarkers and therapeutic targets. Validation of these findings has been, for many years, the bottleneck of translational research. Several biomarkers are proteins, which are expressed in normal and abnormal tissues and are easily identified with immunohistochemistry (IHC) that also identifies their cellular and subcellular localization. This is often important for the function of the biomarker or for a correct targeting of a drug. Moreover, numeric and/or conformational genomic alterations may have diagnostic, prognostic or predictive value. The exact tissue localization of such alterations can be determined by using *in situ* techniques, such as fluorescent *in situ* hybridization (FISH) or chromogenic-ISH (CISH).

Both IHC and ISH are largely used on formalin-fixed paraffin-embedded (FFPE) material (1). The tissue microarray (TMA) (2) technique allows a rapid and cost-effective application of IHC and ISH to the vast majority of archival material retained in all institutes of pathology throughout the world.

## TMA: definition and development

TMAs are "miniaturized pathology archives" (Figure 7.1). Pathology archives contain many thousands of histologic slides and paraffin blocks and are an invaluable resource for translating the results of basic research (both "*in vitro*" and "*in vivo*") into the clinic.

The idea of combining multiple specimens in a single histology block, thus allowing a quick and cost-effective analysis, was first addressed by Hector Battifora in 1986 (3). He wrapped 1 mm thick "rods" of tissue, obtained from different specimens, in a sheet of small intestine. This "sausage" of tissues was then embedded in a paraffin wax block, from which

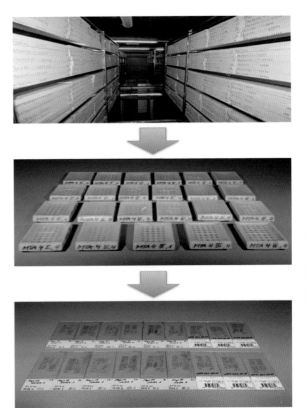

**Figure 7.1** Tissue microarray as miniaturized pathology archive ("tissue chips").

*Molecular Pathology: A Practical Guide for the Surgical Pathologist and Cytopathologist*, ed. John M. S. Bartlett, Abeer Shaaban and Fernando Schmitt. Published by Cambridge University Press. © Cambridge University Press, 2016.

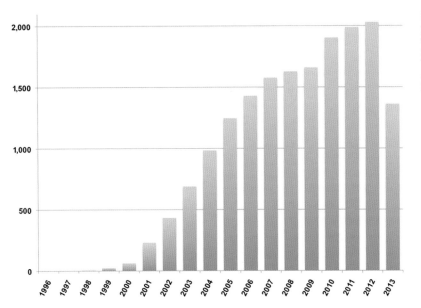

**Figure 7.2 Graphic of number of papers retrieved from the PubMed database by keyword "tissue microarray"**
The total number is 17,262. The last column includes papers published before June 30, 2013.

numerous sections were cut. In this way, up to 100 different specimens could be examined in a single histologic slide. The proposal of Battifora was mainly directed to quality control, testing of new reagents and intra- or inter-laboratory comparison, but did not receive a general acceptance because of the difficulty to identify the different rods in the multi-tissue block.

In 1998, Kononen *et al.* (2) described for the first time the TMA as an economic, reliable and efficient method for the high-throughput *in situ* analysis of large numbers of samples. Compared to the "sausage" technique, TMAs show distinct advantages, namely (4):

- preservation of the morphological integrity of the "donor" tissues (small cylinder, 0.6 to 2 mm diameter);
- possibility of cutting up to 200 slides of a TMA without any significant loss of data;
- exact positioning and orientation of the specimen through a two-dimensional (X-Y) coordinates system.

In summary, 15 years after first description of TMAs, the technology has gained a very important place in research and diagnostic laboratories and is an essential tool for translational research. A search in Pubmed with the "TMA" keyword retrieved more than 15,000 results (Figure 7.2).

## TMA construction

As discussed above, TMAs are miniaturized pathology archives (Figure 7.1). The idea is to collect multiple specimens in one single paraffin block. Every tissue core in a TMA is a "biopsy of a biopsy (block)". Therefore, the most important step of the entire procedure, which needs most of the time and cannot be fully automated, is the identification of the "donor" blocks and the collection of all the pertinent clinicopathological data (Figure 7.3). The production of a TMA can be summarized as follows:

- collection of possibly suitable samples;
- choice of suitable samples ("donor" blocks);
- identification of representative areas on HE slides;
- identification of the corresponding areas on the "donor" block;
- acquiring a cylindrical core (diameter 0.6 to 2 mm) from the "donor" block;
- embedding of the core in a "recipient" block.

To facilitate orientation, it is better to build the TMA asymmetrically (Figure 7.3). The position and identification of the cores within the recipient blocks are recorded. Generally, numbers identify rows and letters identify columns, so that the position of a specific core is identified as, for instance, "3f" (Figure 7.4). It is helpful to include some cores for orientation. Although there are some dedicated

**89**

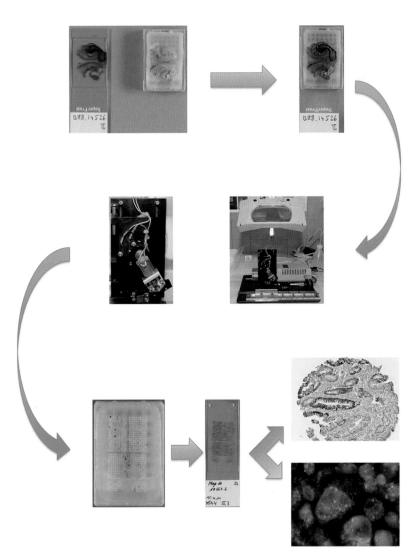

**Figure 7.3 Generation of a TMA**
The donor block is marked according to the slide (upper panel). Punches are taken from the donor block and embedded in the recipient block (middle panel). The recipient block can be cut and the slides can be stained (under panel).

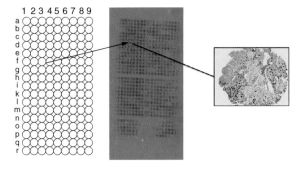

**Figure 7.4** Template of a TMA (left), with the corresponding slide (middle) and a stained core (right).

software packages, the most simple and efficient way to identify the core is, in our opinion, a simple Excel® file (2, 4). The file can be built mirroring the structure of the TMA (as a map) or as a simple table.

## Donor block selection

Defining which type of specimen should be included in the TMA is not a trivial task. It is not uncommon that, after completion of a TMA, the researchers realize that an important type of tumor or a control core is missing. As in all human activities, thorough preparation is the key to success. One of the author's most frustrating experiences was developing a large TMA for the study of progression/prognosis of gastrointestinal stromal tumors and, after months of work, with the final block in hand, to realize that two essential categories of cores were missing.

The critical and most time-consuming steps of the procedure are of course identification and selection of the donor block and of the suitable area on the donor block. We think that a histopathologist with experience in the specific field should perform this step. For instance, if a colon cancer TMA is needed, the selection should be performed by a histopathologist with specific training in gastrointestinal pathology (5). This is for two reasons:

- the need to avoid bias due to, for example, rare entities or difficult morphologic diagnoses; and
- the need to reduce inter-observer variability (for example, staging category pT2 vs. pT3 in colon cancer or carcinoma *in situ* vs. invasive carcinoma of the breast) (6). The revision by an experienced pathologist should indeed ensure that all of the morphological data and pathological diagnoses are consistent.

# Number and diameter of cores – representativity of TMA

In the original paper of Kononen *et al.* (2), only one core/specimen was used, with a diameter of 0.6 mm. The first concern that was raised was obviously one of adequate representation: cancer tissues are essentially heterogeneous, both phenotypically and genetically (7). We could miss heterogeneity using only a small "punch" of tissue. This point has been addressed extensively. First of all, it should be borne in mind that TMAs are tools for high-throughput, population-based studies. Of course, micro-heterogeneity in individual cases cannot be detected, but with a sufficient number of cases (normally more than 200) the relative frequencies of positivity are determined accurately, as shown by the high level of concordance between the immunohistochemical results between TMAs and conventional sections (6). Including more than one core may improve this concordance, although it seems that the addition of more than two cores does not bring any significant change in the final results (8). On the other hand, in selected cases it is probably advisable to use cores from different

areas of a tumor (for example, center and invasive front). Some authors suggest using up to six cores to achieve a good representation of the biology of the specimen (9). In conclusion, we think that a TMA should include at least two cores from functionally different areas of the specimen.

The diameter of the core can vary between 0.6 and 2 mm, depending on the type of TMA and on the aims of the studies. For tumor TMAs, it is probably advisable not to go over 0.8 mm, because there is no added information, while the "noise" (non-malignant cells, other tissues, etc.) increases significantly. Many reports show that known prognostic associations can be reproduced by 0.6 mm cores (10, 11). For normal tissue TMA, it is probably advisable to use larger cores (up to 2 mm) to ensure that all the cellular types of the tissue are included in the core (5).

# Recipient block

TMA recipient blocks are usually cut at room temperature. Therefore, a special type of paraffin is advised (melting temperature 55° to 58°C) (12). It is, of course, very important that the recipient block has no bubbles; therefore, a careful quality control is essential. TMA recipient blocks are normally larger than conventional "routine" blocks, because they are easier to handle. The manufacturing process includes four steps (12):

- punching a hole in a recipient block;
- removing the wax cylinder from the needle;
- removing a cylinder of tissue from the donor block; and
- carefully placing the cylinder in the pre-made hole in the recipient block. It is crucial to place the cylinder neither too deeply, nor too superficially, in the recipient block.

Recipient holes are prepared according to the previously prepared schema, determining the X-Y coordinates on the instrument. For 0.6 mm punches, the distance between the cylinders is usually set at 0.8 mm (Table 7.1, Figure 7.5), but it can be greater if need be (for example, larger punches, particularly with "difficult" tissues).

Sectioning the recipient block is performed using a conventional microtome, but this step requires very good experience and technical skills. Because TMA blocks are heterogeneous, containing different tissues, cutting the slides is difficult. The number of sections that can be obtained from a TMA block depends

Table 7.1 Example of coordinates of TMA

| Punch | Coordinates | Punch | Coordinates |
|-------|-------------|-------|-------------|
| A 1a | 0/0 | A 2a | 0/800 |
| A 1b | 800/0 | A 2b | 800/800 |
| A 1c | 1600/0 | A 2c | 1600/800 |
| A 1d | 2400/0 | A 2d | 2400/800 |
| A 1e | 3200/0 | A 2e | 3200/800 |
| A 1f | 4000/0 | A 2f | 4000/800 |
| A 1g | 4800/0 | A 2g | 4800/800 |
| A 1h | 5600/0 | A 2h | 5600/800 |
| A 1i | 6400/0 | A 2i | 6400/800 |
| A 1k | 7200/0 | A 2k | 7200/800 |
| A 1l | 8000/0 | A 2l | 8000/800 |
| A 1m | 8800/0 | A 2m | 8800/800 |
| A 1n | 9600/0 | A 2n | 9600/800 |
| A 1o | 10400/0 | A 2o | 10400/800 |
| A 1p | 11200/0 | A 2p | 11200/800 |
| A 1q | 12000/0 | A 2q | 12000/800 |
| A 1r | 12800/0 | A 2r | 12800/800 |

Table 7.2 Classification of TMAs

Normal tissue TMA

Multitumor TMA

Prognostic/predictive TMA

Progression TMA

Cell line TMA

Xenograft tissue microarrays

Cryoarray

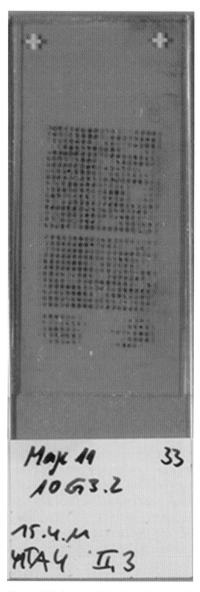

essentially on the donor blocks. In rare cases, up to 400 sections can be cut, but normally the range is 50 to 150 sections. Therefore, it is advisable to minimize loss of tissue during trimming of the block. Because of the heterogeneity of TMA sections, a frequent problem is loss of punches from the sections due to harsh pre-treatment protocols. This problem can partially be solved by using a tape cutting kit (Instrumedics®). This technique maintains the orientation of the TMA grid by preventing individual histospots from floating off the slide, above all when cores are taken from small, thin blocks (8). It has, however, the disadvantage of interfering with staining (for example, strong background in IHC and ISH).

## Type of TMAs

TMA can be classified as shown in Table 7.2.

## Normal tissue TMAs

*Normal tissue TMAs* are useful to study the distribution and expression pattern of a biomarker or of a

Figure 7.5 Stained slide of a multitumor TMA.

diagnostic/therapeutic target in normal tissues/organs of the human body and as quality control.

## Multitumor TMAs

*Multitumor TMAs* are used to state the prevalence of a biomarker in different tumor entities. Generally, data on histotype and grading of the tumors are sufficient and 20 to 50 samples/histotype are sufficient. Our multitumor TMA (Table 7.3) contains more than 3,400 cores, from 79 different histotypes (13). Using this resource, we could state the expression of CDX2 and HEPPAR in human tumors (14, 15).

Small TMAs are often used for quality control and inter-laboratory comparisons (lung.eqascheme.org, www.ukneqas.org.uk, www.quip-ringversuche.de).

## Progression TMAs

*Progression TMAs* contain samples in different stages of the evolution of a disease or of a tumor. The aim of such TMAs is to study the occurrence of a marker, for example, during carcinogenesis, and to associate it with the progression of the tumor. We used such an array to study hepatocarcinogenesis (16).

## Prognostic TMAs

*Prognostic TMAs* are probably the most frequently used TMAs. The idea is to identify a pathologic entity (for example, adenocarcinoma of the colon or ductal carcinoma of the breast) and to collect a sufficient number of cases with clinicopathologic information. This allows research into the association between the level of expression of biomarkers and prognosis. For such TMAs, a thorough collection of the clinical data and a review of the pathological classification is critical, with annotation of all the pathological characteristics. As a guide, we recommend that the following data should be collected/determined as a "minimum data set":

- age;
- sex;
- date of surgery;
- type of surgery;
- type of systemic therapy (if any);
- date of last follow-up;
- date of relapse if any;
- censoring;
- date of death;

**Table 7.3** Composition of a multitumor TMA

| Tumor/tissue type | N |
| --- | --- |
| Adrenal gland, adenoma | 14 |
| Astrocytoma | 48 |
| Benign histiocytoma | 28 |
| Breast, ductal cancer | 45 |
| Breast, lobular cancer | 40 |
| Breast, medullary cancer | 60 |
| Breast, mucinous cancer | 26 |
| Breast, tubular cancer | 20 |
| Carcinoid tumor | 37 |
| Colon adenoma, mild dysplasia | 36 |
| Colon adenoma, moderate dysplasia | 79 |
| Colon adenoma, severe dysplasia | 28 |
| Colon, adenocarcinoma | 49 |
| Endometrium, endometroid carcinoma | 49 |
| Endometrium, serous carcinoma | 32 |
| Gallbladder, adenocarcinoma | 45 |
| Glioblastoma multiforme | 32 |
| Hepatocellular carcinoma | 97 |
| Hodgkin's lymphoma, mixed cell | 17 |
| Hodgkin's lymphoma, nodular sclerosis | 25 |
| Kapillary hemangioma | 21 |
| Kaposi's sarcoma | 25 |
| Kidney, chromophobic cancer | 11 |
| Kidney, clear cell cancer | 58 |
| Kidney, oncocytoma | 24 |
| Kidney, papillary cancer | 38 |
| Larynx, squamous cell carcinoma | 58 |
| Leiomyoma | 57 |
| Leiomyosarcoma | 47 |
| Lipoma | 29 |
| Liposarcoma | 28 |
| Lung, adenocarcinoma | 90 |
| Lung, large cell cancer | 25 |
| Lung, small cell cancer | 49 |
| Lung, squamous cell carcinoma | 45 |

**Table 7.3** (*cont.*)

| Tumor/tissue type | N |
|---|---|
| Malignant fibrous histiocytoma | 30 |
| Malignant mesothelioma | 31 |
| Meningeoma | 48 |
| Neurofibroma | 35 |
| NHL, diffuse large B | 10 |
| NHL, others | 15 |
| Oligodendroglioma | 25 |
| Oral cavity, squamous cell carcinoma | 50 |
| Ovary, endometroid cancer | 43 |
| Ovary, mucinous cancer | 21 |
| Ovary, serous cancer | 47 |
| Pancreas, adenocarcinoma | 49 |
| Pancreas, normal tissue | 49 |
| Paraganglioma | 8 |
| Parathyroid, adenoma | 43 |
| Pheochromocytoma | 28 |
| Prostate cancer, hormone-refractory | 41 |
| Prostate cancer, untreated | 50 |
| Salivary gland, adenolymphoma | 25 |
| Salivary gland, cylindroma | 33 |
| Salivary gland, pleomorphic adenoma | 49 |
| Schwannoma | 49 |
| Skin, basalioma | 73 |
| Skin, benign appendix tumor | 19 |
| Skin, benign nevus | 44 |
| Skin, malignant melanoma | 78 |
| Skin, squamous cell cancer | 38 |
| Small intestine, adenocarcinoma | 22 |
| Stomach, diffuse adenocarcinoma | 25 |
| Stomach, intestinal adenocarcinoma | 51 |
| Submandibular gland, normal | 51 |
| Tendon sheath, giant cell tumor | 28 |
| Testis, non-seminomatous cancer | 48 |
| Testis, seminoma | 49 |
| Thymoma | 37 |

| Tumor/tissue type | N |
|---|---|
| Thyroid, adenoma | 39 |
| Thyroid, follicular cancer | 58 |
| Thyroid, papillary cancer | 34 |
| Urinary bladder cancer, cancer, transitional cell carcinoma invasive (pT2–4) | 78 |
| Urinary bladder cancer, transitional cell carcinoma non-invasive (pTa) | 38 |
| Uterus cervix, squamous cell carcinoma | 4 |
| uterus, cervix, CIN III | 35 |
| Vulva, squamous cell cancer | 28 |
| Breast, normal | 28 |
| Cerebrum, grey substance, normal | 13 |
| Cerebrum, white substance, normal | 5 |
| Colon, mucosa, normal | 5 |
| Endometrium proliferation, normal | 11 |
| Endometrium, secretion, normal | 5 |
| Esophagus, normal tissue | 10 |
| Fat tissue, normal | 3 |
| Gallbladder, normal tissue | 9 |
| Heart, normal | 12 |
| Ileum, mucosa | 4 |
| Kidney, normal | 21 |
| Liver, normal | 20 |
| Lung, normal | 17 |
| Lymph node, normal | 17 |
| Mouth, normal | 10 |
| Myometrium, normal | 12 |
| Pancreas, normal tissue | 10 |
| Parathyroid, normal | 2 |
| Parotis, normal | 5 |
| Prostate, normal | 27 |
| Skin, normal | 29 |
| Striated muscle | 12 |
| Smooth muscle, intestine, normal | 12 |
| Stomach, antrum, normal | 3 |
| Stomach, corpus, normal | 5 |
| Submandibular gland, normal | 8 |

**Table 7.3** (cont.)

| Tumor/tissue type | N |
| --- | --- |
| Testis, normal | 21 |
| Thymus, normal | 3 |
| Thyroid, normal | 17 |
| Urothelium, normal | 3 |
| **Total** | **3,427** |

- cause of death;
- grading;
- histotype;
- pTNM classification; and
- additional descriptors (L, V, Pn).

It is clear that the value of such TMAs is the value of their associated data. Therefore, a good collaboration between pathologists, surgeons and oncologists is essential. Using a large colon cancer TMA (1,400 cases) we could clarify, for instance, the role of ephrin receptor EphB2 (10) and RHAMM (17) in the prognosis of colorectal cancer. Other prognostic associations were found in many different entities, such as breast cancer (7, 18), prostate cancer, (19), lung carcinoma (20) and malignant lymphoma (21).

Prognostic TMAs are also useful to establish the optimal threshold of expression for a clinical application. By searching in the literature, it is clear that there is no rule for the determination of the threshold for IHC positivity. Generally, IHC staining can be evaluated in percentage of stained cells (usually in 5% steps) and intensity on a semi-quantitative scale (from 0 to 3). In most cases, there is absolutely no explanation for the choice, for example, of "a 2+ staining intensity in >10% of the cells," as a cut-off to mark a case as "positive." Sometimes, there is reference to previous work, but most of the time it is simply "common sense." This has two consequences: 1. it is very difficult to compare different studies, because the threshold is different; 2. it is impossible to draw robust clinical conclusions. TMAs allow different thresholds to be tested and the cut-off resulting in the strongest association between target expression and patient prognosis can be used as diagnostic cut-off (22). A more refined and precise way of determining the cut-off is the use of receiver operating characteristic (ROC) curves (23). This measure is independent of disease prevalence and incorporates information from censored patients. ROC curves were used successfully to determine the best cut-offs for several markers in different tumors (for example, 20, 24, 25).

Prognostic TMAs are generally built in a retrospective fashion, hence they share all the disadvantages of retrospective series, first of all selection biases and inhomogeneity of therapy. The best way to overcome these drawbacks is probably to include in clinical trial protocols the generation of TMAs. This has been the case, for example, regarding the Breast Cancer International Research Group 006 (BCIRG) (26). These arrays are probably better designed as *predictive TMAs*. Incorporating data on the therapy, they can give information on the predictive value of the different biomarkers. However, if a TMA database includes information on the therapy used, even if it is not prospectively built, it might be used as a predictive TMA (25).

## Cell line TMAs

*Cell line TMAs* (CMAs) (27) can be used for experimental purposes. CMAs containing a large number of different cell lines would be highly useful for the selection of cell lines with distinct genetic or immunophenotypic features. The expression of a protein can be profiled in more than 60 cell lines (28). It is also possible to set up different experimental settings before fixation of the cells (for example, RNAi experiments) (29). Basically, the procedure of arraying cell culture includes a centrifugation step and the subsequent "embedding" of the pellets in agarose gel. The same method can be used for cell suspension, for example, from the blood or from fine-needle aspirates (FNAs) (30). CMAs are also used as control slides or for inter-laboratory comparison.

## Xenograft TMAs

*Xenograft TMAs* (XMAs) are the incorporation of xenografts in tissue microarrays. This is particularly useful for tumors that do not grow in culture or are rare. Moreover, xenografts are particularly suitable for the identification of possible drug targets, because they are transcriptionally more similar to *in vivo* tumors than cell lines (31). The definitive evidence can then be obtained on conventional TMAs.

## Cryoarrays

*Cryoarrays* are obtained from snap-frozen tissues in OCT. They allow performing studies that are very difficult on FFPE tissues (for example, proteomic studies, RNA hybridization studies). Different methods have been proposed to generate cryoarrays (32). However, generation and handling of cryoarrays is time-demanding and expensive, and as a result this type of TMA has not gained a widespread acceptance.

## IHC and TMAs

The largest application of TMAs is IHC. In IHC, an unlabeled primary antibody, specific for the marker of interest, reacts with the tissue. A secondary labeled antibody then reacts with the primary antibody and the label is then revealed, generally by a bright-field enzymatic method (for example, 3.3-Diaminobenzidine (DAB) or Alkaline Phosphatase-Anti-Alkaline Phosphatase Complex (APAAP)). Although the procedure used for TMAs is roughly the same as for conventional histopathology slides, some important differences do exist. First of all, the pre-treatment has to be adjusted to the TMA and the laboratory conditions. Everyone working with IHC knows that the manufacturer's instruction and the data from the literature often do not apply to every laboratory. In TMAs, there is the added difficulty that the different cores are different in age and fixation conditions. Very old cases (pre-1990, for example) may have been fixed in non-buffered formalin. If they are collected from different institutions, the situation is even trickier. Hence, testing a new antibody on a TMA requires a careful adjusting both of the pre-treatment conditions and of the dilution, maybe on a small "test" array. Inclusion of positive and negative controls is also crucial. Negative controls should be at least omission of the primary and (if the primary is monoclonal) isotype-specific control. Optimally, a blocking pre-absorption with the target should also be performed (13).

The evaluation of staining should include (see also above) intensity on a semi-quantitative scale, generally from 0 (no staining) to 3 (strong staining), percentage of stained cells and subcellular localization (membranous, cytoplasmatic or nuclear). The data can be reported manually on a template or directly in a table at the computer (Figure 7.6). The use of intensity score has been questioned, because of the variability of the staining intensity due to imponderable factors (33). Nevertheless, the registration of intensity is in our opinion advisable, at least as quality control.

Manual evaluation and scoring of IHC is time-consuming and tedious. Many efforts have been dedicated to the development and use of computer-assisted image analysis. TMAs are particularly suitable, because the experimental conditions of the stainings are the same for up to hundreds of samples (same slide). Digital image analysis has been used, for example, for scoring ER, PR and MIB1 in breast cancer (34–38) – with good agreement with manual score and other clinicopathologic factors. The use of such systems will probably allow a more efficient use of TMAs.

## Genomic alterations and TMAs

In the last two decades, fluorescence *in situ* hybridization (FISH) has gained a very important position both in research and in the clinical field. Paradigmatic is, for instance, the use of FISH in the determination of the ERBB2 (HER2) status in breast (39) and stomach cancer (40). ERBB2 amplification is nowadays the most important predictive marker for Trastuzumab. The same is true, for example, for translocations such as ALK and ROS1 translocation in lung adenocarcinoma (41). FISH is also an invaluable diagnostic tool in many fields (for example, CDK4/MDM2 status in adipose tissue tumors or CMYC in the diagnosis of Burkitt's lymphoma). FISH is, however, also a very useful research tool to quantify numeric DNA alterations in a very large set of materials, cells and tissues. Although the best material to perform FISH is fresh or snap-frozen, it has been successfully applied to FFPE tissues (Figure 7.7).

This kind of material is technically demanding, mainly due to fixation. Formalin fixation leads to the formation of methylene bridges between the DNA chains, thus affecting the efficiency of hybridization. Many pre-treatments are nowadays available to enhance FISH performance on FFPE materials and some are applicable to TMAs. The type and efficacy of the pre-treatment is unfortunately influenced by many different parameters, such as age of the tissue, type and length of fixation. Therefore, as for IHC, it is necessary to adjust the protocols for TMA setting (42). We generally use a treatment with protease, adjusting the time according to different experimental settings. It has to be borne in mind that, because of these difficulties, a relatively large number of punches (in the worst case scenario up to 50%, but usually about 10% to 20% depending both on the

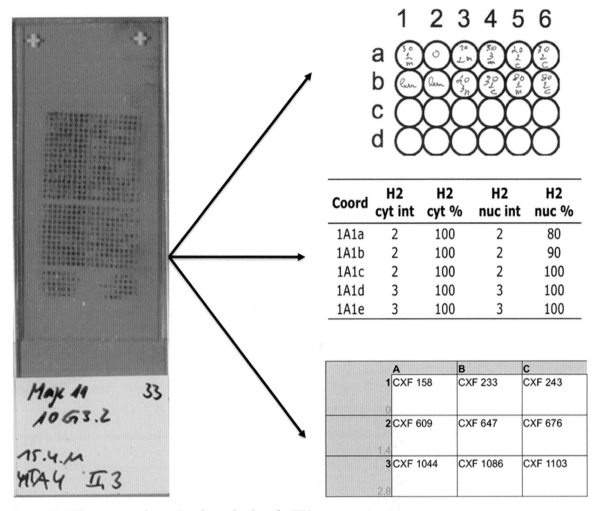

**Figure 7.6 Different ways of reporting the evaluation of a TMA**
Left, stained slide. Upper right, template leaflets. Middle right, Excel® table reporting the coordinates. Bottom right, Excel® table mirroring the structure of the TMA.

| Coord | H2 cyt int | H2 cyt % | H2 nuc int | H2 nuc % |
|---|---|---|---|---|
| 1A1a | 2 | 100 | 2 | 80 |
| 1A1b | 2 | 100 | 2 | 90 |
| 1A1c | 2 | 100 | 2 | 100 |
| 1A1d | 3 | 100 | 3 | 100 |
| 1A1e | 3 | 100 | 3 | 100 |

| | A | B | C |
|---|---|---|---|
| 1 | CXF 158 | CXF 233 | CXF 243 |
| 2 | CXF 609 | CXF 647 | CXF 676 |
| 3 | CXF 1044 | CXF 1086 | CXF 1103 |

probes and on the tissue types) may be unevaluable. Bearing these limitations in mind, TMAs are very useful to determine the incidence and the prognostic/predictive value of genomic alterations (gains, deletions or translocations). Of course, while a wide variety of commercial probes do exist, for most research purposes custom-made probes are needed. In our laboratory, we generally employ bacterial artificial chromosomes (BACs).

The use of FISH on TMAs has allowed us and others to reveal the association between genomic alteration and evolution of many tumors, often translating the results of more demanding technologies such as quantitative PCR (qPCR), aCGH or single nucleotide polymorphism (SNP) and verifying these alterations on large series to explore their possible clinical meaning (for example, 2, 11, 42–44).

## Scoring of FISH on TMAs

Scoring of FISH is in most cases performed manually, with the help of the schemes and tables that have been described above. Normally, at least 50 non-overlapping nuclei are scored. The procedure needs a high-quality fluorescent microscope equipped with a camera and the corresponding software for image capture. Two important things have to be borne in mind:

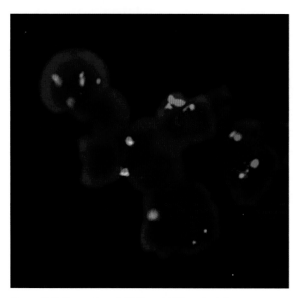 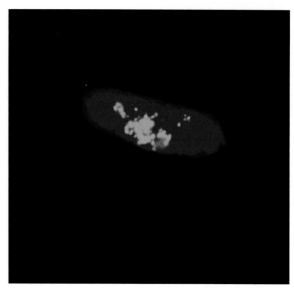

**Figure 7.7 Examples of FISH on FFPE material**
Red, centromere 4, green MDM2 probe. Left, normal. 2 signal each per nucleus. Right, amplification of MDM2. At least 20 green signals and two red signals.

- Histologic sections are normally 4 to 5x μm thick. The diameter of a nucleus is on average 7 to 10x μm, and the diameter of a metabolically very active cell, such as a tumor cell, can be also 40x μm. Therefore, in the evaluation of the results, the so-called "artifact of truncation" should be kept in mind, above all when evaluating losses of genetic material (see Chapter 4).
- Because of the thickness of the section, it is possible that different signals are on different focal planes. That is why automated capture systems take several pictures of the same field with different focal planes.

As for IHC, the manual evaluation of the FISH results is very tedious and time-consuming. Automated scoring systems have, however, been developed and will probably allow a better and more efficient use of this technology (42, 45).

## Ethical aspects

Generation and use of TMAs raises some ethical concerns. The most important step in addressing this is the anonymization of the data. Each patient is usually identified with a unique hospital number, and once the table containing the clinicopathological data is created, the correspondence between number and identification of the patients can be reversibly or irreversibly stripped away, such that data are fully anonymizable. There is no additional invasive procedure to perform, obviously, and the tissue block is available for subsequent diagnostic purposes, in the rare case that the patient needs an additional diagnosis. Because the strength of TMA is due to the number of specimens, there is no exploitation of single patients that could also raise financial concerns. Depending on the local legislation, however, it is always advisable to have a written consent from the patient to utilize the tissue for research purposes and/or appropriate ethical approval by an institutional ethics review board.

## Automation

Although the "classical" manual generation and evaluation of TMAs is very efficient and has produced invaluable results, two major issues remain unsolved:

- The manual manufacture of a TMA is relatively time-consuming, can give rise to errors in the sequence of the cases or the punching could be not satisfactory.
- The manual evaluation is very tedious and subjective, giving rise to problems in the reproducibility of data.

Automated and semi-automated methods for building TMA have been proposed (46). By using digitalization, they allow a precise identification of the region of interest on the slides and on donor blocks and a very precise "punching" of the blocks.

Table 7.4 Tissue image analysis software programs

| Manufacturer | Software |
| --- | --- |
| 3dHistech www.3dhistech.com | MIRAX® |
| Aperio www.aperio.com | Aperio image analysis toolbox |
| Caliper www.caliper.com | inForm® |
| DAKO www.dako.com | ACIS® III |
| Definiens www.definiens.com | Tissue studio® |
| Hamamatsu www.hamamatsu.com | NDP.Analyze® |
| HistoRx www.historx.com | AQUA® |
| Leica www.leica-microsystems.com | Ariol® |
| Ventana www.ventana.com | VIAS® |
| Visiopharm www.visiopharm.com | Tissuemorph® |

In the meantime, there has been a growth of programs for digital image analysis and scoring of slides for use in light microscopy (for example, IHC, bright-field ISH) and in fluorescence setting (for example, FISH, immunofluorescence), some of them developed specially for TMA analysis (reviewed in (47)) (Table 7.4). Some of the image analysis systems also received FDA approval for use in daily diagnostics in breast cancer.

## Conclusions

Fifteen years ago, TMAs were introduced in the practice of pathology (2). They have in some ways revolutionized the way in which pre-clinical and translational research is performed. The ability to analyze in a single experiment up to 1,000 specimens has basically changed the way in which we look at tissue, which can now be considered a "reagent." The mass of data that is produced by other high-throughput technologies (cDNA arrays, protein arrays, aCGH) requires a validation that can often be provided only by a high-throughput *in situ* technology, such as TMAs. Production of poor quality TMA would waste invaluable resources. Guidelines for the correct and successful production of TMA would be of value (48).

TMA production and analysis are not trivial and require careful adaption of technical protocols and standardization of evaluation. The introduction of automated systems will probably improve these aspects, allowing a broader adoption of TMAs in the clinical setting (for example, quality assurance, robust assay controls, optimization of clinically important assays).

The use of TMAs as a component of clinical trials will assist in building correlative projects, which may translate the predictive value of specific markers in the daily clinics, leading to the complete development of tailored/personalized therapies.

## Learning points

- TMAs are an invaluable means to translate the results of basic research to clinical research ("from the bench to the bed").
- To generate a good quality TMA, the crucial step is preparation: identification of donor blocks and collection of all pertinent clinicopathological data. Any weakness in this phase will result in waste of time and resources ("you get what you put in").
- Routine IHC or ISH protocols cannot be used "as they are" for TMAs. Careful adjustment steps are mandatory.

## Acknowledgments

The author thanks Mr. Martin Portmann for taking pictures and Ms. Sandra Schneider for technical assistance.

# References

1. Suvama, K., Layton, C. and Bancroft, J. (eds.), *Theory and Practice of Histological Techniques*, 7th edn. (New York: Churchill & Livingstone, 2008).

2. Kononen, J., Bubendorf, L., Kallioniemi, A., Barlund, M., Schraml, P., Leighton, S. *et al.* Tissue microarrays for high-throughput molecular profiling of tumor specimens. *Nat Med* 1998; 4(7): 844–7. PubMed PMID: 9662379.

3. Battifora, H. The multitumor (sausage) tissue block: novel method for immunohistochemical antibody testing. *Lab Invest* 1986; 55(2): 244–8. PubMed PMID: 3525985.

4. Bubendorf, L., Nocito, A., Moch, H. and Sauter, G. Tissue microarray (TMA) technology: miniaturized pathology archives for high-throughput in situ studies. *J Pathol* 2001; 195(1): 72–9. PubMed PMID: 11568893.

5. Tennstedt, P. and Sauter, G. Quality aspects of TMA analysis. *Methods Mol Biol* 2010; 664: 17–26. PubMed PMID: 20690048.

6. Torhorst, J., Bucher, C., Kononen, J., Haas, P., Zuber, M., Kochli, O. R. *et al.* Tissue microarrays for rapid linking of molecular changes to clinical endpoints. *Am J Path* 2001; 159(6): 2249–56. PubMed PMID: 11733374. Pubmed Central PMCID: 1850582.

7. McCarthy, N. Tumour heterogeneity: Darwin's finches. *Nat Rev Cancer* 2012; 12(5): 317. PubMed PMID: 22495322.

8. Camp, R. L., Charette, L. A. and Rimm, D. L. Validation of tissue microarray technology in breast carcinoma. *Lab Invest* 2000; 80(12): 1943–9. PubMed PMID: 11140706.

9. Graham, A. D., Faratian, D., Rae, F. and Thomas, J. S. Tissue microarray technology in the routine assessment of HER-2 status in invasive breast cancer: a prospective study of the use of immunohistochemistry and fluorescence in situ hybridization. *Histopathology* 2008; 52(7): 847–55. PubMed PMID: 18494613.

10. Lugli, A., Spichtin, H., Maurer, R., Mirlacher, M., Kiefer, J., Huusko, P. *et al.* EphB2 expression across 138 human tumor types in a tissue microarray: high levels of expression in gastrointestinal cancers. *Clin Cancer Res* 2005;

11(18): 6450–8. PubMed PMID: 16166419.

11. Tornillo, L., Duchini, G., Carafa, V., Lugli, A., Dirnhofer, S., Di Vizio, D. *et al.* Patterns of gene amplification in gastrointestinal stromal tumors (GIST). *Lab Invest* 2005; 85(7): 921–31. PubMed PMID: 15864317.

12. Mirlacher, M. and Simon, R. Recipient block TMA technique. *Methods Mol Biol* 2010; 664: 37–44. PubMed PMID: 20690050.

13. Went, P. T., Dirnhofer, S., Bundi, M., Mirlacher, M., Schraml, P., Mangialaio, S. *et al.* Prevalence of KIT expression in human tumors. *J Clin Oncol* 2004; 22(22): 4514–22. PubMed PMID: 15542802.

14. Kaimaktchiev, V., Terracciano, L., Tornillo, L., Spichtin, H., Stoios, D., Bundi, M. *et al.* The homeobox intestinal differentiation factor CDX2 is selectively expressed in gastrointestinal adenocarcinomas. *Modern Pathol* 2004; 17(11): 1392–9. PubMed PMID: 15205684.

15. Lugli, A., Tornillo, L., Mirlacher, M., Bundi, M., Sauter, G. and Terracciano, L. M. Hepatocyte paraffin 1 expression in human normal and neoplastic tissues: tissue microarray analysis on 3,940 tissue samples. *Am J Clin Pathol* 2004; 122(5): 721–7. PubMed PMID: 15491968.

16. Cillo, C., Schiavo, G., Cantile, M., Bihl, M. P., Sorrentino, P., Carafa, V. *et al.* The HOX gene network in hepatocellular carcinoma. *Int J Cancer* 2011; 129(11): 2577–87. PubMed PMID: 21626505.

17. Zlobec, I., Terracciano, L., Tornillo, L., Gunthert, U., Vuong, T., Jass, J. R. *et al.* Role of RHAMM within the hierarchy of well-established prognostic factors in colorectal cancer. *Gut* 2008; 57(10): 1413–19. PubMed PMID: 18436576.

18. Al-Kuraya, K., Schraml, P., Torhorst, J., Tapia, C., Zaharieva, B., Novotny, H. *et al.* Prognostic relevance of gene amplifications and coamplifications in breast cancer. *Cancer Res* 2004; 64(23): 8534–40. PubMed PMID: 15574759.

19. Gannon, P. O., Lessard, L., Stevens, L. M., Forest, V., Begin, L. R., Minner, S. *et al.* Large-scale independent validation of the nuclear factor-kappa B p65 prognostic biomarker in prostate cancer. *Eur J Cancer* 2013; 49(10): 2441–8. PubMed PMID: 23541563.

20. Wu, Y. H., Chang, T. H., Huang, Y. F., Huang, H. D. and Chou, C. Y. COL11A1 promotes tumor progression and predicts poor clinical outcome in ovarian cancer. *Oncogene* 2013; 33(26): 3432–40. PubMed PMID: 23934190.

21. Obermann, E. C., Went, P., Tzankov, A., Pileri, S. A., Hofstaedter, F., Marienhagen, J. *et al.* Cell cycle phase distribution analysis in chronic lymphocytic leukaemia: a significant number of cells reside in early G1-phase. *J Clin Pathol* 2007; 60(7): 794–7. PubMed PMID: 16950856. Pubmed Central PMCID: 1995795.

22. Simon, R., Mirlacher, M. and Sauter, G. Immunohistochemical analysis of tissue microarrays. *Methods Mol Biol* 2010; 664:113–26. PubMed PMID: 20690058.

23. Heagerty, P. J., Lumley, T. and Pepe, M. S. Time-dependent ROC curves for censored survival data and a diagnostic marker. *Biometrics* 2000; 56(2): 337–44. PubMed PMID: 10877287.

24. Chaux, A., Albadine, R., Toubaji, A., Hicks, J., Meeker, A., Platz, E. A. *et al.* Immunohistochemistry for ERG expression as a surrogate for TMPRSS2-ERG fusion detection in prostatic

adenocarcinomas. *Am J Surg Pathol* 2011; 35(7): 1014–20. PubMed PMID: 21677539. Pubmed Central PMCID: 3505676.

25. Fischer, C. A., Zlobec, I., Green, E., Probst, S., Storck, C., Lugli, A. *et al.* Is the improved prognosis of p16 positive oropharyngeal squamous cell carcinoma dependent of the treatment modality? *Int J Cancer* 2010; 126(5): 1256–62. PubMed PMID: 19697324.

26. Press, M. F., Sauter, G., Bernstein, L., Villalobos, I. E., Mirlacher, M., Zhou, J. Y. *et al.* Diagnostic evaluation of HER-2 as a molecular target: an assessment of accuracy and reproducibility of laboratory testing in large, prospective, randomized clinical trials. *Clin Cancer Res* 2005; 11(18): 6598–607. PubMed PMID: 16166438.

27. Hoos, A. and Cordon-Cardo, C. Tissue microarray profiling of cancer specimens and cell lines: opportunities and limitations. *Lab Invest* 2001; 81(10): 1331–8. PubMed PMID: 11598146.

28. Ferrer, B., Bermudo, R., Thomson, T., Nayach, I., Soler, M., Sanchez, M. *et al.* Paraffin-embedded cell line microarray (PECLIMA): development and validation of a high-throughput method for antigen profiling of cell lines. *Pathobiology* 2005; 72(5): 225–32. PubMed PMID: 16374066.

29. Andersson, A. C., Stromberg, S., Backvall, H., Kampf, C., Uhlen, M., Wester, K. *et al.* Analysis of protein expression in cell microarrays: a tool for antibody-based proteomics. *J Histochem Cytochem* 2006; 54(12): 1413–23. PubMed PMID: 16957166.

30. Zhao, S. and Natkunam, Y. Building "tissue" microarrays from suspension cells. *Methods Mol Biol* 2010; 664: 93–101. PubMed PMID: 20690056.

31. Uhlen, M., Bjorling, E., Agaton, C., Szigyarto, C. A., Amini, B., Andersen, E. *et al.* A human protein atlas for normal and cancer tissues based on antibody proteomics. *Mol Cell Proteomics* 2005; 4(12): 1920–32. PubMed PMID: 16127175.

32. Zhou, L., Hodeib, M., Abad, J. D., Mendoza, L., Kore, A. R. and Hu, Z. New tissue microarray technology for analyses of gene expression in frozen pathological samples. *BioTechniques* 2007; 43(1): 101–5. PubMed PMID: 17695259.

33. Zlobec, I., Terracciano, L., Jass, J. R. and Lugli, A. Value of staining intensity in the interpretation of immunohistochemistry for tumor markers in colorectal cancer. *Virchows Archiv* 2007; 451(4): 763–9. PubMed PMID: 17674041.

34. Sundara Rajan, S., Horgan, K., Speirs, V. and Hanby, A. M. External validation of the ImmunoRatio image analysis application for ERalpha determination in breast cancer. *J Clin Pathol* 2014; 67(1): 72–5. PubMed PMID: 23986557.

35. Mohammed, Z. M., McMillan, D. C., Elsberger, B., Going, J. J., Orange, C., Mallon, E. *et al.* Comparison of visual and automated assessment of Ki-67 proliferative activity and their impact on outcome in primary operable invasive ductal breast cancer. *Br J Cancer* 2012; 106(2): 383–8. PubMed PMID: 22251968. Pubmed Central PMCID: 3261670.

36. Mohammed, Z. M., Going, J. J., McMillan, D. C., Orange, C., Mallon, E., Doughty, J. C. *et al.* Comparison of visual and automated assessment of HER2 status and their impact on outcome in primary operable invasive ductal breast cancer. *Histopathology* 2012; 61(4):

675–84. PubMed PMID: 22747525.

37. Mohammed, Z. M., Edwards, J., Orange, C., Mallon, E., Doughty, J. C., McMillan, D. C. *et al.* Breast cancer outcomes by steroid hormone receptor status assessed visually and by computer image analysis. *Histopathology* 2012; 61(2): 283–92. PubMed PMID: 22571413.

38. Ali, H. R., Irwin, M., Morris, L., Dawson, S. J., Blows, F. M., Provenzano, E. *et al.* Astronomical algorithms for automated analysis of tissue protein expression in breast cancer. *Br J Cancer* 2013; 108(3): 602–12. PubMed PMID: 23329232. Pubmed Central PMCID: 3593538.

39. Wolff, A. C., Hammond, M. E., Schwartz, J. N., Hagerty, K. L., Allred, D. C., Cote, R. J. *et al.* American Society of Clinical Oncology/College of American Pathologists guideline recommendations for human epidermal growth factor receptor 2 testing in breast cancer. *J Clin Oncol* 2007; 25(1): 118–45. PubMed PMID: 17159189.

40. Bang, Y. J., Van Cutsem, E., Feyereislova, A., Chung, H. C., Shen, L., Sawaki, A. *et al.* Trastuzumab in combination with chemotherapy versus chemotherapy alone for treatment of HER2-positive advanced gastric or gastro-oesophageal junction cancer (ToGA): a phase 3, open-label, randomised controlled trial. *Lancet* 2010; 376(9742): 687–97. PubMed PMID: 20728210.

41. Takeuchi, K., Soda, M., Togashi, Y., Suzuki, R., Sakata, S., Hatano, S. *et al.* RET, ROS1 and ALK fusions in lung cancer. *Nat Med* 2012; 18(3): 378–81. PubMed PMID: 22327623.

42. Brown, L. A. and Huntsman, D. Fluorescent in situ hybridization on tissue microarrays: challenges

and solutions. *J Mol Histol* 2007; 38(2): 151–7. PubMed PMID: 17216303.

43. Drev, P., Grazio, S. F. and Bracko, M. Tissue microarrays for routine diagnostic assessment of HER2 status in breast carcinoma. Applied immunohistochemistry & molecular morphology. *AIMM* 2008; 16(2): 179–84. PubMed PMID: 18227723.

44. Oeggerli, M., Tian, Y., Ruiz, C., Wijker, B., Sauter, G., Obermann, E. *et al.* Role of KCNMA1 in breast cancer. *PloS ONE* 2012; 7(8): e41664. PubMed PMID: 22899999. Pubmed Central PMCID: 3416802.

45. Turashvili, G., Leung, S., Turbin, D., Montgomery, K., Gilks, B., West, R. *et al.* Inter-observer reproducibility of HER2 immunohistochemical assessment and concordance with fluorescent in situ hybridization (FISH): pathologist assessment compared to quantitative image analysis. *BMC Cancer* 2009; 9: 165. PubMed PMID: 19476653. Pubmed Central PMCID: PMC2698924. Epub 2009/05/30. eng.

46. Zlobec, I., Koelzer, V. H., Dawson, H., Perren, A. and Lugli, A. Next-generation tissue microarray (ngTMA) increases the quality of

biomarker studies: an example using CD3, CD8, and CD45RO in the tumor microenvironment of six different solid tumor types. *J Transl Med* 2013; 11(1): 104. PubMed PMID: 23627766. Pubmed Central PMCID: 3644251.

47. Mulrane, L., Rexhepaj, E., Penney, S., Callanan, J. J. and Gallagher, W. M. Automated image analysis in histopathology: a valuable tool in medical diagnostics. *Expert Rev Mol Diag* 2008; 8(6): 707–25. PubMed PMID: 18999923.

48. www.mged.org/Workgroups/ MIAME/miame_1.1.html.

# Sequencing

Andrew M. K. Brown, Philipe C. Zuzarte and Paul M. Krzyzanowski

## Introduction

The completion of the Human Genome Project marked a milestone event in molecular biology; separating the field into a pre- and post-genomic era. DNA sequencing technology enabled this feat, giving rise to the potential for a modern age of biomedical science. Our understanding of the role of genetics in disease has grown dramatically with modern technological advances, as well as our understanding of the vast amount of inter-individual variation at the molecular level. The field of molecular pathology is utilizing this knowledge to shift traditional population-based medicine to individualized or personalized genomic medicine.

DNA sequencing dates back to 1977 when Walter Gilbert and Frederick Sanger independently developed methods for sequencing DNA, an important milestone that led to the Nobel Prize in Chemistry in 1980.

Sanger's method [1], chain-termination sequencing, proved to be more robust and, eventually, with improvements such as automation and the incorporation of fluorescent labels as opposed to radioactivity, remained the standard method for DNA sequencing until 2005. The process involves the random incorporation of di-deoxynucleosidetriphosphates (ddNTPs) during DNA replication of a template strand of DNA by a DNA polymerase. These ddNTPs lack the 3'-OH group required to form the phosphodiester bond between adjacent nucleotides and thus prevents the polymerase from incorporating additional nucleotides. DNA templates are split into four reactions, each containing DNA polymerase, all four deoxynucleotides (dATP, dCTP, dGTP and dTTP) and one of the ddNTPs. Following rounds of template extension, several DNA products of differing lengths

are produced in each of the four reactions. The ddNTPs are radioactively or fluorescently labeled so that they can be run out on a polyacrylamide gel and visualized. A band in a given lane indicates that the fragment ends at that position with the corresponding nucleotide. By 1987, the method had been updated by the use of four different colored labels, one for each of the four ddNTPs that allowed the sequencing to occur in a single reaction as well as the use of capillary electrophoresis to increase speed and automate detection. Automated chain-termination sequencing machines, sometimes referred to as first generation sequencers, continued to improve throughput over the years and, by 1998, these instruments became the workhorses behind the human genome project completed in 2001 [2].

## Next generation sequencing (NGS) technologies

An immense expansion in DNA sequencing technologies followed in the years after the human genome project. In addition to newer methodologies for sample preparation and signal detection, throughput of second-generation platforms has greatly increased. The fundamental difference between second-generation sequencing platforms and first-generation Sanger sequencing is the improvement to "read" or sample clonally amplified DNA sequences in a massively parallel manner (hundreds of millions simultaneously), as opposed to generating signal from one amplified DNA segment per capillary, per reaction.

Sequencing and analysis of an entire human genome can now readily be done in a matter of days as opposed to years and for a fraction of the price. Before 2008, the annual growth of throughput for DNA sequencing technology roughly followed

*Molecular Pathology: A Practical Guide for the Surgical Pathologist and Cytopathologist*, ed. John M. S. Bartlett, Abeer Shaaban and Fernando Schmitt. Published by Cambridge University Press. © Cambridge University Press, 2016.

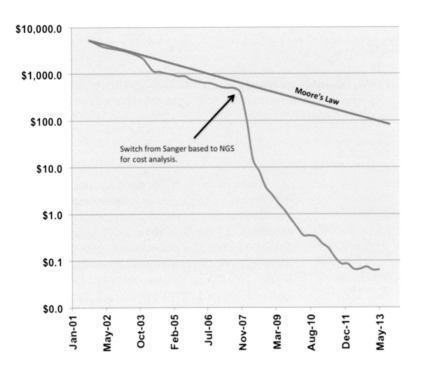

Switch from Sanger based to NGS for cost analysis.

Moore's Law

**Figure 8.1 The cost of DNA sequencing over time**
The blue line represents the total cost associated with generating sequencing data, including labor, reagents and consumables, sequencing instruments (amortized over three years), informatics activities and submission of data to a public database. Beginning in January 2008, the cost is for using NGS. Data source [4].

Moore's law, which was initially used to describe the trends in the computer hardware industry. Originally referring to the doubling of transistors per integrated circuit every 24 months, Moore's law has become a growth benchmark for any developing technology [3]. With the emergence of NGS technologies and the rapid developments in the field, sequencing throughput has dramatically diverged from Moore's law leading to a 40-fold drop in the cost of sequencing 1 million basepairs (1 mb) in 2008 alone. This trend has continued for several years and at the start of 2013 the cost to sequence an entire human genome was almost 20,000 times cheaper than during the human genome project (see Figure 8.1).

For some time, sequencing instrument manufacturers engaged in a sort of "arms race" of delivering greater throughput per machine at lower costs, and while the trend carries on, in 2010 sequencing technology providers began placing an emphasis on platforms that produce smaller amounts of high-quality data with much faster turnaround times. The main drive for this trend has been an effort to make NGS much more applicable in clinical settings.

Numerous sequencing platforms have been and continue to be developed, with third-generation platforms available and on the horizon which are able to interrogate DNA at the single molecule level without the need for clonal amplification. While a thorough discussion of the various NGS platforms is beyond the scope of this chapter, Table 8.1 provides a brief summary of some of the current and past platforms. Furthermore, DNA sequencing technologies have been nicely reviewed elsewhere [5, 6]. Each system has distinct capabilities and weaknesses and it is extremely important to select the appropriate platforms for a given application.

## Capabilities of NGS technologies

NGS platforms are becoming the standard high throughput technology for many genomic applications. This is because NGS platforms have greater sensitivity and a broader dynamic range than other technologies such as microarrays. The digital nature of sequencing reads allows for increased sensitivity simply by generating more data and allows for detection of molecules with extremely low abundance. For example, the detection of single nucleotide variants at a frequency of 1% to 2% is possible compared to traditional Sanger-based sequencing that can detect variants down to 20%. Furthermore, six orders of magnitude of dynamic range of NGS enable a huge range of abundances to be quantified accurately.

**Table 8.1** Brief description of current and past DNA sequencing technologies

| | Sequencing | Year | Principle and method | Comments |
|---|---|---|---|---|
| **First generation** | Sanger sequencing (dideoxy nucleotide chain termination sequencing) | 1977 | Sequencing by synthesis – Incorporation of base-specific dideoxy chain terminators followed by gel read-out of DNA fragments. | The first genome sequenced, that of bacteriophage ΦX174, was completed using Sanger sequencing. The vast majority of the human genome was also sequenced using automated adaptations of this method. |
| | Maxam-Gilbert | 1977 | Chemical base modification of DNA followed by sequence-specific strand cleavage. Gel read-out of fragmented DNA | Developed at the same time as Sanger sequencing, Maxam-Gilbert sequencing was predominant for a short period of time. Walter Gilbert and Frederick Sanger shared the 1980 Nobel Prize for their discovery of DNA sequencing, together with Paul Berg. |
| **Next generation** | 454 FLX (Roche) | 2006 | Sequencing by synthesis/ pyrosequencing | Technologies that employed pyrosequencing were the first "next generation" sequencers commercially available. Instruments such as the Roche 454 FLX are still in common use and produce reads that are longer than other NGS technologies. |
| | HiSeq (Illumina) | 2007 | Sequencing by synthesis | The technology, initially introduced by Solexa and later acquired by Illumina, currently exists in various systems with different throughputs and run times. It is currently the most widely used and robust NGS platform. |
| | SOLiD (Life Technologies) | 2007 | SBL – sequencing by oligonucleotide ligation and detection. Oligonucleotides are fluorescently labeled and read in "colorspace" | A platform release by Applied Biosystems that utilized a unique approach to sequencing: sequencing by ligation. Sequencing was carried using 2-base encoding in "colorspace" before being interpreted as a base sequence. |
| **Third generation** | PacBio RS (Pacific Biosystems) | 2010 | Single molecule real-time sequencing | The first commercially available sequencer capable of single molecule real-time sequencing. It is also the only available instrument capable of generating read lengths greater than 1 kilobase. |
| | Ion Torrent PGM (Life Technologies) | 2010 | Semiconductor mediated sensing of H+ ion release during DNA synthesis | Along with the Illumina MiSeq instrument, Ion Torrent was one of the first "benchtop" next generation sequencers. Ion Proton system is a higher capacity version of semiconductor sequencing. |

Table 8.1 (cont.)

| Sequencing | Year | Principle and method | Comments |
|---|---|---|---|
| Oxford Nanopore Gridion (Oxford Nanopore Technologies Ltd) | 2014 | Single molecules are passed through a biological membrane and current disruptions are detected | An emerging technology available to early access research users as of 2014. |

In addition to simply determining the sequence of nucleotides in endogenous DNA, modifications to sample preparation and analysis allow the same sequencing platforms to produce other types of information relating to gene expression and epigenetic modifications. In short, NGS platforms have become so efficient at producing very large amounts of high-quality data that any experiment capable of transforming an analyte of interest into molecules detectable by NGS platforms can benefit from their use. The following section outlines some of the more common applications for which next generation DNA sequencers are used, and although not all capabilities of NGS technology currently have clinical functions, the goal of this section is to highlight the versatility of the technology that will continue to have expanded utility as new molecular biomarkers are discovered and new targeted agents are developed.

## DNA

The primary application of NGS platforms is to sequence unmodified molecules of DNA to detect mutations or to assemble genomes. DNA is converted into sequencing libraries via addition of specific sequence adaptors to the ends of DNA molecules, which are then used by NGS platforms to prime sequencing reactions. Different sequencing platforms have different adaptors and therefore have various protocols for library construction.

Once raw reads are produced from a sequencer, a common measure of their quality is a Phred score [7], denoted by Q. This score was developed to describe the quality of data produced by Sanger-based sequencers using a logarithmic score related to the probability of error. For example, a Phred score of Q20 indicates that the probability that an incorrect base was called is 1 in 100, or an accuracy of 99%, while a Q30 score indicates a 1 in 1,000 error probability (99.9%). Generally, 90% of the data generated at the read level on current NGS platforms has a Q score of 30 or better. Random sequencing error is overcome by sampling the same region with multiple reads. Each additional overlapping read reduces the chance that an aberrant base call will be made. Furthermore, the amount of data being generated in a single day on a single instrument is far greater than automated Sanger-based sequencers can produce in a year, and it is now possible to sequence an entire human genome, with several fold redundancy (also referred to as "coverage") in a matter of days compared to the years it took to complete the first draft of the Human Genome Project.

The predominant applications of DNA sequencing are whole genome sequencing (WG) and targeted sequencing. WG sequencing, sometimes referred to as shotgun sequencing, involves the random fragmentation of genomic DNA molecules into short pieces, library construction from fragmented DNA and sequencing of the DNA library.

Targeted sequencing adds an enrichment step to the process where a particular region or set of regions of the genome, such as a single gene or the exons of all the genes (known as the exome), are specifically targeted and sequencing is limited to these targets. By restricting sequencing to these regions, dramatic increases of coverage within regions of interest can be obtained. To enrich for regions, PCR can be used to amplify specific regions and resulting amplicons are used for library construction. Many technology providers offer highly multiplexed PCR-based enrichment assays that enable several hundred to thousands of PCR reactions to occur simultaneously by either physically separating them, in emulsion droplets for example, or by modifying the structure of the PCR primers to reduce cross-reactivity. Another common enrichment method, especially utilized for large targets such as an exome, involves the use of biotinylated oligonucleotides complementary to regions of interest that are used to hybridize and pull out desired target molecules from sequencing libraries prior to sequencing.

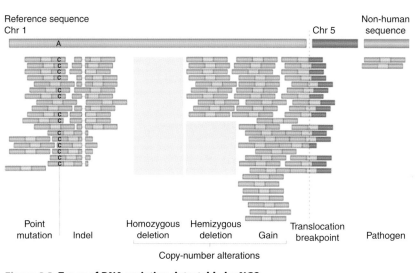

**Figure 8.2 Types of DNA variation detectable by NGS**
Representation of NGS short reads aligned to a reference sequence demonstrating the types of variation that can be detected. Reproduced from [8] with permission from Nature Publishing Group.

The types of variants that can be detected simultaneously by NGS technologies are grouped into three categories: single nucleotide variants (SNVs), short indels and structural changes (see Figure 8.2).

SNVs and short indels are the easiest to detect. Although many algorithms exist to detect these small differences at the basepair level, they all function by comparing sequencing reads to a reference genome. To call these variations with confidence, adequate sequencing depth, or the number of reads that overlap with a given genomic position, is required to observe alternative alleles. In contrast, structural changes, such as copy-number variations (CNVs) and translocations, can be detected due to the type of data generated. The digital nature of NGS data means that the number of reads that map to a region of the genome is proportional to the copy-number of that region. Thus, by comparing read depth across the genome and normalizing for the total number of reads generated, one can determine a genome-wide DNA copy-number profile. Additionally, paired end sequencing, where the same molecule of DNA is sequenced from both ends, allows one to map reads generated from opposite ends of a contiguous molecule independently. Structural variants can be detected if the paired end reads map in unexpected orientations: for example, reads far apart can reveal deleted regions and read pairs mapping across chromosomes can reveal translocations.

Several other genotyping technologies exist to detect different types of DNA variation and are used clinically. For example, microarray-based genotyping methods can detect up to several million single nucleotide polymorphisms in a single experiment and can be used to detect regions of variable copy-number. The downside of genotyping using arrays is that only known variants are included on arrays and therefore have limited ability to detect novel aberrations. Furthermore, DNA input requirements are much higher for genotyping methods compared to NGS and they do not have the ability to detect all types of DNA variation simultaneously.

## RNA

A complement to DNA-based NGS is RNA-based transcriptome sequencing, commonly referred to as RNA-Seq. While the actual reactions used to sequence RNA-Seq libraries are the same as those for DNA sequencing, sequencing libraries for RNA-Seq studies are prepared from cDNA, which is generated from reverse transcribed RNA (see Figure 8.3).

Sequencing libraries generated from RNA yield information unique to the transcriptome level: gene expression levels, information about RNA splicing patterns or evidence that chimeric transcripts (gene fusions) are present in a sample. In addition to protein encoding mRNA, other species of RNA such as

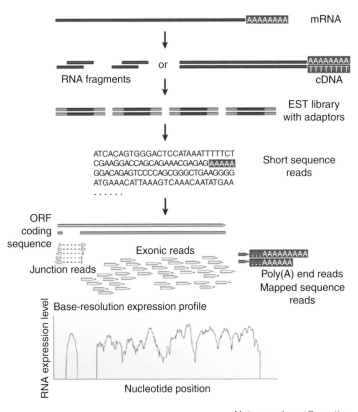

ATCACAGTGGGACTCCATAAATTTTTCT
CGAAGGACCAGCAGAAACGAGAGAAAAA
GGACAGAGTCCCCAGCGGGCTGAAGGGG
ATGAAACATTAAAGTCAAACAATATGAA
. . . . . .

Figure 8.3 **Schematic representation of RNA-Seq**
Representation of the RNA-Seq workflow for the utilization of NGS to detect mRNA expression. Reproduced from [9] with permission from Nature Publishing Group.

Nature reviews|Genetics

regulatory microRNA (miRNA) and long intergenic non-coding RNA (lincRNA) can be profiled when whole RNA is used as input to the assay.

While hybridization-based quantification using microarrays is an established technology to measure gene expression levels and RNA splicing, RNA-Seq has matured to the point that the current cost of sequencing is comparable to well-designed microarray experiments. However, microarray-based analyses are fundamentally limited by the design of the hybridization chip, which generally only includes known transcripts and transcriptomic events, such as spliced RNA species. RNA sequencing is one of the few technologies capable of detecting novel events in the transcriptome, a feature essential for research in a cancer setting where uncharacterized somatic mutations and other genomic alterations are commonly found.

Along this line, there is evidence that RNA sequencing will soon provide value in clinical settings. For example, Oncotype DX is a 21-gene based test used to stratify patients based on recurrence

risk and chemotherapy benefit [10], and while the test is RT-PCR based, RNA-Seq-based quantification of the same gene panel yields similar results in terms of recurrence risk hazard [11], suggesting that RNA sequencing can eventually supplant RT-PCR-based assays. On a practical level, this study showed that RNA sequencing requires approximately one-fifth of the quantity of input RNA as compared with RT-PCR, a significant advantage if RNA is derived from limited samples like FFPE archival tissues.

## Epigenetics

Our understanding of the epigenetic mechanisms underlying the regulation of cellular growth has undergone a transformation with the advent of next generation sequencing technologies. Experiments designed to query the epigenetic state of a population of cells brought a resurgence of interest to the field and epigenetics is now a rapidly growing field of investigation.

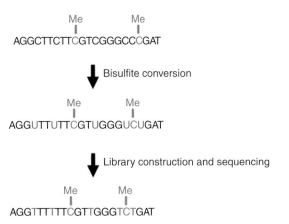

**Figure 8.4 Bisulfite conversion of non-methylated cytosine residues**
Bisulfite treatment of DNA results in the conversion on non-methylated cytosine residues to uracil, which upon sequencing results in the detection of C to T transition.

Epigenetics is commonly subcategorized into two branches: the patterns of cytosine methylation that occur scattered throughout the mammalian genome, and covalent modifications to histone proteins which act to organize and package nuclear DNA. Cytosine residues in genomic regions known as CpG islands can be methylated to produce 5-methylcytosine, yielding methylated CpG regions. The methylation status of CpG motifs are known to regulate gene expression [12]. On the other hand, histone modifications are involved in a variety of cellular processes, including gene silencing, activation and DNA repair mechanisms. These two distinct aspects of epigenetics are critical to our understanding of cancer genetics as each can be commonly dysregulated early on in tumorigenesis. It is possible to discern the genomic patterns of cytosine methylation using various methods. These include the conversion of cytosine residues to uracil with the reducing agent bisulfite (bisulfite-sequencing – see Figure 8.4), immuno-precipitation of 5'-methylcytosine with antibodies or methyl-binding protein (MeDIP), and the use of methylation-sensitive restriction endonucleases.

Bisulfite sequencing of converted DNA provides the highest resolution of 5'-methylcytosine mapping since, theoretically, every cytosine residue can be interrogated for methylation status and mapped precisely to a chromosomal position. DNA is treated with bisulfite, a chemical agent that converts all cytosine residues to uracil, leaving 5-methylcytosine residues unconverted. Upon sequencing, converted cytosine residues are interpreted as C to T transitions after comparing the reads to a reference genome. Although bisulfite sequencing is robust, it is not without shortcomings. Treatment with bisulfite is harsh and can result in mass degradation and cleavage of DNA, and bisulfite itself is unstable and great care must be taken to ensure that fresh reagent is used to ensure complete chemical conversion of cytosine residues. Complicating this approach further is the discovery of 5-hydroxymethylcytosine modifications, a physiologically important cytosine alteration that is indistinguishable from methylcytosine using this method.

Two similar methods of epigenetic analyses are ChIP-seq (Chromatin Immunoprecipitation – sequencing) and MeDIP-seq (Methylated DNA Immunoprecipitation – sequencing). Both methods rely on the specificity of antibodies or proteins with specific binding capabilities (i.e. Methyl DNA binding protein) in order to enrich fragmented DNA that is associated with a desired feature or protein/DNA complex. There are various methods in common use today in order to perform immunoprecipitation of histone-associated DNA and methylated DNA (see Figure 8.5).

The methods used to study DNA methylation and histone modification have existed for decades, but have been reinvigorated since the introduction of next generation sequencing. The introduction of high throughput sequencing technologies resulted in enormous methodological advances. Historically, regions that were interrogated for DNA methylation or nucleosome occupancy were targeted by specific PCR reactions. In this way, only small regions of the genome could be analyzed and the researcher needed to know where to look. With the introduction of next generation sequencing, the experimental read-out of these methods was forever changed, allowing access to the entire genome.

Although there is currently no clinical use of epigenetic profiling, this rapidly advancing field will likely lead to the identification of epigenetic biomarkers that will have an impact on patient care. NGS technologies already established in clinical labs will be able to seamlessly adopt these methods to integrate epigenetic testing.

# Bioinformatics

The bottlenecks of DNA sequencing have shifted away from sequencing and data generation to data

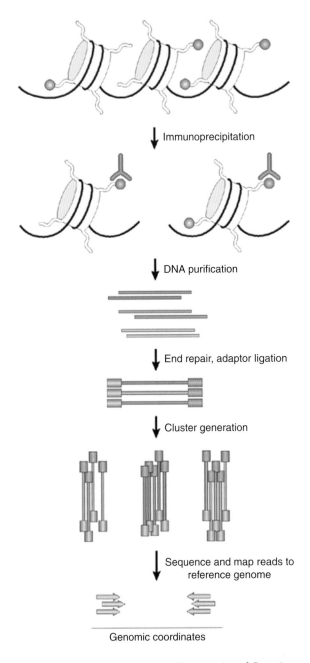

Immunoprecipitation

DNA purification

End repair, adaptor ligation

Cluster generation

Sequence and map reads to reference genome

Genomic coordinates

Nature reviews | Genetics

Figure 8.5 **Chromatin Immunoprecipitation sequencing (ChIP-seq)**
Antibodies are used for the immunoprecipitation of histone-associated DNA. Reproduced from [13] with permission from Nature Publishing Group.

research field is being directed towards improving analytical methods to use computational resources more effectively. Translating NGS data into meaningful information generally involves four steps: conversion of raw signal into DNA sequences or reads; alignment of sequencing reads to a reference genome; calling of genomic variants; and the interpretation of these variants.

Development of software tools to perform these analysis steps and identify and interpret different types of genomic alterations has been a very active and evolving area of research since the emergence of the first NGS technologies. While seemingly straightforward, the simple scenario of calling nucleotides from raw sequencer data and aligning reads is challenging due to regions of homology within the genome, errors and gaps in the reference genome, systematic errors in sequencing chemistries and variability in coverage that can arise in GC-rich regions. Each of these sources of error can influence the ability to call the most simple genomic aberration, a single nucleotide difference, and it has been shown that even with very stringent quality filters, 50-fold coverage is required to achieve a genotyping call error rate of one error in 1 million germline SNP calls [14]. This coverage goes up to 100-fold coverage if variant allele frequencies are much lower than 50%, as frequently happens when detecting somatic variants in cancer genomes [15]. Genomic and technical complexities are an even greater hindrance to more complicated types of analysis such as the detection of inversions and translocations.

In addition to calling variants, there is growing interest in the prediction of the functional consequences of variants. Many software tools exist to use features such as inter-species sequence conservation, the properties of resulting amino acid changes, and mutation frequency to classify novel variants and predict their function. As the breadth of NGS sequencing increases, this will become a more important issue as the number of variants becomes far too large to report on or functionally validate. In a single individual's genome there are on average 3.3 million single nucleotide polymorphisms, of which around 10,000 are in protein coding sequences and can cause amino acid substitutions [16], while cancer genomes harbor between 1,500 and 30,000 somatic alterations [17]. In clinical settings, only a handful of these variants might be actionable to physicians charged with patient care, so automated methods are required to prioritize variant calls so as to distill this

analysis. The computational resources required to store and analyze the vast amount of sequencing data capable of being generated daily are often overlooked, and much effort in the molecular diagnostics and wealth of information down to the most concise and meaningful candidates.

In a clinical setting, software pipelines for NGS analysis need to be validated to assess their sensitivity and specificity and, having done so, accepted processes must be locked down in order to yield reproducible data that are in compliance with the appropriate regulations governing NGS-based clinical tests, which are still evolving.

The final computational component important to NGS is data storage, since a single NGS instrument is capable of generating several gigabases of data at a time. When considering the large amounts of data generated from genomic analyses, huge infrastructure requirements are needed to maintain the accessibility of data for many types of analysis. For example, storing 1 terabyte (approximately the space required to store sequence data for three to four cancer genomes) costs approximately $1,000 per year based on current commercial cloud computing storage prices. In clinical settings, secure computing infrastructure is needed to store and process data that are active and currently being used for patient care or research, but also to maintain them, perhaps indefinitely, for medical records purposes.

## Clinical utilization of NGS

Currently available clinical genetic tests are generally geared towards finding low numbers of variants in particular genes or set of genes, and this low throughput lends itself well to the tests using platforms like capillary sequencing, microarrays or PCR. However, as the utility and success of current clinical tests increases and the number of available tests on the market grows, resources required to conduct testing, both in terms of laboratory resources (such as labor and reagents) and sample availability (tissue, DNA, etc.), will limit the use of low throughput platforms. The greater accuracy, speed and ability to assess multiple variant types in multiple targets simultaneously while using very little amounts of input material will boost the demand for NGS technology in clinical testing, making it the standard tool in molecular pathology laboratories for genetic testing.

One area of medicine where NGS is already having profound effects is for the detection of rare inherited conditions. These monogenic disorders are caused by mutations that do not occur frequently in the general population, and prior to NGS and the completion of the human reference genome,

disease genes were discovered by linkage analysis. This process involved profiling genetic markers, usually short tandem repeats (STRs), spaced across chromosomes in large families with affected and unaffected individuals. While this process successfully identified disease genes for conditions such as cystic fibrosis [18–20], the process was limited to disorders where large pedigrees, clear clinical data, detailed phenotypes and panels of dense genetic markers were available.

With NGS technology, pathogenic mutations, such as those causing rare autosomal recessive disorders, can be detected by broad sequencing (whole genome or exome) of parents and affected children, thus eliminating the need for large pedigrees. Furthermore, mutations underlying monogenic disorders, such as Kabuki syndrome, have even been elucidated by NGS sequencing of multiple cases alone by identifying overlapping genes with rare mutations among cases [21]. While the primary uses of NGS are still discovery efforts, many rare monogenic diseases share extremely similar clinical phenotypes despite arising from genetically heterogeneous causes. In these cases, NGS sequencing holds the promise of making more precise diagnoses by ruling out diseases with known genetic presentations. Furthermore, if it is discovered that the underlying genetic cause of any one of these diseases is targetable by known therapies, sequencing may provide concrete evidence that can be used to decide on a treatment and yield improved clinical outcomes.

A hallmark case of NGS application in the clinic involved two 14-year-old fraternal twins who had been diagnosed with dopa (3,4-dihydroxyphenylalanine)-responsive dystonia (DRD, http://omim.org/entry/128230). DRD is usually treated with L-dopa; however, the treatment was not effective. Whole genome sequencing of the twins identified mutations in the gene encoding sepiapterin reductase, involved in the synthesis of dopamine and serotonin. This information led to the decision to supplement therapy with 5-hydroxytryptophan (which is a precursor to serotonin), resulting in dramatic clinical improvements in both patients [22].

Despite the advances that have been made in NGS technology, the time required to perform and analyze whole genome sequencing data is still too long for clinical situations where results are required quickly to impact therapy. In these situations, a more suitable approach is to restrict sequencing to a subset of genes, an approach called targeted sequencing. However,

Table 8.2 Exemplary set of clinically informative genomic variants

| Gene | Type of genetic alteration | Tumor type | Representative therapeutic agent currently available or in development |
|------|---------------------------|------------|----------------------------------------------------------------------|
| AKT1 | Mutation (E17K) | breast, ovarian | MK-2206, GDC-0068 |
| BRAF | Mutation (V600E) | melanoma, colon, thyroid, lung | vemurafenib, dabrafenib |
| EGFR | Mutation (exons 18-21) | NSCLC | gefitinib, erlotinib, centuximab, panitumumab |
| FLT3 | Internal tandem duplication | AML | midostaurin |
| JAK2 | Mutation (exon 12, V617F) | CML, myeloproliferative disorders | INCB018424, prognostic |
| KIT | Mutation (exons 8,9,11,17) | GIST | imatinib, sunitinib |
| KRAS | Mutation (codons 12,13,61) | PDAC, colon | erlotnib |
| PTCH1/SMO | Mutations | medulloblastoma | vismodegib, erismodegib, saridegib |
| PIK3CA | Mutations (exon 9,10) | colorectal, breast, gastric cancer, glioblastoma | buparlisib, PF-4691502, GSK-2636771 |
| BRCA1/2 | Mutations | breast, ovarian | olaparib |
| ERBB2 (HER2) | Amplification | breast | trastuzumab |
| BCR-ABL1 | Fusion | CML/ALL | imatinib, nilotinib |
| EML4-ALK | Fusion | NSCLC | crizotinib |
| KIF5B-RET | Fusion | lung | vandetanib |
| PDGFRA | Mutation | glioblastoma, GIST | imatinib, sorafenib, sunitinib |
| PDGFRB | Translocation | chronic myelomonocytic leukemia | imatinib, sorafenib, sunitinib |

NSCLC = non-small cell lung cancer; AML = acute myeloid leukemia; CML = chronic myeloid leukemia; GIST = gastrointestinal stromal tumor; PDAC = pancreatic ductal adenocarcinoma; ALL = acute lymphoblastic leukemia.

NGS still becomes the method of choice where many genes and/or many samples need to be processed very quickly. In addition to cost, the biggest determinant for the breadth of sequencing performed in clinical settings is the time required to produce and analyze the data, and to report relevant information back to physicians.

# Cancer

Sequencing technologies will likely have the largest impact in oncology. Cancer is fundamentally a disease of the genome; large-scale cancer genome profiling efforts such as The Cancer Genome Atlas (TCGA; cancergenome.nih.gov) and the International Cancer Genome Consortium (ICGC, www.icgc.org [23]) are characterizing the full spectrum of genomic alterations in hundreds of tumor samples across many

different tumor types. These efforts are leading towards the elucidation of molecular events driving cancer and will yield useful information for clinical applications such as providing more accurate prognoses in newly diagnosed cancer patients. Furthermore, the increased understanding of biological pathways underlying cancer phenotypes is contributing towards the development of targeted agents effective against subsets of molecularly defined tumors. Table 8.2 lists an exemplary set of genomic variants that have clinical utility.

Meanwhile, the list of actionable DNA and RNA variants continues to grow. Some variants, such as those responsible for altered expression of proteins, are currently measured by immunohistochemical methods clinically to guide therapy (HER2 over-expression and trastuzumab [24], for example). Other mutations already have DNA-based tests with

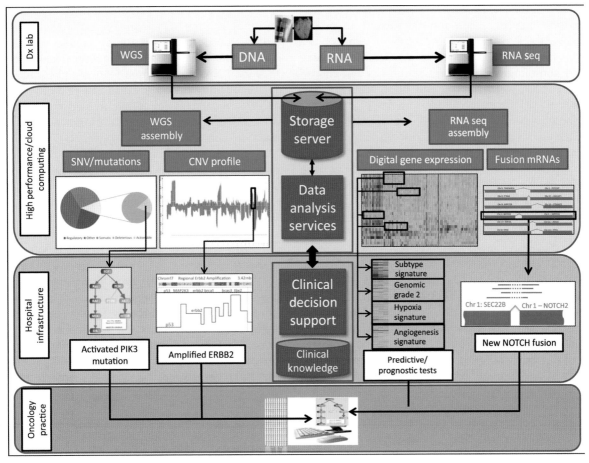

**Figure 8.6 A model for clinical sequencing in oncology**
An overview of the steps required to implement next generation sequencing in clinical oncology. The same process may be applied to other fields of medicine. Reproduced from [29] with permission from Elsevier.

regulatory approval, such as the BRAF V600E mutation that is associated with increased sensitivity to BRAF inhibitors such as vemurafenib in melanoma [25]. The utilization of NGS-targeted sequencing to profile patient tumor samples for many of these variants in a single panel or test is now being carried out in clinical settings [26]. NGS technology will not surpass current histopathological analyses, but rather augment diagnosis by providing more refined characterization of cancer subtypes at the molecular level.

As the list of clinically relevant variants grows, rather than creating additional targeted sequencing assays, one can envision a scenario where every cancer patient has their complete tumor genome and/or transcriptome profiled. Clinical interpretation of whole genome data has been acknowledged as a new problem that requires participation between pathologists, clinicians and experts in biomedical

informatics, with a focus on predicting how genome analyses will replace today's standard molecular diagnostics [27]. Here, Wall and Tonellato estimate that 85% of the 600 tests currently used to interpret tumors for at least 90 conditions can be replaced by whole genome analysis [27]. The adoption of genomics in clinical settings has helped the field to recognize the need to train pathologists in the entire aspect of this discipline. Genomics and personalized medicine curricula were established at major medical training centers as early as 2012 [28]. There will also be a need for automatic software to identify somatic anomalies with clinical relevance, based on current knowledge at the time, that can generate physician-friendly reports that incorporate the growing knowledge base of cancer biology (see Figure 8.6).

Sequencing cancer samples poses distinct challenges that sequencing germline DNA and RNA derived from blood samples does not. First of all, tumors comprise a non-uniform mixture of many different cell types, made up of both tumor cells containing somatic mutations driving the disease and non-tumor cells, such as fibroblasts and endothelial cells, which are by and large genotypically normal. Cellularity of tumor samples is a critical concept, referring to the proportion of the tumor made up of tumor cells. Cellularity can vary dramatically between tumor types and is typically highest in solid tumors with defined margins. While heterozygous germline genetic variants will have allele frequencies of close to 50%, tumor samples with low cellularity exhibit much lower variant allele frequencies and in some cases, such as tumors with less than 20% cellularity, minor allele frequencies can be present at less than 10%. At these low abundances, mutated alleles cannot be reliably detected by Sanger sequencing [30], while NGS sequencing can overcome problems associated with poor cellularity through increased sequencing depth. By sampling the alleles many times, true variants, even those at frequencies close to 1% to 2%, emerge from background noise and can be reliably detected. Additionally, methods such as laser capture micro-dissection and flow cytometry can be used to enrich the sample for tumor cells resulting in increased cellularity that when combined with NGS produces vast amounts of very high-quality data.

The degree of heterogeneity observed within tumors from the same patient further adds to the difficulty of tumor sequencing. It is well accepted that tumors are seldom derived from a single clone and more frequently comprise a mixture of clones evolving independently. Many factors can influence the selective pressures giving rise to growth advantages for particular clones, including: physical location within the tumor; proximity to blood vessels and an oxygen supply; and ongoing therapy which may be ineffective against certain clones carrying drug-resistant mutations. The consequence of tumor heterogeneity is that tumor cells in geographically different locations within the same mass may have a very different genetic background. The implication for sequencing is that different somatic events will occur at different frequencies depending on the abundance of the mutation harboring clones in the sample. If single biopsies or small pieces of tumor are used for testing, it is possible that some mutations end up completely undetected.

Finally, the nature of current clinical samples can cause problems for NGS technologies. Formalin-fixed paraffin-embedded (FFPE) tumor samples are the norm in the current cancer diagnostic realm. The DNA and RNA extracted from FFPE samples is often of lower quantity and quality than that obtained from fresh-frozen samples due to nucleic acid fragmentation and damage during the fixation process, which results in suboptimal library construction and an increased error rate during sequencing. FFPE samples are not likely to disappear as they are required for standard pathological analysis, so the field is currently seeing new improvements in both FFPE fixation processes and in sequencing library construction methods, both contributing to the production of improved NGS data quality when FFPE samples are used.

Despite these challenges, clinical trials have demonstrated that NGS technologies can make personalized cancer therapy a possibility for patients whose tumors carry known actionable mutations [31]. As our understanding of cancer genomes continues to grow and new targeted therapies enter the clinic, the proportion of patients that stand to benefit from NGS analysis of their tumor samples will steadily increase.

## Roadblocks to clinical NGS

While many institutes around the world are beginning to implement some form of NGS into routine clinical practice, it remains, for the most part, limited to larger hospitals that also have large-scale research activities utilizing NGS. Before clinical use of NGS becomes widespread, several issues need to be resolved, notably: regulatory considerations regarding reproducibility of test results, ethical obligations to patients, and education of people making decisions over patient care.

The process for a diagnostic test to enter the clinic first involves analytical validation/verification, followed by regulatory approval by agencies such as the US Food and Drug Administration (FDA). The traditional regulatory approach for diagnostic tests is the approval of the entire systems: assay, instrument and software. This process is time-consuming and is not amenable to the speed of change in fields evolving rapidly, such as with DNA sequencing. These delays can hinder reporting of genetic results to clinicians despite their recognition and acceptance from the scientific and medical community. To cope with the burden of regulations, a short-term strategy for developers of NGS clinical tests has been to package many relevant validated disease genes into single diagnostic tests containing multiple target panels of genes and obtain regulatory approval as a panel. However, future plans to improve the framework of regulatory approval of (novel/individual) NGS-based tests are unclear. Currently, CLIA-waived labs (Clinical Laboratory Improvement Amendment) can conduct NGS-based tests that are classified as Lab Developed Tests (LDT) and do not require FDA approval [32, 33]. Using the standards laid out by CLIA for validation of NGS tests is a first step to ensure that testing is robust and reproducible. A common method for validation is to compare NGS diagnostic test results to a "gold standard" test, such as capillary-based Sanger sequencing. One testing possibility used is to verify NGS findings using Sanger sequencing, but this approach becomes extremely expensive in terms of both reagents and labor for verification of all variants detected in patient exomes or genomes and thus impractical. Another approach is cross-validation tests using multiple NGS platforms that rely on different chemistries, which allow for technical errors to be ruled out. Furthermore, some platforms perform certain analyses better and having multiple platforms available allows the appropriate technology to be selected for a given assay. Finally, there is currently a lack of reference material (RM) for NGS testing and a lack of agreement among clinical users of NGS on what RMs should constitute and how calibration should take place. In other diagnostic areas, RMs are used for equipment calibration and as control samples run concurrently with patient samples, in order to rule out technical and human errors and to ensure that results are reproducible both within labs and between institutes.

One downside to broad-based testing, such as whole genome sequencing, is that genetic variation unrelated to the reason for which sequencing is performed will be uncovered. There is growing concern on how to handle these incidental findings and when they should be reported back to the patient, with three broad categories of incidental findings currently defined: those with clear evidence of adverse but potentially preventable medical outcomes, those without interventions available, and those with unknown significance.

The American College of Medical Genetics and Genomics (ACMG) states that failing to report the first category of findings is unethical [30]. As the other two classes are not currently actionable, the potential for patient distress must be considered and tips the balance against reporting such variants. In addition, pre-test counseling about incidental findings can help patients understand that they generally cannot opt out of labs reporting incidental test results to the ordering physician.

More complex cases of incidental findings also exist, for example whether to report findings of adult onset diseases in children, where no immediate medical benefit to the child is available. In another complex example provided by the ACMG, identification of a child carrying a BRCA1 mutation suggests that at least one parent does as well, and disclosure of the finding may benefit the child by preventing a severe health outcome in a parent [34]. It is important that patients are very well informed when they consent to NGS testing, so that they are aware of the possibility of uncovering that they harbor disease risk or pathogenic variants. There will likely be the involvement of genetic counselors even prior to NGS results being obtained. Having well-informed patients will also ensure that expectations are not exaggerated, as not all patients undergoing molecular analysis will benefit to the same degree.

The final barrier to widespread use of NGS in the clinic is the additional training required for both clinicians and molecular pathologists. The field of NGS is still in its infancy, yet it is expanding rapidly. New molecular biology is being revealed through large-scale genomic studies and technology providers are continuously expanding their capabilities. It is imperative that the advances in the applications, analyses and interpretation of NGS be incorporated into ongoing and continuing medical education that currently only covers the basics of molecular genetics. Only then will the full potential of clinical sequencing be realized.

## Additional reading

As NGS technology becomes more widespread in clinical environments, organizations such as the Association for Molecular Pathology (AMP), the US Centers for Disease Control and Prevention (CDC), the American College of Medical Genetics (ACMG) and the College of American Pathologists have

Table 8.3 Additional resource documents for clinical NGS

| Document | Organization |
| --- | --- |
| Opportunities and challenges associated with clinical diagnostic genome sequencing: a report of the Association for Molecular Pathology [35] | AMP (www.amp.org) |
| Assuring the quality of next generation sequencing in clinical laboratory practice [33] | CDC (www.cdc.gov/) |
| ACMG clinical laboratory standards for next generation sequencing [36] | ACMG (www.acmg.net) |
| Genome Analysis Resource Guide | CAP (www.cap.org) |

established working groups in order to produce guidelines, checklists and white papers to inform and educate various stakeholders. Listed in Table 8.3 are some of the resources currently available from these organizations.

## Learning points

- With the rapid development of genomic tools and their growing availability and applications, it is becoming increasingly important for pathologists to prepare for the inevitable advances on the horizon.

- Methods in genomic analysis are capable of revealing information that goes beyond that seen with classical pathology methods. Molecular markers of prognostic and diagnostic significance are emerging that would otherwise remain invisible on a microscope slide.

- Sequencing technologies will likely have the largest impact in oncology. Understanding the genetic heterogeneity within a tumor is of critical importance for designing effective therapies of the future. The tools afforded by genomic analysis will greatly aid in identifying genetically distinct populations of cells that may respond to therapeutic agents differently within the same tumor.

- Multiple genetic lesions are often at the core of tumor etiology. Complex multi-locus interactions are near impossible to detect without the use of these powerful genetic tools. The ability to identify and understand these complex interactions will inevitably allow great advances in the treatment of cancer.

- The current regulatory framework governing clinical uses of NGS sequencing is ill defined. Governing agencies such as the US-FDA will need to create regulations that are flexible to the rapid advances in this new field while simultaneously protecting patients. Currently, CLIA-waived labs utilize NGS technologies under the category of Lab Developed Tests (LDT), which are exempt from full regulatory approval.

## References

1. Sanger, F., Nicklen, S. and Coulson, A. R. DNA sequencing with chain-terminating inhibitors. *Proc Natl Acad Sci USA* 1977; 74(12): 5463–7.

2. Lander, E. S., Linton, L. M., Birren, B., Nusbaum, C., Zody, M. C., Baldwin, J. *et al.* Initial sequencing and analysis of the human genome. *Nature* 2001; 409(6822): 860–921.

3. Robison, R. A. Moore's law: predictor and driver of the silicon era. *World Neurosurg* 2012; 78(5): 399–403.

4. Wetterstrand, K. DNA sequencing Costs: data from the NHGRI Genome Sequencing Program (GSP), available at www.genome.gov/sequencingcosts.

5. Metzker, M. L. Sequencing technologies – the next generation. *Nat Rev Genet* 2010; 11(1): 31–46.

6. Mardis, E. R. A decade's perspective on DNA sequencing technology. *Nature* 2011; 470(7333): 198–203.

7. Ewing, B. and Green, P. Base-calling of automated sequencer traces using phred. II. Error probabilities. *Genome Res* 1998; 8(3): 186–94.

8. Meyerson, M., Gabriel, S. and Getz, G. Advances in understanding cancer genomes through second-generation sequencing. *Nat Rev Genet* 2010; 11(10): 685–96.

9. Wang, Z., Gerstein, M. and Snyder, M. RNA-Seq: a revolutionary tool for transcriptomics. *Nat Rev Genet* 2009; 10(1): 57–63.

10. Oakman, C., Santarpia, L. and Di Leo, A. Breast cancer assessment tools and optimizing adjuvant

therapy. *Nat Rev Clin Oncol* 2010; 7(12): 725–32.

11. Sinicropi, D., Qu, K., Collin, F., Crager, M., Liu, M.-L., Pelham, R. J. *et al.* Whole transcriptome RNA-Seq analysis of breast cancer recurrence risk using formalin-fixed paraffin-embedded tumor tissue. *PLoS ONE* 2012; 7(7): e40092.

12. Shen, H. and Laird, P. W. Interplay between the cancer genome and epigenome. *Cell* 2013; 153(1): 38–55.

13. Schones, D. E. and Zhao, K. Genome-wide approaches to studying chromatin modifications. *Nat Rev Genet* 2008; 9(3): 179–91.

14. Ajay, S. S., Parker, S. C. J., Abaan, H. O., Fajardo, K. V. F. and Margulies, E. H. Accurate and comprehensive sequencing of personal genomes. *Genome Res* 2011; 21(9): 1498–505.

15. Carter, S. L., Cibulskis, K., Helman, E., McKenna, A., Shen, H., Zack, T. *et al.* Absolute quantification of somatic DNA alterations in human cancer. *Nat Biotechnol* 2012; 30(5): 413–21.

16. Wheeler, D. A., Srinivasan, M., Egholm, M., Shen, Y., Chen, L., McGuire, A. *et al.* The complete genome of an individual by massively parallel DNA sequencing. *Nature* 2008; 452(7189): 872–6.

17. Vogelstein, B., Papadopoulos, N., Velculescu, V. E., Zhou, S., Diaz, L. A. and Kinzler, K. W. Cancer genome landscapes. *Science* 2013; 339(6127): 1546–58.

18. Kerem, B., Rommens, J. M., Buchanan, J. A., Markiewicz, D., Cox, T. K., Chakravarti, A. *et al.* Identification of the cystic fibrosis gene: genetic analysis. *Science* 1989; 245(4922): 1073–80.

19. Riordan, J. R., Rommens, J. M., Kerem, B., Alon, N., Rozmahel, R., Grzelczak, Z. *et al.*

Identification of the cystic fibrosis gene: cloning and characterization of complementary DNA. *Science* 1989; 245(4922): 1066–73.

20. Rommens, J. M., Iannuzzi, M. C., Kerem, B., Drumm, M. L., Melmer, G., Dean, M. *et al.* Identification of the cystic fibrosis gene: chromosome walking and jumping. *Science* 1989; 245(4922): 1059–65.

21. Ng, S. B., Bigham, A. W., Buckingham, K. J., Hannibal, M. C., McMillin, M. J., Gildersleeve, H. I. *et al.* Exome sequencing identifies MLL2 mutations as a cause of Kabuki syndrome. *Nat Genet* 2010; 42(9): 790–3.

22. Bainbridge, M. N., Wiszniewski, W., Murdock, D. R., Friedman, J., Gonzaga-Jauregui, C., Newsham, I. *et al.* Whole-genome sequencing for optimized patient management. *Sci Transl Med* 2011; 3(87): 87re3.

23. Hudson, T. J., Anderson, W., Artez, A., Barker, A. D., Bell, C., Bernabé, R. R. *et al.* International network of cancer genome projects. *Nature* 2010; 464(7291): 993–8.

24. Slamon, D. J., Leyland-Jones, B., Shak, S., Fuchs, H., Paton, V., Bajamonde, A. *et al.* Use of chemotherapy plus a monoclonal antibody against HER2 for metastatic breast cancer that overexpresses HER2. *New Engl J Med* 2001; 344(11): 783–92.

25. Chapman, P. B., Hauschild, A., Robert, C., Haanen, J. B., Ascierto, P., Larkin, J. *et al.* Improved survival with vemurafenib in melanoma with BRAF V600E mutation. *New Engl J Med* 2011; 364(26): 2507–16.

26. Cronin, M. and Ross, J. S. Comprehensive next-generation cancer genome sequencing in the era of targeted therapy and personalized oncology. *Biomark Med* 2011; 5(3): 293–305.

27. Wall, D. P. and Tonellato, P. J. The future of genomics in

pathology. *F1000 Med Rep* 2012 2014:4, available at www.ncbi.nlm. nih.gov/pmc/articles/ PMC3391753/.

28. Haspel, R. L., Arnaout, R., Briere, L., Kantarci, S., Marchand, K., Tonellato, P. *et al.* A call to action: training pathology residents in genomics and personalized medicine. *Am J Clin Pathol* 2010; 133(6): 832–4.

29. Kamalakaran, S., Varadan, V., Janevski, A., Banerjee, N., Tuck, D., McCombie, W. R. *et al.* Translating next generation sequencing to practice: opportunities and necessary steps. *Mol Oncol* 2013; 7(4): 743–55.

30. Kohlmann, A., Klein, H.-U., Weissmann, S., Bresolin, S., Chaplin, T., Cuppens, H. *et al.* The Interlaboratory RObustness of Next-generation sequencing (IRON) study: a deep sequencing investigation of TET2, CBL and KRAS mutations by an international consortium involving 10 laboratories. *Leukemia* 2011; 25(12): 1840–8.

31. Tran, B., Brown, A. M. K., Bedard, P. L., Winquist, E., Goss, G. D., Hotte, S. J. *et al.* Feasibility of real time next generation sequencing of cancer genes linked to drug response: results from a clinical trial. *Int J Cancer* 2013; 132(7): 1547–55.

32. Ferreira-Gonzalez, A., Emmadi, R., Day, S. P., Klees, R. F., Leib, J. R., Lyon, E. *et al.* Revisiting oversight and regulation of molecular-based laboratory-developed tests: a position statement of the Association for Molecular Pathology. *J Mol Diagn* 2014; 16(1): 3–6.

33. Gargis, A. S., Kalman, L., Berry, M. W., Bick, D. P., Dimmock, D. P., Hambuch, T. *et al.* Assuring the quality of next-generation sequencing in clinical laboratory practice. *Nat Biotech* 2012; 30(11): 1033–6.

**117**

34. Green, R. C., Berg, J. S., Grody, W. W., Kalia, S. S., Korf, B. R., Martin, C. L. *et al.* ACMG recommendations for reporting of incidental findings in clinical exome and genome sequencing. *Genet Med* 2013; 15(7): 565–74.

35. Schrijver, I., Aziz, N., Farkas, D. H., Furtado, M., Gonzalez, A. F., Greiner, T. C. *et al.* Opportunities and challenges associated with clinical diagnostic genome sequencing: a report of the Association for Molecular Pathology. *J Mol Diagn* 2012; 14(6): 525–40.

36. Rehm, H. L., Bale, S. J., Bayrak-Toydemir, P., Berg, J. S., Brown, K. K., Deignan, J. L. *et al.* ACMG clinical laboratory standards for next-generation sequencing. *Genet Med* 2013; 15(9): 733–47.

# Chapter 9

# Microsatellite instability in colorectal cancer

Maria Sofia Fernandes, Raquel Seruca and Sérgia Velho

## Microsatellite instability (MSI) – the mutator phenotype

Colorectal cancer (CRC) is one of the most common malignancies and one of the leading causes of cancer mortality worldwide (1). Developing as a multistep process, CRC can be classified in two subclasses according to the type of genetic instability presented, microsatellite instability (MSI) and microsatellite stability (MSS) (2).

About 15% of CRCs are characterized by the accumulation of numerous mutations across the genome mainly in repetitive sequences (microsatellites) due to a defective mismatch repair (MMR) system, and are characterized by a phenotype designated as MSI high (MSI-H) (3). Initially, MSI was associated with a hereditary form of CRC, Lynch syndrome, characterized by germline mutations in MMR genes and in which more than 90% of patients exhibit MSI (3, 4). It was subsequently demonstrated that patients with sporadic CRC can also present with MSI through promoter methylation of MMR genes (5).

The MMR system is composed of at least seven proteins, h-MLH1, h-MLH3, h-MSH2, h-MSH3, h-MSH6, h-PMS1 and h-PMS2, which associate with specific partners to form functional heterodimers that recognize basepair mismatches and small nucleotide insertion/deletions (1 to 4 basepairs) that occur during DNA replication (6, 7, 8). h-MLH1 and h-MSH2 are essential components of the human MMR machinery and form five functional heterodimeric complexes: h-MSH2/h-MSH3; h-MSH2/h-MSH6; h-MLH1/h-PMS1; h-MLH1/h-PMS2; h-MLH1/h-MLH3 (9). The main mechanism by which MMR system failure occurs in MSI-H gastrointestinal cancers involves genetic and epigenetic alterations occurring at these MMR system effectors, namely in h-MLH1 and h-MSH2, and less frequently in h-MSH6 and h-PMS2 (10).

In cells with a deficient MMR system, mutations accumulate not only in repetitive non-coding sequences, but also in coding sequences. Target genes of MMR deficiency include, among many others, TGFBRII, IGFIIR, BAX, TCF-4, MSH3, MSH6, Caspase-5, GRB-14, RHAMM, RAD50, RIZ, E2F4, PTEN, MBD4, CHK1, FAS, APAF-1, BCL-10 and EPHB2 (11). From all described MMR target genes, TGFBRII harbors the highest mutation frequency (about 80%) and these alterations are known to associate with enhanced cell proliferation rates and higher angiogenic potential (12).

## Pathways for colorectal cancer development

The distinct nature of MSI and MSS cancers is highlighted by the observation that they exhibit unique progression pathways associated with distinct mutational spectra (2, 13).

In 1988, Fearon and Vogelstein started to propose a mechanism for CRC development known as the adenoma-carcinoma model (14). This model was a linear, multi-step sequence of accumulation of genetic alterations, in which inactivating mutations of the APC gene were the onset of adenoma formation. Acquisition of further genetic alterations, namely KRAS oncogenic activation and p53 inactivating mutations, would then be the driving force towards progression from adenoma to carcinoma (14).

Currently, it is widely accepted that the above-mentioned adenoma-carcinoma concept over-simplifies the heterogeneity of the molecular, clinical

*Molecular Pathology: A Practical Guide for the Surgical Pathologist and Cytopathologist*, ed. John M. S. Bartlett, Abeer Shaaban and Fernando Schmitt. Published by Cambridge University Press. © Cambridge University Press, 2016.

and pathological basis of colorectal tumors, and therefore cannot explain the development of all types of CRC. For instance, APC, KRAS and p53 mutations, the classic molecular alterations of the Vogelstein pathway, were found to occur in the same tumor in only 7.7% of CRCs (15, 16, 17). A higher percentage of concomitant mutations would be expected if the adenoma-carcinoma pathway was the main sequence leading to CRC initiation and development. The CRCs with MSS are those with higher probability of being originated by the adenoma-carcinoma pathway since APC, or KRAS or p53 alterations are more frequent in this subset of tumors (18, 19, 20, 21). However, in contrast to the Vogelstein model, some MSS carcinomas also exhibit molecular and clinical features commonly found in MSI carcinomas, namely BRAF mutation associated with CpG island methylator phenotype (CIMP) positivity (22, 23) and proximal location (24). In addition, the molecular features of MSI-H / BRAF mutant / CIMP positive CRCs do not fit within the adenoma-carcinoma pathway, since the frequency of KRAS mutations is not very high in this tumor setting and the inactivation of APC and p53 genes is very rare (16, 25). Furthermore, it was also demonstrated that left-sided MSI-H sporadic CRCs show significantly less frequent methylation of MLH1 and CIMP positivity (26). Such evidence demonstrates that MSI and MSS CRCs are not homogenous subsets with regard to the molecular, clinical and pathological features. Therefore, alternative genetic pathways to CRC initiation and development were proposed in order to improve knowledge on the biology of colorectal tumors and to better explain their heterogeneity (27).

In this regard, a serrated neoplasia pathway for CRC origin has emerged (28). The progressive stages of the serrated neoplasia pathway are distinct from those of the classical adenoma-carcinoma sequence (28, 29, 30). In this pathway, hyperplastic polyps (HP), traditional serrated adenomas (TSA) and sessile serrated adenomas (SSA) are assumed to be the precursor lesions of tumor development (29). For a long time, these serrated polyps were considered harmless lesions of the colon with no potential to become malignant. However, molecular studies performed on this type of polyps demonstrated that they already harbor alterations that are commonly found in CRCs, such as BRAF and KRAS mutations, CIMP positivity, MLH1 methylation and MSI-H (29, 31, 32, 33), and thus the possibility of progression to cancer was strengthened.

Mutant BRAF is a specific marker for the serrated polyp pathway that has its origin in a hyperplastic polyp with the potential to originate a MSI-H carcinoma (29, 34). BRAF mutations are frequently associated with the presence of CIMP-H (31, 34), and both events arise early in the serrated sequence (32, 35). Aberrant, widespread methylation of CpG islands increases with the histological progression of serrated adenomas (36). Loss of MSS due to MLH1 promoter hypermethylation develops at late stages and is the key event inducing MSI and malignant transformation (31).

The presence of KRAS mutation in SAs provided a less complete picture for a second serrated pathway (33). KRAS mutations are also found in colonic serrated lesions, although at a lower frequency than BRAF mutations (29, 32, 37) and they are thought to be implicated in the development of CIMP-L and MSS CRCs (33).

## Molecular alterations in colorectal cancer

Activating mutations in genes of the mitogen-activated protein kinase (MAPK) and phosphatidylinositol 3-kinase (PI3K) pathways, including KRAS, BRAF, MLK3 and PIK3CA, are frequent events in CRC (13, 38). Notably, aberrant activation of the MAPK and PI3K pathways will have a major impact in cell behavior as these signaling pathways are involved in a variety of key biological processes, including cell cycle regulation, cell survival and apoptosis (38).

Interestingly, KRAS and BRAF mutation frequencies and patterns differ among the different subsets of CRC. Whereas KRAS mutations are found in both MSS and MSI sporadic and hereditary tumors, BRAF mutations show a more restricted pattern, being mostly found in sporadic MSI CRC (13, 18, 19, 39, 40). A significant percentage of patients with CRC (approximately 30% to 40%) exhibit KRAS mutations mostly affecting codons 12 and 13 of exon 2 and these have been shown to occur early in carcinogenesis (13, 19, 38, 40, 41). Mutations in BRAF occur in about 15% (5% to 45%) of CRCs, with the most frequently reported mutation a valine-to-glutamic acid amino-acid (V600E) substitution in exon 15 (13, 38, 40, 41).

Of particular relevance is the fact that KRAS and BRAF mutations are usually mutually exclusive molecular alterations, suggesting that these oncogenes may play different roles in the development and progression of CRC (13, 42). In contrast, activating mutations involving hotspots on exons 9 and 20 of PIK3CA are found in about 15% of sporadic and hereditary CRC, and occur concomitantly with KRAS or BRAF mutations (38, 43, 44).

MLK3 gene mutations have recently been found in patients with CRC. In 2010, our group described MLK3 mutations in gastrointestinal cancers for the first time and these mutations were significantly associated with MSI phenotype, occurring in 25% of hereditary carcinomas (Lynch) and 19.4% of sporadic CRC (45). Interestingly, MLK3 mutations did not correlate with mutations in any of KRAS, BRAF or PI3K (45). Of relevance is the fact that cells expressing mutant forms of MLK3 exhibited transforming capacity *in vitro* and gave rise to locally invasive tumors upon subcutaneous injection in mice (45).

# Clinical applications of MSI detection
## MSI as a prognostic and predictive marker
The molecular and clinicopathologic features of MSI and MSS CRC tumors have been demonstrated to be distinct. For instance, MSI colorectal tumors are mainly found in the proximal colon, are poorly differentiated and are frequently associated with a mucinous phenotype (46). Furthermore, the presence of tumor infiltrating lymphocytes is prevalent in MSI tumors and it has been suggested as a useful marker in the identification of MSI CRCs (47, 48, 49, 50). Of particular relevance is the fact that, in contrast to MSS tumors, MSI-H tumors have a good prognosis. Moreover, MSI patients have been found to harbor a lower tumor stage at diagnosis, rarely metastasize to the lymph nodes or distant organs (51, 52), and have better overall and relapse-free survival (51, 53). However, despite the reduced aggressiveness of MSI as compared to MSS, several studies demonstrated that patients with MSI-H tumors do not benefit from 5-Fluorouracil (5-FU) based adjuvant chemotherapies (54, 55, 56, 57, 58, 59, 60, 61).

Distal sporadic MSI-H CRCs represent a distinct subgroup with specific clinicopathological and molecular features from proximal MSI-H CRCs. Distal MSI-H CRCs showed significantly more frequent association with younger age, male gender, differentiated histology, small tumor size, distant metastasis, stability in BAT25 and BAT26, and MLH1 expression

on immunohistochemical staining as compared with proximal MSI-H CRCs. In addition, distal MSI-H CRCs demonstrated significantly worse three-year overall and disease-free survival rates than proximal MSI-high CRCs (87.0% vs. 97.4%; 81.6% vs. 95.9%). For stage III-IV CRCs, distal MSI-H CRCs also showed significantly worse three-year overall and disease-free survival rates than proximal MSI-H CRCs (72.2% vs. 90.5%; 58.3% vs. 94.4%) (26, 62).

The large majority of CRCs (about 85%), however, do not harbor the mutator phenotype and are classified as MSS. MSS tumors are mainly aneuploid and are characterized by having multiple chromosomal rearrangements leading to another type of genetic instability known as chromosomal instability (CIN) (63). MSS CRCs are generally observed in the distal colon and rectum, are frequently well/moderately differentiated and are more aggressive than MSI carcinomas. Furthermore, MSS tumors are associated with a poor prognosis, more advanced stage disease and are frequently metastatic to lymph node and distant organs (52).

The recognition of a third group of tumors harboring a milder mutator phenotype (MSI low – MSI-L) is still under debate, being supported by some authors (64, 65, 66) and not accepted by others (67). MSI-L tumors are reported to have instability at some microsatellite markers without evidence of an underlying alteration in MMR genes (68, 69, 70). Furthermore, MSI-L CRCs do not appear to be associated with specific clinicopathological features (69, 71). Therefore, the acceptance of MSI-L as an additional CRC group is still controversial, and MSI-L tumors are often included in the MSS group (72).

# Detection of Lynch syndrome (vs. familial type X syndrome)
Lynch syndrome, also commonly referred to as hereditary non-polyposis colorectal cancer (HNPCC), is an autosomal dominant disorder (73). CRC patients from Lynch families are characterized by early age at onset (approximately 45 years old) and by having an excess of synchronous and metachronous CRC. Frequently, these patients also show extracolonic tumors (endometrium, ovary, stomach, small bowel, pancreas, hepatobiliary tract, brain and upper uroepithelial tract). Patients with Lynch syndrome may also be affected with sebaceous adenomas, sebaceous

carcinomas and multiple keratoacanthomas (Muir-Torre syndrome) (73, 74).

MSI is a molecular hallmark of Lynch syndrome-associated cancers and mutations in the MMR system are the underlying genetic cause for cancer development (73, 74, 75). In particular, MLH1 and MSH2 germline mutations account for almost 90% of all identified mutations, but mutations in other MMR genes, such as MSH6 and PMS2I, may also occur. Therefore, MSI testing is a useful tool for the identification of patients with a defective MMR system. Determination of MSI status has clinical value as it has prognostic and therapeutic implications. The clinical diagnosis of HNPCC can be performed by applying the revised Amsterdam criteria for clinical diagnosis or the revised Bethesda guidelines for molecular testing of suspected patients (74, 76, 77, 78, 79).

Amsterdam criteria and Bethesda guidelines usually point out additional families in which there is no evidence of MMR deficiency, even after screening by MSI analysis and/or immunohistochemistry (IHC) for MMR proteins (80, 81). The term "HNPCC" was formerly used to refer to clinically diagnosed CRC families that might or might not have mismatch repair deficiency, although it has been suggested that it should be replaced by one of the more informative names, such as Lynch syndrome and Familial Colorectal Cancer type X syndrome (FCC-XS), respectively (80–83). FCC-XS is used to designate those HNPCC families that fulfill the clinical criteria, but whose genetic basis remains unknown (83). The designation of Lynch syndrome is more adequate to characterize HNPCC families that fulfill the clinical criteria and have an identified MMR gene alteration (83). This distinction is reasoned by the fact that tumors from XS families were shown to be clinically and molecularly different from Lynch syndrome tumors. XS families are characterized by a smaller number of CRCs and a less frequent spectrum of associated tumors. Furthermore, the tumors were preferentially located at the distal colon/rectum and less often presented mucous production or lymphocytic infiltrate (83).

## Detection methods

A number of methods are available to assess MSI status in patients with CRC or with a CRC familial predisposition and guidelines and recommendations have been issued (84, 85, 86, 87). Over time, these methods have improved and MSI criteria have been adjusted. However, there is not yet consensus as to the best and most cost-effective assay to be routinely used to detect MMR deficiency (78). The following sections summarize the main aspects of each technique being currently used to determine MSI status.

## PCR for MSI markers

Analysis of MSI status has been mainly achieved by evaluating MSI markers, more specifically, a set of mono- and dinucleotide repeat markers. For this purpose, specific primers for each MSI marker are designed and PCR reactions are performed to evaluate allele size variations. In 1998, in an effort to develop uniform international criteria for the determination of MSI in CRC, a National Cancer Institute (NCI) Workshop on MSI recommended the use of a panel of five MSI markers: two mononucleotide repeats (BAT25 and BAT26) and three dinucleotide repeats (D2S123, D5S346 and D17S250) (84). According to these recommendations, tumors could be characterized on the basis of: high-frequency MSI (MSI-H), if two or more of the five markers show instability (insertion/deletion mutations); low-frequency MSI (MSI-L) if only one of the five markers show instability; and MSS if none of the markers presents instability. The cases with MSS and MSI-L could only be truly distinguished if additional markers are tested (84). However, as demonstrated thereafter, the use of this panel of markers presented some limitations, mainly concerning the use of dinucleotide repeat analysis for screening, which occasionally seem to result in misclassification (85). Indeed, when determining MSI status, dinucleotide repeat interpretation can be ambiguous in specific cases and the highly polymorphic nature of these repeats requires comparison of tumor DNA with matching normal DNA from each individual (85, 88). Furthermore, although in the majority of the cases it is suggested that the use of the mononucleotide repeats, BAT-25 and BAT-26, is specific and sensitive for the diagnosis of MSI-H (88, 89), in other cases an additional panel of microsatellite sequences is recommended. Therefore, following a 2002 HNPCC workshop by NCI, a revised version of Bethesda guidelines recommended the use of a secondary panel of mononucleotide markers as BAT40 and/or MYCL in MSI-L cases (85).

As an alternative to the Bethesda markers, other marker panels have been proposed to provide a more standardized and reliable evaluation of MSI status. A panel of five quasimonomorphic mononucleotide repeats in a pentaplex PCR has been proposed and suggested to allow accurate determination of MSI status without the need to match normal DNA and with better specificity and sensitivity than the NCI-panel (90). Subsequent studies were performed to further validate this assay that uses five microsatellite targets (BAT-25, BAT-26, NR-21, NR-24 and NR-27) in a pentaplex PCR system (91, 92, 93, 94). For instance, a cohort of 213 CRC patients was analyzed and results demonstrated that this optimized pentaplex PCR offers a robust, inexpensive, highly sensitive and specific assay (94). Moreover, data suggested that a triplex PCR analyzing the markers BAT-26, NR21 and NR27 was as accurate as the pentaplex PCR (94). In another study, the pentaplex panel was also reported to perform better than the NCI panel for the detection of MMR deficient tumors in a cohort of 1,058 patients (95). Of note is that BAT-25 and BAT-26 were found to be polymorphic in african-americans and special attention has to be made to avoid incorrect classification of patients as MSI (96).

At present, both NCI-recommended panels of markers are accepted and used in clinical practice for determination of MSI status (85, 87). Fluorescent multiplex PCR in commercially available kits are used routinely for detecting MSI status in several diagnostic laboratories. For instance, an MSI analysis kit, which is a fluorescent PCR-based assay, includes the evaluation of five mononucleotide markers (BAT-25, BAT-26, MON0–27, NR-21 and NR-24) and two pentanucleotide markers (Penta C and D to detect potential sample contamination (Promega Corp., Madison, WI)). Studies have confirmed the effectiveness of this commercial assay kit as compared with the Bethesda panel for the determination of MSI in CRC patients (97).

Standardization of MSI status evaluation, as determined by PCR-based assays, has evolved and is extremely valuable for proper and accurate classification of CRC patients. The recommendation of a specific set of markers together with time- and cost-effective aspects has led to the development of simplified assay systems to avoid misdiagnoses.

## Immunohistochemistry for MMR proteins

Immunohistochemistry is also currently used to predict MSI status in CRC patients by analyzing the most commonly affected MMR proteins including MLH1, MSH2, MSH6 and PMS2 (98). In contrast to PCR-based assays, IHC evaluates the localization and expression levels of MMR proteins in tissue sections and the classification is based on the presence/ absence and pattern of expression of these proteins. Immunohistochemical staining for each MMR protein indicates the presence of a detectable protein, although does not distinguish normal and functional protein from mutated non-functional protein that is still recognized by the antibody. Therefore, positive expression of the four proteins does not necessarily exclude Lynch syndrome and no staining suggests the protein is mutated or has been inactivated by another mechanism such as methylation (as occurs in sporadic MSI CRC), and thus is not expressed in tumor cells (assuming that an internal positive control is included) (98, 99). To determine MMR deficiencies by IHC, analysis of four proteins is required and detection is performed by using commercially available antibodies. The four-antibody panel is currently used, but there is also evidence that the analysis of only PMS2 and MSH6 is cost-effective and as effective as the current panel in detecting DNA MMR protein abnormalities (100).

Despite recent advances, it is still unclear whether PCR-based assays and/or IHC should be routinely used to screen CRC patients for MSI. A number of studies have compared the two methods, but no consistent data are yet available. Indeed, while some studies are in favor of IHC, suggesting almost equal sensitivity as PCR-MSI but wider availability (101) and lower cost (102), others argue that IHC is not sensitive and specific enough to be used routinely in detecting MSI in sporadic and hereditary CRC, mainly due to heterogeneity of the tumors, variability in technical protocols for fixation and staining quality and differences in results interpretation (103). Therefore, in many laboratories, IHC or both techniques are routinely used for MSI status screening.

## MLH1 methylation

The molecular mechanisms underlying MSI are distinct in sporadic and hereditary germline CRC patients. In sporadic CRC, in contrast to Lynch syndrome, the instability of microsatellites occurs through epigenetic silencing and the most commonly silenced gene by promoter hypermethylation is MLH1 (104).

The main method for detection of methylated and unmethylated alleles is based on bisulfate

**123**

modification in which unmethylated cytosine is converted to uracil by sodium bisulfate followed by methylation-specific PCR (105, 106). The promoter area of MLH1 has been divided into four regions and the analysis of the "C" and "D" regions is considered to be sufficient for a proper diagnosis (105, 107). For interpretation, a methylation index is determined and deviation from a predetermined normal range will be indicative of disease (87). Determination of MLH1 promoter methylation is a valuable tool as MSI-H HNPCC and MSI-H sporadic CRC patients can be distinguished (108). Indeed, a recent study reported that hypermethylation of MLH1 is an accurate and cost-effective pre-screening method in the selection of patients who are candidates for MLH1 germline analysis when Lynch syndrome is suspected and MLH1 protein expression is absent (109). In clinical practice, MLH1 promoter methylation is performed in specific cases and the guidelines and recommendations for MLH1 methylation testing can be reviewed in Vasen *et al.* (86) and Hegde *et al.* (87). In addition to MLH1 methylation detection,

activating mutations in BRAF have been associated with sporadic MSI and thus evaluation of BRAF mutations further supports the exclusion of HNPCC (110, 111, 112, 113).

## Learning points

- In recent years, our knowledge on colorectal carcinogenesis has evolved. However, despite many efforts, the mechanisms underlying CRC development, namely in the different subsets of patients, are yet to be completely unveiled.
- It is now well established that CRC patients with MSI and CIN result from the accumulation of distinct genetic and/or epigenetic alterations that will result in unique clinical and pathological features. Therefore, stratification of patients based on the molecular and clinico-pathologic characteristics is crucial as it will impact profoundly on the clinical management of patients for both an accurate prognosis and selection of appropriate chemotherapy.

## References

1. Jemal, A., Bray, F., Center, M. M., Ferlay, J., Ward, E. and Forman, D. (2011). "Global cancer statistics." *CA Cancer J Clin* 61(2): 69–90.

2. Vilar, E. and Gruber, S. B. (2010). "Microsatellite instability in colorectal cancer – the stable evidence." *Nat Rev Clin Oncol* 7(3): 153–62.

3. Ionov, Y., Peinado, M. A., Malkhosyan, S., Shibata, D. and Perucho, M. (1993). "Ubiquitous somatic mutations in simple repeated sequences reveal a new mechanism for colonic carcinogenesis." *Nature* 363(6429): 558–61.

4. Thibodeau, S. N., Bren, G. and Schaid, D. (1993). "Microsatellite instability in cancer of the proximal colon." *Science* 260(5109): 816–19.

5. Kane, M. F., Loda, M. , Gaida, G. M., Lipman, J., Mishra, R., Goldman, H. *et al.* (1997). "Methylation of the hMLH1

promoter correlates with lack of expression of hMLH1 in sporadic colon tumors and mismatch repair-defective human tumor cell lines." *Cancer Res* 57(5): 808–11.

6. Jiricny, J. (2006). "The multifaceted mismatch-repair system." *Nat Rev Mol Cell Biol* 7(5): 335–46.

7. Rustgi, A. (2007). "The genetics of hereditary colon cancer." *Genes Dev* 21(20): 2525–38.

8. Jascur, T. and Boland, C. R. (2006). "Structure and function of the components of the human DNA mismatch repair system." *Int J Cancer* 119(9): 2030–5.

9. Jiricny, J. (2006). "MutLalpha: at the cutting edge of mismatch repair." *Cell* 126(2): 239–41.

10. Peltomaki, P. (2001). "DNA mismatch repair and cancer." *Mutat Res* 488(1): 77–85.

11. Duval, A. and Hamelin, R. (2002). "Mutations at coding repeat sequences in mismatch repair-deficient human cancers: toward a

new concept of target genes for instability." *Cancer Res* 62(9): 2447–54.

12. Jakowlew, S. B. (2006). "Transforming growth factor-beta in cancer and metastasis." *Cancer Metastasis Rev* 25(3): 435–57.

13. Velho, S., Corso, G., Oliveira, C. and Seruca, R. (2010). "KRAS signaling pathway alterations in microsatellite unstable gastrointestinal cancers." *Adv Cancer Res* 109: 123–43.

14. Fearon, E. R. and Vogelstein, B. (1990). "A genetic model for colorectal tumorigenesis." *Cell* 61(5): 759–67.

15. Smith, G., Carey, F. A., Beattie, J., Wilkie, M. J., Lightfoot, T. J., Coxhead, J. *et al.* (2002). "Mutations in APC, Kirsten-ras, and p53 – alternative genetic pathways to colorectal cancer." *Proc Natl Acad Sci USA* 99(14): 9433–8.

16. Samowitz, W. S., Slattery, M. L., Sweeney, C., Herrick, J., Wolff, R. K. and Albertsen, H. (2007). "APC

mutations and other genetic and epigenetic changes in colon cancer." *Mol Cancer Res* 5(2): 165–70.

17. Imai, K. and Yamamoto, H. (2008). "Carcinogenesis and microsatellite instability: the interrelationship between genetics and epigenetics." *Carcinogenesis* 29(4): 673–80.

18. Domingo, E., Espin, E., Armengol, M., Oliveira, C., Pinto, M., Duval, A. *et al.* (2004). "Activated BRAF targets proximal colon tumors with mismatch repair deficiency and MLH1 inactivation." *Gene Chromosome Canc* 39(2): 138–42.

19. Oliveira, C., Westra, J., Arango, D., Ollikainen, M., Domingo, E., Ferreira, A. *et al.* (2004). "Distinct patterns of KRAS mutations in colorectal carcinomas according to germline mismatch repair defects and hMLH1 methylation status." *Hum Mol Genet* 13(19): 2303–11.

20. Samowitz, W. (2008). "Genetic and epigenetic changes in colon cancer." *Exp Mol Pathol* 85(1): 64–7.

21. Suehiro, Y., Wong, C. W., Chirieac, L. R., Kondo, Y., Shen, L., Webb, C. R. *et al.* (2008). "Epigenetic-genetic interactions in the APC/WNT, RAS/RAF, and P53 pathways in colorectal carcinoma." *Clin Cancer Res* 14(9): 2560–9.

22. Samowitz, W. S., Sweeney, C., Herrick, J., Albertsen, H., Levin, T. R., Murtaugh, M. A. *et al.* (2005). "Poor survival associated with the BRAF V600E mutation in microsatellite-stable colon cancers." *Cancer Res* 65(14): 6063–9.

23. Sanchez, J. A., Krumroy, L., Plummer, S., Aung, P., Merkulova, A., Skacel, M. *et al.* (2009). "Genetic and epigenetic classifications define clinical phenotypes and determine patient outcomes in colorectal cancer." *Br J Surg* 96(10): 1196–204.

24. Lee, S., Cho, N.-Y., Choi, M., Yoo, E. J., Kim, J. H. and Kang, G. H. (2008). "Clinicopathological features of CpG island methylator phenotype-positive colorectal cancer and its adverse prognosis in relation to KRAS BRAF mutation." *Pathol Int* 58(2): 104–13.

25. Jass, J. R. (2007). "Molecular heterogeneity of colorectal cancer: implications for cancer control." *Surg Oncol* 16(Suppl. 1): S7–9.

26. Tanaka, J., Watanabe, T., Kanazawa, T., Tada, T., Kazama, Y., Tanaka, T. *et al.* (2007). "Left-sided microsatellite unstable colorectal cancers show less frequent methylation of hMLH1 and CpG island methylator phenotype than right-sided ones." *J Surg Oncol* 96(7): 611–18.

27. Jass, J. (2006). "Hereditary non-polyposis colorectal cancer: the rise and fall of a confusing term." *World J Gastroenterol* 12(31): 4943–50.

28. Jass, J. R. (2005). "Serrated adenoma of the colorectum and the DNA-methylator phenotype." *Nat Clin Pract Oncol* 2(8): 398–405.

29. O'Brien, M., Yang, S., Mack, C., Xu, H., Huang, C. S., Mulcahy, E. *et al.* (2006). "Comparison of microsatellite instability, CpG island methylation phenotype, BRAF and KRAS status in serrated polyps and traditional adenomas indicates separate pathways to distinct colorectal carcinoma end points." *Am J Surg Pathol* 30(12): 1491–501.

30. Bettington, M., Walker, N., Clouston, A., Brown, I., Leggett, B. and Whitehall, V. (2013). "The serrated pathway to colorectal carcinoma: current concepts and challenges." *Histopathology* 62(3): 367–86.

31. Kambara, T., Simms, L., Whitehall, V. L., Spring, K. J., Wynter, C. V., Walsh, M. D. *et al.* (2004). "BRAF mutation is associated with DNA methylation in serrated polyps and cancers of the colorectum." *Gut* 53(8): 1137–44.

32. Yang, S., Farraye, F. A., Mack, C., Posnik, O. and O'Brien, M. G. (2004). "BRAF and KRAS mutations in hyperplastic polyps and serrated adenomas of the colorectum: relationship to histology and CpG island methylation status." *Am J Surg Pathol* 28(11): 1452–9.

33. O'Brien, M. J. (2007). "Hyperplastic and serrated polyps of the colorectum." *Gastroenterol Clin North Am* 36(4): 947–68.

34. Kim, Y. H., Kakar, S., Cun, L., Deng, G. and Kim, Y. S. (2008). "Distinct CpG island methylation profiles and *BRAF* mutation status in serrated and adenomatous colorectal polyps." *Int J Cancer* 123(11): 2587–93.

35. Wynter, C., Walsh, M., Higuchi, T., Leggett, B. A., Young, J. and Jass, J. R. (2004). "Methylation patterns define two types of hyperplastic polyp associated with colorectal cancer." *Gut* 53(4): 573–80.

36. Dong, S. M., Lee, E. J., Jeon, E. S., Park, C. K. and Kim, K. M. (2004). "Progressive methylation during the serrated neoplasia pathway of the colorectum." *Mod Pathol* 18(2): 170–8.

37. Rosenberg, D. W., Yang, S., Pleau, D. C., Greenspan, E. J., Stevens, R. G., Rajan, T. V. *et al.* (2007). "Mutations in BRAF and KRAS differentially distinguish serrated versus non-serrated hyperplastic aberrant crypt foci in humans." *Cancer Res* 67(8): 3551–4.

38. De Roock, W., De Vriendt, V., Normanno, M., Ciardiello, F. and Tejpar, S. (2011). "KRAS, BRAF, PIK3CA, and PTEN mutations: implications for targeted therapies in metastatic colorectal cancer." *Lancet Oncol* 12(6): 594–603.

39. Lubomierski, N., Plotz, G., Wormek, M., Engels, K., Kriener,

S., Trojan, J. et al. (2005). "BRAF mutations in colorectal carcinoma suggest two entities of microsatellite-unstable tumors." *Cancer* 104(5): 952–61.

40. Oliveira, C., Velho, S., Moutinho, C., Ferreira, A., Preto, A., Domingo, E. et al. (2007). "KRAS and BRAF oncogenic mutations in MSS colorectal carcinoma progression." *Oncogene* 26(1): 158–63.

41. Velho, S., Moutinho, C., Cirnes, L., Albuquerque, C., Hamelin, R., Schmitt, F. et al. (2008). "BRAF, KRAS and PIK3CA mutations in colorectal serrated polyps and cancer: primary or secondary genetic events in colorectal carcinogenesis?" *BMC Cancer* 8: 255.

42. Rajagopalan, H., Bardelli, A., Lengauer, C., Kinzler, K. W., Vogelstein, B. and Velculescu, V. E. (2002). "Tumorigenesis: RAF/RAS oncogenes and mismatch-repair status." *Nature* 418(6901): 934.

43. Velho, S., Oliveira, C., Ferreira, A., Ferreira, A. C., Suriano, G., Schwartz, S., Jr. et al. (2005). "The prevalence of PIK3CA mutations in gastric and colon cancer." *Eur J Cancer* 41(11): 1649–54.

44. Ekstrand, A. I., Jonsson, M., Lindblom, A., Borg, A. and Nilbert, M. (2010). "Frequent alterations of the PI3K/AKT/mTOR pathways in hereditary nonpolyposis colorectal cancer." *Fam Cancer* 9(2): 125–9.

45. Velho, S., Oliveira, C., Paredes, J., Sousa, S., Leite, M., Matos, P. et al. (2010). "Mixed lineage kinase 3 gene mutations in mismatch repair deficient gastrointestinal tumours." *Hum Mol Genet* 19(4): 697–706.

46. Cai, G., Xu, Y., Lu, H., Shi, Y., Lian, P., Peng, J., Du, X. et al. (2008). "Clinicopathologic and molecular features of sporadic microsatellite- and chromosomal-stable colorectal cancers." *Int J Colorectal Dis* 23(4): 365–73.

47. Banerjea, A., Hands, R. E., Powar, M. P., Bustin, S. A. and Dorudi, S. (2009). "Microsatellite and chromosomal stable colorectal cancers demonstrate poor immunogenicity and early disease recurrence." *Colorectal Dis* 11(6): 601–8.

48. Drescher, K., Sharma, P., Watson, P., Gatalica, Z., Thibodeau, S. N. and Lynch, H. T. (2009). "Lymphocyte recruitment into the tumor site is altered in patients with MSI-H colon cancer." *Fam Cancer* 8(3): 231–9.

49. Greenson, J. K., Huang, S.-C., Herron, C., Moreno, V., Bonner, J. D., Tomsho, L. P. et al. (2009). "Pathologic predictors of microsatellite instability in colorectal cancer." *Am J Surg Pathol* 33(1): 126–33, 110.1097/PAS.1090b1013e31817 ec31812b31811.

50. Chang, E., Dorsey, P., Frankhouse, J., Lee, R. G., Walts, D., Johnson, W. et al. (2009). "Combination of microsatellite instability and lymphocytic infiltrate as a prognostic indicator in colon cancer." *Arch Surg* 144(6): 511–15.

51. Gryfe, R., Kim, H., Hsieh, E. T., Aronson, M. D., Holowaty, E. J., Bull, S. B. et al. (2000). "Tumor microsatellite instability and clinical outcome in young patients with colorectal cancer." *New Engl J Med* 342: 69–77.

52. Malesci, A., Laghi, L., Bianchi, P., Delconte, G., Randolph, A., Torri, V. et al. (2007). "Reduced likelihood of metastases in patients with microsatellite-unstable colorectal cancer." *Clin Cancer Res* 13(13): 3831–9.

53. Clark, A. J., Barnetson, R., Farrington, S. M. and Dunlop, M. G. (2004). "Prognosis in DNA mismatch repair deficient colorectal cancer: are all MSI tumours equivalent?" *Fam Cancer* 3(2): 85–91.

54. Carethers, J., Chauhan, D., Fink, D., Nebel, S., Bresalier, R. S., Howell, S. B. et al. (1999). "Mismatch repair proficiency and in vitro response to 5-fluorouracil." *Gastroenterology* 117(1): 123–31.

55. Arnold, C. N., Goel, A. and Boland, C. R. (2003). "Role of hMLH1 promoter hypermethylation in drug resistance to 5-fluorouracil in colorectal cancer cell lines." *Int J Cancer* 106(1): 66–73.

56. Ribic, C. M., Sargent, D. J., Moore, M. J., Thibodeau, S. N., French, A. J., Goldberg, R. M. et al. (2003). "Tumor microsatellite-instability status as a predictor of benefit from fluorouracil-based adjuvant chemotherapy for colon cancer." *New Engl J Med* 349(3): 247–57.

57. Carethers, J. M., Smith, E. J., Behling, C. A., Nguyen, L., Tajima, A., Doctolero, R. T. et al. (2004). "Use of 5-fluorouracil and survival in patients with microsatellite-unstable colorectal cancer." *Gastroenterology* 126(2): 394–401.

58. Des Guetz, G., Uzzan, B., Nicolas, P., Schischmanoff, O. and Morere, J.-F. (2009). "Microsatellite instability: a predictive marker in metastatic colorectal cancer?" *Target Oncol* 4(1): 57–62.

59. Des Guetz, G. T., Uzzan, B., Nicolas, P., Schischmanoff, O., Perret, G. Y. and Morere, J.-F. (2009). "Microsatellite instability does not predict the efficacy of chemotherapy in metastatic colorectal cancer. A systematic review and meta-analysis." *Anticancer Res* 29(5): 1615–20.

60. Sinicrope, F. A. and Sargent, D. J. (2009). "Clinical implications of microsatellite instability in sporadic colon cancers." *Curr Opin Oncol* 21(4): 369–73, 310.1097/CCO.1090b1013 e32832c32894bd.

61. Jover, R., T. P. Nguyen, Pérez-Carbonell, L., Zapater, P., Payá, A., Alenda, C. et al. (2011). "5-Fluorouracil adjuvant chemotherapy does not increase survival in patients with CpG island methylator phenotype colorectal cancer." *Gastroenterology* 140(4): 1174–81.

62. Kim, Y.-H., Min, B.-H., Kim, S. J., Choi, H. K., Kim, K.-M., Chun, H.-K. et al. (2010). "Difference between proximal and distal microsatellite-unstable sporadic colorectal cancers: analysis of clinicopathological and molecular features and prognoses." *Ann Surg Oncol* 17(5): 1435–41.

63. Trautmann, K., Terdiman, J. P., French, A. J., Roydasgupta, R., Sein, N., Kakar, S. et al. (2006). "Chromosomal instability in microsatellite-unstable and stable colon cancer." *Clin Cancer Res* 12(21): 6379–85.

64. Jass, J., Biden, K., Cummings, M. C., Simms, L. A., Walsh, M., Schoch, E. et al. (1999). "Characterisation of a subtype of colorectal cancer combining features of the suppressor and mild mutator pathways." *J Clin Pathol* 52(6): 455–60.

65. Kambara, T., Matsubara, N., Nakagawa, H., Notohara, K., Nagasaka, T., Yoshino, T. et al. (2001). "High frequency of low-level microsatellite instability in early colorectal cancer." *Cancer Res* 61(21): 7743–6.

66. Mori, Y., Selaru, F. M., Sato, F., Yin, J., Simms, L. A., Xu, Y. et al. (2003). "The impact of microsatellite instability on the molecular phenotype of colorectal tumors." *Cancer Res* 63(15): 4577–82.

67. Graham, T., Halford, S., Page, K. M. and Tomlinson, I. P. (2008). "Most low-level microsatellite instability in colorectal cancers can be explained without an elevated slippage rate." *J Pathol* 215(2): 204–10.

68. Dietmaier, W., Wallinger, S., Bocker, T., Kullmann, F., Fishel, R. and Rüschoff, J. (1997). "Diagnostic microsatellite instability: definition and correlation with mismatch repair protein expression." *Cancer Res* 57(21): 4749–56.

69. Thibodeau, S. N., French, A. J., Cunningham, J. M., Tester, D., Burgart, L.J., Roche, P. C. et al. (1998). "Microsatellite instability in colorectal cancer: different mutator phenotypes and the principal involvement of hMLH1." *Cancer Res* 58(8): 1713–18.

70. Parc, Y. R., Halling, K. C., Wang, L., Christensen, E. R., Cunningham, J. M., French, A. J. et al. (2000). "hMSH6 alterations in patients with microsatellite instability-low colorectal cancer." *Cancer Res* 60(8): 2225–31.

71. Halford, S., Sasieni, P., Rowan, A., Wasan, H., Bodmer, W., Talbot, I. et al. (2002). "Low-level microsatellite instability occurs in most colorectal cancers and is a nonrandomly distributed quantitative trait." *Cancer Res* 62(1): 53–7.

72. Laiho, P., Launonen, V., Lahermo, P., Esteller, M., Guo, M., Herman, J. G. et al. (2002). "Low-level microsatellite instability in most colorectal carcinomas." *Cancer Res* 62(4): 1166–70.

73. Castells, A., Castellví-Bel, S. and Balaguer, F. (2009). "Concepts in familial colorectal cancer: where do we stand and what is the future?" *Gastroenterology* 137(2): 404–9.

74. Lynch, H. T. and de la Chapelle, A. (2003). "Hereditary colorectal cancer." *New Engl J Med* 348(10): 919–32.

75. Peltomäki, P. and Vasen, H. (2004). "Mutations associated with HNPCC predisposition – update of ICG-HNPCC/INSiGHT mutation database." *Dis Markers* 20(4): 269–76.

76. Vasen, H., Watson, P., Mecklin, J. P. and Lynch, H. T. (1999). "New clinical criteria for hereditary nonpolyposis colorectal cancer (HNPCC, Lynch syndrome) proposed by the International Collaborative group on HNPCC." *Gastroenterology* 116(6): 1453–6.

77. Laghi, L., Bianchi, P., Roncalli, M. and Malesci, A. (2004). "Re: revised Bethesda guidelines for hereditary nonpolyposis colorectal cancer (Lynch syndrome) and microsatellite instability." *J Natl Cancer Inst* 96(18): 1403–4.

77. Laghi, L., Bianchi, P. and Malesci, A. (2008). "Differences and evolution of the methods for the assessment of microsatellite instability." *Oncogene* 27(49): 6313–21.

78. Lynch, H., Lynch, P., Lanspa, S. J., Snyder, C. L., Lynch, J. F. and Boland, C. R. (2009). "Review of the Lynch syndrome: history, molecular genetics, screening, differential diagnosis, and medicolegal ramifications." *Clin Genet* 76(1): 1–18.

79. Tops, C. M., Wijnen, J. T. and Hes, F. G. (2009). "Introduction to molecular and clinical genetics of colorectal cancer syndromes." *Best Pract Res Clin Gastroenterol* 23(2): 127–46.

80. Abdel-Rahman, W. and Peltomäki, P. (2008). "Lynch syndrome and related familial colorectal cancers." *Crit Rev Oncog* 14(1): 1–22.

81. Lindor, N. M. (2009). "Familial colorectal cancer type X: the other half of hereditary nonpolyposis colon cancer syndrome." *Surg Oncol Clin North Am* 18(4): 637–45.

82. Jass, J. R. (2006). "Colorectal cancer: a multipathway disease." *Crit Rev Oncog* 12(3–4): 273–87.

83. Ferreira, S., Lage, P., Sousa, R., Claro, I., Francisco, I., Filipe, B. et al. (2009). "Familial colorectal cancer type X: clinical, pathological and molecular

characterization." *Acta Med Port* 22(3): 207–14.

84. Boland, C. R., Thibodeau, S. N., Hamilton, S. R., Sidransky, D., Eshleman, J. R., Burt, R. W. *et al.* (1998). "A National Cancer Institute Workshop on Microsatellite Instability for cancer detection and familial predisposition: development of international criteria for the determination of microsatellite instability in colorectal cancer." *Cancer Res* 58(22): 5248–57.

85. Umar, A., Boland, C. R., Terdiman, J. P., Syngal, S., de la Chapelle, A., Rüschoff, J. *et al.* (2004). "Revised Bethesda Guidelines for hereditary nonpolyposis colorectal cancer (Lynch syndrome) and microsatellite instability." *J Natl Cancer Inst* 96(4): 261–8.

86. Vasen, H. F., Blanco, I., Aktan-Collan, K., Gopie, J. P., Alonso, A., Aretz, S. *et al.* (2013). "Revised guidelines for the clinical management of Lynch syndrome (HNPCC): recommendations by a group of European experts." *Gut* 62(6): 812–23.

87. Hegde, M., Ferber, M., Mao, R., Samowitz, W., Ganguly, A.; Working Group of the ACMG Laboratory Quality Assurance Committee (2014). "ACMG technical standards and guidelines for genetic testing for inherited colorectal cancer (Lynch syndrome, familial adenomatous polyposis, and MYH-associated polyposis)." *Genet Med* 16(1): 101–16.

88. Perucho, M. (1999). "Correspondence re: C.R. Boland et al., A National Cancer Institute workshop on microsatellite instability for cancer detection and familial predisposition: development of international criteria for the determination of microsatellite instability in colorectal cancer. Cancer Res., 58: 5248–5257, 1998." *Cancer Res* 59(1): 249–56.

89. Brennetot, C., Buhard, O., Jourdan, F., Flejou, J. F., Duval, A. and Hamelin, R. (2005). "Mononucleotide repeats BAT-26 and BAT-25 accurately detect MSI-H tumors and predict tumor content: implications for population screening." *Int J Cancer* 113(3): 446–50.

90. Suraweera, N., Duval, A., Reperant, M., Vaury, C., Furlan, D., Leroy, K. *et al.* (2002). "Evaluation of tumor microsatellite instability using five quasimonomorphic mononucleotide repeats and pentaplex PCR." *Gastroenterology* 123(6): 1804–11.

91. Buhard, O., Suraweera, N., Lectard, A., Duval, A. and Hamelin, R. (2004). "Quasimonomorphic mononucleotide repeats for high-level microsatellite instability analysis." *Dis Markers* 20(4–5): 251–7.

92. Ebinger, M., Sotlar, K., Weber, A., Bock, C. T., Bültmann, D. D. and Kandolf, R. (2006). "Simplified detection of microsatellite instability in colorectal cancer without the need for corresponding germline DNA analysis." *J Clin Pathol* 59(10): 1114–15.

93. Soreide, K. (2007). "Molecular testing for microsatellite instability and DNA mismatch repair defects in hereditary and sporadic colorectal cancers – ready for prime time?" *Tumour Biol* 28(5): 290–300.

94. Goel, A., Nagasaka, T., Hamelin, R. and Boland, C. R. (2010). "An optimized pentaplex PCR for detecting DNA mismatch repair-deficient colorectal cancers." *PLoS ONE* 5(2): e9393.

95. Xicola, R. M., Llor, X., Pons, E., Castells, A., Alenda, C., Piñol, V. *et al.* (2007). "Performance of different microsatellite marker panels for detection of mismatch repair-deficient colorectal tumors." *J Natl Cancer Inst* 99(3): 244–52.

96. Pyatt, R., Chadwick, R. B., Johnson, C. K., Adebamowo, C., de la Chapelle, A. and Prior, T. W. (1999). "Polymorphic variation at the BAT-25 and BAT-26 loci in individuals of African origin. Implications for microsatellite instability testing." *Am J Pathol* 155(2): 349–53.

97. Murphy, K. M., Zhang, S., Geiger, T., Hafez, M. J., Bacher, J., Berg, K. D. *et al.* (2006). "Comparison of the microsatellite instability analysis system and the Bethesda panel for the determination of microsatellite instability in colorectal cancers." *J Mol Diagn* 8(3): 305–11.

98. Shi, C. and Washington, K. (2012). "Molecular testing in colorectal cancer: diagnosis of Lynch syndrome and personalized cancer medicine." *Am J Clin Pathol* 137(6): 847–59.

99. Arends, M. J. (2013). "Pathways of colorectal carcinogenesis." *Appl Immunohistochem Mol Morphol* 21(2): 97–102.

100. Shia, J., Tang, L. H., Vakiani, E., Guillem, J. G., Stadler, Z. K., Soslow, R. A. *et al.* (2009). "Immunohistochemistry as first-line screening for detecting colorectal cancer patients at risk for hereditary nonpolyposis colorectal cancer syndrome: a 2-antibody panel may be as predictive as a 4-antibody panel." *Am J Surg Pathol* 33(11): 1639–45.

101. Hampel, H., Frankel, W. L., Martin, E., Arnold, M., Khanduja, K., Kuebler, P. *et al.* (2008). "Feasibility of screening for Lynch syndrome among patients with colorectal cancer." *J Clin Oncol* 26(35): 5783–8.

102. Mvundura, M., Grosse, S. D., Hampel, H. and Palomaki, G. E. (2010). "The cost-effectiveness of genetic testing strategies for Lynch syndrome among newly diagnosed patients with colorectal cancer." *Genet Med* 12(2): 93–104.

103. Soreide, K., Nedrebo, B. S., Knapp, J. C., Glomsaker, T. B., Søreide, J. A. and Kørner, H. (2009). "Evolving molecular classification by genomic and proteomic biomarkers in colorectal cancer: potential implications for the surgical oncologist." *Surg Oncol* 18(1): 31–50.

104. Herman, J. G., Umar, A., Polyak, K., Graff, J. R., Ahuja, N., Issa, J. P. *et al.* (1998). "Incidence and functional consequences of hMLH1 promoter hypermethylation in colorectal carcinoma." *Proc Natl Acad Sci USA* 95(12): 6870–5.

105. Deng, G., Chen, A., Hong, J., Chae, H. S. and Kim, Y. S. (1999). "Methylation of CpG in a small region of the hMLH1 promoter invariably correlates with the absence of gene expression." *Cancer Res* 59(9): 2029–33.

106. Ogino, S., Kawasaki, T., Brahmandam, M., Cantor, M., Kirkner, G. J., Spiegelman, D. *et al.* (2006). "Precision and performance characteristics of bisulfite conversion and real-time PCR (MethyLight) for quantitative DNA methylation analysis." *J Mol Diagn* 8(2): 209–17.

107. Hitchins, M. P. and Ward, R. L. (2009). "Constitutional (germline) MLH1 epimutation as an aetiological mechanism for hereditary non-polyposis colorectal cancer." *J Med Genet* 46(12): 793–802.

108. Bettstetter, M., Dechant, S., Ruemmele, P., Grabowski, M., Keller, G., Holinski-Feder, E. *et al.* (2007). "Distinction of hereditary nonpolyposis colorectal cancer and sporadic microsatellite-unstable colorectal cancer through quantification of MLH1 methylation by real-time PCR." *Clin Cancer Res* 13(11): 3221–8.

109. Gausachs, M., Mur, P., Corral, J., Pineda, M., González, S., Benito, L. *et al.* (2012). "MLH1 promoter hypermethylation in the analytical algorithm of Lynch syndrome: a cost-effectiveness study." *Eur J Hum Genet* 20(7): 762–8.

110. Oliveira, C., Pinto, M., Duval, A., Brennetot, C., Domingo, E., Espín, E. *et al.* (2003). "BRAF mutations characterize colon but not gastric cancer with mismatch repair deficiency." *Oncogene* 22(57): 9192–6.

111. Koinuma, K., Shitoh, K., Miyakura, Y., Furukawa, T., Yamashita, Y., Ota, J. *et al.* (2004). "Mutations of BRAF are associated with extensive hMLH1 promoter methylation in sporadic colorectal carcinomas." *Int J Cancer* 108(2): 237–42.

112. Weisenberger, D. J., Siegmund, K. D., Campan, M., Young, J., Long, T. I., Faasse, M. A. *et al.* (2006). "CpG island methylator phenotype underlies sporadic microsatellite instability and is tightly associated with BRAF mutation in colorectal cancer." *Nat Genet* 38(7): 787–93.

113. Bouzourene, H., Hutter, P., Losi, L., Martin, P. and Benhattar, J. (2010). "Selection of patients with germline MLH1 mutated Lynch syndrome by determination of MLH1 methylation and BRAF mutation." *Fam Cancer* 9(2): 167–72.

# Chapter 10

# Mutational analysis

Aaron R. Hansen, Mahadeo A. Sukhai, Hal K. Berman, Suzanne Kamel-Reid and Philippe L. Bedard

## Introduction

Cancer is a disorder caused by alterations in genomes of tumor cells. These alterations can take the form of sequence variations or mutations in oncogenes, tumor suppressor genes or caretaker genes (1). Multiple cellular protection mechanisms exist to guard against the tumorigenic impact of mutations (2). In the context of solid tumors, no single genetic alteration is sufficient to induce a neoplasm on its own. This is in contrast to other diseases (for example, cystic fibrosis, hemochromatosis and leukemia), where a single genetic aberration can be pathological. An abundance of evidence suggests that the majority of tumors are genetically complex and accumulate multiple mutations that deregulate critical molecular pathways, leading to the growth and development of cancers (3).

Translocations, amplifications and sequence variations can constitutively activate oncogenes in circumstances where the wild-type protein would not be active (4, 5). For example, a common activating mutation in KRAS, glycine to valine at residue 12 (G12V), renders the GTPase domain insensitive to inactivation of GTPase activating proteins (GAPs). This results in continuous activation of KRAS and downstream stimulation of the mitogen-activated protein kinase (MAPK) pathway (6). In contrast, tumor suppressor genes require missense or nonsense mutations, or deletions, to reduce protein activity or produce a non-functional truncated product (7).

Tumor suppressor genes typically must have both alleles inactivated to confer a selective growth advantage to the cell, except in haploinsufficiency cases, where one allele is not sufficient to replace the functionality of two wild-type alleles (8). This has been demonstrated with splice mutations in the ARF gene, leading to familial melanoma in the setting of ARF haploinsufficiency (9). In haploinsufficiency, inactivation of the wild-type allele is required to ensure that there is minimal to no functional levels of resultant protein, which can occur via several mechanisms: widespread chromosomal changes, dual mutations, dominant negative mutations (for example, in TP53, whereby the mutated product can silence the unaffected TP53 allele) and epigenetic silencing (10, 11).

Oncogenes and tumor suppressors facilitate tumor growth by stimulating tumor cell division or preventing tumor cell death, respectively. In contrast, inactivating mutations in DNA repair or caretaker genes yield higher gene mutation rates and genomic instability (12). This can potentiate the development of cancer-driving mutations, as opposed to initiating neoplastic transformation per se. A classic example is mutations in the mismatch repair gene BRCA1, which can increase the predisposition towards breast and ovarian cancer through increased mutational frequency (13).

Since the first publication of the full-length sequence of the human genome in 2001, large-scale sequencing initiatives (for example, the Cancer Genome Atlas project) have characterized the landscape of genomic alterations in common solid tumors (3, 14). These studies highlight the remarkable diversity of genomic alterations from tumors that share the same organ site origin and histology. Recurrent driver genomic alterations, causally implicated in tumorigenesis, have been identified in subsets of common solid tumors (15). The recent successes of molecular targeted agents (for example, erlotinib or gefitinib in epidermal growth factor receptor (EGFR) mutant non small lung cancer (NSCLC); vemurafenib or dabrafenib in BRAF V600E mutant melanoma; and

*Molecular Pathology: A Practical Guide for the Surgical Pathologist and Cytopathologist*, ed. John M. S. Bartlett, Abeer Shaaban and Fernando Schmitt. Published by Cambridge University Press. © Cambridge University Press, 2016.

crizotinib in anaplastic lymphoma kinase (ALK) translocated NSCLC) illustrate the promise of genotype-matched treatment for advanced solid tumors (16–18). With the falling cost of DNA sequencing technology and the increasing application of sequence-derived information to drive therapeutic decision making in oncology, there is a growing demand for mutation analysis of tumor specimens in a clinical setting. The goal of this chapter is to provide an overview of the clinical testing methods for mutation analysis with a focus on high throughput platforms; to review ongoing institutional and national screening programs performing targeted sequencing of tumor specimens obtained from patients with advanced solid tumors; and to discuss the challenges of developing an infrastructure to integrate next generation DNA sequencing into routine clinical care.

## Targeted sequencing methods and technologies

### Optimizing molecular pathology workflow

Optimal pathology workflow is essential for the accuracy, precision and validity of genomic testing. The workflow begins with an optimal tumor biopsy, ideally selected through a multidisciplinary approach involving the anatomic pathologist or cytopathologist, molecular pathologist/geneticist, radiologist and clinician. Review of previous pathologic specimens in advance helps guide sample selection. Tumor multifocality or heterogeneity may require testing of multiple biopsy sites. Adherence to well-defined standard operating procedures minimizes variation in pre-analytical variables from tissue biopsy to DNA isolation. The emerging field of biospecimen sciences seeks evidence-based approaches to control for variability of pre-analytical factors and to ensure the quality and reproducibility of the analysis (19). It is incumbent on the molecular pathologist or geneticist to remain abreast of advances in biospecimen science and incorporate evidence-based standard operating procedures into pathology workflow.

### Rationale for targeted high-throughput platforms

Most diagnostic labs currently utilize single gene assays in mutational analysis. Although testing guidelines exist currently for a comparatively small number of genes in specific malignancies (for example, EGFR, ALK in lung adenocarcinoma; KRAS in colorectal cancer), as pre-clinical and clinical data continue to evolve, the number and complexity of testing guidelines is anticipated to increase. In the future, multiplexed screening approaches, including next generation sequencing, will come into their own as diagnostic tools. Multiplexed screening approaches consolidate a high number of single gene assays and offer several distinct advantages to sequential testing methods. Combining multiple genetic tests simultaneously is a strategy that is parsimonious from a tissue, timing and cost perspective. Panel-based parallel testing has a rapid turnaround time. For instance, the OncoCarta panel (Sequenom, San Diego, CA, USA) is capable of detecting more than 230 mutations in 19 cancer-associated oncogenes, and can run 16 patient samples simultaneously in less than two working days. In contrast, sequentially testing for this number of mutations would be likely to exhaust the tissue specimen, be time inefficient and more expensive. Similarly, with the MiSeq (Illumina, Inc., San Diego, CA, USA) and Ion Torrent Personalized Genome Machine (PGM) (Life Technologies, Guilford, CT, USA), the use of commercially available cancer hotspot panels enables result generation for hundreds of variants in three to five days, not including the time taken to interpret the variant(s) identified. Thus, once a batch of samples is ready to run on these multiplex platforms, a high volume of data can be generated in a relatively short period of time.

Detecting multiple mutations may enable a better understanding of the molecular complexity of cancer and the resultant effect on critical cellular pathways. The impact on sensitivity or resistance to targeted therapies may potentially be predicted from identified mutations. While the value of increased data volume generated from multiplex testing over single gene testing for solid tumors is still being explored, its utility in disciplines such as malignant hematology is more apparent, where, for example, a number of variants can be used for risk stratification in patients with acute myeloid leukemia with normal cytogenetics. It is worth noting two major caveats to the multiplex testing approach described. Firstly, the list of FDA-approved therapies directed against clinically validated mutational targets is still small, although there is a growing portfolio of novel targeted agents at various stages in the development pipeline (20).

**131**

Secondly, tests that identify multiple aberrations are difficult to interpret, as there is limited information about the functional impact of rare or previously unrecognized variants from pre-clinical drug sensitivity testing and concerns have recently been raised about the reproducibility of high-throughput drug sensitivity screening (21).

## Types of high-throughput systems

There are two major types of high-throughput variant detection platforms currently in use: multiplex variant detection systems and next generation sequencing (NGS) systems. Multiplex SNP variant detection systems (for example, the Sequenom MassARRAY system, and the SNaPshot Multiplex chemistry) permit the identification of known variants in characterized gene sequences.

NGS is a technology platform that allows for parallel sequencing of targeted regions of multiple genes. NGS systems designed for panel-based analysis and sequencing of small genomes (for example, the Illumina MiSeq and Life Technologies PGM) operate on the principle of small fragment (150 to 250 basepairs) sequencing generated by PCR or digestion, which are read repeatedly. The post-sequencing bioinformatics pipeline allows for the mapping of each amplicon to the most recent build of the reference human genome; determination of coverage depth for each fragment or amplicon; and identification of sequence variants, through comparison to the reference genome. It is worthwhile noting that the Illumina MiSeq platform is the only FDA cleared high-throughput sequencing device for clinical use that allows laboratories to develop and validate sequencing of any part of a patient's genome (22, 23). Labs are free to develop their own tests, or to utilize the commercially available panels, based on their specific needs.

## Multiplex SNP/variant detection platforms

Multiplex SNP/variant detection platforms are a natural extension of current single-gene assays, in that they rely on established information about sequences of interest. Several different chemistries and platforms are commercially available, including the SNaPShot multiplex chemistry, the Illumina Infinium platform and the Sequenom MassARRAY platform (24–27). Multiplex chemistries are predominantly based on multiplex PCR amplification of regions of interest,

which contain known sequence-base changes, followed by multiplexed primer extension assays to detect those changes. Only the Illumina Infinium platform is based upon hybridization (28). Detection of the mutations of interest is then carried out either by direct sequencing of the primer extension products or by mass spectrometry. A variant on this technology incorporates TaqMan probe-based PCR chemistry to accomplish the variant detection, and can be done on commercially available droplet PCR instruments (29).

Advantages of this set of technologies include the capability of designing highly parallel multiplex assays; the increased information output of these assays compared to single-gene assays; and the savings in time and labor in the application of highly parallel assays in the diagnostic setting. The cost of a single assay can be amortized across the simultaneous application of multiple tests to the same sample. Savings increase when considering time and labor costs are factored in.

Disadvantages to this approach are predominantly technical. Multiplex detection methodologies are only capable of detecting known variants. Detectable variants are limited to single nucleotide variations and small indels or frameshifts, which are less than 10% of the size of the PCR amplicon. Additionally, these indels or frameshifts must result in a sequence change; that is, the first nucleotide of the variant sequence must be different from the first nucleotide of the wild-type sequence, otherwise the change would not be detectable.

The successful application of these technologies depends on several important considerations: throughput, multiplex level, sample quality and quantity, and detection sensitivity or threshold (see Table 10.1). Successful variant detection has been carried out on DNA derived from formalin-fixed paraffin-embedded (FFPE) tissues, fresh-frozen tissues, blood and bone marrow. There has been some success in detecting known variants in circulating free tumor DNA extracted from plasma using Sequenom MassARRAY technology (30). These technologies will also detect SNPs and known variants in RNA, after an initial cDNA synthesis step – although having good quality, intact RNA is a concern, and FFPE samples are less likely to succeed in this analysis. Thus, multiplex detection technologies are extremely versatile in their ability to identify SNPs and known variants, even in samples of poor quality.

**Table 10.1** Factors for consideration in the design of custom high-throughput genotyping panels

| Characteristic | Multiplex SNP/variant detection panels | NGS variant detection panels |
| --- | --- | --- |
| Throughput | • Delimited by size of multiplex assay and maximum reaction capacity of PCR instrument.<br>• Inverse relationship between number of multiplex assays and sample throughput.<br>• In droplet PCR-based methodologies, sample throughput is dictated by detection instruments' capacities (25). | • NGS instruments hardwired to have a ceiling of sequence information collected per run.<br>• Three factors are involved in determining system throughput: library size, sample load and depth of coverage. |
| Library size | N/A | • Total size (in bases) of sequences of interest in panel.<br>• Factors influencing library size include: number of genes in panel; whether panel is intended to cover mutation hotspots only, or whole exons or coding regions; and amount of intronic coverage. |
| Coverage depth | N/A | • Number of reads accumulated for an individual amplicon or fragment.<br>• Average coverage depth refers to the coverage of the entire library. |
| Multiplex level | • Sequencing-based approaches limited by number of discrete sequences analyzable on instrument.<br>• Multiplex level for droplet PCR dependent on ability of instrument to detect multiple fluorophores.<br>• Mass spectrometry-based methodologies have highest theoretical upper limit on multiplex reactions, defined by ability to integrate assays with different molecular weight profiles in one reaction. | N/A |
| Sample quantity | • Dependent on size of assay – i.e. total number of wells required for a complete mutation profile on a given sample. | • Dependent on the instrument used.<br>• Illumina MiSeq: 250 ng optimally.<br>• Life Technologies instruments: as little as 10 ng; optimally 50 ng. |
| Sample quality | • Methods work well on DNA of poor quality.<br>• Quality control carried out during initial optimization can be used to define practical sample quality range. | • Samples of insufficient quality will yield increased levels of sequencing artifact, low coverage and/or difficult-to-interpret variant lists.<br>• DNA extracted from FFPE and fresh-frozen tissues, as well as from blood and bone marrow, can be analyzed by NGS methodologies, as long as they meet an appropriate quality threshold.<br>• The quantity and quality of cell-free DNA extracted from plasma may be limiting. |

**Table 10.1** (*cont.*)

| Characteristic | Multiplex SNP/variant detection panels | NGS variant detection panels |
|---|---|---|
| Detection threshold/ sensitivity | • Sequencing and mass spectrometry-based detection approaches have a practical lower limit of variant detection of approximately 10%; lower variant allele frequencies are often not distinguishable from background, or cannot be verified by an orthogonal method.<br>• Droplet PCR-based systems claim a theoretical lower limit of detection of <0.1% – however, this sensitivity is achievable with higher concentrations of starting material. | • NGS technologies have a lower limit of sensitivity dependent on coverage depth. The higher the coverage, the greater the sensitivity.<br>• Practical limits are imposed by ability to verify the result through an orthogonal method. |
| Variant confirmation | • Important to ensure that all variants identified are verified by orthogonal methods.<br>• Low-frequency variants at or below detection thresholds for established orthogonal methods in the lab may have to be verified by a more sensitive test. | • Important to ensure that all variants identified are verified by orthogonal methods.<br>• Low-frequency variants at or below detection thresholds for established orthogonal methods in the lab may have to be verified by a more sensitive test.<br>• Given the significant differences in chemistry between the Illumina MiSeq/ HiSeq and the Life Technologies instruments, samples can be applied to both platforms to cross-validate results. |

Key: FFPE = formalin-fixed paraffin-embedded; N/A = not applicable; ng = nanograms; NGS = next generation sequencing; PCR = polymerase chain reaction.

## NGS-based variant detection

NGS-based variant detection utilizes high-throughput sequencing of genomic regions of interest. Since the advent of this technology, it has undergone a rapid evolution. Currently, "second-generation" NGS platforms are commercially available and in wide use, while "third-generation" platforms are in active testing or are becoming commercially available (31). Third-generation NGS platforms allow for "single-molecule" sequencing – that is, sequencing without the need for massively parallel clonal amplification of target regions, a characteristic of second-generation sequencers (31). A comparison of the current platforms is shown in Table 10.2 (31–34).

NGS workflows require a target enrichment step, either through PCR amplification and subsequent "capture" and purification of target regions, or through genome shearing/fragmentation, hybridization to "bait" sequences, followed by capture and purification of regions of interest (ROIs). Purified ROIs are "tagged" with sample-specific barcodes and sequencing primers, either as part of the initial amplification step in library preparation, or post-purification, and samples are multiplexed and loaded on the NGS platform for high-throughput sequencing. Post-sequencing analysis is then undertaken to align sequences against the reference sequences for the genes in the panel, and to determine variant calls and read depth. Technical differences between the amplification and capture methods of target enrichment translate to differences in efficiency and region coverage (35). Specific application of a target enrichment method will depend on the laboratory's need for a given panel, and this choice is influenced by some of the factors discussed below.

NGS approaches enable the sequencing of the length of each captured fragment, and allow the identification of all variants, known or unknown, within that region. Thus, these approaches circumvent one key limitation of the multiplex assays previously discussed, in that they are not dependent on prior sequence knowledge. NGS-based variant detection

**Table 10.2** Comparison of second- and third-generation NGS platforms with potential for clinical application

| Company | Illumina | Life Technologies | Roche GS FLX | Pacific Biosciences | Helicos Biosciences |
|---|---|---|---|---|---|
| Platforms | HiSeq 2000 series MiSeq Genome Analyzer IIX, IIE HiScan SQ | Ion Torrent/PGM Ion Proton ABI SOLiD, SOLiD 4 | 454 GS FLX+ 454 GS Junior | SMRT | HeliScope |
| Amplification | Bridge PCR | Emulsion PCR | Emulsion PCR | None | None |
| Sequencing chemistry | Sequencing by synthesis, with reversible terminator dyes | Ion semiconductor sequencing (PGM/Proton) Sequencing by ligation (SOLiD) | Pyrosequencing | Single molecule sequencing | Single molecule sequencing |
| Maximum read length | 100–250 bp | 200 bp (PGM/Proton) 50–75 bp (SOLiD) | 400–1,000 bp | 250 bp–10 kb | 25–55 bp |
| Throughput per run | <10 gb (MiSeq) 10–95 gb (GA II) 105–600 gb (HiSeq) | 300 mb–1 gb (PGM) <10 gb (Proton) 100 gb (SOLiD) | 35–700 mb | N/A | 21–35 gb |
| Run time | 1–14 days | 1–4.5 hr (PGM/Proton) 3.5–16 days (SOLiD) | 10–23 hr | N/A | 8 days |
| Dominant error type | Substitution | Indel (PGM/Proton) Substitution (SOLiD) | Indel | Indel | Deletion |
| Overall error rate | 0.2% | 0.1–1% | 0.5% | 15% | 5% |

Key: bp = base pairs; gb = gigabases; N/A = not applicable; PCR = polymerase chain reaction.

has the ability to detect multiple different kinds of variants – single nucleotide variations, small indels and frameshifts can all be detected. The maximum indel size detectable on NGS platforms is dependent to some degree on the technology being utilized, and some platforms have been reported to have difficulty with homopolymer-associated indels (36). Furthermore, with appropriate bioinformatics approaches, some platforms can detect copy-number variations in analyzed ROIs. More complex analyses – for example, for translocation products – are also possible and have strong bioinformatics components. NGS-based variant detection also allows for sample multiplexing and assay batching. Limitations of NGS-based detection methods are predominantly technical, and involve the complexity of the informatics workflows, and the technology's inability to detect large fragment-spanning indels. The successful application of these platforms depends on several important considerations, including library size, coverage depth, sample throughput, sample quality and quantity, detection threshold and variant confirmation (Table 10.1). Recently, guidelines on the minimum coverage depth required in the diagnostic setting to identify a variant in NGS data have been developed (37). These guidelines focus on validation and monitoring of NGS platforms and tests, and the interpretation and reporting of variants found using these technologies. Of note, interpretation and reporting of multiple somatic variants is still fairly underdeveloped, and available guidelines tend to focus on germline variant interpretation.

## Panel design

Commercially available genotyping panels exist for many platforms discussed herein; perhaps the best known of these are the Sequenom family of panels for mutation hotspots in cancer, for example, Lung-Carta, OncoCarta (26, 27); the Illumina TruSeq Amplicon Cancer Panel (38, 39); and the Life Technologies Ion AmpliSeq Cancer Hotspot Panel

**135**

(40, 41). Custom panels can be designed for each platform, focusing on genes/regions and mutations of interest. It is important to consider several previously identified issues – in particular, panel size, throughput, instrument capacity and the intended use of the panel – to ensure optimal implementation. Larger, more complex assays are more difficult to troubleshoot, can handle lower throughput and may be more expensive.

# Analysis and interpretation

The analysis and interpretation of data generated by high-throughput genotyping platforms is an important aspect of assay design and implementation. Because of the significant multiplex and throughput capacities of the platforms (Tables 10.1 and 10.2), any assay will yield extremely large volumes of data. For example, the Sequenom OncoCarta panels will yield more than 230 discrete sets of data for each sample in the assay; each dataset will contain information for a minimum of two and a maximum of four alleles. The volume of data generated by NGS is orders of magnitude greater in terms of complexity, and requires a more advanced analysis/informatics pipeline (see (42) for a good overview of the available informatics tools for NGS data analysis). In considering the implementation of high-throughput genotyping assays, particularly NGS, it is important to address the issues of run quality control, the fidelity of the informatics pipeline, variant calling sensitivity and the process for variant interpretation.

## Run quality control

Metrics of run quality, unique to the instrument and the assay, and based on experience during assay validation, must be established, in order to determine criteria required to identify a failed run. These metrics can be complex for NGS, and can include basic measures of run quality as output by the instrument, as well as measures of sequence integrity and coverage (43). Some NGS-specific examples include: %GC bias; transition/transversion ratio; first base read success; base call quality; and mapping quality. While several groups have begun to address quality control metrics in establishing NGS assays, there remains no consensus on such metrics for multiplex SNP/variant detection assays, particularly within the clinical diagnostic setting (37, 43).

## Fidelity of informatics pipeline

Newer NGS platforms that produce short DNA sequences or an absence of paired end reads present challenges for analysis software to de-convolute repeat DNA regions and consequently assemble the genome. Hence, different analysis packages can result in discordant and potentially false sequences from the same DNA. The analysis pipeline chosen for any multiplex assay must be reproducible and of high quality. It is important to consider whether a custom pipeline based on individual informatics tools (42) is appropriate, versus commercially available third-party analysis software packages. These software packages such as NextGENe (SoftGenetics), Gene-Spring (Agilent) and Partek Genomics Suite (Partek) have the advantage of streamlining and increasing the user-friendliness of the analysis methodology, at the cost of being able to deconstruct and troubleshoot the pipeline in the event of error. Commercially available NGS platforms also come with their own informatics resources (for example, Life Technologies' Ion Reporter, and Illumina's Variant Studio), which may interpret quality metrics and run data in different ways, and ought to be compared against other tools before their adoption. Thus, the establishment of any analysis framework within the lab must first involve a direct comparison of several suites of tools.

## Variant calling sensitivity

To determine the lower limit of detection of a high-throughput system, one must address two issues: the potential for background signal within the assay (for example, likelihood and presence of sequencing artifact); and the ability to verify the result using an orthogonal technology. Often, the practical limit of sensitivity of variant calling will be dependent on either or both of these factors.

*Whole genome (WGS) and whole exome sequencing (WES).* These approaches have distinct advantages with regard to data volume and human genome coverage over other methods. However, the cost and turnaround time for these approaches remain high, due in part to the instrumentation and informatics requirements necessary to generate and interpret the results. The informatics pipeline, variant interpretation and data storage requirements for WGS and WES are significant, given the volume of sequence generated and the high likelihood of a large number of potential variants.

# Clinical applications of mutational analysis

Technological progress in DNA sequencing has permitted integration of broad molecular profiling of a patient's tumor into the clinic at point of care (44). Results of these investigations can impact treatment decisions for patients by identifying molecular aberrations that may have prognostic and predictive implications. Finding patients whose tumors harbor such alterations is challenging in light of the fact that many unbiased genome sequencing projects across a number of tumor types have reported that the majority of recurrent somatic mutations occur at a low frequency (45–51). Hence, screening large populations of cancer patients is required to detect these aberrations.

A key attraction of this type of approach is to select patients who are most likely to benefit from certain therapies such as molecularly targeted agents. Somatic mutations or aberrations that are in current clinical use that predict response to treatment are listed in Table 10.3. Many agents targeting specific molecular abnormalities are being developed with the prevailing hypothesis being that these drugs will only be effective in patients whose tumors harbor this aberration. Coupling molecular profiling initiatives that screen patients for a wide array of molecular aberrations with programs that have access to a comprehensive portfolio of early phase clinical trials is an appealing strategy to facilitate genotype matched therapy. Organizations attempting to integrate broad targeted variant mutational analysis at point of care have faced logistical, technical, financial, regulatory and scientific barriers (52). A selection of these issues will be discussed in the following section.

## Challenges of clinical assessment

Several pragmatic challenges confront the development of infrastructure for genomic testing in the clinical setting.

## Availability of tumor samples

Surgical resections of primary tumors or metastatic lesions provide large volumes of tumor tissue for mutation testing. Core needle biopsies obtained to establish a cancer diagnosis may also be used. Small needle biopsy specimens from difficult-to-access organ sites (for example, lung or retroperitoneal lymph nodes) may provide limited tumor DNA for mutational analysis, particularly if the diagnostic archival specimens have been previously subjected to multiple immunohistochemical or molecular marker analysis for standard of care testing. After surgical

**Table 10.3** Somatic gene mutations or aberrations that are validated predictive biomarkers in current clinical use

| Gene | Tumor type | Response | Drug(s) |
|---|---|---|---|
| ALK (translocations) | Non-small cell lung cancer | Sensitivity | Crizotinib |
| BRAF | Melanoma | Sensitivity | Vemurafenib |
| EGFR | Non-small cell lung cancer | Sensitivity or Resistance (e.g. T790M) | Gefitinib, Imatinib |
| HER2/ErbB2 amplification | Breast cancer | Sensitivity | Lapatinib, Pertuzumb, Traztuzumab, Trastuzumab emtansine |
| | Gastric cancer | Sensitivity | Traztuzumab |
| c-KIT | Gastrointestinal stromal tumor | Sensitivity* | Imatinib |
| KRAS | Colorectal | Resistance | Cetuximab, Panitumumab |
| PDGFRA | Gastrointestinal stromal tumor | Sensitivity** | Imatinib |

*Notes:*
* certain KIT mutations may confer intermediate sensitivity.
** PDGFRA D842V confers reduced sensitivity.

excision tumor specimens are routinely fixed in formalin and embedded in paraffin to preserve histology. Selecting tissue for macroscopic or microscopic dissection requires expert pathology evaluation. Tumor areas should be marked on the slide and tumor cellularity and degree of necrosis should be recorded. Cores punched from a tumor block are often preferable to select areas of highest viable tumor cellularity and to preserve diagnostic features in the remaining tissue.

It is well recognized that tumor nucleic acids degrade with formalin fixation, which may preclude the use of some archival specimens for NGS applications. The yield of tumor DNA obtained using commercially available kits has improved in recent years. The use of cytology specimens from fine-needle aspiration (FNA) for single-gene (for example, EGFR, BRAF or KRAS) mutation hotspot analysis, using PCR-based techniques, is now routine. Limited reports indicate that NGS of cytology specimens is feasible (53–55), although further studies are required to determine if less invasive cytology sampling methods can be routinely applied for targeted sequencing analysis in a clinical setting.

## Laboratory certification

Clinical laboratories that perform testing on human specimens for the purpose of providing information on diagnosis, prevention or treatment of disease to the supervising physician must adhere to Clinical Laboratory Improvements Amendments (CLIA) standards and be accredited by the College of American Pathologists (CAP) in the United States or similar regulatory agencies in other jurisdictions to ensure ongoing competency and quality control assessment in addition to reimbursement (56). Genome-scale sequencing was previously outside of the purview of a clinical laboratory due to the cost, computing and informatics requirements of the technology. "Benchtop" NGS instruments, such as the Illumina MiSeq and the IonTorrent Proton, which offer high-throughput coverage of large panels (50 to 400 genes) of clinically relevant cancer genes are, however, well suited to the workflow of a clinical laboratory (57). CAP has recently released an 18-requirement checklist for laboratory accreditation standards for NGS, focused on validation and documentation needed for sequence data generation and bioinformatics analysis in a clinical laboratory (58).

## Sequence verification

The Next Generation Sequencing Standardization of Clinical Testing (Nex-StoCT) workgroup recommends that all clinically actionable findings should be confirmed by independent analysis using an alternate method before reporting to the treating clinician (43). This poses a dilemma when high coverage next generation sequencing identifies a low frequency mutation that cannot be confirmed by Sanger or PCR sequencing due to the limitations of sensitivity of direct sequencing methods. Currently, there is no standardized approach to address this problem, although using an orthologous, non-Sanger platform with a similar or lower sensitivity threshold may be a potential solution.

## Reporting standards

The requirement for mutation verification may delay the time to reporting if multiple clinically actionable variants are detected by NGS. Patients with metastatic cancer and their oncologists may not be willing to wait for the return of results to initiate a new treatment if there are prolonged delays for mutation verification (59). An alternative approach to orthologous testing for each individual clinically actionable variant prior to reporting is to perform validation of the testing platform and informatics pipeline for a targeted capture NGS panel.

## Reporting results to clinicians

There are currently no clear standards for reporting; a suggested set of elements to consider including in reporting results from high-throughput and NGS-based tests, is included in Box 10.1. Deciding upon which mutation(s) are clinically relevant and developing a framework to report results to clinicians that can easily be interpreted is complex. There are few mutations that have been validated with a high level of evidence to predict response to treatment (15). Specific mutations may have different clinical implications depending on a cancer's tissue of origin, such as BRAF V600E mutation and response to the BRAF inhibitor vemurafenib in melanoma and colorectal cancer (17, 60). For mutations in tumor-specific contexts where there are no clinical studies available, preclinical drug sensitivity encyclopedias can be mined to infer potential clinical relevance (61, 62). However, there are concerns about the ability to validate

**Box 10.1** Reporting somatic variants in cancer detected through high-throughput approaches to the treating clinician

Technical requirements to consider reporting:

- platform used for sequencing;
- genes and genomic regions sequenced;
- median depth of coverage and range of read depth achieved;
- any genomic regions that did not achieve minimum threshold for coverage depth;
- variant(s) identified and allelic frequency of variant(s); and
- description of whether variant(s) detected were verified by an orthologous sequencing technology.

Elements of clinical annotation to consider reporting:

- prevalence of the specific variant(s) identified (in cancer site of interest, and in cancer generally);
- summary of clinical or pre-clinical studies demonstrating the impact of the variant(s) identified on function and/or patient management;
- predicted effect on protein structure or function for variant(s) identified, but not previously characterized;
- an accompanying framework to provide information to the treating clinician about approved therapeutic agent(s) linked to variant(s) in the same tumor types or in other tumor types; and
- a local context for available clinical trials with matched investigational agent(s) for a particular genotype.

predictive genomic biomarkers across cell line screening datasets (63) and the lack of reproducibility of pre-clinical experiments (64).

## Clinical annotation

Sequencing reports should provide some clinical context for the variant(s) identified. The variant interpretation pipeline must be optimized and validated against available tools, and be implementable in the clinical diagnostic setting. Third-party tools (for example, Alamut, Interactive Biosoftware) and custom variant interpretation packages (for example, MutSig, FunSeq) can be utilized, but must be assessed against the informational requirements for interpretation (see Box 10.1) (65, 66).

## Incidental findings

Another important consideration is the reporting of incidental (or secondary) findings, defined as the results of a deliberate search for pathogenic or likely pathogenic alterations in genes that are not directly relevant to the diagnostic indication for which the sequencing test was ordered (67). In the context of clinical sequencing for somatic tumor alterations, incidental findings usually refer to the discovery of germline variants in genes that are associated with a heritable risk of cancer or other diseases. It is important to ensure that the analysis pipeline is able to differentiate between somatic and germline variants. To that end, NGS-based variant detection may incorporate parallel analysis of patient tumor DNA alongside a germline sample (for example, patient blood or hair follicle). The American College of Medical Genetics and Genomics (ACMG) recently published a minimum list of genes that should be reported to the patient when an incidental constitutional mutation is identified and confirmed (67). Medical genetics and/or affiliated genetic counseling services should be made available to patients with clinically relevant germline findings (67, 68). For patients with advanced disease who may have a limited life expectancy, it is important to identify a delegate, preferably a blood relative, who would be contacted if any clinically relevant incidental germline variants are identified in the event that the patient is unavailable to receive the testing results.

## Multi-disciplinary tumor boards

Many clinical programs that are applying the results of NGS to patient care have established a dedicated forum to discuss genomic testing results from individual patients (15, 69). These meetings may include many different disciplines, such as medical oncologists, pathologists, clinical geneticists, bioinformaticians, genetic counselors, ethicists and laboratory scientists to evaluate the clinical relevance of genomic testing results and devise a personalized treatment recommendation for individual patients. Scalability is an important limitation; as the scope and throughput of clinical genomic testing expand, it may not be feasible for tumor boards at any single institution to meet frequently enough to review all cases sequenced and there may not be sufficient local expertise available to discuss complex testing results.

## Molecular profiling programs

A molecular profiling program is an integrated, multi-disciplinary system focused on implementing personalized cancer medicine (70). The infrastructure of the program facilitates archived tissue retrieval or, in some cases, fresh tumor acquisition for genomic characterization, with these results analyzed and returned to the clinician in a structured molecular report that can be applied to select approved or investigational treatment matched to genotype.

## Clinical molecular profiling

Capitalizing on progress from TCGA, the International Cancer Genome Consortium (ICGC) and other projects would require migration of NGS technologies into the clinic. Realizing the potential benefits of clinical integration of molecular profiling, leading cancer institutions and health agencies have developed institutional molecular screening capabilities. Some of the current programs that have incorporated genomic profiling into clinical service are listed in Table 10.4, Together with key elements of these programs.

### Tumor samples

In the majority of instances, these programs use archival tumor tissue for genomic analysis. Archived samples are accessible and spare the patient from having to undergo an invasive biopsy or surgical excision procedure to obtain tumor tissue for genomic characterization. Initial concerns about yield and quality of tumor DNA from stored FFPE tumor samples for targeted NGS have been addressed by improved DNA extraction protocols, with concordant results between FFPE and fresh or frozen samples of the same tumor (70). Whether routinely stored FFPE archival tumor tissue can be used for clinical WES or WGS remains to be determined, as samples stored for over five years are reported to have more degraded nucleic acids potentially not suitable for such technologies (71). For SNP genotyping or targeted sequencing, there may be limitations related to size of the tumor and age of the sample. Biopsies may have small quantities of tumor and if other molecular tests have already been performed then there is a risk that the sample may either be exhausted or not have sufficient quantities of tumor DNA for mutational analysis. Some profiling initiatives, such as those from Institut Gustav Roussy, Institut Curie and the WIN consortium, require a fresh tumor sample from a primary or metastatic lesion for molecular characterization. The advantage of this approach is that the mutational analysis may be more reflective of a patient's underlying cancer biology at the time the information is needed for clinical decision making. However, spatial heterogeneity is a potential limitation, as there may be intra-tumor heterogeneity within a single tumor or between metastases.

### Sequencing technologies

Genotyping or targeted variant sequencing platforms such as OncoCarta or OncoMap (Sequenom, San Diego, CA, USA) or the SNaPshot™ assay (Applied Biosystems, Foster City, CA, USA) are commonly used. The tumor types that are selected as part of the program guide the genes or variants that are included in the analysis. These technologies are scalable, allowing these institutions to readily increase the number of genes or kilobases of the genome interrogated. Typically, oncogenes or tumor suppressors are selected for inclusion in these panels because there are approved drugs or agents in clinical development known or hypothesized to be more effective in patients whose tumors harbor activating genomic alterations. Targeted NGS technologies are becoming more widely utilized as point-of-care testing platforms. WGS and WES are not yet widely used due to cost and throughput. To date, very few reports have been published of patients having their tumor DNA analyzed by such technologies in a clinical setting (72). It is anticipated that the clinical utilization of WGS and WES will increase as the costs of sequencing fall, bioinformatics pipelines are tailored for clinical applications and DNA input requirements decrease over time.

### Prospectively defined versus opportunistic genotype matched treatment

An important objective of profiling programs is to identify patients with actionable mutations that can be matched to targeted treatments based on their genotype. Since potentially actionable mutations are linked to investigational treatments, the success of this approach is contingent on having access to a large portfolio of phase I and phase II clinical trials. The portfolio of trials accessible through the program will influence treatment selection for patients. Given the inherent dynamic nature of experimental therapeutics, this type of arrangement will be able to evolve

**Table 10.4** A selection of current molecular profiling programs

| Institution, consortium or region | Trial or program name | Profiling platform(s) or technique(s) | Cancer(s) | Tumor samples | Treatment assignment |
|---|---|---|---|---|---|
| Cancer Research UK | Stratified Medicine Programme | PCR FISH | Melanoma, NSCLC, CRC, breast, prostate, ovarian cancer | Archival | NS |
| Dana Farber Cancer Institute | PROFILE | Sequenom | All solid tumors | Archival | NS |
| Institut Curie, Institut National du Cancer | SHIVA (NCT01771458) | Ion Torrent PGM Cytoscan HD | All solid tumors | Fresh biopsy | Prospectively defined |
| Institut Gustav Roussy (non-pediatric trials) | MOSCATO (NCT01566019) | aCGH PCR | Solid tumor phase I patients | Fresh biopsy | Opportunistic |
| | SAFIR01 (NCT01414933) | aCGH PCR | Breast cancer | Fresh biopsy | Opportunistic |
| | MSN | PCR FISH | Melanoma, SCLC, NSCLC | Fresh biopsy | Prospectively defined |
| Massachusetts General Hospital | NS | SNaP Shot | NSCLC, CRC, melanoma, breast cancer | Archival | NS |
| MD Anderson Cancer Center | T9 Program | Sequenom | All solid tumors | Archival | NS |
| | IMPACT (NCT00851032) | PCR FISH | All solid tumors | Archival | Opportunistic |
| | Clearing House Protocol | PCR Illumina NS, Ion Torrent NS | All solid tumors | Archival or fresh biopsy | NS |
| Memorial Sloan-Kettering Cancer Center | IMPACT (NCT01775072) | Illumina HiSeq Sequenom or MiSeq | All solid tumors | Archival or fresh biopsy | NS |
| Netherlands | Centre for Personalized Cancer Treatment | Ion Torrent PGM SOLiD 5500xl | Solid tumors | Fresh biopsy | NS |
| Norwegian Cancer Genomics Consortium | Nationwide program | NS | 9 tumor types both solid and hematopoietic | Archival or fresh biopsy | NS |
| Princess Margaret Cancer Centre | IMPACT (NCT01505400) | MiSeq Sequenom | Selected solid tumors | Archival | Opportunistic |
| Vall D'Hebron Institute of Oncology | NS | Sequenom Illumina GAIIx | Breast cancer, solid tumor phase I patients | Archival | Opportunistic |
| Vanderbilt-Ingram Cancer Center | PCMI | SNaPshot | Melanoma, NSCLC, CRC, Breast cancer | Archival | NS |

Table 10.4 (cont.)

| Institution, consortium or region | Trial or program name | Profiling platform(s) or technique(s) | Cancer(s) | Tumor samples | Treatment assignment |
|---|---|---|---|---|---|
| **WIN Consortium** | WINTHER study (NCT01856296) | NGS CNV CGH | Solid tumors | Fresh biopsy (tumor and matched normal) | Opportunistic |

Key: aCGH = array comparative genomic hybridization; CGH = comparative genomic hybridization; CNV = copy-number variation; CRC = colorectal cancer; FISH = fluorescence *in situ* hybridization; NS = not stipulated; NSCLC = non-small cell lung cancer; PCR = polymerase chain reaction; SCLC = small cell lung cancer.

with new drug trials, giving patients the opportunity to participate in the latest clinical studies. In contrast, some molecular programs, such as the SHIVA trial and the MSN study, pre-specify treatment matching for patients whose tumors harbor specific actionable mutations. Although this strategy is less flexible, it allows for a pre-planned statistical testing of the paradigm of mutational profiling and matching therapy.

## Future directions

Widespread clinical integration of NGS platforms is anticipated as costs of sequencing continue to decline and evidence supporting the clinical benefit of matching treatment to specific molecular aberrations emerges. Furthermore, as these technologies achieve regulatory clearance for use in a CLIA-certified laboratory, it is expected that multiplex testing will become routine. As more therapies enter clinical testing and more genomic variants are identified, more patients will receive genotype-matched treatment. Increasing the depth or number of kilobases sequenced will broaden the genomic coverage and will lead to the identification of multiple somatic mutations within a single tumor and aberrations of unknown significance. Incorporating sophisticated prediction tools and functional analysis software that utilize a systems biology approach may aid in determining the impact and implications of treating such targets. Finally, multi-institutional collaborations to share molecular profiling data as part of a clinically annotated database will enhance knowledge regarding prognostic and predictive effects of these somatic abnormalities and enable clinical trials with investigational treatments in rare cancer subpopulations.

## Learning points

- There is increasing demand for mutational analysis of tumor genomes in a clinical setting to influence treatment decisions. Advances in sequencing technology allow for the consolidation of multiple single-gene assays into targeted sequencing tests that are sensitive, parsimonious and timely.

- At the present time, targeted sequencing is largely restricted to large academic molecular diagnostic laboratories and commercial start-up enterprises. It is likely that the uptake of targeted sequencing will grow to include other laboratories that perform clinical testing of tumor material, as more targeted therapies are approved to treat cancers with specific genomic alterations.

- Mutational analysis in molecular pathology is a rapidly evolving field. In the future, clinical testing will expand beyond SNP genotyping and targeted sequencing to include broader characterization with WES or WGS. A comprehensive molecular pathology assessment may also include evaluation of the epigenome, transcriptome and the immune microenvironment. Detecting somatic and germline mutations are the first steps towards integrated clinical genomics.

- Many challenges still face mutational analysis in routine clinical care, such as utilizing poor quality or scant archival tumor samples for clinical testing; integrating genomic information from multiple informatics databases to select treatment; and collating the outcomes of patients whose tumors harbor genomic alterations that receive matched targeted treatment to create a comprehensive knowledge base that can improve clinical care.

- Mutational tumor analysis identifies somatic alterations that may guide therapeutic decisions. Data are emerging to support the clinical utility of matching treatments to specific molecular aberrations.

- Multiplexed high-throughput sequencing platforms that detect a broad selection of mutations have many advantages over single assay mutation tests, which include improved efficiency, relative low cost and less consumption of tumor tissue.

- There are many challenges to the clinical integration of next generation sequencing (NGS) technologies such as poor quality or low volume of tumor samples, regulatory approval and interpretation of the significance of uncommon or novel mutations.

- Molecular profiling programs that couple mutational analysis with an infrastructure to facilitate genotype-matched treatment is an innovative strategy for personalized cancer medicine.

# References

1. Stratton, M. R., Campbell, P. J. and Futreal, P. A. The cancer genome. *Nature* 2009; 458(7239): 719–24.

2. Vogelstein, B. and Kinzler, K. W. Cancer genes and the pathways they control. *Nat Med* 2004; 10(8): 789–99.

3. Vogelstein, B., Papadopoulos, N., Velculescu, V. E., Zhou, S., Diaz, L. A. and Kinzler, K. W. Cancer genome landscapes. *Science* 2013; 339(6127): 1546–58.

4. Land, H., Parada, L. F. and Weinberg, R. A. Cellular oncogenes and multistep carcinogenesis. *Science* 1983; 222(4625): 771–8.

5. Slamon, D. J., Verma, I. and Cline, M. Expression of cellular oncogenes in human malignancies. *Science* 1984; 224(4646): 256–62.

6. Rodenhuis, S., van de Wetering, M. L., Mooi, W. J., Evers, S. G., van Zandwijk, N. and Bos, J. L. Mutational activation of the k-ras oncogene. *New Engl J Med* 1987; 317(15): 929–35.

7. Weinberg, R. A. Tumor suppressor genes. *Science* 1991; 254(5035): 1138–46.

8. Payne, S. R. and Kemp, C. J. Tumor suppressor genetics. *Carcinogenesis* 2005; 26(12): 2031–45.

9. Hewitt, C., Wu, C. L., Evans, G., Howell, A., Elles, R. G., Jordan, R. et al. Germline mutation of ARF in a melanoma kindred. *Hum Mol Genet* 2002; 11(11): 1273–9.

10. Petitjean, A., Mathe, E., Kato, S., Ishioka, C., Tavtigian, S. V., Hainaut, P. et al. Impact of mutant p53 functional properties on TP53 mutation patterns and tumor phenotype: lessons from recent developments in the IARC TP53 database. *Hum Mutat* 2007; 28(6): 622–9.

11. Jones, P. A. and Laird, P. W. Cancer-epigenetics comes of age. *Nat Genet* 1999; 21(2): 163–7.

12. Negrini, S., Gorgoulis, V. G. and Halazonetis, T. D. Genomic instability – an evolving hallmark of cancer. *Nat Rev Mol Cell Biol* 2010; 11(3): 220–8.

13. King, M.-C., Marks, J. H. and Mandell, J. B. Breast and ovarian cancer risks due to inherited mutations in BRCA1 and BRCA2. *Science* 2003; 302(5645): 643–6.

14. Venter, J. C., Adams, M. D., Myers, E. W., Li, P. W., Mural, R. J., Sutton, G. G. et al. The sequence of the human genome. *Science* 2001; 291(5507): 1304–51.

15. Dancey, J. E., Bedard, P. L., Onetto, N. and Hudson, T. J. The genetic basis for cancer treatment decisions. *Cell* 2012; 148(3): 409–20.

16. Mok, T. S., Wu, Y.-L., Thongprasert, S., Yang, C.-H., Chu, D.-T., Saijo, N. et al. Gefitinib or carboplatin-paclitaxel in pulmonary adenocarcinoma. *New Engl J Med* 2009; 361(10): 947–57.

17. Chapman, P. B., Hauschild, A., Robert, C., Haanen, J. B., Ascierto, P., Larkin, J. et al. Improved survival with vemurafenib in melanoma with BRAF V600E mutation. *New Engl J Med* 2011; 364(26): 2507–16.

18. Kwak, E. L., Bang, Y.-J., Camidge, D. R., Shaw, A. T., Solomon, B., Maki, R. G. et al. Anaplastic lymphoma kinase inhibition in non-small-cell lung cancer. *New Engl J Med* 2010; 363(18): 1693–703.

19. Moore, H. M., Compton, C. C., Alper, J. and Vaught, J. B. International approaches to advancing biospecimen science. *Cancer Epidemiol Biomarkers Prev* 2011; 20(5): 729–32.

20. Tran, B., Dancey, J. E., Kamel-Reid, S., McPherson, J. D., Bedard, P. L., Brown, A. M. K. et al. Cancer genomics: technology, discovery, and translation. *J Clin Oncol* 2012; 30(6): 647–60.

21. Haibe-Kains, B., El-Hacheem, N., Birkbak, N. J., Jin, A. C., Beck, A. H. et al. Inconsistency in large pharmacogenomic studies. *Nature* 2013; 504(7480): 389–93.

22. Collins, F. S. and Hamburg, M. A. First FDA authorization for next-generation sequencer. *New Engl J Med* 2013; 369(25): 2369–71.

**143**

23. FDA allows marketing of four "next generation" gene sequencing devices, Silver Spring Maryland: US Food and Drug Administration; November 19, 2013; available at www.fda.gov/NewsEvents/Newsroom/PressAnnouncements/ucm375742.htm.

24. Gabriel, S., Ziaugra, L. and Tabbaa, D. SNP genotyping using the Sequenom MassARRAY iPLEX platform. *Curr Protoc Hum Genet* 2009; 2–12.

25. Fumagalli, D., Gavin, P. G., Taniyama, Y., Kim, S.-I., Choi, H.-J., Paik, S. *et al.* A rapid, sensitive, reproducible and cost-effective method for mutation profiling of colon cancer and metastatic lymph nodes. *BMC Cancer* 2010; 10(1): 101.

26. Thomas, R. K., Baker, A. C., DeBiasi, R. M., Winckler, W., LaFramboise, T., Lin, W. M. *et al.* High-throughput oncogene mutation profiling in human cancer. *Nat Genet* 2007; 39(3): 347–51.

27. MacConaill, L. E., Campbell, C. D., Kehoe, S. M., Bass, A. J., Hatton, C., Niu, L. *et al.* Profiling critical cancer gene mutations in clinical tumor samples. *PLoS ONE* 2009; 4(11): e7887.

28. Normanno, N., Rachiglio, A. M., Roma, C., Fenizia, F., Esposito, C., Pasquale, R. *et al.* Molecular diagnostics and personalized medicine in oncology: challenges and opportunities. *J Cell Biochem* 2013; 114(3): 514–24.

29. Baker, M. Digital PCR hits its stride. *Nat Methods* 2012; 9(6): 541–4.

30. Perkins, G., Yap, T. A., Pope, L., Cassidy, A. M., Dukes, J. P., Riisnaes, R. *et al.* Multi-purpose utility of circulating plasma DNA testing in patients with advanced cancers. *PLoS ONE* 7(11): e47020.

31. Pareek, C. S., Smoczynski, R. and Tretyn, A. Sequencing technologies and genome sequencing. *J Appl Genetics* 2011; 52(4): 413–35.

32. Quail, M. A., Smith, M., Coupland, P., Otto, T. D., Harris, S. R., Connor, T. R. *et al.* A tale of three next generation sequencing platforms: comparison of Ion Torrent, Pacific Biosciences and Illumina MiSeq sequencers. *BMC Genomics* 2012; 13(1): 341.

33. Desai, A. and Jere, A. Next-generation sequencing: ready for the clinics? *Clin Genet* 2012; 81(6): 503–10.

34. Meldrum, C., Doyle, M. A. and Tothill, R. W. Next-generation sequencing for cancer diagnostics: a practical perspective. *Clin Biochem Rev* 2011; 32(4): 177–95.

35. Wooderchak-Donahue, W. L., O'Fallon, B., Furtado, L. V., Durtschi, J. D., Plant, P., Ridge, P. G. *et al.* A direct comparison of next generation sequencing enrichment methods using an aortopathy gene panel-clinical diagnostics perspective. *BMC Med Genomics* 2012; 5(1): 50.

36. Loman, N. J., Misra, R. V., Dallman, T. J., Constantinidou, C., Gharbia, S. E., Wain, J. *et al.* Performance comparison of benchtop high-throughput sequencing platforms. *Nat Biotech* 2012; 30(5): 434–9.

37. Rehm, H. L., Bale, S. J., Bayrak-Toydemir, P., Berg, J. S., Brown, K. K., Deignan, J. L. *et al.* ACMG clinical laboratory standards for next-generation sequencing. *Genet Med* 2013; 15(9): 733–47.

38. Hubers, A. J., Heideman, D. A., Yatabe, Y., Wood, M. D., Tull, J., Tarón, M. *et al.* EGFR mutation analysis in sputum of lung cancer patients: a multitechnique study. *Lung Cancer* 2013; 82(1): 38–43.

39. Do, H., Wong, S. Q., Li, J. and Dobrovic, A. Reducing sequence artifacts in amplicon-based massively parallel sequencing of formalin-fixed paraffin-embedded DNA by enzymatic depletion of uracil-containing templates. *Clin Chem* 2013; 59(9): 1376–83.

40. Beadling, C., Neff, T. L., Heinrich, M. C., Rhodes, K., Thornton, M., Leamon, J. *et al.* Combining highly multiplexed PCR with semiconductor-based sequencing for rapid cancer genotyping. *J Mol Diagn* 2013; 15(2): 171–6.

41. Yousem, S. A., Dacic, S., Nikiforov, Y. E. and Nikiforova, M. Pulmonary Langerhans cell histiocytosis: profiling of multifocal tumors using next-generation sequencing identifies concordant occurrence of BRAF V600E mutations. *CHEST Journal* 2013; 143(6): 1679–84.

42. Pabinger, S., Dander, A., Fischer, M., Snajder, R., Sperk, M., Efremova, M. *et al.* A survey of tools for variant analysis of next-generation genome sequencing data. *Brief Bioinform* 2013; 15(2): 256–78.

43. Gargis, A. S., Kalman, L., Berry, M. W., Bick, D. P., Dimmock, D. P., Hambuch, T. *et al.* Assuring the quality of next-generation sequencing in clinical laboratory practice. *Nat Biotech* 2012; 30(11): 1033–6.

44. Metzker, M. L. Sequencing technologies – the next generation. *Nat Rev Genet* 2009; 11(1): 31–46.

45. Hudson, T. J., Anderson, W., Aretz, A., Barker, A. D., Bell, C., Bernabé, R. R. *et al.* International network of cancer genome projects. *Nature* 2010; 464(7291): 993–8.

46. Koboldt, D. C., Fulton, R. S., McLellan, M. D., Schmidt, H., Kalicki-Veizer, J., McMichael, J. F. *et al.* Comprehensive molecular portraits of human breast tumours. *Nature* 2012; 490(7418): 61–70. Epub 2012/09/25.

47. Biankin, A. V., Waddell, N., Kassahn, K. S., Gingras, M.-C., Muthuswamy, L. B., Johns, A. L. *et al.* Pancreatic cancer genomes reveal aberrations in axon

guidance pathway genes. *Nature* 2012; 491(7424): 399–405.

48. McLendon, R., Friedman, A., Bigner, D., Van Meir, E. G., Brat, D. J., Mastrogianakis, G. M. *et al.* Comprehensive genomic characterization defines human glioblastoma genes and core pathways. *Nature* 2008; 455(7216): 1061–8.

49. Stransky, N., Egloff, A. M., Tward, A. D., Kostic, A. D., Cibulskis, K., Sivachenko, A. *et al.* The mutational landscape of head and neck squamous cell carcinoma. *Science* 2011; 333(6046): 1157–60.

50. Taylor, B. S., Schultz, N., Hieronymus, H., Gopalan, A., Xiao, Y., Carver, B. S. *et al.* Integrative genomic profiling of human prostate cancer. *Cancer Cell* 2010; 18(1): 11–22.

51. Salvesen, H., Carter, S. L., Mannelqvist, M., Dutt, A., Getz, G., Stefansson, I. *et al.* Integrated genomic profiling of endometrial carcinoma associates aggressive tumors with indicators of PI3 kinase activation. *Proc Natl Acad Sci* 2009; 106(12): 4834–9.

52. Sawyers, C. L. The cancer biomarker problem. *Nature* 2008; 452(7187): 548–52.

53. Buttitta, F., Felicioni, L., Del Grammastro, M., Filice, G., Di Lorito, A., Malatesta, S. *et al.* Effective assessment of egfr mutation status in bronchoalveolar lavage and pleural fluids by next-generation sequencing. *Clin Cancer Res* 2013; 19(3): 691–8.

54. Kanagal-Shamanna, R., Portier, B. P., Singh, R. R., Routbort, M. J., Aldape, K. D., Handal, B. A. *et al.* Next-generation sequencing-based multi-gene mutation profiling of solid tumors using fine needle aspiration samples: promises and challenges for routine clinical diagnostics. *Mod Pathol* 2014; 27(2): 314–27.

55. Young, G., Wang, K., He, J., Otto, G., Hawryluk, M.,

Zwirco, Z. *et al.* Clinical next-generation sequencing successfully applied to fine-needle aspirations of pulmonary and pancreatic neoplasms. *Cancer Cytopathol* 2013; 121(12): 688–94.

56. US Department of Health and Human Services. Medicare, Medicaid and CLIA Programs: regulations implementing the Clinical Laboratory Improvement Amendments of 1988 (CLIA). Final rule. *Fed Regist* 1992; 57(40): 7002–186.

57. Roychowdhury, S., Iyer, M. K., Robinson, D. R., Lonigro, R. J., Wu, Y. M., Cao, X. *et al.* Personalized oncology through integrative high-throughput sequencing: a pilot study. *Sci Transl Med* 2011; 3(111): 111ra21.

58. Accreditation and Laboratory Improvement, Northfield Illinois: College of American Pathologists, 2013; available at www.cap.org/apps/cap.portal%3F_nfpb=true&_pageLabel=accreditation.

59. Tran, B., Brown, A. M. K., Bedard, P. L., Winquist, E., Goss, G. D., Hotte, S. J. *et al.* Feasibility of real time next generation sequencing of cancer genes linked to drug response: results from a clinical trial. *Int J Cancer* 2013; 132(7): 1547–55.

60. Kopetz, S., Desai, J., Chan, E., Hecht, J., O'dwyer, P., Lee, R. *et al.* PLX4032 in metastatic colorectal cancer patients with mutant BRAF tumors. *J Clin Oncol* 2010; 28(15 Suppl.): 3534.

61. Barretina, J., Caponigro, G., Stransky, N., Venkatesan, K., Margolin, A. A., Kim, S. *et al.* The Cancer Cell Line Encyclopedia enables predictive modelling of anticancer drug sensitivity. *Nature* 2012; 483(7391): 603–7.

62. Garnett, M. J., Edelman, E. J., Heidorn, S. J., Greenman, C. D., Dastur, A., Lau, K. W. *et al.* Systematic identification of genomic markers of drug

sensitivity in cancer cells. *Nature* 2012; 483(7391): 570–5.

63. Papillon-Cavanagh, S., De Jay, N., Hachem, N., Olsen, C., Bontempi, G., Aerts, H. J. *et al.* Comparison and validation of genomic predictors for anticancer drug sensitivity. *J Am Med Inform Assoc* 2013; 20(4): 597–602.

64. Begley, C. G. and Ellis, L. M. Drug development: raise standards for preclinical cancer research. *Nature* 2012; 483(7391): 531–3.

65. Khurana, E., Fu, Y., Colonna, V., Mu, X. J., Kang, H. M., Lappalainen, T. *et al.* Integrative annotation of variants from 1092 humans: application to cancer genomics. *Science* 2013; 342(6154): 1235587.

66. Lawrence, M. S., Stojanov, P., Polak, P., Kryukov, G. V., Cibulskis, K., Sivachenko, A. *et al.* Mutational heterogeneity in cancer and the search for new cancer-associated genes. *Nature* 2013; 499(7457): 214–18.

67. Green, R. C., Berg, J. S., Grody, W. W., Kalia, S. S., Korf, B. R., Martin, C. L. *et al.* ACMG recommendations for reporting of incidental findings in clinical exome and genome sequencing. *Genet Med* 2013; 15(7): 565–74.

68. ACMG Board of Directors. Points to consider in the clinical application of genomic sequencing. *Genet Med* 2012; 14(8): 759–61.

69. Roychowdhury, S., Iyer, M. K., Robinson, D. R., Lonigro, R. J., Wu, Y.-M., Cao, X. *et al.* Personalized oncology through integrative high-throughput sequencing: a pilot study. *Sci Transl Med* 2011; 3(111): 111ra21.

70. Tran, B., Brown, A. M. K., Bedard, P. L., Winquist, E., Goss, G. D., Hotte, S. J. *et al.* Feasibility of real time next generation sequencing of cancer genes linked to drug response: results from a clinical

trial. *Int J Cancer* 2013; 132(7): 1547–55.

71. Wang, F., Wang, L., Briggs, C., Sicinska, E., Gaston, S. M., Mamon, H. *et al.* DNA degradation test predicts success in whole-genome amplification from diverse clinical samples. *J Mol Diagn* 2007; 9(4): 441–51. Epub 2007/08/11.

72. Roychowdhury, S., Iyer, M. K., Robinson, D. R., Lonigro, R. J., Wu, Y. M., Cao, X. *et al.* Personalized oncology through integrative high-throughput sequencing: a pilot study. *Sci Transl Med* 2011; 3(111): 111ra21.

# Tumors of the breast

Cathy B. Moelans, Petra van der Groep, Robert Kornegoor,
Jelle Wesseling and Paul J. van Diest

## Introduction

Over the last few decades, breast cancer has become one of the more well-characterized epithelial cancers, particularly at the clinical and molecular levels. Thanks to a series of in-depth genetic analyses, this heterogeneous disease has basically been classified into four distinct molecular subtypes: luminal A, luminal B, basal-like and HER2-driven [1, 2]. Clinically, this classification has been translated to three therapeutic groups. Firstly, the estrogen receptor (ER) positive group, with or without progesterone (PR) expression, mainly representing luminal A and B breast cancer. This is the largest group, for which several molecular tests are available to assist in predicting outcomes [3, 4]. Secondly, the HER2 group, for which much progress has been made because of effective therapeutic targeting of the HER2 receptor. Thirdly, triple-negative breast cancers (TNBCs, lacking expression of ER, PR and HER2), also referred to as basal-like breast cancers, which have an increased incidence in patients with germline BRCA1 mutations or of African ancestry. This type of breast cancer is associated with a poor prognosis and treated with chemotherapy because there is no benefit from endocrine therapy or trastuzumab. Classifying breast cancer into these subtypes thus helps to tailor treatment.

Through the integrated use of multiple different technologies such as genomic DNA copy-number arrays, DNA methylation analysis, exome sequencing, messenger RNA arrays, microRNA sequencing and reverse-phase protein arrays, the Cancer Genome Atlas Network was recently able to collect the most complete picture of breast cancer diversity ever, leading to the detection of multiple novel potential biomarkers for breast cancer diagnosis, prognosis and (individualized) treatment [5].

In this chapter, we will discuss molecular changes that play a key role in breast carcinogenesis, diagnosis, prognosis and prediction of therapy response, while touching on various techniques that have been applied over the years.

## Molecular changes in histological special types of breast cancer

Histological special types of breast cancer have distinctive morphological features and account for up to 25% of all invasive breast cancers. Several studies have provided evidence that some histological special types of breast cancer, including mucinous, neuroendocrine and invasive lobular carcinomas, may constitute entities distinct from histological grade-and/or ER-matched invasive carcinomas of no special type (IC-NST) at the transcriptomic level [6–9]. A recent study performed array CGH and hierarchical clustering on 59 breast cancers of ten histological special types and revealed that samples from each histological special type preferentially clustered together [10]. However, metaplastic and medullary carcinomas were found to have genomic profiles similar to those of grade- and ER-matched IC-NSTs. Integrative aCGH and gene expression profiling led to the identification of 145 transcripts that were significantly over-expressed when amplified in histological special types of breast cancer. Histological special type is thus, together with histological grade and ER status, also associated with the patterns and complexity of gene copy-number aberrations in breast cancer. Adenoid cystic and mucinous carcinomas are examples of ER-negative and ER-positive breast cancers with genomic copy-number patterns distinct from those of other grade- and ER-matched breast cancers, respectively. These

---

*Molecular Pathology: A Practical Guide for the Surgical Pathologist and Cytopathologist*, ed. John M. S. Bartlett, Abeer Shaaban and Fernando Schmitt. Published by Cambridge University Press. © Cambridge University Press, 2016.

results highlight the importance of histological subtyping in breast cancer.

## Intrinsic subtypes of breast cancer

Besides prognostic relevance of tumor stage (tumor size, nodal involvement and metastatic disease), tumor morphology, histological grade and the presence of peritumoral lymphovacular invasion, the routine evaluation of ER, PR and HER2 at diagnosis permits delineation of three major immunophenotypes: ER-positive, ER-negative/HER2-positive and ER-negative/HER2-negative (predominantly PR-negative, i.e. triple-negative). These phenotypes approximate the major intrinsic subtypes of breast cancer, are prognostically relevant and can guide systemic treatment. The intrinsic subtypes (luminal A, luminal B, HER2-enriched, basal-like and normal-like) based on gene expression analysis, first defined by Perou *et al.* and Sorlie *et al.* [1, 2], have gained widespread acceptance as a way of classifying breast tumors. Since gene expression data are often not available, approximations of intrinsic subtypes based on IHC on three to six markers (ER, PR, HER2, EGFR, Ki67 and CK5/6) have been proposed. These subtypes have different epidemiological risk factors, different natural histories, and different responses to systemic and local therapies and may thus be considered when managing breast cancer. The 12th St. Gallen International Breast Cancer Conference (2011) Expert Panel adopted a new approach to the classification of patients for therapeutic purposes based on the recognition of intrinsic biological subtypes within the breast cancer spectrum [11]. In the proposed classification, Ki-67 labeling index is key in the distinction between "Luminal A" and "Luminal B (HER2 negative)" subtypes. If reliable Ki-67 labeling index assessment is not available, some alternative measure of proliferation such as a histological grade may be used in making this distinction. The Panel recommends that systemic therapy should follow the subtype classification. "Luminal A" disease generally requires only endocrine therapy, which also forms part of the treatment of the "Luminal B" subtype. Chemotherapy is considered indicated for most patients with "Luminal B," "Human Epidermal growth factor Receptor 2 (HER2) positive" and "Triple negative" disease, with the addition of trastuzumab in "HER2 positive" disease. Although the immunohistochemical surrogate may generally suffice, different commercial tests have been introduced to establish intrinsic subtypes such as PAM50®, discussed later in this chapter. It has, however, been well established that molecular subtyping based on established gene expression classifiers is poorly reproducible across datasets, classifiers and observers [12], limiting their clinical usefulness at this point.

## HER2 testing

The human epidermal growth factor receptor 2 (HER2, also known as ERBB2) proto-oncogene is amplified in 10% to 15% of human breast cancers [13, 14]. HER2 amplification and over-expression is associated with a worse prognosis, especially in lymph node positive patients [15], and with the response to adjuvant chemotherapy and endocrine therapy [16]. Most importantly, HER2 is a predictive marker for the response to trastuzumab (Herceptin®, Roche), a therapeutic humanized monoclonal antibody directed against the extracellular domain of the HER2-receptor protein. In October 1998, trastuzumab received FDA approval for the treatment of metastasized HER2-positive breast tumors. Trastuzumab significantly increases the survival of HER2-positive patients, both as monotherapy or in combination with chemotherapy [17, 18]. As adjuvant treatment, trastuzumab halves recurrence and reduces mortality by one-third [19–21]. Since the discovery of trastuzumab, many other HER2-targeting agents have been developed. In March 2007, lapatinib (Tyverb® in Europe/Tykerb® in the United States, GlaxoSmithKline) was also registered as combination therapy with capecitabine for the treatment of HER2-positive advanced or metastatic breast cancers [22]. Lapatinib is an inhibitor of the intracellular tyrosine kinase domains of both Epidermal Growth Factor Receptor 1 (EGFR) and HER2. In June 2012, pertuzumab (Perjeta®, Genentech), another HER2 receptor antagonist compound, was FDA-approved for the first-line treatment of HER2 positive metastatic breast cancer in combination with trastuzumab and docetaxel. Pertuzumab targets the extracellular dimerization domain of HER2 and, thereby, blocks ligand-dependent heterodimerization of HER2 with other HER family members, including EGFR, HER3 and HER4. It has been shown to augment anti-tumor activity as a complement to trastuzumab, as the two drugs target different regions on the HER2 receptor. Finally, in

February 2013, the FDA approved yet another drug, ado-trastuzumab emtansine (Kadcyla®, Genentech), a HER2-targeted antibody-drug conjugate (often called T-DM1). Upon binding to the HER2 receptor, ado-trastuzumab emtansine results in intracellular release of DM1-containing cytotoxic catabolites. Binding of DM1 to tubulin disrupts microtubule networks in the cell, which results in cell cycle arrest and apoptotic cell death. Ado-trastuzumab emtansine is specifically indicated for the treatment of patients with HER2-positive, metastatic breast cancer who previously received trastuzumab and a taxane.

In the light of these extensive therapeutic implications, an accurate assessment of HER2 status for breast cancer patients is crucial. Only patients with HER2 over-expression or amplification are eligible for trastuzumab (T-DM1), pertuzumab or lapatinib treatment. A false-positive test outcome could lead to an expensive, ineffective treatment associated with unnecessary side effects, and a false-negative test result will deprive the patient of an important life-extending therapeutic option. HER2 status can be determined at the protein, RNA or DNA level. Traditionally, HER2 status was assessed at the protein level using immunohistochemistry, but nowadays there are many other HER2 testing technologies available, especially at the DNA level [23]. In 2007, the American Society for Clinical Oncology (ASCO) and the College of American Pathologists (CAP) jointly published guidelines to standardize performance and interpretation of HER2 testing in the United States [14]. This guideline was recently updated [24].

## Immunohistochemistry for assessment of HER2 status

Currently, immunohistochemistry (IHC) is the most commonly used primary technique to determine HER2 status. After slides are incubated with an antibody directed against the HER2-receptor protein, the protein is made visible with a chromogen resulting in membrane staining. The degree of membrane staining is usually scored according to the DAKO (Glostrup, Denmark) guidelines as 0 (negative), 1+ (incomplete membrane staining that is faint/barely perceptible within >10% of tumor cells), 2+ (circumferential membrane staining that is incomplete and/or weak/moderate within >10% of tumor cells, or a complete and circumferential membrane staining that is intense and within ≤10% of tumor cells) or 3+

(circumferential membrane staining that is complete, intense, and within >10% of tumor cells) [24]. An IHC 3+ score indicates eligibility for trastuzumab treatment. A patient with a tumor that has an IHC 0 or 1+ score is, however, not eligible. The IHC 2+ equivocal group, comprising 10% to 15% of all breast cancers, is more difficult to interpret since several studies have proven that a significant proportion of the IHC 2+ cancers (approximately 21% [25]) harbor a HER2 amplification. The evaluation of these "non-informative" HER2 IHC 2+ tests therefore requires further molecular analysis. In addition, IHC scoring can be influenced by fixation conditions and false-positive results have been reported, especially in biopsies. In addition, cytological material is not suitable for assessment of HER2 expression [26]. IHC is thus simple, fast, easy to implement and a relatively cheap detection method, but concerns over equivocal and false-positive IHC staining have been raised and described in the ASCO/CAP guidelines. The limitations of IHC testing have required development of *in situ* and PCR-based technologies to more accurately delineate HER2 status.

## *In situ* hybridization techniques for delineation of HER2 status

Nowadays, there are three FDA-approved *in situ* hybridization tests available to assess HER2 gene amplification: fluorescence *in situ* hybridization (FISH), chromogenic *in situ* hybridization (CISH) and silver *in situ* hybridization (SISH). They allow semi-quantitative assessment of gains, amplifications and losses directly on tissue sections and thereby integrate molecular analysis and tumor morphology.

Dual-color FISH (Vysis Pathvysion, DAKO PharmDx) was FDA-approved in 1998. FISH uses fluorescently labeled probes that are complementary to (a part of) the HER2 gene. After hybridization, these probes can be visualized with a fluorescence microscope and the number of copies of the HER2 gene can be estimated. According to current guidelines, a HER2 gene copy-number ratio ≥ 2.0 (a centromere 17 probe (CEP17) is used as a control for polysomy) is considered as HER2 amplification, given that a minimum of 20 tumor cell nuclei are counted. In addition, a dual-probe HER2/CEP17 ratio <2 with an average HER2 copy-number ≥ 6.0 signals/cell is considered ISH positive [24]. Equivocal FISH samples are confirmed or resolved by counting additional cells or repeating the FISH or IHC test. Comparative studies have shown a good correlation between FISH and IHC [27, 28] and conflicting results are predominantly seen in the IHC 2+ group.

FISH, however, is not without limitations as it requires a dedicated fluorescence imaging system and trained personnel. In addition, the scoring process is time-consuming and is often hampered by the presence of autofluorescence and overlapping nuclei. Although image analysis software applications may aid in this process, fluorescence fades over time and slides and kits therefore have a limited half-life and are expensive. Finally, there is limited morphological assessment of overall histology due to the required prior protein digestion and the fluorescence mode, and heterogeneity can easily be missed because the scoring is done using the 100× oil immersion lens. FISH is therefore not a very practical primary screening tool and is usually only performed for clinical decision making in the IHC 2+ group.

Some of the inherent disadvantages of FISH have been addressed through the development of alternative in situ hybridization methodologies that rely on detection strategies that apply bright-field rather than fluorescence microscopy. CISH (Invitrogen, SPOT-Light®) was introduced as an alternative for FISH by Tanner et al. [29] and received its FDA approval in 2008. CISH uses an immunoperoxidase reaction to visualize the HER2 probe that allows scoring with a conventional light microscope. Furthermore, slides can be kept permanently and morphology is better preserved, thereby facilitating the detection of heterogeneity. CISH assays are commercially available as either mono-probe (HER2 only) or dual-probe (HER2 and CEP17 polysomy correction) methodologies. In 2011, a new dual-probe CISH assay, the HER2 CISH pharmDx™ kit (DAKO), was FDA-approved. Several studies showed a good correlation between CISH, FISH and IHC [29–32]. There are a few publications on the combination of bright-field ISH and IHC detection methods [33, 34], which allows simultaneous evaluation of HER2 gene copy-number and protein expression, but such assays are still experimental and have not yet been adopted in clinical practice.

In June 2011, Ventana Medical Systems (Tucson, AZ, USA) received FDA approval for their fully automated INFORM™ HER2 silver in situ hybridization (SISH) technology that allows a diagnosis within 12 hours and uses metallography to produce a black HER2 signal and a red CEP17 signal. SISH scoring is identical to CISH scoring and HER2/CEP17 SISH shows a good correlation with CISH [35] and FISH [36]. Penault-Llorca et al. reported a high concordance between CISH, IHC and FISH and showed that SISH was as reliable as CISH and FISH for the assessment of HER2 status [37]. Furthermore, despite the fact that there is a good inter-observer concordance, a new software application was developed, the Ventana Image Analysis System (VIAS). This system makes a digital image of the microscopic field and counts the HER2 and CEP17 copies in sequential slides. When the minimal number of tumor cells is reached, the VIAS system calculates the HER2/CEP17 ratio.

Using in situ hybridization techniques, high-level HER2 amplifications are easily recognizable, but low-level amplification, a less frequent event, has been proposed to be at least partly due to polysomy of chromosome 17, thereby not reflecting true amplification, and these tumors have been reported to be clinically and morphologically more similar to HER2-negative than to HER2-positive tumors [38]. However, different studies demonstrated that polysomy of chromosome 17 is at best very rare in breast cancer [39, 40], which has caused doubt with regard to the validity of CEP17 correction [41]. Furthermore, FISH-negative patients with polysomy (HER2 amplification but HER2/CEP17 ratio <2) can show a response to trastuzumab monotherapy [42]. This indicates that it may not be justified to deny trastuzumab to patients with an absolute copy-number increase of HER2 in situ signals and a simultaneous CEP17 increase that has led to a normal HER2/CEP17 ratio, and that mono-probe HER2 in situ kits may liberally be used.

## MLPA for assessment of HER2 status

Because more quantitative results are easier to interpret than ISH for the detection of HER2 amplification, PCR-based techniques such as multiplex ligation-dependent probe amplification (MLPA) were introduced. MLPA needs only minute quantities of DNA and works well on DNA isolated from formalin-fixed paraffin-embedded material (50 to 200 ng) [43]. The technique is based on amplification of pairs of hemiprobes that contain specific target sequences (against specific genes) and universal PCR primer sequences. After hybridization to the target sequences, the hemiprobes are ligated and can be PCR amplified. A variable stuffer sequence on one of the hemiprobes determines the length of the PCR product of each probe. Thereby, up to 45 pairs of hemiprobes (directed against different genes or different parts of genes) can be amplified in the same PCR reaction. The PCR products can then be separated according to length using capillary electrophoresis. The probe peak height correlates with the amount of target DNA present, and is normalized against normal reference samples and stable reference probes. Copy-number ratios can be subsequently calculated using a dedicated free software program (MLPAnalyzer). The HER2 MLPA assay (P004-C1, MRC-Holland) contains a probe mix with four sets of hemiprobes that recognize different exons of the HER2 gene, several chromosome 17 probes (such as TOP2A and PPM1D), ESR1, EGFR and a number of control probes located on different chromosomes. This high-throughput PCR-based technique offers an easy-to-perform and easy-to-interpret alternative or supplement to IHC and ISH.

For HER2 assessment, different studies have shown a good correlation between MLPA, IHC, FISH and CISH [44, 45], but MLPA has yet to be clinically validated. The downside of PCR techniques such as MLPA is that tissue morphology is lost, heterogeneity can be missed, and contamination with ductal carcinoma *in situ* (DCIS, often HER2 amplified while the concomitant invasive cancer does not show this amplification) can lead to false-positive results. Furthermore, the tumor percentage should be sufficiently high (>30% [46]). Therefore, a good selection of tumor material in sequential hematoxylin and eosin stain (H&E) slides is essential and (laser) microdissection may be necessary in case of a low tumor percentage or a relevant DCIS component.

## HERmark assay for delineation of HER2 status

The HERmark assay (Monogram Biosciences) is based on Veratag™ technology and is only available in the United States at this time. HERmark uses two monoclonal antibodies directed against unique epitopes on the HER2 receptor. A fluorescent VeraTag™ (V) reporter is conjugated to a first monoclonal antibody (Ab1) specific for HER2. The second HER2-specific monoclonal antibody (Ab2) is conjugated to biotin, which is attached to a photosensitive molecule (FM). Foto-activation of a sample at a specific

wavelength activates the FM, leading to the release of free oxygen radicals that are able to cleave the nearby VeraTag™ reporter. The released reporter is then collected and subsequently quantified using capillary electrophoresis. The amount of cleaved reporter is proportional to the concentration of HER2 in the sample [47]. HERmark accurately quantifies the amount of total HER2 protein and the HER2 homodimer amounts in paraffin-embedded material. The threshold for a positive HERmark test is based on the comparison with HER2 tests performed in 1,090 breast tumor reference samples of the Hershey Medical Center/Medical University of Vienna cohort, the Mayo Clinic cohort and the FinHer Adjuvant Breast Cancer study. The precision, accuracy, reproducibility, linearity, specificity and sensitivity have been validated on a broad dynamic range of HER2 expression. Details of presentations and running clinical trials can be found at http://hermarkassay.com. Monogram Biosciences claims that their test is more accurate than IHC and FISH technology in selecting breast cancer patients who will benefit from trastuzumab. The HERmark assay can detect HER2 at amounts of 2.500 up to more than 1 million receptors per cell, and is thus said to be seven to ten times more sensitive than IHC. The question of course is whether this higher sensitivity is actually clinically useful, since at this time only "over-expression" and not the extent of over-expression matters clinically.

## Is there a best test for HER2?

Except for the necessity for a second-line gene amplification test for all IHC 2+ tumors, there is yet no consensus on which of the above-mentioned techniques is the better one. A clinical diagnostic test for HER2 should accurately determine HER2 status and should be reproducible and precise across multiple sites and users. Most importantly, information about the relative response rates to HER2 targeting agents of patients selected using this assay should be available. For the time being, the choice for a testing strategy will likely be based on local preferences after considering respective practical (availability and ease of application) and economic issues. Therefore, much focus is being directed towards standardization of clinically validated methods such as IHC and ISH, but others believe that the answer clearly lies in applying newer technologies. The latter will probably raise the discussion about whether or not to routinely use these methods alongside IHC or as first-line tests. Although this would seemingly increase the costs initially, it could, however, yield a substantial benefit in time as some of the patients would be spared an expensive therapy associated with significant side effects. It can therefore not be excluded that, after a thorough cost-effectiveness analysis, high-throughput amplification tests may be able to cost-effectively complement or even substitute IHC and ISH.

## Metastatic patients: testing of primary tumors or metastases?

Treatment of breast cancer metastases was traditionally based on the HER2 status of the primary tumor since metastases are rarely biopsied due to the often limited accessibility, but also because it is not considered necessary for further therapeutic decision making. However, different studies have shown that HER2 status can differ between primary tumor and metastasis, a process named "receptor conversion" [48, 49]. HER2 receptor conversion has important clinical consequences, since a number of patients may be withheld adequate systemic treatment for their metastases when the indication is based on the primary tumor status. The percentage of patients converting varies between studies from 0% to 58.3%, where conversion from negative in the primary tumor to positive in the metastases and vice versa are seen about equally often [50–53]. This probably indicates that metastases should be biopsied as often as possible to reassess HER2 status (as well as ERα/PR status), maybe even more than just one metastasis, since heterogeneity between metastases occurs as well [54]. Fine-needle aspiration cytology (FNAC) has the potential to become an excellent method to sample different metastasis with minimal discomfort for the patients. There are some concerns about the use of FNAC to study markers such as ER, PR and HER2. Different types of fixatives and cytological specimens can reduce the biomarker detection sensitivity. However, for many years, we and others have been demonstrating that the rate of detection of biomarkers on cytological specimens correlates with the respective histological resection [55, 56]. For HER2 assessment, only in situ hybridization (ISH) is valid for cytological material. Although FISH and SISH can be used in smears and liquid-based cytology, we prefer the use of cell blocks.

## HER2 mutation testing

In breast cancer, the potential therapeutic opportunities offered by rare (1% to 3%) HER2 somatic mutations was long neglected, given the high prevalence of HER2 gene amplification [57]. The development of massive parallel sequencing has shed new light on these activating mutations, mostly present in the tyrosine kinase domain (68%, exons 19 to 20) and the extracellular domain (20%, exon 8) [58]. Tumors considered to be HER2-negative based on current guidelines may still be "addicted" to HER2 signaling due to HER2 activating mutations and hence may also benefit from HER2 targeting agents. Bose *et al.* (2013) have functionally characterized 13 HER2 mutations using *in vitro* kinase assays, protein structure analysis, cell culture and xenograft experiments. Seven of these mutations were activating mutations and all of these mutations were sensitive to the irreversible HER2/EGFR tyrosine kinase inhibitor neratinib, thus validating HER2 somatic mutations as drug targets for breast cancer treatment [58]. This finding may very well lead to a new era for breast cancer management, where HER2 status is no longer solely determined by immunohistochemistry and ISH techniques. However, clinical trials are first needed to test whether HER2-mutated tumors are responsive to HER2-targeted drugs and, if so, which mutations are predictive of sensitivity to which agent.

## Predicting resistance to HER2 targeted therapy

All of the technologies described above focus on the detection of HER2 over-expression/amplification or mutation in order to predict trastuzumab response, but many tumors are primary resistant to this therapy or develop resistance during treatment. Therefore, a whole new set of testing methods for some of these resistance mechanisms is currently under development to provide a more accurate prediction to anti-HER2 therapy. Several mechanisms of resistance to anti-HER2 therapy have been described, including impaired antibody dependent cellular cytotoxicity via CD44 over-expression, aberrant downstream signaling via PTEN down-regulation, activating PIK3CA mutations (see next paragraph) and p27 down-regulation, alternative receptor tyrosine kinase signaling via over-expression of IGF1R, impaired access to the HER2 receptor via MUC4 over-expression, and expression of truncated isoforms of HER2 lacking the extracellular domain (p95-HER2) [23]. Interestingly, it seems that some of the mechanisms leading to trastuzumab resistance do not necessarily lead to lapatinib resistance. For example, testing for the presence of p95-HER2 might predict worse response to trastuzumab but seemingly not to lapatinib, which could stimulate the development of p95-HER2 testing.

## Prognostic and predictive assays

In addition to established markers such as HER2 and ER, there are some emerging single IHC markers (Ki-67, cyclin D1 and E, ERβ, topoisomerase IIα, urokinase-type plasminogen activator (uPA) and inhibitor (PAI-1), p53, HER2 extracellular domain (ECD), circulating and disseminated tumor cells) and combinatorial indices to classify breast cancer based on prognosis and/or therapeutic response. The latter include Oncotype DX®, Mammaprint®, PAM50®, Genomic Grade Index (GGI) and IHC4 [59]. Although the gene sets comprising these combinatorial indices have limited overlap, key functional groups are consistently represented, including estrogen response and proliferation.

## Oncotype DX

The Oncotype DX recurrence score (RS) (Genomic Health Institute) is applicable to formalin-fixed samples and involves reverse transcription-PCR of 21 genes, including ER, PR, HER2 and Ki67. A complex algorithm generates RS values (0 to 100) with independent prognostic utility for recurrence (low, intermediate or high ten-year distant relapse risk) and overall survival in tamoxifen-treated, node-negative, ER-positive patients [4, 60]. The RS permits a subgroup to be defined with sufficiently low residual risk to safely omit chemotherapy [60, 61]. In addition, high-risk patients appear to benefit proportionately more from adjuvant chemotherapy [61, 62]. The optimal management (hormonal therapy alone or in combination with chemotherapy) of node-negative steroid receptor positive patients with a RS between 11 and 25 is currently being evaluated in the trial assigning individualized options for treatment (TAILORx) [60]. Despite the obvious benefit of avoiding unnecessary chemotherapy, and inclusion in the ASCO, National Cancer Center Network (NCCN) and St Gallen clinical practice guidelines, its application into routine

practice has yet to be recommended at the national level in many countries. The high costs of this test obviously play a role here, as well as the fact that the cost-effectiveness of Oncotype DX-directed chemotherapy has been doubted [63].

## MammaPrint

The 70-gene MammaPrint signature (Agendia BV) comprises 70 genes identified by supervised analyses of gene-expression data from 78 node-negative primary breast cancers. Thirty-four of these patients relapsed within five years, while forty-four remained disease-free in the absence of adjuvant chemotherapy [3]. Patients were under 55 years of age and had ER-positive as well as ER-negative tumors. The ability to distinguish good from poor prognosis, in terms of risk of distant recurrence, has been extensively validated in multiple studies [64, 65]. MammaPrint was the first *in vitro* diagnostic multivariate index assay to be cleared by the FDA as a prognostic factor.

High-risk or poor-prognosis patients benefit significantly from the addition of chemotherapy to endocrine treatment, in contrast to their low-risk or good-prognosis counterparts [66]. Whether chemotherapy can indeed safely be omitted in case of a low-risk MammaPrint even in the presence of poor clinicopathological factors is the subject of the microarray in node-negative disease may avoid chemotherapy (MINDACT) trial [67]. The results of this randomized, multicenter trial are still awaited. Results from the prospective, observational RASTER study are, however, promising [68]. At first, the test could only be performed on fresh frozen tissue. Recently, however, the test was methodologically validated for formalin-fixed material [69]. Experience with the paraffin test is limited, and important methodological issues like the sensitivity for intra-tumor heterogeneity and fixation delay have not yet been addressed. Results of a recent study show that MammaPrint is cost-effective [70].

## PAM50

The PAM50 signature was developed as a single-sample predictor of intrinsic subtype, and employs 50 genes that incorporate the gene expression-based intrinsic subtypes [71]. The subtype-predictor can be applied on formalin-fixed paraffin-embedded material and generates a risk of recurrence score (ROR), when weighted for proliferation associated genes and tumor size [71, 72]. Although derived from systemically untreated node-negative patients, the score has been proven useful to recognize a very low-risk prognostic group among women receiving tamoxifen and no chemotherapy, similar to the Oncotype DX assay [72]. A predictive effect has also been demonstrated for the response of node-negative patients to neoadjuvant chemotherapy [71, 73].

## GGI

The genomic grade index (GGI) consists of 97 genes, including many associated with cell cycle control and proliferation. The GGI allows stratification of grade II tumors into those with a grade I-like or grade III-like risk of distant relapse [74]. Prognostic utility and concordance with Oncotype DX and MammaPrint has been demonstrated in both untreated and endocrine-treated ER-positive patients [75, 76].

## IHC4

Four markers, ERα, PR, HER2 and Ki67, evaluated by IHC, were each found to have independent prognostic utility and their integration, expressed as the IHC4 score, provided at least as much prognostic information, in terms of distant recurrence, as the Oncotype DX recurrence score in a study of ER-positive patients from the ATAC trial who did not receive adjuvant chemotherapy [77]. In addition, relatively similar prognostic information was added by the PAM50 ROR score and the IHC4 score in all patients, but more by ROR in the HER2-negative/node-negative group [78]. This raises the possibility that IHC4 may have utility for informing adjuvant chemotherapy decisions in endocrine-treated, node-negative women based on their residual risk. Furthermore, this may offer a viable alternative to the more expensive Oncotype DX and MammaPrint tests, given that the three receptor components are routinely evaluated and many centers assess Ki67 in other contexts. Quantitative evaluation of ER, PR and HER2 status is rigorously standardized and recommendations from the International Ki67 in breast cancer working group have recently been published [79]. This approach could provide an opportunity to significantly improve the routine availability of prognostic information in a cost-effective manner.

The above-mentioned combinatorial tests seem to be generally reproducible as well as precise, and may improve the prognostic and predictive information derived from histopathology and IHC assessment. These multigene assays cannot, however, replace routine pathological work-up, often lack direct morphological correlation, have hardly been studied for sensitivity to intra-tumor heterogeneity, remain prohibitively expensive and are therefore only endorsed in specific cases. Their proper place in breast cancer management remains to be determined by clinical trials and costs-effectiveness studies.

## The integrative molecular approach

Besides the development of prognostic and predictive classifiers, recent integrative molecular approaches have led to the discovery of new driver mutations as well as key epigenetic processes involved in breast carcinogenesis. Most of the elaborate molecular studies of breast cancer have focused on just one or two profiling platforms, most frequently mRNA expression profiling or DNA copy-number analysis, and more recently next generation sequencing. mRNA expression profiling has reproducibly established that breast cancers encompass several distinct disease entities, often referred to as the intrinsic subtypes of breast cancer. The recent development of additional high information content assays, focused on epigenetic abnormalities such as DNA methylation and microRNA (miRNA) expression, as well as on protein expression, provides further opportunities to characterize more thoroughly the molecular portrait of breast cancer.

In 2012, The Cancer Genome Atlas Network published their work on the analysis of a diverse set of primary breast cancers assayed by six different technology platforms: genomic DNA copy-number arrays, DNA methylation, exome sequencing, messenger RNA arrays, microRNA sequencing and reverse-phase protein arrays. This has by far provided the most complete molecular portrait of breast cancer diversity ever [5].

This study provided a near complete framework for the genetic driver events of breast cancer, which will significantly impact clinical medicine in the coming years as these genetic markers are evaluated as possible markers of prognosis or therapeutic responsiveness. The ability to integrate information across platforms provided key insights into previously defined gene expression (intrinsic) subtypes and confirmed the existence of four main breast cancer classes when combining data from five platforms, each of which showed significant molecular heterogeneity. Somatic mutations in only three genes (TP53, PIK3CA and GATA3) occurred at >10% incidence across all breast cancers. In addition, there were numerous subtype-specific and novel gene mutations, including the enrichment of specific mutations in GATA3, PIK3CA and MAP3K1 with the ER positive/luminal A subtype. Two novel protein-expression-defined subgroups were identified, possibly produced by stromal/microenvironmental factors. And a stunning similarity was discovered between basal-like breast cancers and high-grade serous ovarian tumors, indicating a related aetiology and similar therapeutic opportunities.

Despite these interesting findings, this enormous amount of new data on the breast cancer genomic landscape proved yet again that breast cancer is a heterogeneous disease that, clinically, can still roughly be classified into ER-positive (luminal A/B, better prognosis) and ER-negative disease (triple negative/basal-like and HER2 driven, worse prognosis), phenotypes that can be easily be established by immunohistochemistry. Only time will tell which of the above findings will be translated to the clinic.

# New developments
## PIK3CA mutation testing

PIK3CA is an oncogene exhibiting gain-of-function mutations in several cancers, including breast, colorectal and endometrial cancer. PIK3CA mutations occur at high frequency in 20% to 40% (25% by COSMIC; July 2013) of breast cancers and cluster in two major hotspots located in its helical (E542K and E545K in exon 9) and catalytic (H1047R in exon 20) domains. These mutations have been shown to be oncogenic in mammary epithelial cells by driving constitutive, growth factor-independent PI3K pathway activation. In addition, retrospective as well as prospective studies have suggested that phosphatidylinositol 3-kinase (PI3K) pathway activation can negatively influence response to trastuzumab therapy [80–82] and endocrine therapy [83, 84].

Given their frequency, oncogenic capabilities and the potential to induce resistance to commonly prescribed breast cancer treatments, the clinical relevance of PIK3CA mutations needs to be further clarified. In light of the emergence of a broadening array of anti-HER2 agents, determination of *PIK3CA* mutational

status could have important clinical utility. In addition, inhibitors of the PI3K pathway that may reverse acquired and *de novo* drug resistance are currently in clinical development.

# Mutations in other genes

Most breast cancer cases are sporadic, with many different oncogenes and tumor suppressor genes involved, while 5% to 10% is estimated to be due to an inherited predisposition. Germline mutations in two genes, BRCA1 and BRCA2, are likely to account for most familial cases of early-onset breast cancer, and for 3% to 4% of all breast cancers. Mutations in several other genes, including TP53, PTEN, STK11/LKB1, CDH1, CHEK2, ATM, MLH1 and MSH2, have also been associated with hereditary breast tumors [85]. Hereditary breast cancer will be discussed in more detail in the section entitled "Hereditary versus sporadic breast cancer," which appears later in this chapter.

## BRCA1

BRCA1, located on chromosome 17q21, has several cellular roles. It has been implicated in DNA repair, cell-cycle regulation, transcriptional regulation and chromatin remodeling.

Somatic mutations of the BRCA1 coding sequence are very rare in breast cancers. In contrast, more than 300 sequence variations have been reported at the germline level (a list is available on the BIC website: http://research.nhgri.nih.gov/bic/). BRCA1 germline mutations are dispersed throughout its coding sequence. Although a majority of these variations are unique, recurrent mutations such as 185delAG and 5382insC were initially described in the Ashkenazy Jewish population. More than 80% of the sequence variants lead to a truncated protein. In contrast, the majority of BRCA1 missense mutations are of unknown clinical significance, except those in the RING finger region. Women carrying a germline BRCA1 mutation have a 57% to 65% chance of developing breast cancer and a 39% to 59% ovarian cancer risk before the age of 70 years [86, 87].

A comprehensive BRCA1/2 mutation analysis in 193 breast cancer patients without a family history for the disease identified a deleterious germline BRCA1/2 mutation in 8.8%, and therefore suggested that the prevalence of BRCA1/2 mutations may be underestimated, especially in sporadic patients who developed breast and ovarian cancer [88].

BRCA1-associated breast cancers have specific morphological features: they are highly proliferative, poorly differentiated tumors characterized by high frequencies of p53 alterations and receptor negativity (triple-negative/basal-like subtype) [89].

### BRCA2

BRCA2, located on chromosome 13q12, is another well-known breast cancer susceptibility gene that plays a role in DNA recombination and repair processes. More than 100 unique germline mutations have been reported to be dispersed throughout the coding sequence (a list is available at the BIC website). Recurrent mutations are seen: 6174delT (of Ashkenazy Jewish origin), 999del5 (Icelandic) and 6503delTT (in France and in the United Kingdom). The majority of BRCA2 mutations lead to a truncated protein. The cumulative risks for BRCA2 mutation carriers are 45% to 55% for breast cancer and 11% to 18% for ovarian cancer [86, 87, 90].

BRCA2-mutated breast cancers seem to be different from both BRCA1-associated breast cancers and sporadic cases, with a poor differentiation, but low proliferation rate. Their frequency of ER and PR positivity and p53 mutation rate is not significantly different from sporadic breast cancers [89].

### E-cadherin

Cadherins are transmembrane receptors that function through calcium-dependent interactions that provide cell-cell contact and communication. Inherited mutations in the CDH1 (E-Cadherin) gene, located on chromosome arm 16q, increase a woman's lifetime risk of developing lobular breast cancer (39% to 52%). In many cases, this increased risk occurs as part of hereditary diffuse gastric cancer (HDGC), a condition characterized by a very high risk of developing cancer of the stomach lining as well as an increased risk of lobular breast cancer [91].

The incidence of somatic CDH1 mutations in invasive lobular carcinoma varies significantly in public databases and literature from 31% (COSMIC; July 2013; http://cancer.sanger.ac.uk/cancergenome/projects/cosmic/) to 62% [92]. Most investigators consider a mutation in CDH1 to represent a genomic alteration characteristic of the lobular subtype of breast cancer. Other mechanisms that lead to loss of E-cadherin function include methylation of CDH1

[93]. The resulting loss of E-cadherin may not only allow cells to grow and divide unchecked, but may also facilitate cells to detach from the primary tumor and metastasize.

### TP53

The tumor suppressor gene TP53, located on chromosome 17p13, encodes a ubiquitous nuclear protein involved in the control of genome integrity by preventing cells from dividing before DNA damage is repaired. 20% to 25% (23% by COSMIC) of breast cancers show TP53 mutations and these correspond to aggressive (ER-negative) breast tumors. As much as 90% of TP53 mutations are found within exons 5 through 9. The majority of *TP53* mutations (80%) in breast cancer are missense, while nonsense mutations, deletions, insertions or splice site mutations make the rest (20%). Prolonged half-life of the protein leads to accumulation that can also be detected by IHC and shows correlation with missense mutations. At the same time, p53 staining may be completely negative when the mutant protein is too short to be detected by IHC.

### PTEN

The protein encoded by this gene is a phosphatidylinositol-3,4,5-trisphosphate 3-phosphatase that antagonizes the PI3K-AKT signaling pathway and thereby modulates cell cycle progression and cell survival. About 25% to 50% of women with Cowden disease, a syndrome associated with germline mutations of the PTEN gene (at 10q23), develop breast cancer, but PTEN mutations have been found in only 5% of sporadic breast cancers. However, 29% to 48% of breast cancers display loss of heterozygosity at 10q23, about 40% of breast cancers show a decrease or absence of PTEN protein levels at the time of diagnosis and PTEN promoter hypermethylation was reported to be a common event in sporadic breast cancer, occurring in 20% to 50% of breast cancers [94]. PTEN not only antagonizes tumorigenesis, but also sensitizes breast cancers to targeted therapy with trastuzumab. Its loss has therefore been associated with trastuzumab resistance [95].

### GATA3

Somatic mutations in the dual zinc-finger transcription factor, GATA3, have been reported in approximately 7% of breast tumors (COSMIC). These mutations are particularly associated with luminal breast cancers: approximately 20% of ER-positive breast cancers have somatic GATA3 mutations (mostly frameshift) that lead to a loss of GATA3 transactivation activity and altered cell invasiveness [96]. Many of these mutations occur in tumors that retain GATA3 immunostaining, indicating that absence of GATA3 immunostaining is an unreliable predictor of the presence of GATA3 mutations [96].

A series of recent next generation sequencing studies have further underlined the genetic diversity of breast cancer. Beyond confirming recurrent somatic mutations in PIK3CA, TP53, PTEN, CDH1, AKT1, GATA3, MLL3, CDKN1B and MAP3K1, potential driver mutations were identified in several new cancer genes, including AKT2, ARID1B, CASP8, MAP3K13, NCOR1, SMARCD1, TBX3, MTAP, PPP2R2A, CBFB, TBX3, RUNX1, CBFB, AFF2, PIK3R1, PTPN22, PTPRD, NF1, SF3B1, CCND3 and MAP2K3 [5, 94]. Their clinical significance needs to be further clarified.

## ESR1 testing
### ESR1 amplification testing
There is an ongoing debate concerning the prevalence and the clinical relevance of ESR1 amplification in breast cancer after an initial report showing that ESR1 amplified cases had an excellent response to tamoxifen treatment [97]. Three further studies from three other groups confirmed the presence of ESR1 gain and amplification in some 20% of cases [98–100]. Other studies, however, reported significantly lower rates [101, 102], probably related to different cut-offs, different technologies, contamination with non-tumor cells, intratumoral heterogeneity of copy-number status [103, 104] and pre-mRNA contamination [105]. Although the technological problems have probably been solved now, ESR1 amplification testing that can be done by FISH or MLPA has not found its way to clinical applications yet.

### ESR1 mutation testing
Two independent teams have now discovered that mutations in ESR1 could be an important route to endocrine resistance [106, 107]. Both groups analyzed tumor samples from patients with metastatic breast cancer who had relapsed after months of hormonal therapy, and found that these tumors frequently had mutations in ESR1, all of which affected the part of ER that recognizes estrogen, the ligand-binding

domain. Patients generally do not have ESR1 mutations when their tumors are confined to their breasts, and these mutations are generally rare among primary tumors. ESR1 mutation analysis in metastatic breast tumors will probably become mainstream and will be used to make decisions about hormonal treatments, as more potent ER antagonists may be of substantial therapeutic benefit.

## Translocations
Chromosomal translocations that form fusion products and/or activate gene expression by promoter insertion are key events in hematological malignancies and soft tissue tumors, but have been reported to be less common in epithelial cancers such as breast cancer. However, this view is currently being challenged by array painting and next generation sequencing studies. Reciprocal and more complex balanced translocations seem to be far more frequent than expected. The NRG1 gene on chromosome 8p12, for example, seems to be translocated in 6% of breast cancers [108, 109] and, furthermore, several translocation breakpoints are located within known cancer-critical genes such as EP300/p300 and CTCF [110, 111].

### Secretory carcinoma
Secretory carcinoma is a rare but distinct subtype of breast carcinoma that has been shown to harbor a recurrent balanced chromosomal translocation t(12;15) (p13;q25), which leads to the formation of an ETV6-NTRK3 fusion gene encoding a chimeric tyrosine kinase. Identification of these tumors is of clinical significance because secretory carcinomas occur mainly at a young age and have a favorable prognosis [112]. ETV6 split signal FISH DNA probes are commercially available.

### Adenoid cystic carcinoma
Adenoid cystic carcinomas of the breast account for 0.1% to 1% of all breast cancers and are, in contrast to adenoid cystic carcinomas of the salivary gland, associated with an excellent long-term prognosis, despite their triple negative or basal-like phenotype [113]. These carcinomas consistently display the recurrent chromosomal translocation t(6;9) (q22e23;p23e24), which generates fusion transcripts involving the two transcription factor genes MYB and NFIB. In the t(6;9)(q22eq23;p23ep24), the exon 14 of MYB is fused

to the last coding exons of NFIB, most often due to breakpoints in MYB intron 14 and in NFIB intron 8. The fusion results in loss of the 3'-end of MYB, including several conserved binding sites for micro-RNAs that regulate MYB expression negatively.

Due to the characteristic histological features of adenoid cystic carcinoma, the use of split-apart FISH probes for the identification of this characteristic translocation are unlikely to be frequently used in diagnostic practice. The fusion gene may, however, lead to new therapeutic avenues for the management of advanced adenoid cystic carcinoma.

## Methylation

Methylation of a cytosine base located upstream of a guanosine base can occur across the genome, but most notably within CpG dinucleotide rich regions, known as CpG islands. Under normal conditions, the vast majority of CpG sites in the genome are methylated, with the exception of CpG islands located in gene promoter regions. During carcinogenesis, these normal methylation patterns are frequently disordered. In general, a shift towards local promoter CpG island hypermethylation is seen within the context of an overall loss of methylation (hypomethylation). While global hypomethylation is thought to play a role in carcinogenesis primarily by increasing genetic instability, local hypermethylation alters gene expression as it is tightly linked to histone modifications and chromosome remodeling mechanisms that lead to gene silencing.

Aberrant promoter hypermethylation is a common and early event in carcinogenesis, thought to provide a selective growth advantage to neoplastic cells and contributing to the overall genetic instability of the tumor. It occurs at least as frequently as genetic mutations in somatic cells, so that hundreds of genes may be inactivated by DNA methylation in a single tumor. Breast tumors show frequent methylation of genes involved in cell cycle regulation (p16$^{INK4A}$, p14$^{ARF}$, CCDN2, RASSF1A), DNA repair (BRCA1, MGMT, MLH1), apoptosis (DAPK1, TWIST), transformation (GSTP1), signal transduction (RARβ2, APC, ERβ) and adhesion and metastasis (CDH1, CDH13). Promoter hypermethylation in breast cancer has been associated with patient prognosis, and with response to chemotherapeutic, targeted and demethylating drugs [114]. Hypermethylation of the homeodomain transcription factor PITX2, for

example, has proven to be a consistent prognostic biomarker in breast as well as prostate cancer. Node-negative, estrogen receptor positive breast cancer patients with a methylated PITX2 promoter have been associated with worse prognosis, and with increased risk of recurrence upon tamoxifen treatment. In addition, node-positive, estrogen receptor positive breast cancers methylated at the PITX2 promotor respond worse to adjuvant anthracycline-based chemotherapy. Demethylating drugs have not yet proceeded to the clinical trial setting for breast cancer despite promising results of an increasing number of *in vitro* studies. Demethylating drugs such as 5-aza-(deoxy)cytidine (Vidaza®) are cytosine analogs that have been approved by the FDA for treatment of myelodysplastic syndromes. Once incorporated into the DNA, these analogs can inhibit DNA methyltransferases, the enzymes responsible for DNA methylation. Both drugs showed promising results at low doses in clinical trials, either as single agents or in combination with other drugs, for the treatment of hematologic as well as solid malignancies.

The high frequency and early appearance of promoter hypermethylation in breast cancer, as well as the fact that changes in methylation patterns observed in tumors are also detectable in the circulation and nipple fluid of women with breast cancer, further underlines its potential as biomarker for early minimally invasive tumor detection.

A wide range of techniques is available to determine tumor and biofluid DNA methylation at different levels, spanning from genome-wide methylation analysis to methylation of single residues in specific genes. Different methodologies vary in their sensitivity and limitations. Some techniques such as quantitative multiplex methylation specific PCR (QM-MSP) are very sensitive, but allow a focused approach only, and often require bisulfite conversion prior to analysis, a critical step that not only leads to degradation of DNA, but can also lead to misinterpretation of results when not adequately controlled. Other techniques of lower resolution such as methylation specific multiplex ligation-dependent probe amplification (MS-MLPA) allow a multi-targeted approach and do not require bisulfite conversion since they are restriction enzyme based.

### Methylation as a biomarker in nipple fluid

The high prevalence of breast cancer motivates the development of better screening and diagnostic technologies. Mammography screening has moderate sensitivity and specificity, and low positive-predictive value in younger women. Although MRI is a very sensitive breast cancer detection tool that has become standard for women at very high risk, it lacks sufficient specificity and cost-effectiveness for use as a general screening method. To complement current screening methods for early breast cancer detection, there is a substantial need for novel non-invasive biomarkers. The greatest opportunity for these biomarker tools to improve breast cancer screening is within a subset of high-risk, younger women who would benefit from intensive surveillance or preventive interventions.

Biomarker discovery studies so far have mainly relied on tissue samples obtained from patients with relatively advanced disease. However, to be meaningful in a screening population, diagnostic biomarkers must preferably be discovered in non-invasive biological samples from early-stage, non-metastatic cancers since biomarker expression can change over the course of the disease and can be very different depending on the type of sample investigated (blood, nipple fluid, tissue). Most early biomarkers such as "methylation" are generally not breast specific, rather, aberrant methylation of the same genes exists in several types of cancer. One direct approach is therefore to evaluate those markers using sample sources from the breast itself: nipple fluid.

The nipple fluid aspiration procedure offers a minimally invasive method to obtain material from the ductal system, where most breast cancers arise. Nipple fluid contains cells, RNA, DNA and proteins directly derived from the breast ducts and is thereby a rich source of highly specific breast cancer biomarkers that can aid individualized risk assessment. Nipple fluid can be non-invasively obtained from both breasts by aspiration under vacuum and can be harvested from virtually all women under intranasal stimulation with oxytocin spray [115, 116]. The high success rate of the procedure (90%) is not restricted by age, reproductive factors or previous therapy, suggesting that a new tool for biomarker detection in nipple fluid of women at increased risk for breast cancer is at hand [117]. Using quantitative multiplex methylation-specific PCR (QMMSP), a method that encompasses a nested multiplex PCR method, methylation levels can be assessed in very small volumes of nipple fluid (generally 10–20 µl) [118, 119].

Fackler *et al.* showed that, compared to cytology, analyzing promoter methylation using QMMSP in ductal lavage cells doubled the detection rate of breast cancer [118]. Thus, epigenetic aberrations in nipple fluid may predict the presence of tumor, irrespective of the amount of ducts or area of the breast that it is derived from. The combined methylation status of a panel of 11 tumor suppressor genes (RARB, RASSF1, TWIST1, CCND2, ESR1, SCGB3A1, BRCA1, BRCA2, CDKN2A, APC, CDH1) in breast tumor tissue predicts sporadic as well as hereditary breast cancer with high accuracy (92% and 86%, respectively), and can be very useful for early detection of cancer in nipple fluid of high-risk women [120].

Besides methylation assessment, the analysis of microRNAs, genomics and proteomics in these aspirates might soon become feasible and provide new diagnostic opportunities.

## Methylation as blood-based breast cancer screening

Assessment of promoter hypermethylation in easily accessible bodily fluids such as serum or plasma is a rapidly growing research field in early breast cancer detection, based on the fact that tumors release significant amounts of circulating free DNA into the bloodstream through cellular necrosis, apoptosis or spontaneous detachment. The diagnostic potential of, for example, RASSF1A and APC promoter methylation in circulating DNA from breast cancer patients has been investigated by several studies. While RASSF1A methylation predicted the presence of breast cancer with a sensitivity ranging from 15% to 75%, APC showed sensitivities ranging from 2% to 47%. Next to RASSF1A and APC, other genes such as ITIH5 and DKK3 have also been shown to be differentially methylated in cell-free DNA of breast cancer patients and healthy individuals [121]. In most studies, a combination of a panel of methylated genes lead to the highest sensitivity.

Nevertheless, at present, none of these gene panels has reached clinical practice. Major limitations to further development for clinical use have been the relatively small sample sizes, and the lack of large (prospective) validation studies. Furthermore, investigation of the methylation patterns in circulating DNA from non-breast cancers or different benign breast diseases such as fibroadenomas to identify potential specificity issues is lacking in most of these studies.

In April 2013, the largest genome-wide prospective blood-based methylation study so far evaluated methylation in blood samples from 298 women at

27,578 CpG sites, and discovered 250 differentially methylated CpGs between women that had developed breast cancer zero to five years after enrolment and women who remained cancer-free [122]. The use of a 57-CpG panel led to a prediction accuracy of 65.8%, compared with 56.0% for the Gail model, the best breast cancer risk prediction method currently available for populations. The differences in methylation were evident even among women whose blood sample was collected more than one year before diagnosis. Particularly encouraging was the fact that these predictions could be validated in a small independent set of 81 women of different ethnicities. In addition to this study, a growing number of case-control studies have investigated known breast cancer susceptibility genes, showing differences in BRCA1 promoter methylation and intragenic ATM methylation [123, 124].

Serial monitoring of DNA-methylation markers in blood during neo-adjuvant chemotherapy is yet another potential application. Patients with large or non-operable breast tumors often receive neo-adjuvant chemotherapy to downsize their tumor and facilitate full tumor resection, enabling radical surgery and conservation of the breast in some cases. However, currently available methods for evaluation of response during therapy are limited and the actual treatment effect can only be assessed by pathological evaluation of the resection specimen. Timely assessment of treatment efficacy could allow individual tailoring of the treatment and save ineffective drugs and unnecessary toxicity. Two studies were able to show that circulating tumor-derived DNA methylation of RASSF1A and BRCA1 reflected changes in tumor burden in response to chemotherapy and allowed stratification of responders and non-responders [125, 126].

### BRCA1 promoter hypermethylation

The pathologist may play a role in detecting hereditary breast cancer. BRCA1-associated breast cancers are associated with particular morphological and immunohistochemical features such as early onset, poor histological differentiation, solid histology, pushing borders, prominent lymphocytic infiltrate and hormone receptor negativity (ER, PR and HER2 "triple negative" subtype). In addition, molecular pathology may aid in further characterizing these BRCA1-suspect breast tumors, as it was recently shown that BRCA1 promoter hypermethylation and

BRCA1 germline mutations are mutually exclusive events [127]. In a large cohort of 377 triple negative breast carcinomas, Lips et al. demonstrated that 27% to 37% showed BRCA1 promoter hypermethylation, a phenomenon that was never seen in BRCA1-mutated carcinomas. The analysis of BRCA1 promoter hypermethylation in morphologically BRCA1-suspect breast tumors may thus function as a pre-screening tool, stratifying patients for referral to the clinical geneticist for BRCA1 mutation analysis and those patients who need no BRCA1 sequencing because of the sporadic nature of their cancer.

Furthermore, methylation of the BRCA1 promoter region, regardless of any hereditary factor, has been associated with unfavorable prognosis in women with early-stage breast cancer and has been shown to sensitize breast cancer cell lines to treatment with poly(adenosine diphosphate)-ribose polymerase (PARP) inhibitors such as olaparib (AZD2281).

## MicroRNAs

MicroRNAs are a class of small (around 22 nucleotide), non-protein-encoding RNAs that post-transcriptionally regulate gene expression by targeting specific mRNAs and triggering either their translational repression or their degradation. MicroRNAs regulate more than 60% of all protein-encoding genes and have been implicated in control of a wide range of biological processes such as cell proliferation, differentiation and apoptosis. Dysregulation of microRNA function is a common feature of multiple cancers, including breast cancer. Many microRNAs map to genomic regions that are frequently deleted or amplified in human cancers. Despite the complexities of understanding how microRNAs influence tumorigenesis, aberrantly expressed microRNAs have considerable potential as biomarkers for the early detection, diagnosis, classification and treatment of breast cancer.

### MicroRNAs as minimally invasive biomarkers

Owing to their small sizes, microRNAs are highly resistant to degradation and can be easily extracted from nearly every cell and tissue type. MicroRNAs have been shown to be well preserved in archived formalin-fixed paraffin-embedded sections up to ten years old, allowing retrospective analysis of patient samples. Moreover, circulating microRNAs can easily be measured in plasma or serum. Circulating microRNAs have been found to be significantly elevated in the blood of cancer patients compared with healthy controls, and these levels are reflected in the primary tumors. Moreover, the removal of the primary tumor leads to the loss of elevated circulating microRNAs, suggesting that many of these elevated circulating microRNAs are "tumor-derived" and thus cancer-specific. Reports on the existence of stable circulating microRNAs (free or within microvesicles such as exosomes) associated with cancer have emerged only within the past five years.

To date, only a few studies have begun to profile and validate circulating microRNAs in whole blood, serum or plasma of breast cancer patients. A review of the five genome-wide circulating microRNA studies to date showed that only 6 of the 158 (4%) candidate microRNAs reported to be differentially expressed between breast cancer cases and healthy controls overlapped consistently between two of these studies (miR-497 up, miR-451 up, miR-25 up, miR-222 up, miR-31 down, miR-151–5p down) [128]. The lack of reproducibility of published studies on circulating microRNAs in breast cancer might have several reasons: (1) sample type (plasma vs. serum vs. whole blood); (2) differences in blood processing protocols (for example, blood cell contamination); (3) differences in study populations; and (4) differences in time-points of sample collection.

### Early detection and diagnosis

MicroRNA dysregulation has been shown to be an early event during breast cancer progression. Their potential use as screening biomarkers was mainly shown in other cancer types, such as lung cancer, where for example analysis of specific microRNAs in sputum or plasma was able to predict the presence of adenocarcinoma or squamous cell carcinoma and even discriminate between these two types. Furthermore, a large screening study could show that testing expression levels of ten serum microRNAs could identify non-small cell lung carcinoma (NSCLC) up to 33 months ahead of clinical diagnosis [129]. There have been no prospective circulating microRNA screening studies in breast cancer yet. First, sensitive as well as breast-cancer-specific microRNAs or microRNA panels need to be discovered and validated in large independent study populations. As mentioned before, the discovery of microRNAs in nipple fluid might lead to more specific biomarkers.

### Monitoring disease progression and predicting treatment response

As removal of the primary tumor leads to loss of elevated circulating microRNAs, they can be used to monitor disease progression and measure minimal residual disease. In addition, microRNAs may be used to predict treatment response. Several trials are now ongoing and recruiting breast cancer patients to evaluate circulating microRNAs as biomarkers of hormone sensitivity (NCT01612871) and bevacizumab sensitivity (NCT01598285, in the metastatic setting). Other trials aim to identify microRNA markers of prognosis, and predictors for response to neoadjuvant or adjuvant treatment (NCT01231386, inflammatory breast cancer) and to evaluate their use as circulating biomarkers for guiding and monitoring chemotherapy response (NCT01722851).

### MicroRNAs as therapeutic agents and targets

The growing list of reports indicating the significance of microRNAs in diagnosis and prognosis of breast cancer has led to the exploration of their potential relevance as therapeutics. Because microRNA expression is often altered in cancer cells, agents that modulate microRNA activity could potentially produce cancer-specific effects. One of the most appealing properties of microRNAs as therapeutic agents is their ability to target multiple mRNAs, making them extremely efficient in regulating distinct biological cell processes relevant to tumorigenesis and tumor progression. There are two main strategies to target microRNA expression in (breast) cancer: direct strategies involve the use of antisense oligonucleotides or virus-based constructs to either block or substitute the loss of expression of a particular microRNA, and indirect strategies involve the use of drugs to modulate microRNA expression by targeting their transcription and processing (extensively reviewed by Garzon et al. [130]). Despite the progress that has been made in this new era of microRNA therapeutics, there is still a gap between basic research and clinical application. Current challenges of microRNA-based therapies include tissue-specific delivery, potential off-target effects, biological instability and cellular uptake.

Besides tumor-specific and tissue-specific delivery of tumor-suppressive microRNAs and silencing oncogenic microRNAs with so-called "antagomirs," microRNAs are also being evaluated for their ability to sensitize tumors to chemotherapy and endocrine therapy. For example, tamoxifen-resistant breast tumors are known to repress microRNAs miR-15a and miR-16, thereby restoring anti-apoptotic BCL2 function. Re-expression of miR-15a/16 decreased BCL2 expression and cells became sensitized to tamoxifen [131], and miR-21 knock-down in breast cancer cell lines has been associated with increased sensitivity to topotecan and taxol *in vitro* and the limitation of lung metastasis *in vivo* [132]. These emerging data give hope that panels of microRNAs will be identified that can contribute to predicting and influencing treatment response in breast cancer.

In conclusion, given their extensive biomarker potential (diagnostic, prognostic, as well as predictive), the measurement of microRNAs in tumor biopsies, excisions, blood and perhaps nipple fluid might become standard practice in each (molecular) pathology lab.

## Hereditary versus sporadic breast cancer

In about 5% to 10% of all the breast cancer cases, the disease will occur as part of a hereditary cancer susceptibility syndrome, caused by mutations in high penetrance susceptibility genes. About 16% of these can be attributed to germline mutations in either of the BRCA (breast cancer 1 and 2) genes. Various other genes conferring an increased hereditary risk of breast cancer include CHEK2, PTEN (Cowden syndrome), TP53 (Li-Fraumeni syndrome), ATM, STK11/LKB1 (Peutz-Jeghers syndrome), CDH1, NBS1, RAD50, BRIP1 and PALB2. Since BRCA1 and BRCA2 cancers are most prevalent, breast cancers within the framework of these syndromes have now been fairly well characterized, but knowledge on cancers related to the other genes is scarce.

Female BRCA1 mutation related breast cancers are more frequently ductal, medullary or metaplastic, poorly differentiated (grade 3), have a high mitotic count and show a high frequency of necrotic areas. Tubule formation is decreased, and a higher degree of nuclear pleomorphism is observed, all aspects pointing to a more aggressive phenotype [133–136]. In addition, tumors are often well demarcated and show a remarkable degree of lymphoplasmocytic infiltration, and a high frequency of lymphovascular invasion [137]. Their immunophenotype is characterized by low expression of HER2 and luminal proteins like ERα and PR, cell cycle regulators like cyclin D1, and p27$^{kip1}$, and low expression of the apoptosis-

related proteins BAX and BCL2. In contrast, over-expression of p53, estrogen receptor beta (ERβ), cyclin E, as well as high expression of basal proteins such as EGFR, CK5/CK6, CK14, caveolin 1, vimentin, laminin and p-cadherin, high levels of active caspase 3, HIF-1α and the stem cell marker ALDH1 is observed [137]. By gene expression analysis, female BRCA1-associated breast cancers were classified as basal, thereby confirming the basal subtype by immunohistochemistry as described above [137]. Promotor hypermethylation of tumor suppressor genes is somewhat less abundant than in sporadic cancers [120] and copy-number analysis by CGH showed frequently occurring gains of 3q, 7p, 8q 10p, 12p, 16p and 17q and loss of 2q, 3p, 4p, 4q, 5q, 12q, 16q and 18q [137]. The morphology and immunophenotype of DCIS in BRCA1 mutation carriers is similar to that of their accompanying invasive cancers [138]. The non-malignant breast shows many pre-malignant changes and T-cell lobulitis [137]. Although male BRCA1 germline mutation related breast cancers have been described, little is known about the morphological aspects of these tumors [139].

Female BRCA2 mutation related cancers are mostly invasive ductal carcinoma, but also show a higher incidence of invasive (pleomorphic) lobular, tubular and cribriform carcinomas compared to sporadic cancers. BRCA2 mutation related tumors are more frequently grade 2 and 3, show more nuclear pleomorphism, higher mitotic rates, and more often pushing margins compared to sporadic breast cancers. The immunophenotype of female BRCA2 mutation related breast cancers is similar to sporadic breast cancers (and thereby different from BRCA1 related cancers) except for more frequent expression of FGF1 and FGFR2 [137]. Male BRCA2 mutation related breast cancers have been described to have frequent HER2 over-expression and high histological grade, suggesting an aggressive behavior of these tumors [138]. By gene expression analysis, also high expression of FGF1 and FGFR2 was observed and most *BRCA2* related breast cancers were classified as luminal. By CGH, BRCA2 related breast cancers show more frequently gains of 8q, 17q22-q24 and 20q13 and loss of 8p, 6q, 11q and 13q compared to BRCA1-related cancers [137]. In female BRCA2 mutation carriers, DCIS and LCIS lesions occur in about the same frequency as in BRCA1 mutation carriers. The non-malignant breast shows frequent pre-malignant lesions like DCIS, LCIS, ADH, ALH and columnar cell lesions, and T-cell lobulitis [137]. Probably, a significant proportion of male breast cancer is BRCA2 related and seems to be preferentially of micropapillary type [140], but it is yet unclear if these cancers have other specific characteristics.

Morphologic and immunophenotypic studies of female CHEK2-related breast cancer in patients have yielded conflicting results, probably largely due to the limited cases of breast cancers that have been found being related to this mutation. Studies on ER and PR expression have reported contradictory results, ranging from similar to over-expression of ER and PR. Breast cancer in patients with a U157T mutation seems to be more often of lobular type [137]. Male CHEK2-related breast cancer cases have been reported, but the total number of cases is so low that clinicopathological characteristics are unclear [141]. Female TP53 germline-related breast cancers appear to be very often over-expressing HER2 [142, 143].

Only a few female PALB2-related cancers have been studied, most exhibiting a phenotype of high grade mostly of ductal type and ER, PR and HER2 negativity. They were mostly CK5/6, CK14 and CK17 negative, showed high expression of Ki67 and low expression of Cyclin D1 as compared with other familial and sporadic patients [137]. Female ATM-related breast cancers did not appear to be associated with distinctive histopathological features [134, 144].

CDH1 germline mutations specifically give rise to invasive lobular breast cancer [135, 145]. PTEN germline mutations are often of the apocrine histological type, and in concordance with this, show often expression of AR and BRST2 [146]. The tumor characteristics, hormone receptor status and grade of female NBS1 mutation related breast cancer were similar to non-NBS1 mutation related breast cancer in one study [147]. Little to no histopathological characteristics have been described of STK11/LKB1, RAD50 and BRIP1 mutation related breast cancer.

## Male breast cancer: a different genetic entity

Male breast cancer is a rare disease and most of the knowledge has been extrapolated from females. However, it had already been demonstrated that there are differences between male and female breast cancer, and experts agree that male breast cancer should be considered a unique disease, rather than a male variant of female breast cancer [148]. Approximately 15%

to 20% of the male breast cancer patients report a family history of breast / ovarian cancer and probably at least 10% of the men have a genetic predisposition [148]. BRCA2 mutation carriers have the highest chance of developing male breast cancer with a 6.8% cumulative breast cancer risk at age 70 years [149–151]. In females, BRCA1 germline mutations are more important, while in male BRCA1 mutation carriers the cumulative breast cancer risk is relatively low (<2%) [150]. There is yet little knowledge on the genetic make-up of male breast cancer and most of the few available studies are based on small, single institutional series, and results therefore have to be interpreted with care.

Using comparative genomic hybridization analyses, Johansson et al. found more frequent genomic gains in male breast cancer than in female breast cancer which often involved whole chromosome arms, while losses of genomic material were less frequent [152]. Male breast cancer is very often and more frequently ER and PR positive, while (over-) expression of HER2 and accumulation of p53 is rare. As a consequence, the vast majority is of the luminal A intrinsic subtype, followed by the luminal B subtype. HER2 driven and basal-like are very rare [153–158]. On the molecular level, several genes have been identified which seem to play an important role in male breast carcinogenesis (CCND1, TRAF4, CDC6 and MTDH) and CCND1 amplification seems to be an independent predictor of adverse survival [156]. Several studies indicate that there are differences in the genetic profile of male and female breast cancer. EGFR and CCND1 copy-number gain were more often seen in male breast cancer, while gain of EMSY and CPD, amplification of TRAF4 and EMSY and copy-number loss on 16q were less frequent [156, 159]. Androgen receptor related genes play a more prominent role in male breast cancer, while genes correlated with progesterone receptor and HER2 are less important and expression profiles of estrogen-induced genes are different compared to female breast cancer, illustrating the different hormonal balance between the two [160, 161].

In addition, there are differences in hypermethylation status of CpG islands in promoter regions of several genes. In a study on promoter hypermethylation of 25 tumor suppressor genes using methylation-specific MLPA (MS-MLPA), hypermethylation of the genes MSH6, WT1, PAX5, CDH13, GATA5 and PAX6 was seen in more than 50% of the cases, while uncommon or absent in normal male breast tissue, indicating that promoter hypermethylation of these genes is important in the carcinogenesis of male breast cancer. High overall methylation status was correlated with high grade and was an independent predictor of poor survival. ESR1 and GTSP1 were the only individual genes for which promoter hypermethylation correlated with tumor phenotype (high mitotic count and high grade). Compared to female breast cancers, promoter hypermethylation was less common for ESR1, MGMT, BRCA1, BRCA2, VHL, RARB, ATM, PTEN and STK11. The most frequently hypermethylated genes (MSH6, CDH13, PAX5, PAX6 and WT1) were similar for male and female breast cancer [162].

Three studies have evaluated microRNA expression in male breast cancer [151, 163, 164]. In the first, miR-21, miR519d, miR-183, miR-197 and miR-493-5p were identified as most prominently up-regulated, miR-145 and miR-497 as most prominently down-regulated [163]. In another study, RASSF1A was more frequently methylated in men than women, while miR17 and let-7a expression frequency was higher in women than in men. RASSF1A seemed to be involved in familial MBC, while miR17 and let-7a seemed to be implicated in familial FBC [151]. Fassan et al. did microRNA microarrays in MBC versus FBC and found 17 significantly deregulated miRNAs, with four up-regulated (miR-663, miR-618, miR-605 and miR-616) and 13 down-regulated (miR-200b, miR-181c, miR-106a, miR-125a-5p, miR-16, miR-25, miR-100, has-let-7f, miR-125b, miR-15b, miR-425, miR-199a-5p and miR-223 in MBC) [164].

Collaborative efforts are essential in moving forward and to study more complex issues and elucidate the molecular signature of male breast cancer and confirm important differences between male and female breast cancer in the (near) future, especially by applying next generation sequencing techniques.

## Future perspectives

Molecular pathology is one of the most rapidly growing areas in medicine. Molecular diagnostic applications are now available in virtually all of the traditional areas of breast pathology. These provide highly accurate diagnostic, prognostic and even therapeutic information for clinicians and researchers. These developments are both exciting as well as a challenge for diagnostic pathologists, since they pose many new demands with regard to knowledge, infrastructure, workflow and staffing. In order not to lag behind and prevent molecular diagnostics from drifting to the periphery, additional training, investments in infrastructure and an innovative flexible mind set will remain crucial for decades to come.

Integrative genetic, epigenetic and expression profiling studies as well as whole-genome or whole-exome sequencing of breast cancers is exposing the complexity of tumor diversity and intratumor heterogeneity, and helping to pinpoint avenues for precise diagnostics and targeted therapies while avoiding resistance mechanisms. Speed of clinical adoption of newly discovered diagnostic, prognostic and predictive signatures or panels hinges on several factors, including assay costs and reproducibility, speed, bioinformatics, clinical usefulness (additional value), payment uncertainty and regulatory uncertainty. For example, initial concerns of whole-genome sequencing studies were cost and data accuracy, but the major challenge has turned out to be the logistics of delivering genome sequence information to clinicians and patients in a manner that is understandable and comprehensive without being overwhelming. Many unanswered questions remain. What genetic information should go into the medical record? What should be done with unrelated, secondary genetic findings like unexpected germline aberrations? What kind of reimbursement strategy is optimal as clinical adoption becomes more widespread? Should we be sampling all of the metastatic sites to measure clonal heterogeneity? The implementation of methods of sequencing and clonal analysis coupled with simple methods to collect cells from the metastatic sites like fine-needle aspiration cytology may aid this practice [55, 165].

Although many challenges remain, there is no doubt that new technological breakthroughs in genetic testing and automation such as next generation sequencing will expand the field of molecular pathology, and that these developments will influence the diagnosis and treatment of breast cancer.

## Learning points

- The breast cancer intrinsic subtypes (luminal A, luminal B, HER2-enriched, basal-like and normal-like) have gained widespread acceptance as a way of classifying breast cancers with prognostic relevance. Approximations of intrinsic subtypes based on immunohistochemistry on three to six markers (ER, PR, HER2, EGFR, Ki67 and CK5/6) have been proposed.

- Combinatorial molecular indices to (further) classify breast cancer in terms of prognosis and/or therapeutic response such as Oncotype DX®, Mammaprint®, PAM50® and Genomic Grade Index (GGI) are rapidly emerging and are likely to become more widely adopted in daily pathology when they prove to be methodologically and clinically robust.

- Male and hereditary breast cancers are different genetic entities, where molecular analysis by the

pathologist will play an increasingly important role.

- Analysis of methylation, microRNAs and next generation sequencing (NGS) are emerging technologies that are likely to shed more light on tumor heterogeneity and resistance mechanisms, and may refine prognosis prediction. As such, they will contribute to individualized targeted treatment and will be routinely applied in molecular pathology to determine prognostic and predictive profiles of each breast cancer.

# References

1. Perou, C. M., Sorlie, T., Eisen, M. B., van de Rijn, M., Jeffrey, S. S., Rees, C. A. et al. Molecular portraits of human breast tumours. Nature 2000; 406: 747–52.

2. Sorlie, T., Perou, C. M., Tibshirani, R., Aas, T., Geisler, S., Johnsen, H. et al. Gene expression patterns of breast carcinomas distinguish tumor subclasses with clinical implications. Proc Natl Acad Sci USA 2001; 98(19): 10869–74.

3. Van't Veer, L. J., Dai, H., van de Vijver, M. J., He, Y. D., Hart, A. A., Mao, M. et al. Gene expression profiling predicts clinical outcome of breast cancer. Nature 2002; 415: 530–6.

4. Paik, S., Shak, S., Tang, G., Kim, C., Baker, J., Cronin, M. et al. A multigene assay to predict recurrence of tamoxifen-treated, node-negative breast cancer. New Engl J Med 2004; 351(27): 2817–26.

5. The Cancer Genome Atlas Network. Comprehensive molecular portraits of human breast tumours. Nature 2012; 490: 61–70.

6. Weigelt, B., Horlings, H. M., Kreike, B., Hayes, M. M., Hauptmann, M., Wessels, L. F. et al. Refinement of breast cancer classification by molecular

characterization of histological special types. J Pathol 2008; 216(2): 141–50.

7. Weigelt, B., Geyer, F. C., Horlings, H. M., Kreike, B., Halfwerk, H. and Reis-Filho, J. S. Mucinous and neuroendocrine breast carcinomas are transcriptionally distinct from invasive ductal carcinomas of no special type. Mod Pathol 2009; 22(11): 1401–14.

8. Weigelt, B., Geyer, F. C., Natrajan, R., Lopez-Garcia, M. A., Ahmad, A. S., Savage, K. et al. The molecular underpinning of lobular histological growth pattern: a genome-wide transcriptomic analysis of invasive lobular carcinomas and grade- and molecular subtype-matched invasive ductal carcinomas of no special type. J Pathol 2010; 220(1): 45–57.

9. Gruel, N., Lucchesi, C., Raynal, V., Rodrigues, M. J., Pierron, G., Goudefroye, R. et al. Lobular invasive carcinoma of the breast is a molecular entity distinct from luminal invasive ductal carcinoma. Eur J Cancer 2010; 46(13): 2399–407.

10. Horlings, H. M., Weigelt, B., Anderson, E. M., Lambros, M. B., Mackay, A., Natrajan, R. et al. Genomic profiling of histological special types of breast cancer. Breast Cancer Res Treat 2013; 142(2): 257–69.

11. Goldhirsch, A., Wood, W. C., Coates, A. S., Gelber, R. D., Thurlimann, B. and Senn, H. J. Strategies for subtypes – dealing with the diversity of breast cancer: highlights of the St. Gallen International Expert Consensus on the Primary Therapy of Early Breast Cancer 2011. Ann Oncol 2011; 22(8): 1736–47.

12. Mackay, A., Weigelt, B., Grigoriadis, A., Kreike, B., Natrajan, R., A'Hern, R. et al. Microarray-based class discovery for molecular classification of breast cancer: analysis of interobserver agreement. J Natl Cancer Inst 2011; 103(8): 662–73.

13. Owens, M. A., Horten, B. C. and Da Silva, M. M. HER2 amplification ratios by fluorescence in situ hybridization and correlation with immunohistochemistry in a cohort of 6556 breast cancer tissues. Clin Breast Cancer 2004; 5(1): 63–9.

14. Wolff, A. C., Hammond, M. E., Schwartz, J. N., Hagerty, K. L., Allred, D. C., Cote, R. J. et al. American Society of Clinical Oncology/College of American Pathologists guideline recommendations for human epidermal growth factor receptor 2 testing in breast cancer. J Clin Oncol 2007; 25(1): 118–45.

15. Zemzoum, I., Kates, R. E., Ross, J. S., Dettmar, P., Dutta, M.,

Henrichs, C. *et al.* Invasion factors uPA/PAI-1 and HER2 status provide independent and complementary information on patient outcome in node-negative breast cancer. *J Clin Oncol* 2003; 21(6): 1022–8.

16. Ross, J. S., Fletcher, J. A., Bloom, K. J., Linette, G. P., Stec, J., Symmans, W. F. *et al.* Targeted therapy in breast cancer: the HER-2/neu gene and protein. *Mol Cell Proteomics* 2004; 3(4): 379–98.

17. Vogel, C. L., Cobleigh, M. A., Tripathy, D., Gutheil, J. C., Harris, L. N., Fehrenbacher, L. *et al.* Efficacy and safety of trastuzumab as a single agent in first-line treatment of HER2-overexpressing metastatic breast cancer. *J Clin Oncol* 2002; 20(3): 719–26.

18. Slamon, D. J., Leyland-Jones, B., Shak, S., Fuchs, H., Paton, V., Bajamonde, A. *et al.* Use of chemotherapy plus a monoclonal antibody against HER2 for metastatic breast cancer that overexpresses HER2. *New Engl J Med* 2001; 344(11): 783–92.

19. Smith, I. Future directions in the adjuvant treatment of breast cancer: the role of trastuzumab. *Ann Oncol* 2001; 12(Suppl. 1): S75–9.

20. Piccart-Gebhart, M. J., Procter, M., Leyland-Jones, B., Goldhirsch, A., Untch, M., Smith, I. *et al.* Trastuzumab after adjuvant chemotherapy in HER2-positive breast cancer. *New Engl J Med* 2005; 353(16): 1659–72.

21. Romond, E. H., Perez, E. A., Bryant, J., Suman, V. J., Geyer, C. E. Jr., Davidson, N. E. *et al.* Trastuzumab plus adjuvant chemotherapy for operable HER2-positive breast cancer. *New Engl J Med* 2005; 353(16): 1673–84.

22. Esteva, F. J., Yu, D., Hung, M. C. and Hortobagyi, G. N. Molecular predictors of response to trastuzumab and lapatinib in breast cancer. *Nat Rev Clin Oncol* 2010; 7(2): 98–107.

23. Moelans, C. B., de Weger, R. A., van der Wall, E. and van Diest, P. J. Current technologies for HER2 testing in breast cancer. *Crit Rev Oncol Hematol* 2011; 80: 380–92.

24. Wolff, A. C., Hammond, M. E., Hicks, D. G., Dowsett, M., McShane, L. M., Allison, K. H. *et al.* Recommendations for human epidermal growth factor receptor 2 testing in breast cancer: american society of clinical oncology/college of american pathologists clinical practice guideline update. *J Clin Oncol* 2013; 31(31): 3997–4013.

25. Kostopoulou, E., Vageli, D., Kaisaridou, D., Nakou, M., Netsika, M., Vladica, N. *et al.* Comparative evaluation of non-informative HER-2 immunoreactions (2+) in breast carcinomas with FISH, CISH and QRT-PCR. *Breast* 2007; 16(6): 615–24.

26. Bedard, Y. C., Pollett, A. F., Leung, S. W. and O'Malley, F. P. Assessment of thin-layer breast aspirates for immunocytochemical evaluation of HER2 status. *Acta Cytol* 2003; 47(6): 979–84.

27. Pauletti, G., Dandekar, S., Rong, H., Ramos, L., Peng, H., Seshadri, R. *et al.* Assessment of methods for tissue-based detection of the HER-2/neu alteration in human breast cancer: a direct comparison of fluorescence in situ hybridization and immunohistochemistry. *J Clin Oncol* 2000; 18(21): 3651–64.

28. Lebeau, A., Deimling, D., Kaltz, C., Sendelhofert, A., Iff, A., Luthardt, B. *et al.* HER-2/neu analysis in archival tissue samples of human breast cancer: comparison of immunohistochemistry and fluorescence in situ hybridization. *J Clin Oncol* 2001; 19(2): 354–63.

29. Tanner, M., Gancberg, D., Di, L. A., Larsimont, D., Rouas, G., Piccart, M. J. *et al.* Chromogenic in situ hybridization: a practical alternative for fluorescence in situ hybridization to detect HER-2/ neu oncogene amplification in archival breast cancer samples. *Am J Pathol* 2000; 157(5): 1467–72.

30. Arnould, L., Denoux, Y., MacGrogan, G., Penault-Llorca, F., Fiche, M., Treilleux, I. *et al.* Agreement between chromogenic in situ hybridisation (CISH) and FISH in the determination of HER2 status in breast cancer. *Br J Cancer* 2003; 88(10): 1587–91.

31. Hanna, W. M. and Kwok, K. Chromogenic in-situ hybridization: a viable alternative to fluorescence in-situ hybridization in the HER2 testing algorithm. *Mod Pathol* 2006; 19(4): 481–7.

32. Gruver, A. M., Peerwani, Z. and Tubbs, R. R. Out of the darkness and into the light: bright field in situ hybridisation for delineation of ERBB2 (HER2) status in breast carcinoma. *J Clin Pathol* 2010; 63(3): 210–19.

33. Ni, R., Mulligan, A. M., Have, C. and O'Malley, F. P. PGDS, a novel technique combining chromogenic in situ hybridization and immunohistochemistry for the assessment of ErbB2 (HER2/neu) status in breast cancer. *Appl Immunohistochem Mol Morphol* 2007; 15(3): 316–24.

34. Downs-Kelly, E., Pettay, J., Hicks, D., Skacel, M., Yoder, B., Rybicki, L. *et al.* Analytical validation and interobserver reproducibility of EnzMet GenePro: a second-generation bright-field metallography assay for concomitant detection of HER2 gene status and protein expression in invasive carcinoma of the breast. *Am J Surg Pathol* 2005; 29(11): 1505–11.

35. Francis, G. D., Jones, M. A., Beadle, G. F. and Stein, S. R. Bright-field in situ hybridization for HER2 gene amplification in breast cancer using tissue microarrays: correlation between chromogenic (CISH) and automated silver-enhanced (SISH) methods with patient outcome. *Diagn Mol Pathol* 2009; 18(2): 88–95.

36. Bartlett, J. M., Campbell, F. M., Ibrahim, M., Wencyk, P., Ellis, I., Kay, E. *et al.* Chromogenic in situ hybridization: a multicenter study comparing silver in situ hybridization with FISH. *Am J Clin Pathol* 2009; 132(4): 514–20.

37. Penault-Llorca, F., Bilous, M., Dowsett, M., Hanna, W., Osamura, R. Y., Ruschoff, J. *et al.* Emerging technologies for assessing HER2 amplification. *Am J Clin Pathol* 2009; 132(4): 539–48.

38. Van den Bempt, I., Van Loo, P., Drijkoningen, M., Neven, P., Smeets, A., Christiaens, M. R. *et al.* Polysomy 17 in breast cancer: clinicopathologic significance and impact on HER-2 testing. *J Clin Oncol* 2008; 26(30): 4869–74.

39. Moelans, C. B., de Weger, R. A. and van Diest, P. J. Absence of chromosome 17 polysomy in breast cancer: analysis by CEP17 chromogenic in situ hybridization and multiplex ligation-dependent probe amplification. *Breast Cancer Res Treat* 2010; 120(1): 1–7.

40. Yeh, I. T., Martin, M. A., Robetorye, R. S., Bolla, A. R., McCaskill, C., Shah, R. K. *et al.* Clinical validation of an array CGH test for HER2 status in breast cancer reveals that polysomy 17 is a rare event. *Mod Pathol* 2009; 22(9): 1169–75.

41. Moelans, C. B., Reis-Filho, J. S. and van Diest, P. J. Implications of rarity of chromosome 17 polysomy in breast cancer.

*Lancet Oncol* 2011; 12(12): 1087–9.

42. Hofmann, M., Stoss, O., Gaiser, T., Kneitz, H., Heinmoller, P., Gutjahr, T. *et al.* Central HER2 IHC and FISH analysis in a trastuzumab (Herceptin) phase II monotherapy study: assessment of test sensitivity and impact of chromosome 17 polysomy. *J Clin Pathol* 2008; 61(1): 89–94.

43. Schouten, J. P., McElgunn, C. J., Waaijer, R., Zwijnenburg, D., Diepvens, F. and Pals, G. Relative quantification of 40 nucleic acid sequences by multiplex ligation-dependent probe amplification. *Nucleic Acids Res* 2002; 30(12): e57.

44. Moelans, C. B., de Weger, R. A., van Blokland, M. T., Ezendam, C., Elshof, S., Tilanus, M. G. *et al.* HER-2/neu amplification testing in breast cancer by multiplex ligation-dependent probe amplification in comparison with immunohistochemistry and in situ hybridization. *Cell Oncol* 2009; 31(1): 1–10.

45. Moerland, E., van Hezik, R. L., van der Aa, T. C., van Beek, M. W. and van den Brule, A. J. Detection of HER2 amplification in breast carcinomas: comparison of Multiplex Ligation-dependent Probe Amplification (MLPA) and Fluorescence In Situ Hybridization (FISH) combined with automated spot counting. *Cell Oncol* 2006; 28(4): 151–9.

46. Moelans, C. B., de Weger, R. A., Ezendam, C. and van Diest, P. J. HER-2/neu amplification testing in breast cancer by Multiplex Ligation-dependent Probe Amplification: influence of manual- and laser microdissection. *BMC Cancer* 2009; 9: 4.

47. Shi, Y., Huang, W., Tan, Y., Jin, X., Dua, R., Penuel, E. *et al.* A novel proximity assay for the detection of proteins and protein complexes: quantitation of HER1

and HER2 total protein expression and homodimerization in formalin-fixed, paraffin-embedded cell lines and breast cancer tissue. *Diagn Mol Pathol* 2009; 18(1): 11–21.

48. Hoefnagel, L. D., van de Vijver, M. J., van Slooten, H. J., Wesseling, P., Wesseling, J., Westenend, P. J. *et al.* Receptor conversion in distant breast cancer metastases. *Breast Cancer Res* 2010; 12(5): R75.

49. Hoefnagel, L. D., Moelans, C. B., Meijer, S. L., van Slooten, H. J., Wesseling, P., Wesseling, J. *et al.* Prognostic value of estrogen receptor alpha and progesterone receptor conversion in distant breast cancer metastases. *Cancer* 2012; 118(20): 4929–35.

50. Broom, R. J., Tang, P. A., Simmons, C., Bordeleau, L., Mulligan, A. M., O'Malley, F. P. *et al.* Changes in estrogen receptor, progesterone receptor and HER-2/neu status with time: discordance rates between primary and metastatic breast cancer. *Anticancer Res* 2009; 29(5): 1557–62.

51. Tapia, C., Savic, S., Wagner, U., Schonegg, R., Novotny, H., Grilli, B. *et al.* HER2 gene status in primary breast cancers and matched distant metastases. *Breast Cancer Res* 2007; 9: R31.

52. Santinelli, A., Pisa, E., Stramazzotti, D. and Fabris, G. HER-2 status discrepancy between primary breast cancer and metastatic sites. Impact on target therapy. *Int J Cancer* 2008; 122(5): 999–1004.

53. Gancberg, D., Di, L. A., Cardoso, F., Rouas, G., Pedrocchi, M., Paesmans, M. *et al.* Comparison of HER-2 status between primary breast cancer and corresponding distant metastatic sites. *Ann Oncol* 2002; 13(7): 1036–43.

54. Hoefnagel, L. D., van der Groep, P., van de Vijver, M. DJ, Boers, J. E., Wesseling, P., Wesseling, J.

*et al.* Discordance in ER alpha, PR and HER2 receptor status across different distant breast cancer metastases within the same patient. *Ann Oncol* 2013; 24(12): 3017–23.

55. Beca, F. and Schmitt, F. Growing indication for FNA to study and analyze tumor heterogeneity at metastatic sites. *Cancer Cytopathol* 2014; 122(7): 504–11; doi: 10.1002/cncy.21395.

56. Gu, M., Ghafari, S. and Zhao, M. Fluorescence in situ hybridization for HER-2/neu amplification of breast carcinoma in archival fine needle aspiration biopsy specimens. *Acta Cytologica* 2005: 49: 471–6.

57. Weigelt, B. and Reis-Filho, J. S. Activating mutations in HER2: neu opportunities and neu challenges. *Cancer Discov* 2013; 3(2): 145–7.

58. Bose, R., Kavuri, S. M., Searleman, A. C., Shen, W., Shen, D., Koboldt, D. C. *et al.* Activating HER2 mutations in HER2 gene amplification negative breast cancer. *Cancer Discov* 2013; 3(2): 224–37.

59. Patani, N., Martin, L. A. and Dowsett, M. Biomarkers for the clinical management of breast cancer: international perspective. *Int J Cancer* 2013; 133(1): 1–13.

60. Sparano, J. A. and Paik, S. Development of the 21-gene assay and its application in clinical practice and clinical trials. *J Clin Oncol* 2008; 26(5): 721–8.

61. Paik, S., Tang, G., Shak, S., Kim, C., Baker, J., Kim, W. *et al.* Gene expression and benefit of chemotherapy in women with node-negative, estrogen receptor-positive breast cancer. *J Clin Oncol* 2006; 24(23): 3726–34.

62. Albain, K. S., Barlow, W. E., Shak, S., Hortobagyi, G. N., Livingston, R. B., Yeh, I. T. *et al.* Prognostic and predictive value of the 21-gene recurrence score assay in postmenopausal women with

node-positive, oestrogen-receptor-positive breast cancer on chemotherapy: a retrospective analysis of a randomised trial. *Lancet Oncol* 2010; 11(1): 55–65.

63. Hall, P. S., McCabe, C., Stein, R. C. and Cameron, D. Economic evaluation of genomic test-directed chemotherapy for early-stage lymph node-positive breast cancer. *J Natl Cancer Inst* 2012; 104(1): 56–66.

64. Buyse, M., Loi, S., van't Veer, L., Viale, G., Delorenzi, M., Glas, A. M. *et al.* Validation and clinical utility of a 70-gene prognostic signature for women with node-negative breast cancer. *J Natl Cancer Inst* 2006; 98(17): 1183–92.

65. van de Vijver, M. J., He, Y. D., Van't Veer, L. J., Dai, H., Hart, A. A., Voskuil, D. W. *et al.* A gene-expression signature as a predictor of survival in breast cancer. *New Engl J Med* 2002; 347(25): 1999–2009.

66. Knauer, M., Mook, S., Rutgers, E. J., Bender, R. A., Hauptmann, M., van de Vijver, M. J. *et al.* The predictive value of the 70-gene signature for adjuvant chemotherapy in early breast cancer. *Breast Cancer Res Treat* 2010; 120(3): 655–61.

67. Bogaerts, J., Cardoso, F., Buyse, M., Braga, S., Loi, S., Harrison, J. A. *et al.* Gene signature evaluation as a prognostic tool: challenges in the design of the MINDACT trial. *Nat Clin Pract Oncol* 2006; 3(10): 540–51.

68. Drukker, C. A., Bueno-de-Mesquita, J. M., Retel, V. P., van Harten, W. H., van Tinteren, H., Wesseling, J. *et al.* A prospective evaluation of a breast cancer prognosis signature in the observational RASTER study. *Int J Cancer* 2013; 133(4): 929–36.

69. Sapino, A., Roepman, P., Linn, S. C., Snel, M. H., Delahaye, L. J., van den Akker, J. *et al.* MammaPrint molecular diagnostics on formalin-fixed,

paraffin-embedded tissue. *J Mol Diagn* 2013; 16(2): 190–7

70. Retel, V. P., Joore, M. A., Drukker, C. A., Bueno-de-Mesquita, J. M., Knauer, M., van Tinteren, H. *et al.* Prospective cost-effectiveness analysis of genomic profiling in breast cancer. *Eur J Cancer* 2013; 49(18): 3773–9.

71. Parker, J. S., Mullins, M., Cheang, M. C., Leung, S., Voduc, D., Vickery, T. *et al.* Supervised risk predictor of breast cancer based on intrinsic subtypes. *J Clin Oncol* 2009; 27(8): 1160–7.

72. Nielsen, T. O., Parker, J. S., Leung, S., Voduc, D., Ebbert, M., Vickery, T. *et al.* A comparison of PAM50 intrinsic subtyping with immunohistochemistry and clinical prognostic factors in tamoxifen-treated estrogen receptor-positive breast cancer. *Clin Cancer Res* 2010; 16(21): 5222–32.

73. Esserman, L. J., Berry, D. A., Cheang, M. C., Yau, C., Perou, C. M., Carey, L. *et al.* Chemotherapy response and recurrence-free survival in neoadjuvant breast cancer depends on biomarker profiles: results from the I-SPY 1 TRIAL (CALGB 150007/150012; ACRIN 6657). *Breast Cancer Res Treat* 2012; 132(3): 1049–62.

74. Sotiriou, C., Wirapati, P., Loi, S., Harris, A., Fox, S., Smeds, J. *et al.* Gene expression profiling in breast cancer: understanding the molecular basis of histologic grade to improve prognosis. *J Natl Cancer Inst* 2006; 98(4): 262–72.

75. Loi, S., Haibe-Kains, B., Desmedt, C., Lallemand, F., Tutt, A. M., Gillet, C. *et al.* Definition of clinically distinct molecular subtypes in estrogen receptor-positive breast carcinomas through genomic grade. *J Clin Oncol* 2007; 25(10): 1239–46.

76. Desmedt, C., Giobbie-Hurder, A., Neven, P., Paridaens, R., Christiaens, M. R., Smeets, A. *et al.* The Gene expression Grade

Index: a potential predictor of relapse for endocrine-treated breast cancer patients in the BIG 1–98 trial. *BMC Med Genomics* 2009; 2: 40.

77. Cuzick, J., Dowsett, M., Pineda, S., Wale, C., Salter, J., Quinn, E. *et al.* Prognostic value of a combined estrogen receptor, progesterone receptor, Ki-67, and human epidermal growth factor receptor 2 immunohistochemical score and comparison with the Genomic Health recurrence score in early breast cancer. *J Clin Oncol* 2011; 29(32): 4273–8.

78. Dowsett, M., Sestak, I., Lopez-Knowles, E., Sidhu, K., Dunbier, A. K., Cowens, J. W. *et al.* Comparison of PAM50 risk of recurrence score with oncotype DX and IHC4 for predicting risk of distant recurrence after endocrine therapy. *J Clin Oncol* 2013; 31(22): 2783–90.

79. Dowsett, M., Nielsen, T. O., A'Hern, R., Bartlett, J., Coombes, R. C., Cuzick, J. *et al.* Assessment of Ki67 in breast cancer: recommendations from the International Ki67 in Breast Cancer working group. *J Natl Cancer Inst* 2011; 103(22): 1656–64.

80. Dave, B., Migliaccio, I., Gutierrez, M. C., Wu, M. F., Chamness, G. C., Wong, H. *et al.* Loss of phosphatase and tensin homolog or phosphoinositol-3 kinase activation and response to trastuzumab or lapatinib in human epidermal growth factor receptor 2-overexpressing locally advanced breast cancers. *J Clin Oncol* 2011; 29(2): 166–73.

81. Wang, L., Zhang, Q., Zhang, J., Sun, S., Guo, H., Jia, Z. *et al.* PI3K pathway activation results in low efficacy of both trastuzumab and lapatinib. *BMC Cancer* 2011; 11: 248.

82. Jensen, J. D., Knoop, A., Laenkholm, A. V., Grauslund, M., Jensen, M. B., Santoni-Rugiu, E. *et al.* PIK3CA mutations, PTEN,

and pHER2 expression and impact on outcome in HER2-positive early-stage breast cancer patients treated with adjuvant chemotherapy and trastuzumab. *Ann Oncol* 2012; 23(8): 2034–42.

83. Cizkova, M., Dujaric, M. E., Lehmann-Che, J., Scott, V., Tembo, O., Asselain, B. *et al.* Outcome impact of PIK3CA mutations in HER2-positive breast cancer patients treated with trastuzumab. *Br J Cancer* 2013; 108(9): 1807–9.

84. Ma, C. X., Crowder, R. J. and Ellis, M. J. Importance of PI3-kinase pathway in response/resistance to aromatase inhibitors. *Steroids* 2011; 76(8): 750–2.

85. Campeau, P. M., Foulkes, W. D. and Tischkowitz, M. D. Hereditary breast cancer: new genetic developments, new therapeutic avenues. *Hum Genet* 2008; 124(1): 31–42.

86. Mavaddat, N., Peock, S., Frost, D., Ellis, S., Platte, R., Fineberg, E. *et al.* Cancer risks for BRCA1 and BRCA2 mutation carriers: results from prospective analysis of EMBRACE. *J Natl Cancer Inst* 2013; 105(11): 812–22.

87. Antoniou, A., Pharoah, P. D., Narod, S., Risch, H. A., Eyfjord, J. E., Hopper, J. L. *et al.* Average risks of breast and ovarian cancer associated with BRCA1 or BRCA2 mutations detected in case Series unselected for family history: a combined analysis of 22 studies. *Am J Hum Genet* 2003; 72(5): 1117–30.

88. De Leeneer, K., Coene, I., Crombez, B., Simkens, J., Van den Broecke, R., Bols, A. *et al.* Prevalence of BRCA1/2 mutations in sporadic breast/ovarian cancer patients and identification of a novel de novo BRCA1 mutation in a patient diagnosed with late onset breast and ovarian cancer: implications for genetic testing. *Breast Cancer Res Treat* 2012; 132(1): 87–95.

89. Da, S. L. and Lakhani, S. R. Pathology of hereditary breast cancer. *Mod Pathol* 2010; 23(Suppl. 2): S46–51.

90. Chen, S. and Parmigiani, G. Meta-analysis of BRCA1 and BRCA2 penetrance. *J Clin Oncol* 2007; 25(11): 1329–33.

91. Schrader, K. A., Masciari, S., Boyd, N., Wiyrick, S., Kaurah, P., Senz, J. *et al.* Hereditary diffuse gastric cancer: association with lobular breast cancer. *Fam Cancer* 2008; 7: 73–82.

92. Bertucci, F., Orsetti, B., Negre, V., Finetti, P., Rouge, C., Ahomadegbe, J. C. *et al.* Lobular and ductal carcinomas of the breast have distinct genomic and expression profiles. *Oncogene* 2008; 27(40): 5359–72.

93. Morrogh, M., Andrade, V. P., Giri, D., Sakr, R. A., Paik, W., Qin, L. X. *et al.* Cadherin-catenin complex dissociation in lobular neoplasia of the breast. *Breast Cancer Res Treat* 2012; 132(2): 641–52.

94. Moelans, C. B. and van Diest, P. J. Breast: ductal carcinoma. *Atlas Genet Cytogenet Oncol Haematol* 2013; 17(3): 209–20.

95. Nahta, R. and O'Regan, R. M. Evolving strategies for overcoming resistance to HER2-directed therapy: targeting the PI3K/Akt/mTOR pathway. *Clin Breast Cancer* 2010; 10(Suppl. 3): S72–8.

96. Gaynor, K. U., Grigorieva, I. V., Allen, M. D., Esapa, C. T., Head, R. A., Gopinath, P. *et al.* GATA3 mutations found in breast cancers may be associated with aberrant nuclear localization, reduced transactivation and cell invasiveness. *Horm Cancer* 2013; 4(3): 123–39.

97. Holst, F., Stahl, P. R., Ruiz, C., Hellwinkel, O., Jehan, Z., Wendland, M. *et al.* Estrogen receptor alpha (ESR1) gene amplification is frequent in breast

cancer. *Nat Genet* 2007; 39(5): 655–60.

98. Tomita, S., Zhang, Z., Nakano, M., Ibusuki, M., Kawazoe, T., Yamamoto, Y. *et al.* Estrogen receptor alpha gene ESR1 amplification may predict endocrine therapy responsiveness in breast cancer patients. *Cancer Sci* 2009; 100(6): 1012–17.

99. Tsiambas, E., Georgiannos, S. N., Salemis, N., Alexopoulou, D., Lambropoulou, S., Dimo, B. *et al.* Significance of estrogen receptor 1 (ESR-1) gene imbalances in colon and hepatocellular carcinomas based on tissue microarrays analysis. *Med Oncol* 2011; 28(4): 934–40.

100. Moelans, C. B., de Weger, R. A., Monsuur, H. N., Maes, A. H. and van Diest, P. J. Molecular differences between ductal carcinoma in situ and adjacent invasive breast carcinoma: a multiplex ligation-dependent probe amplification study. *Anal Cell Pathol (Amst)* 2010; 33(3): 165–73.

101. Moelans, C. B., Monsuur, H. N., de Pinth, J. H., Radersma, R. D., de Weger, R. A. and van Diest, P. J. ESR1 amplification is rare in breast cancer and is associated with high grade and high proliferation: a multiplex ligation-dependent probe amplification study. *Anal Cell Pathol (Amst)* 2010; 33(1): 13–18.

102. Lin, C. H., Liu, J. M., Lu, Y. S., Lan, C., Lee, W. C., Kuo, K. T. *et al.* Clinical significance of ESR1 gene copy number changes in breast cancer as measured by fluorescence in situ hybridisation. *J Clin Pathol* 2013; 66(2): 140–5.

103. Holst, F., Moelans, C. B., Filipits, M., Singer, C. F., Simon, R. and van Diest, P. J. On the evidence for ESR1 amplification in breast cancer. *Nat Rev Cancer* 2012; 12(2): 149.

104. Nessling, M., Richter, K., Schwaenen, C., Roerig, P.,

Wrobel, G., Wessendorf, S. *et al.* Candidate genes in breast cancer revealed by microarray-based comparative genomic hybridization of archived tissue. *Cancer Res* 2005; 65(2): 439–47.

105. Ooi, A., Inokuchi, M., Harada, S., Inazawa, J., Tajiri, R., Kitamura, S. S. *et al.* Gene amplification of ESR1 in breast cancers–fact or fiction? A fluorescence in situ hybridization and multiplex ligation-dependent probe amplification study. *J Pathol* 2012; 227(1): 8–16.

106. Robinson, D. R., Wu, Y. M., Vats, P., Su, F., Lonigro, R. J., Cao, X. *et al.* Activating ESR1 mutations in hormone-resistant metastatic breast cancer. *Nat Genet* 2013; 45: 1446–51.

107. Toy, W., Shen, Y., Won, H., Green, B., Sakr, R. A., Will, M. *et al.* ESR1 ligand-binding domain mutations in hormone-resistant breast cancer. *Nat Genet* 2013; 45(12): 1439–45.

108. Huang, H. E., Chin, S. F., Ginestier, C., Bardou, V. J., Adelaide, J., Iyer, N. G. *et al.* A recurrent chromosome breakpoint in breast cancer at the NRG1/neuregulin 1/heregulin gene. *Cancer Res* 2004; 64(19): 6840–4.

109. Chua, Y. L., Ito, Y., Pole, J. C., Newman, S., Chin, S. F., Stein, R. C. *et al.* The NRG1 gene is frequently silenced by methylation in breast cancers and is a strong candidate for the 8p tumour suppressor gene. *Oncogene* 2009; 28(46): 4041–52.

110. Edwards, P. A. Fusion genes and chromosome translocations in the common epithelial cancers. *J Pathol* 2010; 220(2): 244–54.

111. Howarth, K. D., Blood, K. A., Ng, B. L., Beavis, J. C., Chua, Y., Cooke, S. L. *et al.* Array painting reveals a high frequency of balanced translocations in breast cancer cell lines that break in

cancer-relevant genes. *Oncogene* 2008; 27(23): 3345–59.

112. Vasudev, P. and Onuma, K. Secretory breast carcinoma: unique, triple-negative carcinoma with a favorable prognosis and characteristic molecular expression. *Arch Pathol Lab Med* 2011; 135(12): 1606–10.

113. Marchio, C., Weigelt, B. and Reis-Filho, J. S. Adenoid cystic carcinomas of the breast and salivary glands (or "The strange case of Dr Jekyll and Mr Hyde" of exocrine gland carcinomas). *J Clin Pathol* 2010; 63(3): 220–8.

114. Mikeska, T., Bock, C., Do, H. and Dobrovic, A. DNA methylation biomarkers in cancer: progress towards clinical implementation. *Expert Rev Mol Diagn* 2012; 12(5): 473–87.

115. Suijkerbuijk, K. P., van der Wall, E. and van Diest, P. J. Oxytocin: bringing magic into nipple aspiration. *Ann Oncol* 2007; 18(10): 1743–4.

116. Suijkerbuijk, K. P., van der Wall, E., Vooijs, M. and van Diest, P. J. Molecular analysis of nipple fluid for breast cancer screening. *Pathobiology* 2008; 75(2): 149–52.

117. Suijkerbuijk, K. P., van der Wall, E., Meijrink, H., Pan, X., Borel, R. Ausems, M. G. *et al.* Successful oxytocin-assisted nipple aspiration in women at increased risk for breast cancer. *Fam Cancer* 2010; 9(3): 321–5.

118. Fackler, M. J., Malone, K., Zhang, Z., Schilling, E., Garrett-Mayer, E., Swift-Scanlan, T. *et al.* Quantitative multiplex methylation-specific PCR analysis doubles detection of tumor cells in breast ductal fluid. *Clin Cancer Res* 2006; 12(11 Pt. 1): 3306–10.

119. Suijkerbuijk, K. P., Pan, X., van der Wall, E., van Diest, P. J. and Vooijs, M. Comparison of different promoter methylation assays in breast cancer. *Anal Cell*

*Pathol (Amst)* 2010; 33(3): 133–41.

120. Suijkerbuijk, K. P., Fackler, M. J., Sukumar, S., van Gils, C. H., van Laar, T., van der Wall, E. et al. Methylation is less abundant in BRCA1-associated compared with sporadic breast cancer. *Ann Oncol* 2008; 19(11): 1870–4.

121. Kloten, V., Becker, B., Winner, K., Schrauder, M. G., Fasching, P. A., Anzeneder, T. et al. Promoter hypermethylation of the tumor-suppressor genes ITIH5, DKK3, and RASSF1A as novel biomarkers for blood-based breast cancer screening. *Breast Cancer Res* 2013; 15(1): R4.

122. Xu, Z., Bolick, S. C., Deroo, L. A., Weinberg, C. R., Sandler, D. P. and Taylor, J. A. Epigenome-wide association study of breast cancer using prospectively collected sister study samples. *J Natl Cancer Inst* 2013; 105(10): 694–700.

123. Iwamoto, T., Yamamoto, N., Taguchi, T., Tamaki, Y. and Noguchi, S. BRCA1 promoter methylation in peripheral blood cells is associated with increased risk of breast cancer with BRCA1 promoter methylation. *Breast Cancer Res Treat* 2011; 129(1): 69–77.

124. Brennan, K., Garcia-Closas, M., Orr, N., Fletcher, O., Jones, M., Ashworth, A. et al. Intragenic ATM methylation in peripheral blood DNA as a biomarker of breast cancer risk. *Cancer Res* 2012; 72(9): 2304–13.

125. Sharma, G., Mirza, S., Parshad, R., Gupta, S. D. and Ralhan, R. DNA methylation of circulating DNA: a marker for monitoring efficacy of neoadjuvant chemotherapy in breast cancer patients. *Tumour Biol* 2012; 33(6): 1837–43.

126. Avraham, A., Uhlmann, R., Shperber, A., Birnbaum, M., Sandbank, J., Sella, A. et al. Serum DNA methylation for monitoring response to neoadjuvant chemotherapy in breast cancer

patients. *Int J Cancer* 2012; 131(7): E1166–72.

127. Lips, E. H., Mulder, L., Oonk, A., van der Kolk, L. E., Hogervorst, F. B., Imholz, A. L. et al. Triple-negative breast cancer: BRCAness and concordance of clinical features with BRCA1-mutation carriers. *Br J Cancer* 2013; 108(10): 2172–7.

128. Leidner, R. S., Li, L. and Thompson, C. L. Dampening enthusiasm for circulating microRNA in breast cancer. *PLoS ONE* 2013; 8(3): e57841.

129. Chen, X., Hu, Z., Wang, W., Ba, Y., Ma, L., Zhang, C. et al. Identification of ten serum microRNAs from a genome-wide serum microRNA expression profile as novel noninvasive biomarkers for non-small cell lung cancer diagnosis. *Int J Cancer* 2012; 130(7): 1620–8.

130. Garzon, R., Marcucci, G. and Croce, C. M. Targeting microRNAs in cancer: rationale, strategies and challenges. *Nat Rev Drug Discov* 2010; 9(10): 775–89.

131. Cittelly, D. M., Das, P. M., Salvo, V. A., Fonseca, J. P., Burow, M. E. and Jones, F. E. Oncogenic HER2 {Delta}16 suppresses miR-15a/16 and deregulates BCL-2 to promote endocrine resistance of breast tumors. *Carcinogenesis* 2010; 31(12): 2049–57.

132. Mei, M., Ren, Y., Zhou, X., Yuan, X. B., Han, L., Wang, G. X. et al. Downregulation of miR-21 enhances chemotherapeutic effect of taxol in breast carcinoma cells. *Technol Cancer Res Treat* 2010; 9(1): 77–86.

133. Marcus, J. N., Watson, P., Page, D. L., Narod, S. A., Lenoir, G. M., Tonin, P. et al. Hereditary breast cancer: pathobiology, prognosis, and BRCA1 and BRCA2 gene linkage. *Cancer* 1996; 77(4): 697–709.

134. Honrado, E., Osorio, A., Milne, R. L., Paz, M. F., Melchor, L., Cascon, A. et al.

Immunohistochemical classification of non-BRCA1/2 tumors identifies different groups that demonstrate the heterogeneity of BRCAX families. *Mod Pathol* 2007; 20(12): 1298–306.

135. Lakhani, S. R., Jacquemier, J., Sloane, J. P., Gusterson, B. A., Anderson, T. J., van de Vijver, M. J. et al. Multifactorial analysis of differences between sporadic breast cancers and cancers involving BRCA1 and BRCA2 mutations. *J Natl Cancer Inst* 1998; 90(15): 1138–45.

136. Armes, J. E., Egan, A. J., Southey, M. C., Dite, G. S., McCredie, M. R., Giles, G. G. et al. The histologic phenotypes of breast carcinoma occurring before age 40 years in women with and without BRCA1 or BRCA2 germline mutations: a population-based study. *Cancer* 1998; 83(11): 2335–45.

137. van der Groep, P., van der Wall, E. and van Diest, P. J. Pathology of hereditary breast cancer. *Cell Oncol (Dordr)* 2011; 34(2): 71–88.

138. van der Groep, P., van Diest, P. J., Menko, F. H., Bart, J., de Vries, E. G. and van der Wall, E. Molecular profile of ductal carcinoma in situ of the breast in BRCA1 and BRCA2 germline mutation carriers. *J Clin Pathol* 2009; 62(10): 926–30.

139. Ottini, L., Silvestri, V., Rizzolo, P., Falchetti, M., Zanna, I., Saieva, C. et al. Clinical and pathologic characteristics of BRCA-positive and BRCA-negative male breast cancer patients: results from a collaborative multicenter study in Italy. *Breast Cancer Res Treat* 2012; 134(1): 411–18.

140. Deb, S., Jene, N. and Fox, S. B. Genotypic and phenotypic analysis of familial male breast cancer shows under representation of the HER2 and basal subtypes in BRCA-associated carcinomas. *BMC Cancer* 2012; 12: 510.

141. Wasielewski, M., den Bakker, M. A., van den Ouweland, A., Meijer-van Gelder, M. E., Portengen, H., Klijn, J. G. *et al.* CHEK2 1100delC and male breast cancer in the Netherlands. *Breast Cancer Res Treat* 2009; 116(2): 397–400.

142. Melhem-Bertrandt, A., Bojadzieva, J., Ready, K. J., Obeid, E., Liu, D. D., Gutierrez-Barrera, A. M. *et al.* Early onset HER2-positive breast cancer is associated with germline TP53 mutations. *Cancer* 2012; 118(4): 908–13.

143. Wilson, J. R., Bateman, A. C., Hanson, H., An, Q., Evans, G., Rahman, N. *et al.* A novel HER2-positive breast cancer phenotype arising from germline TP53 mutations. *J Med Genet* 2010; 47(11): 771–4.

144. Balleine, R. L., Murali, R., Bilous, A. M., Farshid, G., Waring, P., Provan, P. *et al.* Histopathological features of breast cancer in carriers of ATM gene variants. *Histopathology* 2006; 49(5): 523–32.

145. Keller, G., Vogelsang, H., Becker, I., Hutter, J., Ott, K., Candidus, S. *et al.* Diffuse type gastric and lobular breast carcinoma in a familial gastric cancer patient with an E-cadherin germline mutation. *Am J Pathol* 1999; 155(2): 337–42.

146. Banneau, G., Guedj, M., MacGrogan, G., de Mascarel, I., Velasco, V., Schiappa, R. *et al.* Molecular apocrine differentiation is a common feature of breast cancer in patients with germline PTEN mutations. *Breast Cancer Res* 2010; 12(4): R63.

147. Huzarski, T., Cybulski, C., Jakubowska, A., Byrski, T., Gronwald, J., Domagala, P. *et al.* Clinical characteristics of breast cancer in patients with an NBS1 mutation. *Breast Cancer Res Treat* 2013; 141(3): 471–6.

148. Korde, L. A., Zujewski, J. A., Kamin, L., Giordano, S., Domchek, S., Anderson, W. F. *et al.* Multidisciplinary meeting on male breast cancer: summary and research recommendations. *J Clin Oncol* 2010; 28(12): 2114–22.

149. Thompson, D. and Easton, D. Variation in cancer risks, by mutation position, in BRCA2 mutation carriers. *Am J Hum Genet* 2001; 68(2): 410–19.

150. Tai, Y. C., Domchek, S., Parmigiani, G. and Chen, S. Breast cancer risk among male BRCA1 and BRCA2 mutation carriers. *J Natl Cancer Inst* 2007; 99(23): 1811–14.

151. Pinto, R., Pilato, B., Ottini, L., Lambo, R., Simone, G., Paradiso, A. *et al.* Different methylation and microRNA expression pattern in male and female familial breast cancer. *J Cell Physiol* 2013; 228(6): 1264–9.

152. Johansson, I., Nilsson, C., Berglund, P., Strand, C., Jonsson, G., Staaf, J. *et al.* High-resolution genomic profiling of male breast cancer reveals differences hidden behind the similarities with female breast cancer. *Breast Cancer Res Treat* 2011; 129(3): 747–60.

153. Anderson, W. F., Jatoi, I., Tse, J. and Rosenberg, P. S. Male breast cancer: a population-based comparison with female breast cancer. *J Clin Oncol* 2010; 28: 232–9.

154. Giordano, S. H., Cohen, D. S., Buzdar, A. U., Perkins, G. and Hortobagyi, G. N. Breast carcinoma in men: a population-based study. *Cancer* 2004; 101(1): 51–7.

155. Muir, D., Kanthan, R. and Kanthan, S. C. Male versus female breast cancers. A population-based comparative immunohistochemical analysis. *Arch Pathol Lab Med* 2003; 127(1): 36–41.

156. Kornegoor, R., Moelans, C. B., Verschuur-Maes, A. H., Hogenes, M. C., de Bruin, P. C., Oudejans, J. J. *et al.* Oncogene amplification in male breast cancer: analysis by multiplex ligation-dependent probe amplification. *Breast Cancer Res Treat* 2012; 135(1): 49–58.

157. Kornegoor, R., Verschuur-Maes, A. H., Buerger, H., Hogenes, M. C., de Bruin, P. C., Oudejans, J. J. *et al.* Molecular subtyping of male breast cancer by immunohistochemistry. *Mod Pathol* 2012; 25(3): 398–404.

158. Kornegoor, R., Verschuur-Maes, A. H., Buerger, H., Hogenes, M. C., de Bruin, P. C., Oudejans, J. J. *et al.* Immunophenotyping of male breast cancer. *Histopathology* 2012; 61(6): 1145–55.

159. Lacle, M. M., Kornegoor, R., Moelans, C. B., Maes-Verschuur, A. H., van der Pol, C., Witkamp, A. J. *et al.* Analysis of copy number changes on chromosome 16q in male breast cancer by multiplex ligation-dependent probe amplification. *Mod Pathol* 2013; 26(11): 1461–7.

160. Callari, M., Cappelletti, V., De Cecco, L., Musella, V., Miodini, P., Veneroni, S. *et al.* Gene expression analysis reveals a different transcriptomic landscape in female and male breast cancer. *Breast Cancer Res Treat* 2011; 127(3): 601–10.

161. Takagi, K., Moriya, T., Kurosumi, M., Oka, K., Miki, Y., Ebata, A. *et al.* Intratumoral estrogen concentration and expression of estrogen-induced genes in male breast carcinoma: comparison with female breast carcinoma. *Horm Cancer* 2013; 4(1): 1–11.

162. Kornegoor, R., Moelans, C. B., Verschuur-Maes, A. H., Hogenes, M. C., de Bruin, P. C., Oudejans, J. J. *et al.* Promoter hypermethylation in male breast cancer: analysis by multiplex ligation-dependent probe amplification. *Breast Cancer Res* 2012; 14(4): R101.

163. Lehmann, U., Streichert, T., Otto, B., Albat, C., Hasemeier, B., Christgen, H. *et al.* Identification

of differentially expressed microRNAs in human male breast cancer. *BMC Cancer* 2010; 10: 109.

164. Fassan, M., Baffa, R., Palazzo, J. P., Lloyd, J., Crosariol, M., Liu, C. G.

*et al.* MicroRNA expression profiling of male breast cancer. *Breast Cancer Res* 2009; 11(4): R58.

165. Costa, J., Gerhard, R., Rossi, E., Cirnes, L., Justino, A., Machado, J.

C. *et al.* Massive parallel sequencing to assess the mutational landscape of fine needle aspirate samples: a pilot study. *Lab Invest* 2013; 93: 87A.

# Chapter 12

# Tumors of the female genital system

Adhemar Longatto Filho, Sigurd F. Lax and Bin Yang

Tumors of the female genital tract system encompass a number of neoplasias of different origins that are in common in the anatomic region. Most of these tumors are now associated to persistent infections of human papillomavirus (HPV) and others related to varied conditions of complex molecular events that culminate in cancer progression. This chapter will be restricted to the principal molecular oncogenic alterations that induce the tumor development and has no intention of being a comprehensive overview of all interfaces related to the female genital tract cancers.

## Uterine cervical cancer

Uterine cervical cancer is importantly prevalent in developing countries with high indexes of mortality; developed countries that incorporated systematic and well-controlled programs of cancer control or have consistent opportunistic scenarios to screen women at risk, have low prevalence of invasive cancer and consequently a reduced number of mortality associated with cervical cancer development. The development of uterine cervical cancer is related to the persistent infection HPV. The natural history of cervical cancer development depends on essentially high-risk HPV biological behavior and the plethora of intricate molecular signaling pathways involved with cervical carcinogenesis. The following section will focus primarily on HPV characterization, the mechanisms related to the cervical cancer development and the role of HPV testing in cervical cancer screening.

## Human papillomavirus (HPV)

HPV contains approximately 8 kb double-stranded circular DNA genomes which are encapsulated by

capsid proteins and form 52 to 55 nm diameter viral particles. The genome of HPV is relatively stable since it has undergone relatively few changes in genetic composition over thousands of years cohabiting with humans. To date, more than 120 types of HPV have been discovered. HPV can be classified as either cutaneotropic or mucosotropic based on its characteristic tissue/organ tropism. Infections with cutaneotropic HPV types often do not cause symptoms or are not linked to human diseases. Most common cutaneotropic papillomavirus types include HPV 1, 2, 3, 4, 5, 8, 26, 27, 28, 41, 49 and 57. They are often associated with cutaneous plantar warts, verruciform epidermodysplasia and rarely with cutaneous neoplasms. Approximately 40 types of HPV have been linked to human mucosal infection, especially in the anogenital region. Most common mucosotropic papillomavirus types include HPV 6, 11, 30, 16, 18, 31, 33, 35, 39, 45, 51, 52, 56, 58, 59, 68 and 69. Traditionally, these HPV types are identified in benign and malignant anogenital tract lesions (1). Recently, these viral types have also been isolated in lesions of the oral cavity, oropharynx, larynx and esophagus. Mucosotropic HPV types are further classified as low-risk and high-risk malignant potential groups according to their ability to induce malignant transformation. Low-risk HPV types are typically involved in non-malignant and non-dysplastic lesions such as condyloma acuminatum in the vulva, vagina and perianal regions. HPV 6 and 11 are the prototypes of low-risk HPV. In contrast, high-risk strains are capable of inducing of malignant transformation and are also the most frequently seen types in human malignancies in different regions and ethnic populations worldwide (2). HPV 16 and 18 are the prototypes of high-risk HPV and are also the most virulent strains and most isolated HPV types in high-grade dysplasia and cancer. More than 50% of cervical squamous cell carcinomas harbor HPV16 and nearly 40% of cervical adenocarcinomas are associated with HPV 18 infection.

## Characteristics of HPV viral genome

Understanding HPV molecular characteristics will facilitate the comprehension of the pathways responsible for malignant transformation of infected cells and also the mechanisms behind HPV detection and vaccination. The genome of HPV virus is organized in three regions: the early genes, the late genes (Table 12.1) and a region called long control region (LCR) or upstream non-coding regulatory region (URR) (3). The early region has eight genes named E1 to E8. The E1 and E2 genes are responsible for DNA replication and transcription of HPV. The E3 gene transcribes an ubiquitin ligase which is involved in regulation of E6-AP induced p53 stability. The E4 gene is involved in maturation and release of viral particles. The E5 gene encodes a short transmembrane protein which is involved in modulating the activity of cellular proteins, such as PDGF and EGF. The E6 and E7 genes encode two viral oncoproteins which are involved directly in cell proliferation, transformation and immortalization. These proteins stimulate cell proliferation by interacting and suppressing the functions of two important tumor suppressor proteins – p53 and pRb. It is important to remember that only the E6/E7 proteins of high-risk HPVs, but not those of low-risk HPVs, are capable of immortalizing primary human keratinocytes (4). The E5, E6 and E7 proteins have become the targets for studying therapeutic HPV vaccines in treating those women who have already developed squamous dysplasia. The late region encodes a major (L1) and a minor (L2) capsid protein. The L1 gene is the most conserved among the HPV types. The L1 protein represents 80% of the viral capsid proteins and is the most abundant protein detected at the episomal stage, but gradually disappeared when the HPV genome is integrated into the host genome. The L1 capsid protein is highly immunogenic and is the main antigen utilized in producing HPV vaccine. The L2 protein, together with L1, contributes to the incorporation of viral DNA into the virion. The LCR region is between L1 and E6 and is not well conserved among the HPVs. The LCR or URR region is involved in the gene expression and viral replication that occurs in the nucleus of the host cell.

## Molecular basis of HPV-related tumorigenesis

HPVs are the causative agents for cervical cancer and pre-cancerous lesions. HPV infection in human tissue can be divided into two biological stages: the episomal stage and the integrated stage. Most of early and transient HPV infection stays at the episomal stage in which the virus forms circular viral particles coated with L1 and L2 capsid proteins. The episomal stage of HPV infection is usually seen in those women with normal cervical cytology, low-grade squamous intraepithelial lesions (LSIL), mild squamous dysplasia (CIN1) or in condyloma acuminatum. The initial HPV infection usually occurs at the basal layer cells at the transformational zone, usually associated with microtrauma. The circular viral particles are produced and released using host nucleic acid and protein synthesis apparatuses during the maturation process of the squamous epithelium. Due to the high number of HPV viral particles produced in the episomal state, women with low-grade lesions (LSIL/CIN1 or condyloma) are often highly contagious clinically. The good news is that most of these early and low-grade lesions can be reversed and even undergo spontaneous regression in most immune-competent individuals. Immunocompromised status

**Table 12.1** Principal characteristics of HPV genes

| HPV gene(s) | Function |
| --- | --- |
| E1 and E2 | DNA replication and transcription of HPV |
| E3 | Transcribes a ubiquitin ligase which is involved in the regulation of E6-AP induced p53 stability |
| E4 | Maturation and release of viral particles |
| E5 | Encodes a short transmembrane protein which is involved in modulating the activity of cellular proteins, such as PDGF and EGF |
| E6, and E7 | Encodes two viral oncoproteins that are directly involved in cell proliferation, transformation and immortalization |
| L1 and L2 | Contributes to the incorporation of viral DNA into the virion |

175

not only facilitates viral production and is widespread, seen in papillomatosis or condylomatosis, but is also vulnerable for viral integration and malignant transformation of the infected host cells.

The persistent HPV infection and/or immunocompromised state are often the prerequisite for viral DNA becoming integrated into the host genome. Once integrated, viral DNA will actively transcribe and translate E6 and E7, which are invariably expressed in HPV-positive cervical cancer cells (5). Expression of E6 and E7 oncoproteins are necessary for malignant transformation, and this is thought to be due to their ability to interrupt functions of two most important tumor suppressors, p53 and pRB, in host cells (Table 12.2). The E6 protein encoded by the high-risk type HPVs, such as HPV 16 and HPV 18, promotes cell proliferation by stimulating ubiquitin-dependent degradation of the tumor suppressor p53 protein via the formation of a trimeric complex comprising E6, p53 and E6-AP (6). The degradation of p53 protein mediated by E6 will compromise and perturb the control of cell cycle progression, leading finally to increased tumor cell growth. Importantly, E6 proteins of low-risk HPV 6 and 11 are unable to target p53 protein degradation, and therefore confer no or minimal malignant transformation potential. Although E6-induced loss of p53 protein is an important element of E6-induced cellular transformation, it is also clear that the E6 protein has oncogenic activities that are independent of p53,

such as involvement in telomere activation, DNA repair and apoptosis. The expression of E7 protein is necessary in HPV-induced tumorigenesis. The E7 protein binds to a region of the pRb protein and forms a trimeric protein complex of E7, pRb and E7-AP. It triggers the ubiquitin-dependent degradation of pRb protein (7). One of the major biochemical functions of pRb is to bind E2F-family transcription factors and repress the expressions of replication enzyme genes. The ability to repress the expressions of replication enzyme genes correlates with the tumor suppression function of pRb. E7 disrupts the interaction between pRb and E2F, resulting in the activation of E2F. This E7-mediated conversion of E2Fs to their activator forms stimulates replication and cell division, which is consistent with the observation that keratinocytes constitutively expressing E7 remain replication competent, even after differentiation (8). Therefore, complex formation between the products of oncogenes and tumor suppressor genes is believed to be important in the cellular transformation that leads to the disruption of the normal physiological functions of the specific tumor suppressor gene products. Like E6, E7 protein produced by HPV high-risk types binds pRb with a much higher affinity compared to those encoded by the low-risk HPV types. Recent studies suggest that E6 and E7 cooperate to effectively immortalize human primary epithelial cells. Although expression of E6 and E7 is itself not sufficient for cancer development, it seems to be either directly or indirectly involved in every stage of multistep carcinogenesis. Indeed, it has been shown that only one or two genetic alterations in addition to the expression of E6 and E7 are experimentally sufficient to confer tumorigenicity to normal human cervical keratinocytes.

A final HPV gene product that is important to mention in order to understand HPV-related tumorigenesis is the CDKN2A gene product, p16INK4A. This is a tumor suppressor protein that inhibits cyclin-dependent kinases CDK4 and CDK6, which phosphorylate the retinoblastoma (pRb) protein. A reciprocal association between p16INK4A and pRb expression has been found, suggesting the presence of a negative feedback loop that allows pRb to limit levels of p16 expression (9). In normal cells, the activity of CDK4 and CDK6 is tightly regulated by several cyclin-dependent kinase inhibitors, including p16INK4a. p16INK4a protein is inactivated in many

Table 12.2 Principal molecular pathways for cellular malignization induced by HPV

| HPV oncogene proteins | Function |
| --- | --- |
| E6 | Cell proliferation by stimulating ubiquitin-dependent degradation of the tumor suppressor p53 protein via the formation of a trimeric complex comprising E6, p53 and E6-AP |
| E7 | Binds to a region of the pRb protein and forms a trimeric protein complex of E7, pRb and E7-AP and triggers the ubiquitin-dependent degradation of pRb protein. pRb binds E2F-family transcription factors and represses the expressions of replication enzyme genes |

cancers through deletion or hypermethylation of the gene, resulting in reduced or absent expression of the p16INK4a protein. This leads to enhanced activity of CDK4 and CDK6 and consequently to premature phosphorylation and thus inactivation of pRB. In cells infected with HPV, particularly after HPV genome integrated into human cells, E6 and E7 oncoproteins are over-expressed, and pRB protein was reduced through the E7-induced ubiquitin-dependent protein degradation pathway (10). A low level of pRb in turn decreases the inhibitory efforts of p16 expression. p16INK4A can also be directly induced by the transcription factor E2F, which is released from the pRb protein after the binding of HPV E7. Based on the above molecular mechanism, over-expression of p16 in HPV-related squamous cells has been considered as a surrogate biomarker for HPV integration, viral oncoprotein expression and malignant transformation. Indeed, strong and diffuse p16INK4A expression has been immunohistochemically demonstrated in invasive cervical cancers and high-grade squamous dysplasia (11). It is now widely accepted that p16INK4A is a sensitive and specific surrogate biomarker of HPV-related high-grade squamous dysplasia. This is further reflected in the recently released Lower Anogenital Squamous Terminology (LAST) guidelines proposed jointly by the College of American Pathologists (CAP) and the American Society for Colposcopy and Cervical Pathology (ASCCP) (12). These guidelines recommend using p16 immunohistochemistry in facilitating accurate identification of high-grade intraepithelial neoplasia of the cervix, vulva and anus.

## Learning points

- Persistent high-risk HPV is a necessary, but not sufficient, cause of cervical cancer development.
- E6 and E7 HPV oncogenes have synergic activities for cervical carcinogenesis.
- E6 oncogene promotes cell proliferation by stimulating ubiquitin-dependent degradation of the tumor suppressor p53 protein.
- The expression of E7 protein is necessary in HPV-induced tumorigenesis.
- The E7 protein binds to a region of the pRb protein and forms a trimeric protein complex of E7. It triggers the ubiquitin-dependent degradation of pRb protein.

## Molecular tests for HPV for cervical cancer screening

Currently, most of the molecular steps of HPV-induced cancer have been used, or are intended to be used, in routine conditions, facilitating diagnoses and screening, and integrating basic research knowledge and medical assistance. What exactly have we learned about the combination of HPV testing and Pap test evaluation in the last 20 years? The HPV tests are more sensitive than cytology, and less specific. Contradictorily, for some authors, the HPV test is supposed to be more expensive and for others more cost beneficial. Has the HPV test really influenced the reduction of cytotechnologists' schools? Moreover, has the introduction of HPV tests caused a fall in the number of cytologists in the gynecological field? The arguments in this area are quite impressive and provoking, but are far from being in agreement.

We are positively convinced that many new novelties are improving the quality of morphological evaluation and offering opportunities to transform cytology in a new bridge between microscopy and molecular assays. The field of cytologists was gradually augmented, combining the computer-assisted screening and molecular evaluation of several players of cervical carcinogenesis (including the detection of human papillomavirus), and placing the cytologist in the spotlight, forcing him to live with old-fashioned remembrance, or seize historic opportunities and cross the Rubicon (13).

## The limits of cytology – the beginning of DNA analysis

Cytological examination presents important limitations, which include intense training of the cytotechnologists and cytopathologists (one or two years, or more), a limited number of slides examined daily (40 to 50? Perhaps even 70?) and a very stringent system for internal quality control of the diagnoses. The Pap test is indeed very expensive for countries with huge populations where the cervical cancer incidence is highly prevalent, because these countries need more human resources to justify the workload of 40 to 50 slides per day. Not surprisingly, the efficiency of the Pap test as a methodological tool for primary screening was more prominently observed in developed countries where the organizations of the screening programs were always superior to

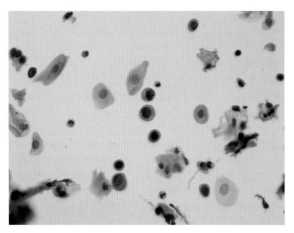

**Figure 12.1** Isolated dyskariotic cells morphologically representative of high-grade lesion (Papanicolaou, Surepath liquid-based cytology preparation, original magnification x20).

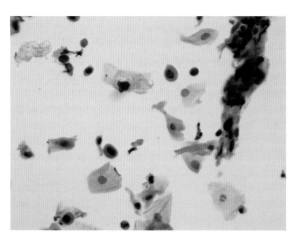

**Figure 12.2** Group of atypical dyskariotic cells and single cell characteristic of high-grade lesion (Papanicolaou, Surepath liquid-based cytology preparation, original magnification x20).

specificity. Taking into account the commercial options that exist for HPV testing, the principal goal is how to plan and implement an organizational system which can evaluate the best options to optimize the identification of women who must be selected for colposcopy examination and subsequent clinical conduction (15). There are official guidelines from different countries and continents that try to adjust their comprehension about the problem with the human and financial resources available to implement the best options with regard to their systems. Very briefly, cytology is still the recommended standard test for women, with screening taking place with three- or five-year intervals until the age of 60 for many countries. Stopping the screening in older women is probably appropriate among women who have had three or more consecutive (recent) normal cytology results. Several applications for HPV DNA detection have been proposed by European guidelines (15). They are: 1. primary screening for oncogenic HPV types alone or in combination with cytology; 2. triage of women with equivocal cytological results; and 3. follow-up of women treated for CIN to predict success or failure of treatment. HPV infections are very common and usually clear spontaneously. Detection of HPV DNA thus carries a risk of unnecessary colposcopies, psychological distress and possibly over-diagnosis. The need to perform CC screening in an organized program, rather than in an opportunistic setting, therefore applies particularly to screening based on HPV testing. However, as cytology examination necessitates well-structured laboratorial facilities and well-trained professionals, low-income countries do not reap similar benefits from cytology as developed countries.

## American societies' recommendations for cervical screening

Recently, the American Cancer Society, the American Society for Colposcopy and Cervical Pathology and the American Society for Clinical Pathology joined forces to make recommendations for cervical screening based on the accumulated information about the biological natural history of HPV-induced lesions, carcinogenic markers and new technologies for improvements in testing. Currently, HPV testing is acceptable as a co-test or the primary option for screening, but judiciously options should be considered as outlined below. The principal goal of the

developing countries, but public health authorities will probably criticize the huge amounts of money needed to maintain this strategy. The current option is to invest in primary screening based on HPV testing and for the positive cases evaluate the cytological preparation. This combination has been judiciously considered based on very robust data worldwide, and favors an early detection of CIN 2 or worse (Figures 12.1 and 12.2) (14).

The current concern is to define the strategy and what HPV tests are better to be used. The variety of HPV-DNA tests that can be performed is not really significant. All of the tests commercially available have similar sensitivity and specificity; however, RNA tests still lack sensitivity, despite the best screening is to avoid critical lesions developing, and the intervals between screening are calculated to result in the minimum probability of invasive cancer developing before the subsequent screen. Details of this important publication are freely available on the internet. A summary of the main points is provided below (15).

## Age for starting screening

The age for starting screening is critical for Public Health Authorities, since HPV infection is predominant in young women and most of the high-grade lesions are known to develop in women with persistent high-risk HPV. For this reason, screening for women under 21 years of age is not recommended.

## The periodicity for screening

Liquid-based cytology and conventional cytology are both accepted for organized or opportunistic screening programs. For women aged 21 to 29, only cytology is recommended, with 3-year intervals. HPV testing alone or in combination with cytology is not endorsed for these women. For women aged 30 to 65, the combination of a Pap test and HPV testing every five years is desired; however, the use of Pap testing alone every three years is also suitable. Women older than 65 years of age should continue screening only in cases of high-grade lesion (or invasive cancer) history (20 years after the treatment); no screening is recommended for women who have undergone a hysterectomy (no cervix) and who have no high-grade lesion (or invasive cancer) history in the previous 20 years (15).

## The use of ancillary techniques for screening

Recently, additional techniques were developed in order to improve the quality of cytological examination. Among several proposals, immunocytochemical reaction using p16 protein has been qualified as one of the most promising tools to determine lesions with the potential for progression and to differentiate abnormal, non-intraepithelial lesions from real lesions with a dubious appearance. The participation of p16 in HPV-induced carcinogenesis, as explained previously, is the rationale behind its use in daily routine. The use of biomarkers as p16 enhanced the positive predictive value of cervical screening results, mainly when associated with the Ki-67 double staining (CINtec, mtm laboratories AG, Heidelberg, Germany). As a marker of cell-cycle activity, Ki-67 has importantly improved the performance of p16 staining. Similarly, BD ProEx C (BD Diagnostics, Burlington, NC, USA) was developed to reduce diagnoses of uncertain significance. Antibodies against two proteins were associated in ProExC: nuclear proteins minichromosome maintenance protein 2 (MCM 2) and topoisomerase II alpha (TOP2A), which were identified as accumulating in cells transformed by high-risk HPV. BD ProEx C is intensely augmented as a consequence of the aberrant S-phase induced by HPV E7 protein in a number of intraepithelial and invasive lesions of the cervix (16).

## Learning points

- Cytology has low sensitivity, but high specificity to detect HSIL.
- HPV testing has high sensitivity, but lower specificity to detect HSIL.
- HPV testing is suggested for screening in women aged 30 and older.
- P16 and ProExC are two ancillary markers to enhance the detection of HSIL.

## Endometrial carcinoma

### Histopathological classification of endometrial carcinoma

The recently published WHO classification of tumors of the female reproductive organs distinguishes between several histologically and biologically distinctive types (Table 12.3) (17). The most frequent type is endometrioid carcinoma, which resembles in its well-differentiated, glandular appearance proliferative phase endometrium. The neoplastic glands consist of strongly cohesive columnar cells and show well-defined luminal borders. They may be admixed with solid non-squamous areas, which account for less than 5% of tumoral tissue in grade 1, 5% to 50% in grade 2 and greater than 50% in grade 3 endometrioid carcinomas. A subset of endometrioid carcinomas shows a variety of squamous, secretory and mucinous as well as ciliated cell differentiation. Pure mucinous carcinoma is defined by a mucinous differentiation of more than 50% of the tumor. Serous carcinoma is characterized by a discrepancy between a well-differentiated papillary or glandular architecture and a high degree of nuclear atypia. Since serous carcinomas may also show a solid pattern, the term

**179**

"serous papillary carcinoma" should definitely be avoided. There is a strong phenotypical resemblance to high-grade serous carcinoma of the ovary. Distinctive cytological features define clear cell carcinoma, in particular, polygonal- or hobnail-shaped cells with either clear or eosinophilic cytoplasm, and may reveal a solid, tubulo-cystic or papillary architecture. Serous and clear cell carcinomas are characterized by high-grade nuclear atypia and particularly serous carcinoma by frequent mitosis.

**Table 12.3** 2013 WHO classification of endometrial carcinoma (18)

### Histological type

Endometrioid carcinoma, usual type

Endometrioid carcinoma, variants (with squamous differentiation, secretory, ciliated type, villoglandular)

Mucinous carcinoma

Serous endometrial intraepithelial carcinoma

Serous carcinoma

Clear cell carcinoma

Undifferentiated carcinoma

Neuroendocrine carcinoma

Mixed carcinomas

Undifferentiated carcinoma is rare and consists of two subtypes – monomorphic undifferentiated carcinoma, which lack any differentiation, and dedifferentiated carcinoma. The latter is characterized by a collision of a usually smaller well- or moderately-differentiated component and a larger undifferentiated component. There may be some overlap between undifferentiated and poorly differentiated neuroendocrine carcinoma. The neuroendocrine tumors and carcinomas, respectively, have been newly categorized according to the proposal of the EURONET group for the gastrointestinal tract (19). The problem is that most tumors are very rare and there is very little if any evidence for this classification in the literature.

### A current model for endometrial tumorigenesis

Currently, endometrial carcinoma is considered to develop along two different pathways, one driven by estrogens, the other unrelated to estrogen (Table 12.4) (20). This model is based on clinico-pathological observations and originally goes back to Jan Bokhman, but was later developed particularly by Sherman *et al.* (21). By its ability to stimulate growth of the endometrium, estrogen is considered an important co-factor for the development of the vast majority of endometrial neoplasms. However, a subset of endometrial carcinoma develops through an estrogen-independent pathway driven by so far unknown tumorigenic factors.

**Table 12.4** Dualistic model of endometrial carcinoma

|  | Type I carcinoma | Type II carcinoma |
| --- | --- | --- |
| **Adjacent endometrium** | Frequently hyperplastic | Atrophic/inactive |
| **Uterine size** | Enlarged | Small |
| **Patient's age** | Peri-/postmenopausal (55–65) | Postmenopausal (70) |
| **Tumor stage at diagnosis** | Low (mostly stage I) | High (frequent stage III) |
| **Prognosis** | Favorable | Poor |
| **Serum hormone level** | Elevated | Normal |
| **Histological types** | Endometrioid and variants | Serous, clear cell |
| **ER, PR** | High | Low/intermediate or negative |
| **Genes involved** | KRAS, PTEN, CTNNB1, FGFR2 | TP53, cyclin E, PIK3CA |
| **Types of genetic alteration** | Low LOH and SCNA, MSI, frequent nucleotide changes | Frequent LOH and SCNA |
| **Molecular subtype (TCGA)** | Ultra-, hypermutated, MSI | Serous-like |

Endometrial carcinomas with association to estrogens are also designated type I carcinomas. They mostly develop from atypical endometrial hyperplasia (AEH) in a non-atrophic uterus at a median age of about 60 to 65 years. AEH, which was recently also designated as endometrioid intraepithelial neoplasia (EIN), is considered to be the immediate precursor lesion of type I carcinomas (17). AEH/EIN may occur superimposed on endometrial hyperplasia without atypia or within inactive endometrium. Type I carcinomas are mostly of usual endometrioid types or variants, rarely of mucinous type. Histopathological grade is typically low, either grade 1 or grade 2, and only about 10% to 20% are high grade. In particular, low-grade type I carcinomas frequently express estrogen and progesterone receptors, a characteristic which is decreased in high-grade carcinomas (22). In addition, most type I carcinomas are diagnosed at stages I or II and show a favorable clinical course.

In contrast, type II endometrial carcinomas arise within atrophic endometrium and a small uterus. They typically occur at a median age of about 65 to 75 years, which is five to ten years later than type I tumors. Histologically, type II carcinomas are of serous or clear cell type or are undifferentiated carcinomas, high grade (grade 3) by definition and frequently diagnosed at the advanced stage. Estrogen and progesterone receptor expression is usually low or absent. Thus, they are considered to be unrelated to estrogen.

This dualistic model has been widely accepted, but at the same time intensely criticized, particularly for its simplistic approach. However, it seems to be a practically useful and easily understandable model both for clinical work and research. In addition, during the last two decades, molecular studies did consider this pathogenetic model and linked molecular genetic findings to it.

## Molecular tumorigenesis of endometrial carcinoma based on the proposed model

It is more or less well established that type I and type II carcinomas develop through distinct molecular genetic pathways (23). For type I carcinoma, the molecular changes of endometrioid carcinoma and its variants have been extensively studied, whereas most investigations on type II carcinoma focused on serous carcinoma. Endometrioid carcinoma seems to develop stepwise from its precursor lesion atypical endometrial hyperplasia/endometrioid intraepithelial neoplasia (AEH/EIN) and progress into well-differentiated endometrioid and subsequently into moderately and poorly differentiated carcinoma (24). This tumor progression is accompanied by various molecular genetic alterations, similar to the usual colorectal adenocarcinoma. So far, a sequential model has been favored for the molecular pathogenesis of the adenoma-carcinoma sequence based on the interpretation of an established model for colorectal carcinoma. A sequential theory would propose that driver mutations occur at different steps of tumor development. In contrast, driver mutations may occur early in tumor development and remain stable during tumor progression (25). This so-called "big bang model" has recently been favored for colorectal tumorigenesis (26). Thus, this hypothesis may be applied for type I endometrial carcinoma, but, so far, is not well established. In contrast, type II carcinomas seem to arise "de novo" from flat, highly atypical lesions that are designated as intraepithelial carcinoma. Therefore, in type II carcinomas, the "big bang" clearly occurs at an early stage.

Type I and type II carcinomas are characterized by different molecular genetic alterations, most of which are statistically significant. The most important genetic alterations are listed in Table 12.5. For endometrioid carcinoma and its variants, several key molecular alterations are well known and may be considered as driver mutations. In fact, the most frequent genetic alterations in endometrioid carcinoma involve the genes PTEN and ß-catenin. PTEN is a putative tumor gene that encodes for a cytoplasmic protein involved in several important cell functions such as proliferation, growth and survival of the cell. It is crucially involved in the PI3K pathway by antagonizing PIK3CA (27–29). Alterations of PTEN caused by mutation, allelic loss or promoter methylation lead to a loss of the protein expression and occur in about 50% of type I carcinomas (30, 31). Loss of PTEN is frequently associated with a mutator phenotype which is found in about 25% to 40% of type I carcinomas (15). Loss of PTEN is an early event that is found in about 50% of AEH and seems to be associated with progression into endometrioid adenocarcinoma (32, 33). In addition to alteration and loss of PTEN, Pax-2 – a nuclear transcription factor – seems to be involved in endometrial tumorigenesis, since it is lost in up to 80% of AEH and endometrioid adenocarcinomas, respectively (34). Another important genetic alteration of type I

**Table 12.5** Type I and type II endometrial carcinomas are characterized by distinctive molecular genetic alterations

| Genetic alteration | Type I carcinomas | Type II carcinomas |
|---|---|---|
| Genomic disorder | Minor | Major (frequent LOH, SCNA) |
| Microsatellite instability | 20–40% | 0–5% |
| Single nucleotide changes | Frequent in a subset | Most likely absent |
| ß-catenin mutations | 25–40% | 0<5% |
| PTEN inactivation | 35–50% | 10% |
| KRAS mutation | 15–30% | <5% |
| PIK3CA mutation | 15–40% | 25% |
| P53 mutation | 5–10% (30% in G3) | 90% |
| Her2/neu amplification | 30% | <5% |
| e-cadherin inactivation | 10–20% | 80–90% |

carcinomas relates to mutations of the ß-catenin (CTNNB1) gene, which is part of the e-cadherin-catenin unit and, therefore, important for cell differentiation and maintenance of normal cell architecture. CTNNB1 mutations typically within exon 3 occur in about 14% to 44% of type I carcinomas and lead to stabilization and nuclear accumulation of the protein (35). CTNNB1 mutations are frequently found in AEH with squamous metaplasia and thus seem to be an early event in endometrial tumorigenesis (36). In addition, the fibroblast growth factor (FGF) pathway seems to be altered in a subset of endometrioid carcinoma by either inactivation of the negative regulator SPRY-2 (in about 20% of type I carcinomas) or FGFR2 mutations (in 6% to 12% of type I carcinomas), which occur mutually exclusively with KRAS mutations (37).

KRAS mutations were detected in about 25% to 30% of AEH, but also in grade 2 and 3 endometrioid carcinomas (38). Alterations of the mismatch repair system leading to a mutator phenotype

with microsatellite instability were found in 25% to 40% of endometrioid carcinomas (15, 39). Microsatellite instability in endometrioid carcinoma is most frequently caused by methylation of the MLH1 promoter, followed by mutations of MSH2 and MSH6. Whereas the former alteration is only present in the tumor, the latter is usually also found in the germline. TP53 mutations were found mostly in grade 3 endometrioid carcinomas and, thus, have been considered as a late event during tumor development (38). However, it remains to be unraveled whether p53 mutations may occur early, for example, in AEH, and lead to the rapid development of a grade 3 carcinoma.

TP53 mutation is definitely the most frequent molecular alteration of type II carcinomas, in particular as regards serous carcinomas, and is associated with a severe degree of genomic instability (40). Further important molecular genetic alterations of type II/ serous carcinoma involve the e-cadherin gene with mutations and reduced protein expression, her2/neu with amplification and over-expression, p16 with deregulation and over-expression, and genes involved in the regulation of the mitotic spindle checkpoint (STK15) (3, 41, 42). However, a mutator phenotype is very rare in serous carcinoma of the endometrium (43). Recently detected alterations of the genes PIK3CA, FBXW7 and PPP2R1A involve about 20% uterine serous carcinoma (44). In particular, PIK3CA, a counterpart of PTEN, is altered in both endometrioid and serous carcinoma, but exon 20 m-RNA over-expression due to amplification or mutation is only found in high-grade carcinoma, of which a subset may show a mixed endometrioid and serous histology. Serous intraepithelial carcinoma (SEIC), representing the earliest stage of serous carcinoma, harbors mutant TP53 partially with retained wild-type allele. Recently, over-expression of cyclin E due to amplification of the CCNE1 gene was detected in SEIC and invasive serous carcinoma. Alternatively, the activation of cyclin E may be caused by the mutation of FBXW7 (45).

Only a few studies focused on clear cell carcinoma of the endometrium and revealed molecular changes similar both to high-grade endometrioid carcinoma and serous carcinoma. In particular, less than 10% of clear cell carcinomas harbor microsatellite instability and mutation of KRAS and PTEN, whereas about 30% reveal TP53 mutations (46). Mutations of the ARID1A (BAT250a) gene, which are frequently present in clear cell and endometrioid carcinomas of the ovary, were found both in low-grade and high-grade endometrioid carcinoma, as well as clear cell carcinoma of the endometrium and, therefore, seem to be associated both with the type I and type II pathways (47, 48).

The Cancer Genome Atlas (TCGA) Research Network found a correlation between the outcome of endometrial carcinoma and the frequency of somatic copy-number alterations (SCNA) (49). The combination between somatic nucleotide substitutions, microsatellite instability (MSI) and SCNA led to the stratification of endometrial carcinoma into four distinctive prognostic groups: 1. an ultra-mutated group with an unusually high number of mutations, stable microsatellites and low SCNA with excellent prognosis; 2. a hypermutated group of tumors with MSI mostly by methylated MLH1 promoter; 3. a group of mostly endometrioid carcinomas with stable microsatellites and a low mutation rate, both with intermediate outcome; and 4. a group of serous-like cancers with a high number of SCNA, but low mutation rate and poor prognosis. The ultra-mutated group was characterized by mutations in the exonuclease domain of POLE, which is a catalytic subunit of DNA polymerase epsilon and is involved in nuclear DNA replication and repair. The MSI group showed mutations among others in KRAS and less frequently in CTNNB1. Interestingly, a coincidence of non-silent TP53 and PTEN mutations, which is considered a distinctive molecular pathway, was found in a subset of endometrioid carcinomas.

This very recent development and progress in endometrial cancer research has the potential to usher in new therapeutic perspectives. In addition to a prognostic stratification, contemporary and future molecular techniques will be able to unravel effective therapeutic targets, in particular for highly aggressive cancer types. It remains to be clarified whether targeted therapy is able to effectively fight the broad spectrum of genetic alterations that accompanies the enormous clonal evolution within aggressive carcinomas. With regard to pathogenesis, it is interesting that the recently developed high throughput methods mostly confirm older data detected by single gene analyses. Moreover, the results of modern molecular research will continuously transform our histological tumor classification in molecular-based classifications by integrating the geno- and phenotype of the tumor.

## Learning points

- Type I and type II endometrial carcinomas have a favorable and unfavorable clinical outcome, respectively.
- Peritumoral endometrium in type I carcinoma is frequently hyperplastic and type 2 is atrophic.
- Type II carcinoma is more frequent in postmenopausal women.
- P53 mutation and e-cadherin inaction is highly frequent in type II carcinoma.
- Microsatellite instability, single nucleotide changes and ß-catenin mutations are highly frequent in type I carcinoma, but not in type II.

## Ovary and fallopian tube tumors

Ovarian cancer is moderately prevalent for women worldwide, oscillating from 6 to 9 cases in 100,000 women, and is highest in high-resource countries (9.3 per 100,000 women) (50). The vast majority of ovarian cancers are carcinomas, which are divided into high-grade serous carcinomas and low-grade serous carcinomas; endometrioid carcinomas; mucinous carcinomas and clear cell carcinomas. These cancers have different natural histories of development and origin, which demands accurate identification of these tumors to optimize the potential treatment of them; relevant but infrequent, the ovarian types (around 3%) also include the germ cell tumors, dysgerminomas, yolk sac tumors and teratomas sex cord-stromal tumors.

A number of genetic and molecular alterations recently described have been offering a remarkable opportunity to study ovarian cancers through different perspectives for these very complex tumors in women that, despite lesser frequency in comparison with breast and uterine cervix cancer, have very high rates of mortality (50). These molecular alterations supported the classification of ovarian tumors in two distinct types: type I and type II, as described below (51) (Table 12.6). However, the origin of ovarian tumors is still controversial and the risk factors currently associated with ovarian malignancy do not clarify sufficiently the cascade of events that leads to cancer development. A reduced number of ovulation cycles during a woman's lifetime is supposedly associated with a lower risk of ovarian cancer development. Continued replication, in this case, is supposed to favor DNA alterations and mutations.

**183**

**Table 12.6** Main characteristics of types I and II ovarian carcinomas

| Characteristics | Ovarian carcinoma types | |
| --- | --- | --- |
| | Type I | Type II |
| Histopathology classification | Low-grade serous, mucinous, endometrioid, clear cell and transitional cell carcinomas | High-grade serous carcinomas and undifferentiated carcinomas |
| Genetic | PTEN, PIK3CA, KRAS, BRAF and b-catenin mutations. | TP53 mutations and BRCA 1/2 gene alterations, hypermethylations |
| Clinical outcome | Indolent | Highly aggressive |

However, women with polycystic syndrome of the ovaries have an augmented risk of developing ovarian cancer and have reduced ovulatory cycles, which contradict in part this hypothesis.

Based on the histopathological and molecular characteristics, type I tumors comprise low-grade serous, mucinous, endometrioid, clear cell and transitional cell carcinomas, while type II tumors comprise high-grade serous carcinomas and undifferentiated carcinomas. Clinically, type I tumors have an indolent behavior and are supposedly part of a biological continuum from benign tumors that later progress to borderline lesions and invasive tumors. On the other hand, type II tumors have a more aggressive behavior, and result in more pronounced genetic alterations.

## Ovarian cancer genetic alterations
### High- and low-grade serous carcinomas

High-grade serous carcinomas are associated with TP53 mutations and BRCA gene alterations; conversely, low-grade serous carcinomas are more frequently associated with KRAS and BRAF mutations. Interestingly, both are currently believed to originate from the fallopian tube precursor epithelium and/or lesions (51). Indeed, the TP53 mutation is very common in all ovarian carcinomas. Most high-grade serous carcinomas stain positively for an immunohistochemical reaction for p53, BRCA1, WT1 and p16, with constant Ki-67 high index. The hereditary variant of ovarian carcinomas represents circa 15% of all cases and has very high penetrance regarding not only BRCA1 (risk of 40% to 50% during the lifetime of women who have the mutation), but also BRCA2 (the risk of developing ovary carcinoma is 20% to 30% for women with the mutation), since they are associated with 90% of all ovarian carcinomas of hereditary origin. Additionally, estrogen receptor (ER) stains high-grade carcinomas in circa 70% of all cases. Interestingly, the low-grade carcinomas have quite similar immunohistochemical patterns, except for Ki-67, which stained a significantly lower number of cells than the high-grade counterpart.

### Endometrioid carcinomas

A proportion of the endometrioid carcinomas are originated from the ovarian atypical endometriosis. Relevant evidence associates similar genetic alteration in ovarian endometrioid carcinoma associated with endometriosis. PTEN inactivation, for example, is believed to be associated with endometrial carcinoma development in these cases. The ARID1A (AT-rich interactive domain 1A) gene mutation was recognized in ovarian cancer associated with the endometriosis. Endometrioid carcinomas positively react with vimentin, cytokeratins 7 and 20, EMA, estrogen and progesterone receptors.

## Mucinous carcinoma

Mucinous carcinoma has a non-identified origin. Its name indicates that its appearance generally resembles gastrointestinal differentiation. Not surprisingly, these tumors have the expression of CDX2 and KRAS, which are usually expressed in intestinal differentiation. Of note, KRAS mutation is frequently found in mucinous ovarian cancer type, and is sometimes associated with the TP53 mutation (51). Mucinous carcinomas mostly stain for cytokeratin 7 (strongly) and keratin 20 (weakly). Furthermore, nuclear-positive immune-stain for CDX-2, a homeobox gene necessary for intestinal organogenesis, can be observed.

## Clear cell ovarian carcinoma

Finally, the clear cell ovarian carcinoma is also associated with the endometriosis and ARID1A mutations, and Hepatocyte nuclear factor-1beta up-regulation. Clear cell carcinoma is immunohisto-chemically positive for Hepatocyte nuclear factors Beta, but consistently negative for WT1 and estrogen receptor.

## The role of homeobox genes in ovarian carcinogenesis

The different ovarian carcinomas re-express abnormally the homeobox (Hox) genes expressed during embryological development. HOXA9, for example, is expressed in the fallopian tube and serous ovarian cancer (52). Recently, Toss and colleagues reported a very interesting revision of molecular state-of-the-art ovarian carcinomas. According to the status of knowledge of ovarian cancer, the genetic profile of these tumors allows the identification of two groups based on genetic alterations; however, not everyone agrees about this division (50). The type I ovarian cancers include low-grade and borderline serous cancers, endometrioid, mucinous and clear cell cancers, and are frequently characterized with PTEN, PIK3CA, KRAS, BRAF and b-catenin mutations, with infrequent genomic stability and TP53 mutations as anticipated. The type II ovarian cancers comprise high-grade serous carcinomas, mixed malignant mesodermal tumors, carcinosarcomas and undifferentiated cancers. Different from type I, these neoplasias are frequently associated with TP53 mutations and accentuated genomic instability and most of them emerge from the fallopian tubes and the peritoneum and in cases where BRCA1 and BRCA2 mutation have occurred (52).

The familial history of ovarian cancer is a powerful risk factor for ovarian cancer development. Mutations in BRCA1 and BRCA2 are also associated with an augmented risk of ovarian cancer.

In additional, hereditary ovarian cancers are linked to the Lynch syndrome, which is associated with several carcinomas, including colorectal, endometrial and ovarian (52).

## Fallopian tube tumors

Tumors arising primarily from the fallopian tubes are infrequent. Benign tumor originate from the sub-serosal area and are named adenomatoid tumors. Tubal adenocarcinomas are rare and currently their origin is associated with the BRCA germline mutation (53). The pivotal role of fallopian tube secretory cells in ovarian carcinoma indicates that the fallopian tubes can be at the center of further studies intending to address the origins of ovarian carcinoma and also the potential targets for specific therapies involving the connection ovary tubes. Recent evidence demonstrated that high-grade serous tumors of the ovaries originate from fallopian tubal secretory epithelial cells; moreover, serous tubal intraepithelial carcinoma have been defined as the precursor to high-grade serous ovarian and peritoneal carcinomas in animal models involving the genes BRCA (1 and 2), Tp53 and Pten. Interestingly, experimental model Tp53-/-Pten-/-do not develop high-grade ovarian cancer (53).

## Learning points

- Type I ovarian carcinoma is clinically indolent.
- Type II ovarian carcinoma is clinically aggressive.
- Type II ovarian carcinoma is frequently associated with TP53 mutations and BRCA 1/2 gene alterations.
- Type I ovarian carcinoma is more frequently associated with KRAS and BRAF mutations.

## References

1. Munoz, N., Bosch, F. X., de Sanjose, S., Herrero, R., Castellsague, X., Shah, K.V. *et al.* Epidemiologic classification of human papillomavirus types associated with cervical cancer. *New Engl J Med* 2003; 348(6): 518–27.

2. Schiffman, M. H., Bauer, H. M., Hoover, R. N., Glass, A. G., Cadell, D. M., Rush, B. B. *et al.*

Epidemiologic evidence showing that human papillomavirus infection causes most cervical intraepithelial neoplasia. *J Natl Cancer Inst* 1993; 85(12): 958–64.

3. zur Hausen, H. and de Villiers, E. M. Human papillomaviruses. *Annu Rev Microbiol* 1994; 48: 427–47.

4. Klingelhutz, A. J. and Roman, A. Cellular transformation by human

papillomaviruses: lessons learned by comparing high- and low-risk viruses. *Virology* 2012; 424(2): 77–98.

5. Wentzensen, N., Vinokurova, S. and von Knebel Doeberitz, M. Systematic review of genomic integration sites of human papillomavirus genomes in epithelial dysplasia and invasive cancer of the female lower genital tract. *Cancer Res* 2004; 64(11): 3878–84.

6. Wise-Draper, T. M. and Wells, S. I. Papillomavirus E6 and E7 proteins and their cellular targets. *Front Biosci* 2008; 13: 1003–17.

7. Munger, K. and Phelps, W. C. The human papillomavirus E7 protein as a transforming and transactivating factor. *Biochim Biophys Acta* 1993; 1155(1): 111–23.

8. Liu, X., Clements, A., Zhao, K. and Marmorstein, R. Structure of the human Papillomavirus E7 oncoprotein and its mechanism for inactivation of the retinoblastoma tumor suppressor. *J Biol Chem* 2006; 281(1): 578–86.

9. Sano, T., Oyama, T., Kashiwabara, K., Fukuda, T. and Nakajima, T. Expression status of p16 protein is associated with human papillomavirus oncogenic potential in cervical and genital lesions. *Am J Pathol* 1998; 153(6): 1741–8.

10. Sano, T., Oyama, T., Kashiwabara, K., Fukuda, T. and Nakajima, T. Immunohistochemical overexpression of p16 protein associated with intact retinoblastoma protein expression in cervical cancer and cervical intraepithelial neoplasia. *Pathol Int* 1998; 48(8): 580–5.

11. Agoff, S. N., Lin, P., Morihara, J., Mao, C., Kiviat, N. B. and Koutsky, L. A. p16(INK4a) expression correlates with degree of cervical neoplasia: a comparison with Ki-67 expression and detection of high-risk HPV types. *Mod Pathol* 2003; 16(7): 665–73.

12. Darragh, T. M., Colgan, T. J., Cox, J. T., Heller, D. S., Henry, M. R. and Luff, R. D. *et al.* The lower anogenital squamous terminology standardization project for HPV-associated lesions: background and consensus recommendations from the College of American Pathologists and the American Society for Colposcopy and Cervical Pathology. *J Low Genit Tract Dis* 2012; 16(3): 205–42.

13. Longatto-Filho, A. and Schmitt, F. C. Cytology education in the 21st century: living in the past or crossing the Rubicon? *Acta Cytol* 2010; 54(4): 654–6.

14. Arbyn, M., Anttila, A., Jordan, J., Ronco, G., Schenck, U., Segnan, N. *et al.* (eds.), *European Guidelines for Quality Assurance in Cervical Cancer Screening*, 2nd edn (City of Luxembourg, Grand Duchy of Luxembourg: Office for Official Publications of the European Communities, 2008).

15. Saslow, D., Solomon, D., Herschel, W., Killackey, M., Kulasingam, S., Cain, J., Garcia, F. A. R. *et al.* ACS-ASCCP-ASCP Cervical Cancer Guideline Committee. American Cancer Society, American Society for Colposcopy and Cervical Pathology, and American Society for Clinical Pathology screening guidelines for the prevention and early detection of cervical cancer. *CA Cancer J Clin* 2012; 62(3): 147–72.

16. Brown, C. A., Bogers, J., S. Sahebali, Depuydt, C. E., De Prins, F. and Malinowski, D. P. *et al.* Role of protein biomarkers in the detection of high-grade disease in cervical cancer screening programs. *J Oncol* 2012; 2012:289315.

17. Carcangiu, M. L., Herrington, S., Kurman, R. J. and Young, R. H. (eds.), *Tumours of the Female Genital Organs* (Lyon: IARC Press, 2014).

18. Conklin, C. M. and Longacre, T. A. Endometrial stromal tumors: the new WHO classification. *Adv Anat Pathol* 2014; 21(6): 383–93.

19. Kloppel, G., Couvelard, A., Perren, A., Komminoth, P., McNicol, A. M., Nilsson, O. *et al.* ENETS Consensus Guidelines for the Standards of Care in Neuroendocrine Tumors: towards a standardized approach to the diagnosis of gastroenteropancreatic neuroendocrine tumors and their prognostic stratification. *Neuroendocrinology* 2009; 90(2): 162–6.

20. Lax, S. F. Molecular genetic pathways in various types of endometrial carcinoma: from a phenotypical to a molecular-based classification. *Virchows Arch* 2004; 444(3): 213–23.

21. Sherman, M. E., Bur, M. E. and Kurman, R. J. p53 in endometrial cancer and its putative precursors: evidence for diverse pathways of tumorigenesis. *Hum Pathol* 1995; 26(11): 1268–74.

22. Lax, S. F., Pizer, E. S., Ronnett, B. M. and Kurman, R. J. Clear cell carcinoma of the endometrium is characterized by a distinctive profile of p53, Ki-67, estrogen, and progesterone receptor expression. *Hum Pathol* 1998; 29(6): 551–8.

23. Lax, S. F. Molecular genetic changes in epithelial, stromal and mixed neoplasms of the endometrium. *Pathology* 2007; 39(1): 46–54.

24. Kurman, R. J., Ellenson, L. H. and Ronnett, B. M. (eds.), *Blaustein's Pathology of the Female Genital Tract*, 6th edn. (New York: Springer Verlag, 2011).

25. Bozic, I., Antal, T., Ohtsuki, H., Carter, H., Kim, D., Chen, S. *et al.* Accumulation of driver and passenger mutations during tumor progression. *Proc Natl Acad Sci USA* 2010; 107(43): 18545–50.

26. Humphries, A., Cereser, B., Gay, L. J., Miller, D. S., Das, B., Gutteridge, A. *et al.* Lineage tracing reveals multipotent stem cells maintain human adenomas and the pattern of clonal expansion in tumor evolution. *Proc Natl Acad Sci USA* 2013; 110(27): E2490–9.

27. Baker, S. J. PTEN enters the nuclear age. *Cell* 2007; 128(1): 25–8.

28. Chow, L. M. and Baker, S. J. PTEN function in normal and neoplastic growth. *Cancer Lett* 2006; 241(2): 184–96.

29. Mutter, G. L. Pten, a protean tumor suppressor. *Am J Pathol* 2001; 158(6): 1895–8.

30. Tashiro, H., Blazes, M. S., Wu, R., Cho, K. R., Bose, S., Wang, S. I. *et al.* Mutations in PTEN are frequent in endometrial carcinoma but rare in other common gynecological malignancies. *Cancer Res* 1997; 57(18): 3935–40.

31. Bussaglia, E., del Rio, E., Matias-Guiu, X. and Prat, J. PTEN mutations in endometrial carcinomas: a molecular and clinicopathologic analysis of 38 cases. *Hum Pathol* 2000; 31(3): 312–17.

32. Diaz-Padilla, I., Romero, N., Amir, E., Matias-Guiu, X., Vilar, E., Muggia, F. *et al.* Mismatch repair status and clinical outcome in endometrial cancer: a systematic review and meta-analysis. *Crit Rev Oncol Hematol* 2013; 88(1): 154–67.

33. Baak, J. P., Van Diermen, B., Steinbakk, A., Janssen, E., Skaland, I., Mutter, G. L. *et al.* Lack of PTEN expression in endometrial intraepithelial neoplasia is correlated with cancer progression. *Hum Pathol* 2005; 36(5): 555–61.

34. Mutter, G. L., Lin, M. C., Fitzgerald, J. T., Kum, J. B., Baak, J. P., Lees, J. A. *et al.* Altered PTEN expression as a diagnostic marker for the earliest endometrial precancers. *J Natl Cancer Inst* 2000; 92(11): 924–30.

35. Monte, N. M., Webster, K. A., Neuberg, D., Dressler, G. R. and Mutter, G. L. Joint loss of PAX2 and PTEN expression in endometrial precancers and cancer. *Cancer Res* 2010; 70(15): 6225–32.

36. Scholten, A. N., Creutzberg, C. L., van den Broek, L. J., Noordijk, E. M. and Smit, V. T. Nuclear beta-catenin is a molecular feature of type I endometrial carcinoma. *J Pathol* 2003; 201(3): 460–5.

37. Machin, P., Catasus, L., Pons, C., Munoz, J., Matias-Guiu, X. and Prat, J. CTNNB1 mutations and beta-catenin expression in endometrial carcinomas. *Hum Pathol* 2002; 33(2): 206–12.

38. Gatius, S., Velasco, A., Azueta, A., Santacana, M., Pallares, J., Valls, J. *et al.* FGFR2 alterations in endometrial carcinoma. *Modern Pathol* 2011; 24(11): 1500–10.

39. Lax, S. F., Kendall, B., Tashiro, H., Slebos, R. J. and Hedrick, L. The frequency of p53, K-ras mutations, and microsatellite instability differs in uterine endometrioid and serous carcinoma: evidence of distinct molecular genetic pathways. *Cancer* 2000; 88(4): 814–24.

40. Esteller, M., Catasus, L., Matias-Guiu, X., Mutter, G. L., Prat, J., Baylin, S. B. *et al.* hMLH1 promoter hypermethylation is an early event in human endometrial tumorigenesis. *Am J Pathol* 1999; 155(5): 1767–72.

41. Tashiro, H., Isacson, C., Levine, R., Kurman, R. J., Cho, K. R. and Hedrick, L. p53 gene mutations are common in uterine serous carcinoma and occur early in their pathogenesis. *Am J Pathol* 1997; 150(1): 177–85.

42. Hayes, M. P. and Ellenson, L. H. Molecular alterations in uterine serous carcinoma. *Gynecol Oncol* 2010; 116(2): 286–9.

43. Morrison, C., Zanagnolo, V., Ramirez, N., Cohn, D. E., Kelbick, N., Copeland, L. *et al.* HER-2 is an independent prognostic factor in endometrial cancer: association with outcome in a large cohort of surgically staged patients. *J Clin Oncol* 2006; 24(15): 2376–85.

44. Tashiro, H., Lax, S. F., Gaudin, P. B., Isacson, C., Cho, K. R. and Hedrick, L. Microsatellite instability is uncommon in uterine serous carcinoma. *Am J Pathol* 1997; 150(1): 75–9.

45. Kuhn, E., Bahadirli-Talbott, A. and Shih, I. M. Frequent CCNE1 amplification in endometrial intraepithelial carcinoma and uterine serous carcinoma. *Mod Pathol* 2013; 27(7): 1014–19.

46. An, H. J., Logani, S., Isacson, C. and Ellenson, L. H. Molecular characterization of uterine clear cell carcinoma. *Mod Pathol* 2004; 17(5): 530–7.

47. Guan, B., Mao, T. L., Panuganti, P. K., Kuhn, E., Kurman, R. J., Maeda, D. *et al.* Mutation and loss of expression of ARID1A in uterine low-grade endometrioid carcinoma. *Am J Surg Pathol* 2011; 35(5): 625–32.

48. Wiegand, K. C., Lee, A. F., Al-Agha, O. M., Chow, C., Kalloger, S. E., Scott, D. W. *et al.* Loss of BAF250a (ARID1A) is frequent in high-grade endometrial carcinomas. *J Pathol* 2011; 224(3): 328–33.

49. Cancer Genome Atlas Research Network, Kandoth, C., Schultz, N., Cherniack, A. D., Akbani, R., Liu, Y. *et al.* Integrated genomic characterization of endometrial carcinoma. *Nature* 2013; 497(7447): 67–73.

50. Ferlay, J., Shin, H. R., Bray, F., Forman, D., Mathers, C. and Parkin, D. M. Estimates of worldwide burden of cancer in 2008: GLOBOCAN 2008. *Int J Cancer* 2010; 127(12): 2893–917.

51. Prat, J. Ovarian carcinomas: five distinct diseases with different origins, genetic alterations, and clinicopathological features. *Virchows Arch* 2012; 460(3): 237–49.

52. Rechsteiner, M., Zimmermann, A. K., Wild, P. J., Caduff, R., von

Teichman, A., Fink, D. *et al.* TP53 mutations are common in all subtypes of epithelial ovarian cancer and occur concomitantly with KRAS mutations in the mucinous type. *Exp Mol Pathol* 2013; 95(2): 235–41.

53. Perets, R., Wyant, G. A., Muto, K. W., Bijron, J. G., Poole, B. B., Chin, K. T. *et al.* Transformation of the fallopian tube secretory epithelium leads to high-grade serous ovarian cancer in Brca; Tp53;Pten models. *Cancer Cell* 2013; 24(6): 751–65.

# Chapter 13

# Tumors of the male urogenital system

Kirsten D. Mertz and Lukas Bubendorf

Despite recent advances in individualized targeted therapy, (male) urogenital cancers remain some of the most challenging diseases. Knowledge of the molecular changes of the various types of urogenital tumors has increased dramatically over the past decade. The ultimate goal of current research is the identification of biomarkers with utility in establishing diagnosis, predicting prognosis, guiding treatment, as well as identifying novel therapeutic targets. The broad application of high-throughput techniques for the analysis of genome-wide patterns of structural (copy-number alterations, single nucleotide polymorphisms, methylation pattern) and functional (gene expression profiling, proteomics, microRNA) alterations in cancer tissues will not only lead to a better understanding of the tumor biology, but also to the definition of cancer subtypes beyond histology-based stratification systems. In this chapter, we give an overview on the current status of molecular diagnostic, prognostic and predictive markers for urogenital tumors.

## Prostate cancer

### Introduction

Prostate cancer (PCA) is the most common non-skin malignancy among men and is the second leading cause of cancer deaths in Europe and the United States. The high incidence and prevalence of PCA is reflected in the diagnostic routine workload in surgical pathology, where prostate needle biopsies and radical prostatectomies account for a steadily rising part of the workload.

The spectrum of PCA ranges from relatively indolent tumors to cancers with rapid metastatic progression. It has been recognized that early detection of prostate cancers due to serum PSA testing has led to

over-treatment of many patients in the past two decades. Therefore, an increasing proportion of patients with early detected, low-risk prostate cancer are now considered as candidates for active surveillance. However, there remains a sizeable subset of PCA patients who require aggressive therapeutic intervention. Patient management mainly depends on morphological findings in prostate biopsies. However, histological features alone including Gleason Score and tumor quantification remain imperfect in predicting the biological behavior, calling for molecular markers that can better stratify the risk of progression in individual patients.

Complex molecular alterations have recently been identified in PCA, involving many different genes, multiple gene translocations, epigenetic changes and microRNA species (1). Despite these increasing insights and the countless prognostic markers that have been proposed in the past, there are no uniformly recommended ancillary tests in prostate cancer. However, a number of promising molecular tests have recently emerged. Here, we review several novel areas in the molecular diagnostics of PCA, including state-of-the-art tissue-based molecular biomarkers, with the potential for further development and implementation in routine clinical diagnostics in the near future. PCA biomarkers of the future could avoid unnecessary biopsies, reduce the number of prostatectomies and radiotherapy, stratify organ-confined tumors curable by surgery, monitor progression during watchful waiting, detect metastases below the limit of imaging techniques and lower overall mortality from PCA. It is foreseeable that a rational approach to biomarker discovery, combined with modern molecular methods and bioinformatics, will eventually allow clinicians to better diagnose and treat those patients who are most likely to benefit.

*Molecular Pathology: A Practical Guide for the Surgical Pathologist and Cytopathologist*, ed. John M. S. Bartlett, Abeer Shaaban and Fernando Schmitt. Published by Cambridge University Press. © Cambridge University Press, 2016.

# Immunohistochemical markers in prostate cancer

The conventional diagnosis of PCA is based on three criteria: a haphazard glandular pattern, lack of basal cells and nuclear atypia with prominent nucleoli. However, conventional morphology is prone to subjective interpretation and clearly benefits from additional information for more objective and reproducible conclusions.

### Immunohistochemical basal cell markers for diagnosis of prostatic intraepithelial neoplasia (PIN) and cancer

A hallmark feature of PCA is the loss of basal cells. Therefore, basal cell markers are a cornerstone of immunohistochemistry in PCA diagnostics. Commonly used antibodies to identify basal cells include high-molecular weight cytokeratins (34βE12, CK5/6) and p63. Thereby, PIN retains an intact or fragmented basal cell layer, whereas cancer glands are devoid of basal cells. Basal-cell specific anti-keratins 34βE12 and CK5/6 stain the cytoplasm of normal basal cells of the prostate, with continuous intact circumferential staining in most cases. P63 is a nuclear protein that is as sensitive and specific for the identification of basal cells in prostate specimens as high molecular weight cytokeratin staining. Multiple stain combinations (multiplex immunohistochemistry) such as double or triple stainings with α-methylacyl-CoA racemase (AMACR), which is helpful in discriminating benign and malignant acini, a high molecular weight cytokeratin and p63 are commonly used in routine diagnostic settings to confirm the diagnosis of PCA, especially in challenging cases.

### Immunohistochemical markers for determination of prostatic origin

Determination of tissue origin (prostatic versus non-prostatic) relies mainly on three markers: prostate-specific antigen (PSA); prostate-specific membrane antigen (PSMA); and prostatic acid phosphatase (PAP).

PSA is a 34-kDa serine protease produced almost exclusively by prostatic epithelial cells. It is not entirely prostate-specific and has also been detected in carcinomas of ovary, salivary glands, breast and other tissues, but it is still the most commonly used immunohistochemical marker for tumors of prostatic origin. This is very useful in the differential diagnosis of poorly differentiated or undifferentiated carcinomas. Earlier detection through screening for elevated PSA serum levels has been shown to decrease PCA mortality (2). Serum PSA accurately predicts cancer status and can detect recurrence several months before detection by any other method. However, serum PSA may become elevated by conditions other than PCA, including prostatitis, benign prostatic hyperplasia or urinary retention. Thus, testing for serum PSA is hampered by its low specificity.

PSMA is a membrane-bound antigen that is highly specific for benign and malignant prostatic epithelial cells. It is also strongly expressed by most PCA metastases. In contrast to PSA, PSMA is generally up-regulated during PCA progression. However, similar to PSA, it is also not prostate-specific, but is widely expressed in other solid tumors. PSMA can be detected in the serum of normal men, and an elevated concentration is associated with the presence of PCA, clinical progression of PCA and hormone-refractory PCA.

PAP is another prostate-specific immunohistochemical marker that seems to be more sensitive than PSA in difficult cases of advanced PCA and is routinely employed to confirm prostatic identity.

AMACR has demonstrated high sensitivity and specificity (each >90%) as a diagnostic biomarker on prostate tissues. However, as the other markers, it is also not entirely specific to PCA and is also not suitable for non-invasive detection in urine, rendering it most useful as a tissue biomarker when prostate needle biopsies yield ambiguous pathological results.

### Proliferation markers

Increased proliferation is a common feature of malignant tumors. The proliferative fraction of tumor cells can be measured by immunohistochemistry for Ki-67. Numerous studies have analyzed Ki-67 expression levels in PCA and many of these studies have found a prognostic value of the proliferation index (3, 4). However, Ki-67 adds little predictive information for patient outcome above the traditional parameters such as Gleason score and pathologic stage. The Ki-67 labeling index appears to be particularly helpful in the discrimination between organ-confined and metastatic cancer, as elevation in the Ki-67 proliferation index can reflect PCA progression. Studies to clarify whether Ki-67 can be employed to guide treatment are still needed.

# Molecular-genetic markers and alterations in prostate cancer

Prostate carcinogenesis involves multiple genetic changes, including loss of specific genomic sequences that may lead to inactivation of tumor suppressor genes and gain of specific chromosome regions that may activate oncogenes. High-grade PIN and PCA share similar molecular genetic alterations. The most common chromosomal aberrations in PIN and PCA are TMPRSS2-ETS gene fusions, gain of chromosome 7 (particular 7q31), loss of 8p, gain of 8q and loss of 10q, 16q and 18q.

The principal hurdle in defining a unified molecular classification of PCA is the enormous complexity of this cancer – even very early or small cancers already contain hundreds of deregulated, aberrantly expressed and/or mutated genes. Thus, it is extremely difficult to identify gene-signaling pathways as potential drivers of carcinogenesis suitable for therapeutic intervention. Furthermore, marked heterogeneity of PCA at both the cellular level and the level of different cancer foci hampers efforts to stratify PCA based on molecular-genetic changes.

## TMPRSS2 and ETS family gene fusions

In 2005, Tomlins *et al.* developed a bioinformatics approach to discover oncogenic chromosomal aberrations based on outlier gene expression (Cancer Outlier Profile Analysis, COPA). This analysis identified recurrent gene fusions between the 5'-noncoding region of the androgen-responsive gene TMPRSS2 and members of the ETS family of DNA-binding transcription factors in approximately half of PCAs and in about 20% of cases of high-grade PIN (Figure 13.1) (5). These fusions are the driving force for over-expression of members of the ETS transcription factor family, including ERG (21q22.3), ETV1 (7p21.2) and ETV4 (17q21). Considering the high incidence of prostate cancer and the high frequency of this gene fusion, the TMPRSS2-ETS gene fusions are the most common genetic aberrations in human malignancies described to date.

TMPRSS2-ERG gene fusions represent the most common genetic events and account for around 90% of known PCA fusions (6). There is still some debate whether the presence of a TMPRSS2-ERG fusion itself is a prognostic biomarker when detected in tissues. Several groups have reported an association between TMPRSS2-ERG and higher Gleason grade, higher stage and poorer survival compared to fusion-negative tumors. Other studies failed to observe this association. TMPRSS2-ERG gene fusions might arise independently in different foci (7). ERG immunohistochemistry has emerged as a reliable and highly specific surrogate marker for ERG rearrangements and can facilitate the diagnosis of small foci of prostate cancer, together with AMACR and high-molecular cytokeratin (Figure 13.1). Physiological ERG expression in endothelial cells serves as a positive internal control. Interestingly, recent data suggest that ERG protein expression of PCA at diagnosis might identify patients with an increased risk of disease progression during active surveillance (8).

The detection of TMPRSS2-ERG RNA in patient urine has also been investigated (9). However, TMPRSS2-ERG is absent in about 50% of PCAs, and therefore its potential use lies in multiplexed assays with other biomarkers.

## Prostate cancer antigen 3 (PCA3)

The most prominent non-PSA based diagnostic biomarker for PCA is prostate cancer antigen 3 (PCA3). PCA3 is a non-coding RNA that is elevated in >90% of PCAs, but not in normal or hyperplastic tissues (10). The high sensitivity and specificity of PCA3 in tissues have led to its evaluation as a non-invasive biomarker. Numerous assays have been developed to detect PCA3 in urine samples of PCA patients, containing cells shed from the prostate during urination. Urine PCA3 measurements add to the diagnostic information obtained from PSA testing. In addition, combining a serum PSA value with a urine PCA3 analysis improves both measurements. In 2012, PCA3 was approved by the FDA as a diagnostic test for PCA in the setting of a previous negative prostate biopsy.

## Germline risk loci

Genomic analyses have identified single-nucleotide polymorphisms (SNPs) associated with PCA, which may serve as germline indications of a patient's risk for developing cancer. To date, more than 50 SNPs have been proposed as putative risk loci for PCA, of which around 30 have been validated in multiple studies. Zheng *et al.* have defined a core set of five disease-associated SNPs that were combined with family history to predict risk for developing PCA (11).

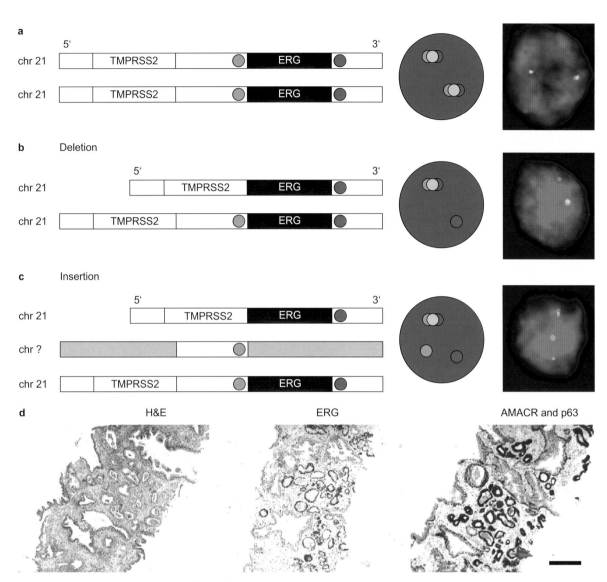

**Figure 13.1 The TMPRSS2-ERG gene fusion in PCA**
(a) *Left:* Schematic representation of chromosome 21 with the androgen-regulated TMPRSS2 gene and the ERG gene, located approximately 3 megabases apart. *Right:* Schematic representation of FISH results and representative FISH pictures are shown, with a green 5′-probe (5′ of ERG) and a red 3′-probe (3′ of ERG). Co-localization of the 5′- and 3′-probes is observed in cells without gene fusion and appears yellow. (b) Fusion of TMPRSS2 and ERG can occur through deletion of the genomic region between the two genes. (c) Alternatively, the genomic material between TMPRSS2 and ERG can insert in another region in the genome, outside of chromosome 21. (d) The TMPRSS2-ERG gene fusion results in ERG over-expression in fusion-positive PCA cells, which can be visualized immunohistochemically using a specific anti-ERG antibody. *Left:* H&E staining of a prostate core needle biopsy with infiltrating PCA glands. *Middle:* ERG immunohistochemistry. ERG is strongly expressed exclusively in the nucleus of PCA glands. *Right:* double immunohistochemistry for AMACR (brown) and the basal cell marker p63 (red). Note that the PCA glands lack basal cells, but strongly express cytoplasmic AMACR. Scale bar, 200 μm.

# Next generation of prostate cancer biomarkers

Advances in DNA sequencing and RNA transcriptome profiling have enabled detailed dissections of cancer biology at a level previously unattainable. As a result, biomarker research has shifted to use these "-omics" methods, leading to profiling of tumors for aberrations in DNA, RNA or epigenetic DNA methylation states. It is important to consider the role of tissue-based biomarkers reviewed above in disease diagnosis and staging. Here, we focus on discovery and characterization of emerging biomarker assays for PCA, including blood- and urine-based diagnostics.

## Circulating tumor cells

Circulating tumor cells (CTCs) in the bloodstream represent an area of expanding interest. The number of CTCs present in whole blood can be used as a biomarker for cancer detection, and the cells themselves are a source of molecular information, such as TMPRSS2-ERG gene fusion, androgen receptor and PTEN copy-number status (12). Since an increased abundance of CTCs in the blood of castration-resistant PCA patients predicts worse overall survival, CTC enumeration using the CELLSEARCH® system has received FDA clearance for use in monitoring advanced prostate cancer (13). However, detecting CTCs and extracting molecular information are currently labor-intensive and expensive, and it is yet unknown if CTC abundance in blood represents aggressive disease undergoing hematogenous spread or if they are simply cells that have dislodged from the bulk tumor.

## Exosomes

Prostate-derived exosomes (prostatosomes) are small vesicles generated from internalized parts of the cellular membrane, which are subsequently secreted into the blood, semen or urine (14). PCA patients have increased numbers of exosomes in their serum compared to men without the disease, and elevated levels of exosomes may also correlate with increasing Gleason score. PCA biomarkers, including PCA3 and TMPRSS2-ERG, can also be detected in urine-derived exosomes from PCA patients. Although these efforts remain mainly research-oriented at this point, they may provide promising directions for future biomarker research and molecular PCA diagnostics.

## Conclusions and future directions

Although currently PCA can be detected very early on, the high prevalence of latent cancers detected by PSA screening argues for adjunctive biomarkers better refining disease risk. Molecular genetics underlying PCA is exceptionally complex, with many different genetic events playing a role in its development and progression. Despite the abundance of knowledge

already known as described above, current PCA molecular diagnostic applications are clearly limited and there is an urgent need for more sensitive and specific diagnostic and prognostic tests. The emergence of new technologies such as next generation sequencing holds great promise for significant breakthroughs that will contribute to patient care. Furthermore, the combination of diagnostics linked to therapy has not yet found a role in PCA treatment, but is likely to happen in the near future. Within the years to come, molecular diagnostics will very likely be applied to PCA on a routine basis and prove a useful tool for patient risk stratification and personalized therapeutic approaches to individual patients.

# Penile, scrotal and testicular cancer
## Introduction

Malignant tumors of the penis, scrotum and testes are rare, accounting for approximately 0.5% of all male tumors. At present, the diagnosis of these tumors depends on histologic examination, supported by immunohistochemistry. Over the past decades, genetic changes have been identified that are largely specific to different tumors and tumor classes, such as 12p gains in testicular germ cell tumors. Molecular genetic testing is available for these tumors and is becoming an adjunct in their diagnosis and treatment, although not commonly employed in daily routine diagnostics. Here, we focus on the few molecular testing modalities currently available and used. We also briefly elucidate possible future molecular diagnostic and maybe therapeutic approaches for these tumors.

## HPV molecular diagnostics

Approximately half of penile squamous cell carcinomas (SCC) are caused by human papilloma virus (HPV) infection, with HPV types 16 and 18 accounting for around 70% of tumors (15). A limited number of HPV types have been identified as conferring a probable or definite high oncogenic risk. Although successful HPV vaccines have been developed, HPV infection remains common. Thus, molecular diagnostics for HPV, especially the high oncogenic risk types, is often clinically warranted. The detection and analysis of HPV types are mainly performed on cervical specimens, and only a few studies examined HPV infection in men. As in the case of cervical HPV infections, the detection of HPV alone is not clinically significant, as many HPV infections are benign and do not produce significant pathology. Cellular HPV infections produce specific cytological changes often seen by the surgical pathologist in routine light microscopy examination. Similar to the analysis of HPV-induced cervical dysplasia, p16 and Ki-67 are used as surrogate markers for HPV-induced dysplasia in penile cancer.

PCR amplification is commonly used for HPV nucleic acid detection and subtype identification. Although useful for detecting HPV, PCR cannot distinguish between clinically irrelevant transient infections and infections related to significant pathology and oncogenesis. Therefore, PCR-based HPV analysis must be interpreted with caution and only in the context of histologic findings and patient history.

## Molecular diagnostic tests in other tumors

A number of extremely rare scrotal tumors are associated with specific molecular alterations. These include specific chromosomal translocations in aggressive angiomyxoma, desmoplastic small round cell tumors, liposarcoma and rhabdomyosarcoma (refer to Chapter 15 for more details).

The diagnosis of testicular tumors is usually accomplished by conventional histology, supplemented with immunohistochemistry. Molecular diagnostic testing is not necessary and is therefore currently limited to research settings. The main molecular test used to detect seminomas and other testicular germ cell tumors is fluorescent *in situ* hybridization (FISH) to identify gain of chromosome 12p, typically isochromosome 12, which is consistently present in testicular germ cell neoplasms (16).

## Future directions

Molecular diagnostics are not part of the routine work-up of penile, scrotal and testicular malignancies. This is due to the rarity of most of these tumors and also because diagnosis can usually be successfully made by combining clinical presentation, histology and immunohistochemistry. As new molecular therapies are developed, the identification of specific molecular alterations will likely play a role prior to initiation of therapy also in these rare male neoplasms in the future.

# Tumors of the urinary bladder

## Introduction

Bladder cancer is the second most common genitourinary malignancy. The vast majority of malignant tumors arising in the bladder are urothelial carcinomas. The central diagnostic procedures are cystoscopy and transurethral biopsy or resection. In contrast to the clinical management of tumors of lung, colon and breast, molecular biomarkers are not yet an integral component for diagnosis, risk stratification and treatment of urinary bladder cancers. However, recent major advances in cancer genetics and genomics will undoubtedly affect the management of these cancers in the near future.

Most urothelial carcinomas (around 70%) are superficial and include non-invasive low-grade papillary carcinoma (pTa), carcinoma *in situ* (pTis) and urothelial carcinomas with invasion of the subepithelial lamina propria (pT1). The remaining urothelial carcinomas are muscularis propria invasive tumors ($\geq$ pT2), which have a poor prognosis (17). Patients with low-grade and lower stage tumors have lower rates of progression and mortality than high-grade and higher stage tumors, suggesting two different categories of urothelial carcinomas with a different biology. Two main pathways are believed to be involved in urothelial carcinogenesis (18). One pathway involves mutation of the fibroblast growth factor receptor 3 gene (FGFR3). This pathway seems to give rise to low-grade, non-invasive papillary tumors that may recur, but rarely invade. The second pathway involves mutations or deletions in the TP53 gene. Tumors with TP53 gene mutations are high-grade and include high-grade papillary urothelial carcinoma and urothelial carcinoma *in situ* (19). In addition, several chromosomal abnormalities may occur in high-grade urothelial carcinoma. The most frequent chromosomal alterations involve chromosome 9, including monosomy, and deletions of 9p and 9q. Deletion of 9p21, affecting the tumor suppressor gene p16 (INK4a), occurs particularly frequently (19). Loss of chromosomes 4 and 8, deletions of 2q, 8p, 11p, 13q, 14q and 17p, and gains of chromosomes 3, 7 and 17 are also reported. In support of this molecular genetic classification, cDNA expression analysis reveals specific mRNA signatures that are associated with these two pathways (20).

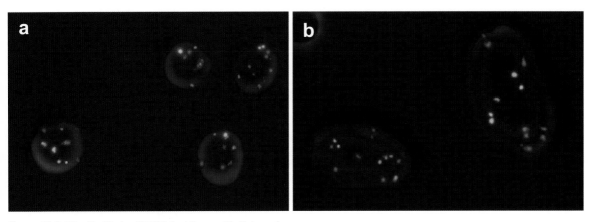

**Figure 13.2 The UroVysion™ FISH test for urothelial carcinoma**
(a) On the *right*: three cells of a low-grade urothelial carcinoma with isolated homozygous deletion of 9p21 (gold) but normal copy-numbers for chromosomes 3 (red), 7 (green) and 17 (blue). One normal cell with retained 9p21 signals on the *left* (UroVysion™ test). (b) Two cells of a urothelial carcinoma with increased copy-number of chromosomes 3 (red), 7 (green) and 17 (blue), but a normal copy-number of 9p21 (gold), consistent with heterozygous 9p21 deletion (UroVysion™ test).

In current daily routine, urine cytology is the initial test of choice for early diagnosis, screening and follow-up of urothelial carcinomas. It is a reliable, sensitive and specific test for diagnosing high-grade urothelial carcinoma. However, urine cytology yields equivocal or negative results in a large proportion of patients with low-grade urothelial neoplasms. In addition, the diagnosis is difficult in cases of upper urinary tract neoplasms and in urothelial carcinomas treated with BCG (21). Therefore, there is a clear need to develop ancillary tests to identify urothelial carcinoma by non-invasive methods.

## UroVysion™ fluorescent *in situ* hybridization (FISH) test for urothelial carcinoma

The FISH technique allows for the visualization of specific DNA sequences within the cell nucleus by the precise annealing of fluorescently labeled DNA probes to its complementary DNA target sequence on chromosomes. Hybridization of the probes becomes visible as fluorescent dots, and each dot represents a copy of the targeted sequence.

UroVysion™ fluorescence *in situ* hybridization (FISH) has become a useful ancillary technique for better detection of urothelial carcinoma in routine cytologic urine specimens. Multiple studies have shown that UroVysion™ FISH in voided urine and washing specimens can support patient management due to its superior sensitivity over cytology in ambiguous situations (21). The commercially available UroVysion™ FISH multiprobe test (Abbott, DesPlaines, IL) is Food and Drug Administration (FDA-) approved for the detection of urothelial carcinoma in voided urine specimens from patients with hematuria without a history of urothelial carcinoma, and for the detection of recurrent urothelial carcinoma in voided urine specimens from patients with a prior history of urothelial carcinoma (22). The UroVysion™ FISH kit consists of a four-color/four-probe mixture of DNA probes to detect specific regions on chromosomes 3, 7, 9 and 17, including three Chromosome Enumeration Probes (CEP), CEP 3 SpectrumRed, CEP 7 SpectrumGreen and CEP 17 SpectrumAqua, plus a locus specific identifier (LSI) 9p21 Spectrum-Gold (Figure 13.2) (22). Abnormal cells are defined as cells with a gain of multiple chromosomes (three or more signals of CEP 3, CEP 7, CEP 17) or a homozygous loss of 9p21. A minimum of 25 morphologically abnormal cells have to be analyzed, and the total number of chromosomally abnormal cells are reported. A positive result is defined when either four or more cells with multiple chromosomal gains or 12 or more cells with loss of both 9p21 signals are observed.

The UroVysion™ FISH test may detect more abnormalities than cytology and is particularly useful in clarifying equivocal cytological findings (21). Although the UroVysion™ test has a higher sensitivity than cytology, the specificity of cytology is similar or higher. Therefore, as with any test, correlation of all results with the clinical picture is always recommended.

## Other tests for urothelial carcinoma

The following assays are not used in daily routine at this time, but represent promising possibilities for future diagnostic strategies. The combination of Uro-Vysion™ FISH and FGFR3 mutation analysis is under investigation (23). In addition to the UroVysion™ FISH multiprobe test (Abbott, DesPlaines, IL), ImmunoCyt™/uCyt+™ (Scimedx, Denville, New Jersey), Bladder Tumour Antigen (BTA stat® und BTA TRAK®; polyMedco, Radmond, WA) and Nuclear Matrix Protein 22 (NMP22® Bladder Check®; Inverness Medical Innovation, Bedford, UK) have also been approved by the FDA for bladder cancer surveillance (24). Although numerous other molecular markers for urothelial cancers have been published, their use is still limited to research studies and their clinical relevance in daily routine diagnostics has not been established (19, 25).

## Future directions

Recent advances in the knowledge of the molecular pathways and pathogenesis of bladder cancer have moved the field towards personalized targeted therapy directed towards a specific molecular profile of the tumor. The future of bladder cancer management will likely involve the use of molecular studies and biomarkers to determine the diagnosis, individual therapy and prognosis, as is already common practice for many other cancer types (26).

## Tumors of the kidney

### Introduction

Currently, the molecular diagnosis of kidney tumors is still evolving. Gene expression and sequencing studies have revealed that renal cell carcinoma (RCC), by far the most frequent type of kidney cancer, is a heterogeneous disease at the histological, morphological and molecular level. However, these approaches have so far failed to improve molecular stratification or to establish a classification system that predicts which patients are likely to relapse or respond to targeted therapy. Prognostic and predictive molecular tests for RCC remain elusive and histopathology remains the gold standard for determining prognosis. Several gene expression profiling studies

have attempted to take a global approach to the analysis of the molecules and pathways intrinsic to RCC and the interaction between them. However, translation of these results into clinical practice has proven challenging and is still evolving (27). Clearly, novel approaches are required to resolve the complexity of RCC prognostication and prediction of treatment response.

## Molecular diagnostic tests

Within the group of renal neoplasms, molecular tests have not become routine. Molecular diagnostic analyses mainly involve the identification of Xp11.2 translocations/TFE fusions in renal cell carcinomas, which typically affect children and young adults and show a papillary architecture with clear cells or cells with granular eosinophilic cytoplasm (Figure 13.3) (28). The Xp11.2 translocations all involve the TFE3 gene and include t(X;1)(p11.2;q21) with fusion of PRCC and TFE3 genes, t(X;17)(p11.2;p25) with fusion of ASPL (RCC17) and TFE3 genes, t(X;1)(p11.2;p34) with fusion of PSF and TFE3 genes, and inv(X)(p11;q12) with fusion of NonO (p54$^{nrb}$) and TFE3 genes. The diagnosis of these tumors can be established based on morphology and confirmation by immunohistochemistry for TFE3. FISH may be applied to confirm the specific molecular change in these tumors, but these tests are currently limited to specialized centers (Figure 13.3).

Molecular analyses have shown some utility in pediatric kidney tumors such as the cellular variant of congenital mesoblastic nephroma (but not the classic variant). This tumor shows the same t(12;15)(p13;q25) and ETV6-NTRK3 gene fusion as infantile fibrosarcoma. Rhabdoïd tumor of the kidney shows a deletion of the hSNF5/INI1 gene. As with molecular tests for renal cell carcinoma, these assays are not routinely used.

## Genetic predisposition

A number of genetic syndromes predispose to the development of RCC, and several genes associated with such syndromes have been identified (VHL, MET, FH, BHD and HRPT2) (29). Approximately 4% of all RCCs are inherited. Knowledge of the hereditary forms of RCC has also improved our understanding of the pathophysiology of sporadic RCC (30). The two main pathways that are deregulated in both hereditary and sporadic RCC and that have

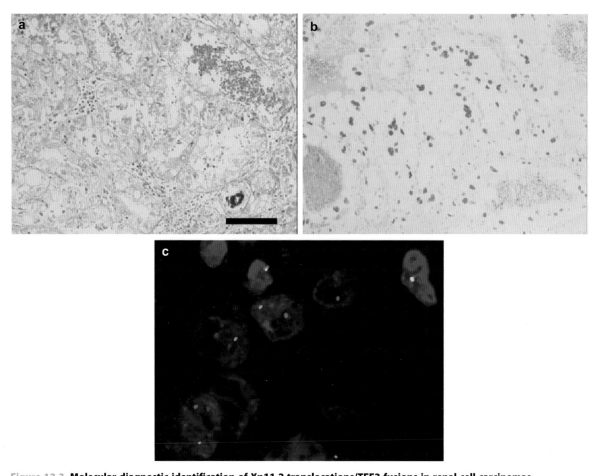

**Figure 13.3 Molecular diagnostic identification of Xp11.2 translocations/TFE3 fusions in renal cell carcinomas**
(a) Xp11.2 translocation-associated renal cell carcinoma in a 27-year-old male patient. The tumor shows clear cells and cells with granular eosinophilic cytoplasm. One Psammom body is visible in the lower-right corner. Scale bar for (a) and (b), 100 μm. (b) The tumor shows diffuse nuclear over-expression of TFE3. (c) The translocation is confirmed by a FISH assay using TFE3 break-apart probes. Normal cells in this male patient (XY) show one yellow signal (co-localization of red and green probes), whereas tumor cells are characterized by separated red and green signals.

become of interest for therapeutic targeting are the von Hippel-Lindau (VHL) pathway and that of the membrane-bound receptor tyrosine kinase MET. Loss-of-function mutations of the VHL tumor suppressor gene (3p25–26), which are responsible for inherited cases of clear cell RCC (ccRCC), are also involved in at least two-thirds of sporadic ccRCC cases. Papillary RCC (pRCC) is the second most common subtype of inherited RCC and can be subdivided into hereditary pRCC (HPRCC) and hereditary leiomyomatosis RCC. HPRC – the MET proto-oncogene (7q31.3) that is responsible for HPRCC – is mutated in 5% to 13% of sporadic papillary type I RCCs. Deregulation of MET results in increased mitogenesis and morphogenesis. Several

other pathways that provide potential targets for RCC treatment have been identified through study of inherited RCC, including the mammalian target of rapamycin (mTOR) pathway, growth factor signaling pathways and the Wnt/β-catenin pathway (31). However, the advanced understanding of these pathways still contributes little to the current clinical management of patients with RCC.

# Future directions

Gene expression and next generation sequencing studies have increased our understanding of the genetic basis of RCC, but have so far failed to establish a unified classification system to improve molecular stratification or to predict patient outcome or response to therapy. However, they have highlighted that RCC is a heterogeneous disease at histological, morphological and molecular levels. In view of the limited options, poor outcomes and narrow therapeutic windows, there has been a drive to use targeted therapy to improve patient outcomes in RCC, but targeted therapy has so far contributed little to patient management and yet awaits implementation in clinical practice.

# References

1. Beltran, H. and Rubin, M. A. New strategies in prostate cancer: translating genomics into the clinic. *Clin Cancer Res* 2013; 19(3): 517–23.

2. Schröder, F. H., Hugosson, J., Roobol, M. J., Tammela, T. L., Ciatto, S., Nelen, V. *et al.* Screening and prostate-cancer mortality in a randomized European study. *New Engl J Med* 2009; 360(13): 1320–8.

3. Jhavar, S., Bartlett, J., Kovacs, G., Corbishley, C., Dearnaley, D., Eeles, R. *et al.* Biopsy tissue microarray study of Ki-67 expression in untreated, localized prostate cancer managed by active surveillance. *Prostate Cancer P D* 2009; 12(2): 143–7.

4. Zellweger, T., Gunther, S., Zlobec, I., Savic, S., Sauter, G., Moch, H. *et al.* Tumour growth fraction measured by immunohistochemical staining of Ki67 is an independent prognostic factor in preoperative prostate biopsies with small-volume or low-grade prostate cancer. *Int J Cancer* 2009; 124(9): 2116–23.

5. Tomlins, S. A., Rhodes, D. R., Perner, S., Dhanasekaran, S. M., Mehra, R., Sun, X. W. *et al.* Recurrent fusion of TMPRSS2 and ETS transcription factor genes in prostate cancer. *Science* 2005; 310(5748): 644–8.

6. Prensner, J. R. and Chinnaiyan, A. M. Oncogenic gene fusions in epithelial carcinomas. *Curr Opin Genet Dev* 2009; 19(1): 82–91.

7. Mertz, K. D., Horcic, M., Hailemariam, S., D'Antonio, A., Dirnhofer, S., Hartmann, A. *et al.* Heterogeneity of ERG expression in core needle biopsies of patients with early prostate cancer. *Hum Pathol* 2013; 44(12): 2727–35.

8. Berg, K. D., Vainer, B., Thomsen, F. B., Roder, M. A., Gerds, T. A., Toft, B. G. *et al.* ERG protein expression in diagnostic specimens is associated with increased risk of progression during active surveillance for prostate cancer. *Eur Urol* 2014 Mar. 7 (e-pub ahead of print).

9. Tomlins, S. A., Aubin, S. M., Siddiqui, J., Lonigro, R. J., Sefton-Miller, L., Miick, S. *et al.* Urine TMPRSS2:ERG fusion transcript stratifies prostate cancer risk in men with elevated serum PSA. *Sci Transl Med* 2011; 3(94): 94ra72.

10. Hessels, D. and Schalken, J. A. The use of PCA3 in the diagnosis of prostate cancer. *Nat Rev Urol* 2009; 6(5): 255–61.

11. Zheng, S. L., Sun, J., Wiklund, F., Smith, S., Stattin, P., Li, G. *et al.* Cumulative association of five genetic variants with prostate cancer. *New Engl J Med* 2008; 358(9): 910–19.

12. Attard, G., Swennenhuis, J. F., Olmos, D., Reid, A. H., Vickers, E., A'Hern, R. *et al.* Characterization of ERG, AR and PTEN gene status in circulating tumor cells from patients with castration-resistant prostate cancer. *Cancer Res* 2009; 69(7): 2912–18.

13. Hu, B., Rochefort, H. and Goldkorn, A. Circulating tumor cells in prostate cancer. *Cancers* 2013; 5(4): 1676–90.

14. Duijvesz, D., Luider, T., Bangma, C. H. and Jenster, G. Exosomes as biomarker treasure chests for prostate cancer. *Eur Urol* 2011; 59(5): 823–31.

15. Daling, J. R., Madeleine, M. M., Johnson, L. G., Schwartz, S. M., Shera, K. A., Wurscher, M. A. *et al.* Penile cancer: importance of circumcision, human papillomavirus and smoking in in situ and invasive disease. *Int J Cancer* 2005; 116(4): 606–16.

16. Boublikova, L., Buchler, T., Stary, J., Abrahamova, J. and Trka, J. Molecular biology of testicular germ cell tumors: unique features awaiting clinical application. *Crit Rev Oncol Hematol* 2014; 89(3): 366–85.

17. Kaufman, D. S., Shipley, W. U. and Feldman, A. S. Bladder cancer. *Lancet* 2009; 374(9685): 239–49.

18. Cheng, L., Davidson, D. D., Maclennan, G. T., Williamson, S. R., Zhang, S., Koch, M. O. *et al.* The origins of urothelial carcinoma. *Expert Rev Anticancer Ther* 2010; 10(6): 865–80.

19. Cheng, L., Zhang, S., MacLennan, G. T., Williamson, S. R., Lopez-Beltran, A. and Montironi, R. Bladder cancer: translating molecular genetic insights into clinical practice. *Hum Pathol* 2011; 42(4): 455–81.

20. van der Kwast, T. H. and Bapat, B. Predicting favourable prognosis of urothelial carcinoma: gene expression and genome profiling. *Curr Opin Urol* 2009; 19(5): 516–21.

21. Bubendorf, L. Multiprobe fluorescence in situ hybridization (UroVysion) for the detection of urothelial carcinoma – FISHing for the right catch. *Acta Cytol* 2011; 55(2): 113–19.

22. Halling, K. C. and Kipp, B. R. Bladder cancer detection using FISH (UroVysion assay). *Adv Anat Pathol* 2008; 15(5): 279–86.

23. Wild, P. J., Fuchs, T., Stoehr, R., Zimmermann, D., Frigerio, S., Padberg, B. *et al.* Detection of urothelial bladder cancer cells in voided urine can be improved by a combination of cytology and standardized microsatellite analysis. *Cancer Epidemiol Biomarkers Prev* 2009; 18(6): 1798–806.

24. Mitra, A. P. and Cote, R. J. Molecular screening for bladder cancer: progress and potential. *Nat Rev Urol* 2010; 7(1): 11–20.

25. Netto, G. J. Molecular biomarkers in urothelial carcinoma of the bladder: are we there yet? *Nat Rev Urol* 2012; 9(1): 41–51.

26. Mitra, A. P. and Cote, R. J. Molecular pathogenesis and diagnostics of bladder cancer. *Ann Rev Pathol* 2009; 4: 251–85.

27. Stewart, G. D., O'Mahony, F. C., Powles, T., Riddick, A. C., Harrison, D. J. and Faratian, D. What can molecular pathology contribute to the management of renal cell carcinoma? *Nat Rev Urol* 2011; 8(5): 255–65.

28. Hodge, J. C., Pearce, K. E., Wang, X., Wiktor, A. E., Oliveira, A. M. and Greipp, P. T. Molecular cytogenetic analysis for TFE3 rearrangement in Xp11.2 renal cell carcinoma and alveolar soft part sarcoma: validation and clinical experience with 75 cases. *Mod Pathol* 2014; 27(1): 113–27.

29. Pavlovich, C. P. and Schmidt, L. S. Searching for the hereditary causes of renal-cell carcinoma. *Nat Rev Cancer* 2004; 4(5): 381–93.

30. Verine, J., Pluvinage, A., Bousquet, G., Lehmann-Che, J., de Bazelaire, C., Soufir, N. *et al.* Hereditary renal cancer syndromes: an update of a systematic review. *Eur Urol* 2010; 58(5): 701–10.

31. Linehan, W. M., Srinivasan, R. and Schmidt, L. S. The genetic basis of kidney cancer: a metabolic disease. *Nat Rev Urol* 2010; 7(5): 277–85.

# Tumors of the gastrointestinal system

Manuel Salto-Tellez, Benedict Yan, Roseann I. Wu
and Martha Bishop Pitman

## Gastrointestinal

### Introduction

Molecular diagnostics is the application of molecular biology techniques, and our knowledge of the molecular basis of diseases, to diagnose, prognosticate or treat patients (1). In the area of tissue molecular diagnosis, pertinent to the focus of this book, most tests are related to cancer. Of all the organ systems, the gastrointestinal (GI) tract is, together with breast and lung, an area that generates a higher volume of tissue- and cell-based molecular tests for the analysis of cancers in these organs. Within the GI tract, most of the interest in molecular diagnostics to date has been focused on colorectal cancer (CRC), with the notable exceptions of HER2 amplification testing in gastric cancer and KIT/PDGFRA mutational testing in gastrointestinal stromal tumor (GIST). CRC is one of the top three most common cancers worldwide, with 1 million new cases each year, and it represents the second most common cause of cancer death in the Western world. With a five-year survival rate of 65% in the United States only, it remains one of the main healthcare problems in modern oncology.

Despite extensive knowledge of the molecular biology of CRC, a comprehensive molecular classification of the disease is lacking. The well-known adenoma-carcinoma sequence by Vogelstein and colleagues has been subsequently complemented by the Epidermal Growth Factor Receptor (EGFR) pathway, the chromosomal instability pathway (the one more closely associated with Vogelstein's original morpho-molecular sequence), the APC-β catenin-Wnt signaling pathway, the microsatellite instability pathway and the description of the "methylator" genotype. Unfortunately, these categories are far from

exclusive and overlap in a significant manner, not allowing mutually exclusive diagnostic and therapeutic subgroups that are the backbone of other molecular classifications with strong therapeutic value, such as with adenocarcinoma of the lung. In parallel with this unresolved taxonomical issue, there are single biomarkers in CRC that are tested routinely in molecular diagnostic laboratories to make key diagnoses, as well as more complex genetic signatures that allow prognostication, and these will be the subject of this chapter. Gastrointestinal stromal tumors (the most common form of sarcoma across the GI tract) and gastric adenocarcinomas are the other two main cancer types having specific tests with a clear therapeutic value, and these will also be reviewed in this chapter. Regardless of the cancer type, we have divided this section of the chapter into two main subsections, namely those with a primary diagnostic/genetic value, and those tests with a predominantly therapeutic value. The former group is composed of tests aiming to make a diagnosis of an entity, usually inherited/genetic in nature, while the latter comprises a series of tests performed for the selection of specific therapeutic interventions (see Table 14.1).

### Tests with a predominant diagnostic value – diagnosis on inherited colorectal cancer patient

While some of the therapeutic tests in molecular onco-pathology may have an additional diagnostic utility on top of their predictive/therapeutic value, the bulk of the diagnostic molecular tests that we perform in the context of GI pathology are aimed towards making the diagnosis of inherited colorectal cancer. Approximately 20% of CRC can be considered familial in nature, and 1% to 5% are clearly syndromic. The molecular diagnosis of such syndromes

**Table 14.1**

**Test with a predominant diagnostic value**

1. APC mutation detection

2. MMR IHC

3. MSI analysis

4. *MYH* mutation detection

**Test with a predominant therapeutic value**

1. KRAS mutation detection

2. BRAF mutation detection

3. Thymidylate synthase expression

4. MSI analysis

5. PIK3CA mutation detection

6. Gene expression signatures

7. HER2 amplification

8. KIT and PDGFRA mutation detection

allows the clinical management of these patients and their close relatives, following established international recommendations. In this chapter, we will consider Familial Adenomatous Polyposis (FAP), Hereditary Nonpolyposis Colorectal Cancer (HNPCC), MYH-associated polyposis (MAP) and the hamartomatous polyposis syndromes. Occasionally, these syndromes will be accompanied by neoplasias outside the colon or GI tract, and will be discussed accordingly. The tissue pathologist's role in this scenario is to be fully aware of: (1) the histological presentations of these disorders; and (2) the tissue-based molecular tests that can be carried out before the patient is labeled as a "high-risk individual" and undergoes genetic counseling and further genetic testing.

## Familial adenomatous polyposis (FAP)

FAP is an autosomal dominant disorder. Patients develop hundreds to thousands of adenomas of the colon prior to adenocarcinoma formation, usually in early adult life if prophylactic colectomy is not performed before then (2, 3). In addition, these patients have a tendency to develop polyps in the upper GI tract, in addition to other malignancies in the upper GI tract, thyroid and brain. Prophylactic colectomy is the treatment of choice once colonic polyposis is manifested.

Patients with FAP have mutations in the Adenoma Polyposis Coli (APC) gene, on chromosome 5q21. The APC gene is composed of 15 exons, encoding for a protein of 2,843 amino acids. APC mutations are detectable in 85% of FAP patients, 90% of which lead to protein truncation.

As the key cause of this inherited disease, APC is germline-mutated in FAP and, as such, must be detected in the patient's peripheral blood. In general, this falls in the realm of departments of molecular genetics. Obtaining a full sequence of the APC gene is, like in many other cancer-inherited disorders, a very laborious endeavor. Although there are "hot-spots" in the APC gene where the mutation, if present, is more likely to be identified (such as the mutation located on codon 1307 of the APC gene, which is present in up to 5% of the American Ashkenazi Jewish population), the mutation profile can be very widespread over this large gene, hence the difficulty in the analysis. This process is likely to be significantly facilitated in the near future by the regular use of next generation sequencing technology, which is able to deliver a much better turnaround time and a much more affordable way of testing by its capacity to sequence multiple targets and multiple samples concomitantly.

The main task of the histopathologist still remains being aware of the histological findings that are associated with a diagnosis of FAP. These diagnostic features are:

- More than 100 polyps, usually thousands, leading to predominantly left-sided colorectal cancer if unresected. The morphology of these polyps is that of traditional tubular adenomas.

- Periampullary duodenal adenomas, usually multiple. These may be tubular, tubulovillous or villous, and they frequently recur after resection.

- Desmoid fibromatosis, mesenteric/abdominal in location, is usually a consequence of surgery. This can represent a source of significant complications in management if other aspects of the disease are well controlled.

- In the context of Gardner syndrome – osteomas, fibromatosis and cutaneous epidermoid cysts.

- Rare, isolated associations: thyroid carcinoma, particularly of the distinctive cribriform-morular variant; hepatoblastoma; pancreatobiliary neoplasms.

- In the context of Turcot syndrome – CNS neoplasms, more likely medulloblastomas.

**201**

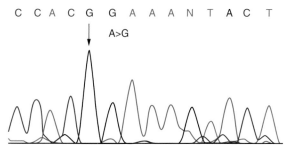

C C A C G G A A A N T A C T

A>G

**Figure 14.1** ACG>ACA (Thr>Thr) sequence variant at codon 1493 seen in all tumoral components of a case of cribriform-morular thyroid cancer. For further details, see (4).

- Attenuated FAP, a phenotypically milder form of the disease, also APC mutation-related, may be especially difficult to recognize as the adenomas are fewer in number and appear later, usually less than 100 in number and typically smaller than 1 cm until adulthood; they have a tendency to be right-sided. The main differential diagnosis here would be MYH-associated polyposis syndrome (see below).

It should not be forgotten that the APC gene is mutated in many cancer types, the vast majority of which are not syndromic in nature. Figure 14.1 depicts a mutation detected in DNA extracted from the formalin-fixed paraffin-embedded material of a cribriform-morular subtype of thyroid carcinoma, sporadic in nature.

### HNPCC

*Clinico-pathological background* –– Hereditary non-polyposis colorectal cancer (HNPCC) is the most important known hereditary CRC syndrome, accounting for approximately 3% of all CRCs (5). HNPCC is caused by a mutation in the mismatch repairs genes, the best known ones being hMSH2, hMLH1, hPMS1, PMS2 and hMSH6. These genes are key players in the repair of failures occurring during the DNA replication process. Individuals with such mutations and suboptimal replication repair machinery will have a tendency to accumulate mutations throughout the genome which, eventually, will lead to the HNPCC or Lynch syndromes. The HNPCC/Lynch syndromes can also be associated with cancers of the endometrium, ovaries and stomach, among others. Once the diagnosis is proven by the detection of the mutation, colonoscopic

surveillance usually takes place at annual intervals, with extra surveillance in the case of female mutation carriers for gynecological malignancies.

The diagnosis of HNPCC is, to start, a clinico-pathological one, based on the Amsterdam criteria and the revised Bethesda guidelines. The Amsterdam criteria require that at least three relatives have colorectal cancer and all of the following criteria are present: (1) one is a first-degree relative (parent, sibling or child) of the other two; (2) at least two successive generations are involved; (3) at least one relative had colorectal cancer when they were younger than 50 years of age; and (4) familial adenomatous polyposis has been excluded. The revised Bethesda Guidelines aim to detect CRCs that need to undergo one of the tests associated with HNPCC described below (the microsatellite instability test), and one of the following is sufficient to start the process of testing: (1) colorectal cancer in a patient younger than age 50 years of age; (2) a second synchronous or metachronous colorectal cancer or cancer associated with HNPCC (as described above); (3) presence of colorectal cancer with high-level microsatellite instability in a patient younger than 60 years of age; (4) one or more first-degree relative(s) with either colorectal cancer or HNPCC-associated tumor diagnosed younger than 50 years of age; or (5) colorectal cancer in two or more first- or second-degree relatives with HNPCC-related tumors at any age. In our experience, the confirmation of some of these criteria often involves the review of pathology records and pathology materials from other family members.

*The testing for HNPCC* –– The logical approach to HNPCC diagnosis would be to test up-front for mutations in the mismatch repair genes. Logical as it seems, this approach has a series of logistical barriers that would make it impractical, the most important being that we are faced with four to five genes that are very large and typically lack well-defined "hot-spots"; as such, the test has a very large turnaround time and a high cost. Hence, a more practical approach is to consider the Amsterdam criteria, the Bethesda guidelines and three analytical surrogates of mismatch repair proteins to decide who should be tested. These surrogates are: (1) the expression of the MMR proteins hMSH2, hMLH1, hPMS1, PMS2 and hMSH6by immunohistochemistry (IHC); (2) the analysis of microsatellite instability (MSI); and (3) the analysis of BRAF mutations.

Approximately 15% of CRCs have lost the expression of one of the MMR proteins, which is largely correlated with the presence of microsatellite instability. More than two-thirds of cancers with MMR protein expression loss by IHC are due to somatic (not germline/inherited) mutations in the MMR genes, and less than one-third (3% to 5% of the total) are due to an inherited mutation in the context of HNPCC. Hence, a "negative" test for MMR IHC or MSI excludes a diagnosis of HNPCC, but only one-third of patients with a "positive" test will have HNPCC. In an ideal world, the results of MMR IHC and MSI should be concordant, except for those cases in which the mutation leads to a protein that is still structurally detectable by IHC but functionally inactive, which are very few in number. Unfortunately, more discordances than those expected do exist that, in many cases, can be attributed to technical rather than biological reasons. As such, it is recommended that both tests be carried out in parallel. One of these possible technical issues relates to the interpretation of the IHC. Here, the pathologist is looking for loss of expression of the MMR protein as a sign of a mutation in the concordant MMR gene. Unfortunately, variations in the staining intensity secondary to manually performed IHC or suboptimal fixation of the material may lead to partial loss of expression in the tumor, which is reported by the pathologist accordingly; this, in our experience, represents the vast majority of the cases that, once submitted for full genetic analysis, are diagnosed as non-HNPCC-related tumors.

The mechanism of how we perform MSI testing is described in some detail in the section entitled "MSI," and depicted in Figure 14.2. Microsatellite instability is a representation of the accumulation of mutations throughout the CRC genome that result from the suboptimal activity of the MMR machinery. For this test, pathologists need to identify areas of cancer (and, for some versions of this test, also normal tissue from the same patient as a control). Typically, the MSI tests have a sensitivity of 20%. As such, it is recommended that, whenever possible, the pathologist submits tissue blocks or marked tissue areas where there is a substantial high tumor to non-tumor ratio.

If, as indicated before, only one-third of MSI-positive CRC cases are HNPCC, is there any way of narrowing this number down? In this context, testing for BRAF mutations may be of help. In general, the detection of BRAF mutations is becoming of

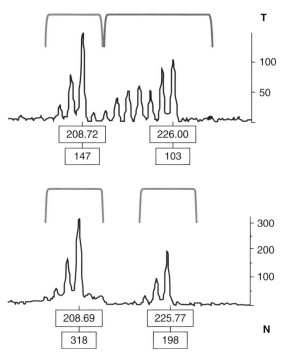

**Figure 14.2 Microsatellite instability**
Analysis of a dinucleotide microsatellite in a colorectal cancer (T) and the normal mucosa (N). Note the regular cadence of the stutter peaks in both alleles in N and the left allele in T (all highlighted in blue), and the change in the stutter cadence in the right allele in T (red).

significant diagnostic help in modern pathology – for example, in the diagnosis of pilocytic astrocytomas, hairy cell leukemias, thyroid cancer and malignant melanoma, among others. In CRC, the detection of BRAF mutations can help in treatment decisions, as patients with a BRAF mutation do not benefit from cetuximab therapy (see "CRC – response to cetuximab," below). In the context of HNPCC diagnosis, it appears that MSI-positive CRC that are BRAF mutant are more likely to be sporadic; HNPCC-associated CRCs are usually BRAF wild-type. Hence, there are groups that have advocated incorporating BRAF mutational analysis as part of a screening panel for the diagnosis of HNPCC. The test type and the histopathological requirements for BRAF testing are similar for both diagnostic and therapeutic purposes, and are described below.

In summary, the clinical background (Amsterdam and Bethesda) and the specific testing for MMR IHC, MSI and BRAF can confidently identify patients with a very high likelihood of HNPCC who need to be referred for genetic analysis. These tests are either part of the pathologist's armamentarium (MMR IHC) or require well-annotated FFPE material for successful molecular testing (MSI and BRAF).

Indeed, due to the robustness of the molecular tests currently available, and a heightened awareness of HNPCC in general, it has been suggested that screening patients for HNPCC should be performed in all patients with CRC.

### CRC – MYH-associated polyposis syndrome (MAP)

*Clinico-pathological background –*– The MYH gene, similar to the MMR genes in HNPCC, is involved in the DNA proof-reading machinery of the genome, and MYH mutations will result in the accumulation of further genomic mutations (5). Perhaps because one of the genes most likely to be affected is APC, the morphological expression of MAP is the presence of colorectal polyps, usually small tubular adenomas, and occasionally some extra-colonic manifestations not dissimilar to FAP. The polyps in MAP are usually less in number compared with FAP and, as such, are closer to the attenuated FAP phenotype. MAP is an autosomal recessive disease, where both parental alleles must be mutated for the disease to manifest. Perhaps because of this, these patients usually do not undergo adequate surveillance. However, once diagnosis is established in a family member, relatives at risk should benefit from preventive measures.

*Testing strategies –*– When a patient appears with a polyposis phenotypic appearance as described before, but no clear-cut family history of CRC, a diagnosis of MAP should be suspected. Although the number of germline mutations recorded to date is high, there appear to be two common mutations (Y165C and G382D) causing up to 80% of CRCs in patients with Northern European descent. Thus, this provides a cost-effective and relatively simple way of detecting the germline mutation. Should this first-line mutation analysis be negative and MAP remains in the differential diagnosis, a full-gene mutation screening will be necessary. For the routine diagnostic pathologist, the same provisos as with FAP apply – for example, awareness of the phenotypic features and the need for peripheral blood for a reliable diagnosis.

### Tests with a predominant therapeutic value

Cancer molecular tests can be divided into two main types, namely diagnostic (sometimes genetic) and therapeutic (6–11).

Pathologists are the taxonomist of diseases. The main aim of this exercise is to place cancers within entities with a clear diagnostic value and therapeutic course of action. It is increasingly obvious that such taxonomy cannot be morphological only and, indeed, many of the new classifications of diseases are morpho-molecular in nature. As indicated earlier, most of the molecular tests with a predominant diagnostic value in the GI tract are used to identify an inherited cause of disease.

Therapeutic tests are at the core of so-called therapeutic pathology, personalized medicine or precision medicine. The field of oncology is increasingly populated by a series of antibodies and small molecule inhibitors targeting specific molecules (actionable targets) involved in clearly defined oncogenic signaling pathways. One of the hallmarks of this process is the existence of biomarkers able to predict which patients are more likely to respond to these targeted therapies. This transformation in oncology is also rapidly changing the world of pathology and molecular diagnostics. In fact, the bulk of molecular diagnostics applied to GI cancer is related to therapeutic pathology and, in particular, the prediction of response to three main drugs: cetuximab in colon cancer, trastuzumab in gastric cancer and imatinib in gastrointestinal stromal tumors.

### CRC – response to cetuximab

Cetuximab (for the purpose of CRC treatment) is, together with erlotinib/gefitinib in lung cancer and trastuzumab in breast cancer, the most commonly used drug in the area of personalized medicine of solid tumors. Consequently, predictive profiling of CRCs for response to cetuximab represents one of the major efforts of a conventional molecular diagnostic laboratory currently.

*KRAS testing*

**Brief molecular background** KRAS belongs to the family of RAS oncogenes that serve as transducers coupling cell surface receptor signaling to intracellular effector pathways. KRAS is one of the most frequently mutated genes in human cancers. In colorectal carcinomas, the prevalence of KRAS mutations is around 30%, with most of these (around 90%) occurring in codons 12 and 13; less commonly affected sites include codons 61 and 146. These mutations lead to constitutive activation of KRAS, independent of upstream signaling receptors such as the epidermal growth factor receptor (EGFR). Several studies, although not all, have documented a correlation between the presence of KRAS mutations and poorer survival in colorectal carcinomas.

**Clinical and diagnostic utility** Cetuximab and panitumumab are monoclonal antibodies directed against the extracellular domain of EGFR. These antibodies prevent EGFR dimerization and subsequent downstream oncogenic signaling pathways. Clinical trials, reported between 2004 and 2007, documented clinically significant activity of cetuximab and panitumumab therapy against a subset of metastatic CRC. Further retrospective analyses showed that the presence of KRAS codon 12 and 13 mutations generally correlated with resistance to cetuximab and panitumumab therapy.

Currently, this observation forms the premise for KRAS mutational testing in the major guidelines – all CRC patients who are candidates for anti-EGFR monoclonal antibody therapy should undergo KRAS mutational analysis, and if KRAS mutations in codons 12 or 13 are detected, these patients should not receive cetuximab or panitumumab therapy.

More recent studies also suggest that KRAS mutations in codon 61, but not codon 146, correlate with lower response rates. Hence, routine testing of codon 61, in addition to codons 12 and 13, is advocated.

Of note, there is an emerging school of thought that different KRAS mutations are biologically distinct with regard to their oncogenicity and, as a corollary, their role in mediating resistance to cetuximab/panitumumab therapy. Some investigators have reported that the presence of codon 13 mutations, unlike codon 12 mutations, is associated with benefit in response to cetuximab therapy. Studies are still ongoing, and more evidence is required before this observation can be incorporated into routine practice.

It is also necessary to point out that, while there is a high concordance in the KRAS mutational profile between the primary colorectal tumor and metastasis, reportedly up to 30% of cases may show discordant results. This phenomenon might be due to several factors, including intratumoral heterogeneity or clonal evolution. It is therefore in the interest of the patient and managing team to evaluate the KRAS mutational status on both the primary and metastatic tumor if feasible.

Various assays exist for the detection of KRAS mutations (see an illustration of three of them in Figure 14.3). The most widely used method, at present, is direct sequencing of KRAS polymerase chain reaction (PCR) products. The sensitivity of this method is fairly low, and requires that mutant DNA copies have a concentration that is at least 20% to 50% of the wild-type sequences. This translates to a working rule of thumb that at least 30% of the sample submitted for KRAS sequencing should comprise tumor cells. Other newer, and purportedly more sensitive and specific, assays employ restriction fragment length polymorphism, allele-specific oligonucleotide hybridization, high-resolution melting analysis, amplification refractory mutation system and pyrosequencing. Selecting the right technology to detect a certain genotype is an important component of assay validation in molecular diagnostics, and a discussion of this subject is well beyond the scope of this chapter. However, it is important to indicate that up to 10% of cases would be genotyped differently for KRAS depending on the choice of technology. This explains the large number of publications advocating different testing platforms, both for KRAS mutational analysis and other tests in molecular diagnostics.

*BRAF testing*

**Brief molecular background** BRAF is a well-studied oncogene that belongs to the family of RAF serine/threonine kinases. RAF kinases function as downstream effectors of the RAS signaling pathway. Somatic BRAF mutations were first reported in diverse cancer types, including colorectal cancer, in 2002. The most common BRAF mutation occurs in exon 15, in which a T > A transversion at position 1799 results in a substitution of valine by glutamate at position 600 of the protein. This mutation, V600E, leads to constitutive activation of the BRAF protein. See Figure 14.4 for an example.

In colorectal carcinomas, the prevalence of BRAF V600E mutations, as documented in most studies, is less than 10%. The presence of this mutation has been reported in some studies to be an adverse prognostic marker. BRAF and KRAS mutations are generally mutually exclusive.

**Clinical and diagnostic utility** As stated in the previous section, there is strong evidence that patients with KRAS mutations do not benefit from cetuximab/panitumumab therapy. Therefore, to date, the major guidelines state that only patients with wild-type KRAS codon 12 or 13 mutations should be considered eligible for anti-EGFR monoclonal antibody therapy.

**205**

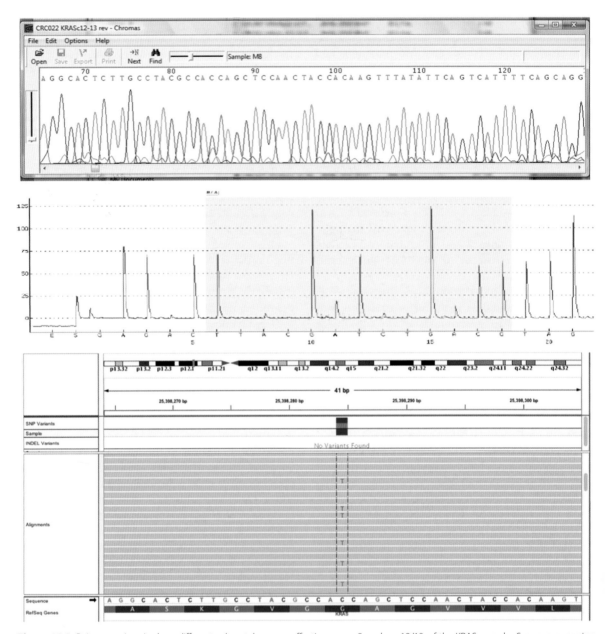

**Figure 14.3** Point mutations in three different colorectal cancers affecting exons 2, codons 12/13, of the KRAS gene by Sanger sequencing (top), pyrosequencing (middle) and next generation sequencing (bottom). We thank Drs. Catherwood and McCourt, from our laboratory, for these images.

However, approximately 60% of patients with KRAS wild-type tumors are resistant to anti-EGFR monoclonal antibody therapy, prompting the need to evaluate and identify more predictive biomarkers. One potential biomarker that has received much scrutiny is BRAF. Although the evidence is less conclusive at present, due in part to the low prevalence of BRAF

mutations in colorectal carcinomas, several studies have reported that patients with BRAF V600E mutations similarly do not benefit from cetuximab therapy.

Besides being an indirect predictive biomarker (for EGFR-targeted therapeutics), the BRAF V600E mutation may, in the future, be a direct predictive biomarker for BRAF V600E-targeted therapeutics in

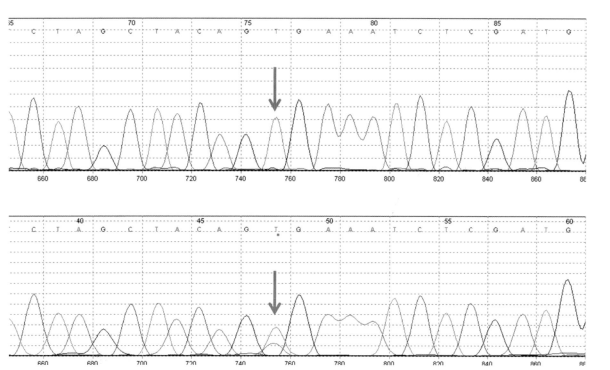

**Figure 14.4** BRAF wild-type (top) and mutant (bottom). Note the partial change of the GTG sequence into a GAT in the mutant trace. We thank Dr. Catherwood, from our laboratory, for these images.

colorectal carcinomas. These therapeutics include vemurafenib, which has demonstrated significant clinical activity against BRAF V600E-mutant melanomas, and dabrafenib. At the time of writing, both agents have already been tested in phase I clinical trials, with documented clinical activity against colorectal carcinoma.

The methods used to detect BRAF mutations are similar to those stated in the earlier section for the detection of KRAS mutations, and include direct sequencing and pyrosequencing (8). There is also a BRAF V600E mutation-specific monoclonal antibody that can be utilized for immunohistochemistry. To date, most studies report a high concordance between this immunohistochemical assay and genotyping.

*CRC – response to 5-FU*

**Thymidylate synthase**    *Brief molecular background –* thymidylate synthase is involved in the sole *de novo* pathway of thymidine production that is vital for DNA replication and repair. 5-fluorouracil (5-FU), a standard chemotherapeutic agent used in the treatment of colorectal carcinoma, acts by inhibiting thymidylate synthase (11). This leads to cessation of DNA synthesis and activation of cell death.

*Clinical and diagnostic utility –* although conflicting results have been reported, it is generally thought that higher thymidylate synthase expression levels correlate with resistance to 5-FU-based chemotherapeutic regimes. A meta-analysis by Popat *et al.* (11) reported that colorectal carcinomas with higher thymidylate synthase expression were linked to a poorer overall survival rate than those with low expression. However, to date, the major guidelines have not advocated routine thymidylate synthase expression analysis.

*Test method –* at present, the optimal method of evaluating thymidylate synthase expression is not ascertained. Most studies have performed IHC and/ or reverse transcriptase polymerase chain reaction (RTPCR). RTPCR requires fresh tissue and a more sophisticated diagnostic set-up, while IHC is more practical for a routine diagnostic service. A smaller number of studies have employed enzyme assay, which is technically tedious and unsuitable for implementation into routine molecular diagnostics. Finally, there has also been interest in correlating thymidylate synthase gene polymorphisms with 5-FU response and toxicity. This genotyping can be performed on genomic DNA extracted from normal colon. Similar to that of thymidylate synthase expression levels, to date, the evidence for a genotype-response relationship is inconclusive.

**MSI**   Brief molecular background – microsatellites are simple repetitive sequences occurring in the genome (12, 13). Microsatellite instability refers to increases or decreases in the number of repeats in these microsatellites, typically occurring as a result of defects in mismatch repair (see earlier section and Figure 14.2). Approximately 15% of sporadic colorectal cancers display MSI.

*Detection rational* – MSI is detected by polymerase chain reaction (PCR) of specific microsatellite repeats. Originally, five microsatellite markers were typically evaluated: three dinucleotide (D2S123, D5S346 and D17S250) and two mononucleotide (BAT25 and BAT26) repeats; this panel of five markers is referred to as the Bethesda Panel. With these markers, MSI is categorized as high-frequency MSI (MSI-H) if two or more of five markers show instability, and low-frequency MSI (MSI-L) if one of five markers shows instability. Tumors that do not display instability in any of the markers are categorized as microsatellite stable (MSS). Subsequently, it was perceived that the MSI-L category was of little clinical use, and that a different choice of markers (all mononucleotide) would be able to discern between MSI and MSS more efficiently. Hence, many laboratories have adopted the all-mononucleotide approach, which is also the preferred design in many off-the-shelf kits for this analysis.

*Clinical and diagnostic utility* – in addition to its prognostic value described previously, MSI status is thought to provide predictive information for response to adjuvant chemotherapy, in particular 5-fluorouracil (5-FU). To date, the data are still conflicting, and there are differing schools of thought. Most studies, including randomized clinical trials, retrospective studies and a meta-analysis, have reported a lack of benefit from adjuvant 5-FU in MSI-H colorectal carcinomas. This is supported by *in vitro* experimental studies that have shown that a competent mismatch repair system enhances the toxicity of 5-FU in human colorectal carcinoma cell lines. There are also more recent and ongoing efforts to

evaluate the utility of MSI status as a predictive biomarker of response to irinotecan and other chemotherapeutic agents.

### PIK3CA, aspirin and colorectal carcinoma

*Brief molecular background* –– Although still early days for this theme, brief mention is made of PIK3CA mutations as a potential predictive biomarker for adjuvant aspirin therapy in colorectal carcinomas, in view of a recent major molecular pathological epidemiology study by Liao *et al.* (14).

Many earlier studies reported that regular aspirin use lowers the risk of colorectal neoplasia development. Some investigators advanced the idea that this protective effect of aspirin might be due, in part, to its inhibition of cyclooxgenase-2 (COX-2, also termed PTGS2), an enzyme involved in prostaglandin synthesis. Prostaglandins are known to have tumorigenic properties through mechanisms such as angiogenesis and immune modulation. COX-2 is widely regarded as an important oncogenic player in colorectal carcinogenesis.

The phosphatidylinositol 3-kinase (PI3K) signaling pathway is another significant oncogenic driver in colorectal carcinomas. Up to 20% of colorectal carcinomas harbor mutations in PIK3CA, the gene that codes for phosphatidylinositol 3-kinase (PI3K). Given that PI3K signaling has been reported to enhance COX-2 activity, Liao *et al.* investigated the relationship between colorectal carcinoma survival, aspirin consumption and the presence of PIK3CA mutations. They found that regular aspirin use after diagnosis was associated with longer survival among patients with PIK3CA-mutant colorectal carcinomas, but not among patients with wild-type PIK3CA tumors. Their findings suggest that PIK3CA mutations may serve as a predictive biomarker for adjuvant aspirin therapy in colorectal carcinomas.

### Gene expression signatures

*Brief molecular background* –– Gene expression profiling, the quantitation of mRNA expression levels of multiple genes simultaneously, first came to prominence in oncology in 2004, when a multigene assay was shown to predict recurrence of tamoxifen-treated, node-negative breast cancer (15–17). The Onco*type* DX Breast Cancer 21-gene assay (marketed by Genomic Health, Inc., Redwood City, CA) is now included in many breast cancer consensus guidelines as an adjunct for chemotherapeutic decision making.

There has been recent interest in applying this strategy to colorectal cancer, specifically with regard to assessment of recurrence risk and benefits from chemotherapy in stage II CRC patients.

*Clinical and diagnostic utility* –– At present, there is sufficient evidence to recommend adjuvant chemotherapy for stage III (node-positive) CRC patients. However, adjuvant chemotherapy offers very modest benefit in stage II (node-negative) CRC patients, with survival improvement of less than 5% at five years. Some investigators opine that better prognostic markers, beyond traditional clinicopathological parameters such as intestinal perforation, high tumor grade, etc., are needed to identify stage II CRC patients who have higher recurrence risk, and who are therefore more likely to benefit from adjuvant chemotherapy.

*Testing approaches* –– The Oncotype DX Colon Cancer test evaluates the expression levels of 12 genes (seven cancer-related, five reference) from formalin-fixed paraffin-embedded tissue and generates a recurrence score, scaled from 0 to 100. This recurrence score is significantly associated with recurrence risk at three years post-surgical resection. Patients can also be classified as low- (score <30), intermediate- (score 30 to 40) and high-risk (score ≥41). In multivariate analysis, the recurrence score is prognostically significant, independent of conventional clinicopathological parameters. However, the presence of either T4 tumor stage or mismatch repair protein deficiency reportedly outweighs the prognostic significance of the recurrence score. At present, the recurrence score, or another treatment score generated from a separate gene panel, has not been shown to be predictive of benefit from adjuvant chemotherapy.

Other high-throughput gene expression profiling technologies (such as the CRC DSA™ tool) are following a similar path of development as prognostication assays.

These tests are "single laboratory tests," performed by a central laboratory to which pathologists submit samples according to protocols established by the companies. Controversy has not abated in relation to the use of tests provided by single, central laboratories that, because of commercial reasons or because of the difficulty of validating the test, do not have test designs that can be utilized in other accredited laboratories.

## Gastric cancer – HER2

### HER2, trastuzumab and gastric cancer

*Brief molecular background* –– HER2 is a member of the oncogenic epidermal growth factor receptor (EGFR) family of tyrosine kinase receptors (18–19). HER2 genomic amplification and protein over-expression, first identified in breast cancers in the 1980s, have been reported in diverse cancer types, including gastric cancer. The prevalence of HER2 genomic amplification and protein over-expression in gastric cancers is between 10% and 30%.

Trastuzumab, a monoclonal antibody targeting HER2, is efficacious against HER2-positive breast cancers. The landmark 2010 Trastuzumab for Gastric Cancer (ToGA) trial showed that addition of trastuzumab to conventional chemotherapy significantly improved overall survival in patients with HER2-positive advanced gastric cancers, setting the stage for routine HER2 testing in gastric cancer diagnostics.

*Clinical and diagnostic utility* –– HER2 status serves as a predictive biomarker for response to trastuzumab in gastric cancers, and this is determined both at the genomic and protein level by *in situ* hybridization and IHC respectively.

HER2 genomic amplification, as assessed by fluorescence *in situ* hybridization, is defined as a HER2: CEP17 ratio >2 according to the ToGA trial. The immunohistochemical scoring criteria, as stated in the ToGA trial, are as shown in Table 14.2.

The ToGA trial reported that trastuzumab benefit was limited to patients with IHC 2+ and HER2 amplified-, or IHC 3+ gastric cancers. Hence, most major guidelines now recommend IHC as the first line for HER2 diagnostics in gastric cancer, with a confirmatory fluorescence *in situ* hybridization (FISH) for IHC equivocal cases, similar to that in breast cancer. Whether such an algorithm is ideal is subject to debate.

It is necessary to point out that although FISH is currently the most widely used technique to determine HER2 genomic status, other brightfield-based assays, such as chromogenic and silver *in situ* hybridization, show accuracy equivalent to FISH, and offer more advantages including greater ease of use, durability of records and enhanced correlation with morphological features.

Given the increasingly recognized phenomenon that considerable intratumoral heterogeneity in the HER2 genomic and protein expression status exists in gastric cancers, brightfield-based assays may be

Table 14.2

|  | Surgical specimen | Biopsy specimen | Assessment |
|---|---|---|---|
| 0 | No reactivity or membranous reactivity in <10% of tumor cells | No reactivity or no membranous reactivity in any tumor cell | Negative |
| 1+ | Faint or barely perceptible membranous reactivity in ≥ 10% of tumor cells; cells are reactive only in part of their membrane | Tumor cell cluster with a faint or barely perceptible membranous reactivity irrespective of percentage of tumor cells stained | Negative |
| 2+ | Weak to moderate complete, basolateral or lateral membranous reactivity in ≥ 10% of tumor cells | Tumor cell cluster with a weak to moderate complete, basolateral or lateral membranous reactivity irrespective of percentage of tumor cells stained | Equivocal |
| 3+ | Strong complete, basolateral or lateral membranous reactivity in ≥ 10% of tumor cells | Tumor cell cluster with a strong complete, basolateral or lateral membranous reactivity irrespective of percentage of tumor cells stained | Positive |

more desirable than fluorescence-based assays, as screening for amplification at low-power is rendered easier on a light microscope. Figure 14.5 provides illustrations of HER2 genomic amplification (on two different platforms) and protein over-expression in gastric cancer.

Also, intratumoral heterogeneity poses a challenge when evaluating HER2 status on small biopsy specimens, as these samples may not be representative of the entire tumor. This issue has been highlighted by several groups, including our own. It is therefore necessary for the pathologist to include this caveat when reporting the HER2 status on small biopsy specimens.

## KIT and PDGFRA

### Brief molecular background

The presence of activating KIT and platelet-derived growth factor receptor alpha (PDGFRA) mutations in gastrointestinal tumors (GISTs) was reported in 1998 and 2003 respectively (20). Shortly after the discovery of KIT mutations, imatinib, a tyrosine kinase inhibitor that inhibits both KIT and PDGFR, was demonstrated to be efficacious against GISTs. The significance of this development cannot be over-stated; prior to this, the median survival for advanced GISTs was less than 20 months for metastatic and/or locally recurrent tumors. Since the advent of imatinib therapy, the median survival for advanced GISTs has increased to more than 50 months.

### KIT and PDGFRA mutational analyses – clinical and diagnostic utility

KIT and PDGFRA mutational analyses primarily serve as diagnostic (i.e. to confirm the diagnosis of

GIST) and predictive (i.e. to predict therapeutic response) biomarkers. Approximately 85% of GISTs harbor primary KIT mutations, that is, KIT mutations occurring prior to imatinib therapy. Around 70% of GISTs harbor *KIT* mutations in exon 11, which encodes the juxtamembrane domain. Around 10% to 15% of GISTs harbor KIT mutations in exon 9, which encodes part of the extracellular domain. Other less common KIT mutations involve exons 13 and 17, which encode the kinase domain; and exon 8, which encodes part of the extracellular domain. Approximately 5% to 7% of GISTs have an activating mutation of PDGFRA, homologous to those of KIT. KIT and PDGFRA mutations are, thus far, mutually exclusive. PDGFRA-mutant GISTs arise most commonly in the stomach, and are associated with an epithelioid morphology. The most common mutation site is exon 18, which encodes for the second kinase domain in PDGFRA. The single most common primary PDGFRA mutation is the D842V substitution in exon 18, accounting for around two-thirds of PDGFRA mutations.

The identification of KIT and PDGFRA mutations, together with the development of imatinib, ushered in a target molecule genotype-drug response paradigm in oncology. Patients whose tumors contained exon 11 KIT mutations have a higher response rate to imatinib than those with exon 9 KIT mutations or wild-type KIT. Patients with tumors containing exon 9 KIT mutations have improved response rates when treated with a higher dose of imatinib. Tumors harboring the PDGFRA D842V mutation are reportedly resistant to imatinib.

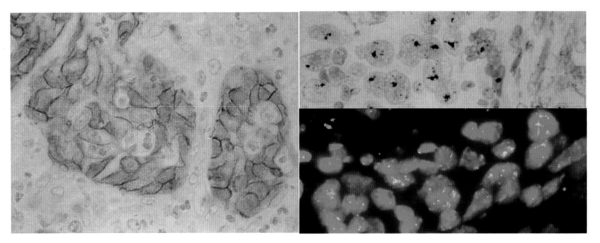

**Figure 14.5** Gastric cancer with HER2 protein over-expression by immunohistochemistry (left, note the characteristic basolateral membrane reactivity), and HER2 genomic amplification by chromogenic *in situ* hybridization (right top) and fluorescent *in situ* hybridization (bottom right).

Although the majority of GISTs show response to imatinib, approximately 10% will progress within six months of therapy initiation, indicating primary resistance. PDGFRA D842V and KIT exon 9 mutations account for the majority of primary imatinib resistance. Another 40% to 50% will develop imatinib resistance within two years, indicating secondary resistance. KIT mutations account for the majority of secondary imatinib resistance. These mutations cluster in exons 13, 14, 17 and 18. PDGFRA mutations account for a minority of secondary imatinib resistance.

The molecular analysis of GISTs as a purely diagnostic (and not therapeutic) tool can be useful, particularly in those GISTs without immunohistochemical expression of c-kit/CD117, where a differential diagnosis with other spindle cell lesions (for example, leiomyoma, leiomyosarcoma) still remains. Leiomyomatous lesions do not harbor KIT or PDGFRA mutations.

**Detection methods**

KIT or PDGFRA mutations are usually identified by PCR-based tests on FFPE material, designed to detect either the common mutation sites ("hot-spots") or covering all the exons of interest. It is a DNA-based test, for which the histopathologist will need to provide material from the most representative tissue block. An example is provided in Figure 14.6.

**Molecular cytopathology in the gastrointestinal tract**

Paraphrasing the general definition offered at the beginning of this chapter, molecular cytopathology is the application of molecular biology techniques to cytopathology samples, including both exfoliative and interventional (for example, FNA) specimens (21–23). The advances in tissue procurement, nucleic acid isolation and test sensitivity have led to the dictum that cytology samples are as good as tissue samples for molecular testing. Thus, the same rules for adequacy of samples for histopathology apply to cytopathology, such as appropriate fixation, adequate cellularity and optimal *tumor: non-tumor* ratio, which are important factors in determining the sensitivity of the test. Analysis with varying levels of tumor burden in the diagnostic sample is recommended for each test that is validated in a molecular diagnostic laboratory, and cytology samples should be included so that the technical feasibility of using such samples can be documented in the laboratory records.

The use of cytology samples for molecular testing is becoming increasingly common and is not restricted to GI pathology. Indeed, reports are available in the literature supporting the use of PCR-based techniques in cytology samples of all types and from all organ systems (see Figure 14.7).

1. KRAS and BRAF testing – KRAS mutations can be confidently detected in FNA samples. The first diagnosis of adenocarcinoma of the colon is seldom done on cytology samples, but there are

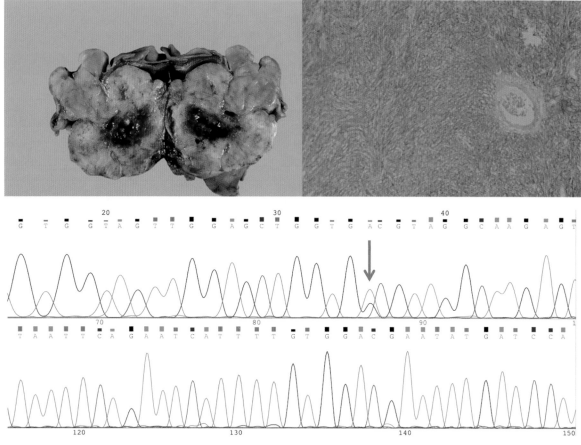

**Figure 14.6** Classic example of a GIST, with a characteristic central necrosis (top left), CD117 protein expression by IHC (top right) and point mutation in the c-kit gene (bottom). In collaboration with Dr. Brendan Pang, National University of Singapore.

occasions where the FNA material of a metastatic lesion (primarily in the liver) is the only material available in a referral hospital, with the primary material housed in another center and difficult to track. Those studies looking at the tissue-cytology concordance have shown excellent correlation, but with some discrepancies, usually attributed to clonal evolution or tumor heterogeneity rather than to technical reasons.

2. CKIT and PGDFRA testing – GISTs are not uncommonly diagnosed on a cytology sample, primarily in those cases in which the lesion is still clearly submucosal and the endoscopic examination demonstrates a smooth epithelial surface; on those occasions, endoscopic ultrasound and fine-needle aspirate is a reliable method. Mutational analysis is possible with these samples, delivering both predictive and diagnostic information.

3. Other PCR-based tests – microsatellite analyses of FNA materials have been done successfully in several cancer types. However, in view of the relatively high ratio of tumor vs. non-tumor needed for this test, and the need for some protocols to analyze a normal sample from the same patient for comparison, this is not a recommended way of detecting the microsatellite status of cancers. Equally so, the detection of mutations of APC, MYH and others is possible in FFPE cytology material, but the germline nature of these mutations (in the patient's normal genome), the availability of normal samples (typically peripheral blood) and the significance of the result to the patient and to many of the family members mean that such analyses should fall under the purview of a genetics department.

4. Therapeutic immunohistochemistry – HER2 IHC/ISH and thymidylate synthase IHC can be

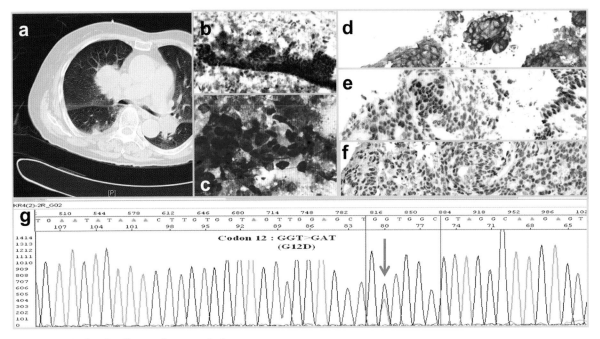

**Figure 14.7 Molecular diagnostic cytopathology**
Patient with a right hilar mass in the lower lobe of the lung (a); FNA appearances of adenocarcinoma with a necrotic background (b) and (c); IHC suggestive of a CRC primary, including expression of Villin (d) and CDX2 (e) and lack of TTF-1 expression (f); and mutation in KRAS, exon 2 codon 12 (g). The patient has a rectal carcinoma resected two years prior to this lung mass. In collaboration with Dr. Brendan Pang, National University of Singapore.

technically performed on cell block cytology samples. However, the very specific rules of scoring for these biomarkers and the increasing relevance of heterogeneity (particularly in the context of HER2) do not support this practice.

5. The use of cytology samples for high-throughput molecular testing is, to date, in the realm of research endeavors only.

## Future directions

Future predictions in molecular pathology and molecular diagnostics are not easy. However, if we accept the premise that the future of molecular medicine will be dictated by (1) the development of molecular medicine and (2) the pace of technological development, then we can presume that molecular pathology will be one of the key areas of development in the foreseeable future. In the area of the GI tract, the following trends are likely to happen:

### Colon cancer – the need for new discoveries

It is paradoxical that there are less options for personalized medicine/targeted therapy in CRC, the most studied cancer type worldwide, than lung or breast cancer. The current paradigm of discovery is leading to the characterization of actionable targets that are applicable to a small percentage of each cancer type. Hence, many more tests will be available in the future.

### Cancers of unmet needs

While there is only one biomarker in gastric cancer that is currently standard of care (HER2), full-genome analysis of this disease has identified subgroups that are potentially actionable therapeutically: detection of MET, EGFR or FGFR2 mutations may become standard of care in gastric cancer. Equally, cancer types in which personalized medicine is currently not a prominent feature, such as eosophageal or small bowel carcinomas, are likely to have new molecular biomarkers of therapeutic utility.

### New technologies

The increasing number of available biomarkers will result in the need to detect more than one biomarker for diagnosis or therapeutic decision making in a single cancer. This requires a change of technology from one currently centered on single-biomarker analyses, to one capable of detecting multiple targets in a single experiment. In view of this, next generation sequencing technologies, which are already used for mutation analysis in genomic DNA for inherited diseases, will also be fully validated and readily available for FFPE material, increasing exponentially the availability of clinically valuable information. This will pose a challenge to pathologists (*how do we report results related to a significant portion of the cancer's genome?*) and to clinicians (*how do we make use of the plethora of possible therapeutic options generated by large amounts of information?*).

### The pathologist's role

How will the practice of traditional morphology-based pathology survive the increasing relevance of molecular diagnostics? Is awareness of the molecular diagnostics provided by others, based on FFPE materials, enough to maintain full clinical relevance? Or do we need to become active players in the provision of molecular testing beyond "therapeutic immunohisto-chemistry"? Some of these questions are addressed in Chapter 21.

## Pancreas and bile duct
## Introduction

Pancreatic and biliary tract lesions are among the most challenging of human neoplasias to screen for in a population, accurately diagnose, successfully treat and appropriately manage. Surgical pathologists and cytopathologists who review pancreatic and biliary tract specimens should be familiar with their role within the healthcare team and well aware of the implications of their diagnoses. Pancreatic carcinoma carries a poor prognosis and is one of the leading causes of cancer death, partially because the disease is often undetected until advanced stages. Although more pancreatic and biliary lesions are now being detected incidentally during abdominal imaging procedures for other reasons, definitive diagnosis and prognosis usually relies upon tissue sampling.

Pancreatic and biliary specimen types vary from cyst fluid and cytology obtained by endoscopic ultrasound-guided fine-needle aspiration (EUS-FNA) and biliary brushings to tissue biopsies from upper endoscopy procedures to histologic examination following partial or complete surgical resection. While more tissue is generally preferable for definitive

diagnosis and clear margins, patient comorbidities and the risks of more invasive procedures may necessitate limited sampling. Cytologic and histologic examinations for morphology remain paramount in clinical practice, but refined or more specific diagnoses can now be achieved with the help of ancillary studies.

Molecular testing may be added to the armamentarium of available studies, although triaging the specimen and selective use of these tests will ensure optimal efficiency and effectiveness within a healthcare system. Specimens enriched with tumor cells are generally more amenable to successful molecular tests. However, there is continued pressure to extract more information from ever-smaller samples and less invasive procedures. Furthermore, sampling and contamination issues become magnified in molecular testing, highlighting the importance of the pathologist's role in correlating morphologic findings and ensuring quality control. Currently, there is insufficient evidence that any molecular test should be used as a definitive or stand-alone method of evaluating pancreatic and biliary disease.

Thus far, molecular pathology has demonstrated only limited utility in supplementing current diagnostic modalities in pancreatic and biliary specimens, but there is significant potential for growth (Table 14.3). This section will review the molecular landscape of pancreatic and biliary pathology with a focus on clinically relevant alterations and tests that may be readily incorporated into a molecular laboratory. In addition to reviewing a practical approach to molecular testing for specimens from the pancreas and biliary tree, we address the clinical utility of various tests and indicate future directions.

## Molecular alterations
### Opportunities and challenges

Molecular diagnostics has brought a number of opportunities and challenges to the area of pancreatic and biliary pathology. While understanding these molecular changes may help with earlier detection and diagnosis of neoplastic lesions, sampling issues and the overlap between diagnostic entities will continue to frustrate pathologists. The earlier we screen for neoplastic conditions using sensitive molecular tests, the more questions arise regarding how to manage these patients. And while molecular diagnostics may better guide the development and utilization

Table 14.3 Molecular alterations and testing in pancreatic and biliary neoplasia

|  | Select molecular alteration(s) | Molecular test(s) with clinical utility |
|---|---|---|
| **PDAC** | KRAS, telomere shortening, CDKN2A, TP53, SMAD4, BRAF, STK11/LKB1 | KRAS mutational analysis |
| **SCA** | VHL (3p) | N/A |
| **MCN** | KRAS, RNF43, TP53, SMAD4 | KRAS mutational analysis |
| **IPMN** | KRAS, GNAS, RNF43, TP53, SMAD4 | KRAS and GNAS mutational analysis |
| **SPN** | CTNNB1 | N/A |
| **PanNET** | MSI | N/A |
| **CC** | KRAS, polysomy | KRAS mutational analysis, FISH for polysomy |

Key: N/A = not applicable; PDAC = pancreatic ductal adenocarcinoma; SCA = serous cystadenoma; MCN = mucinous cystic neoplasm; IPMN = intraductal papillary mucinous neoplasm; SPN = solid pseudo-papillary neoplasm; PanNET = pancreatic neuroendocrine tumor; MSI = microsatellite instability; CC = cholangiocarcinoma

of targeted therapies, tumors are known to develop new pathways of resistance. Even with the promise of whole genome sequencing of tumors, there are questions of how to interpret the molecular alterations and how to integrate this information with the rest of the patient's clinical picture.

## Molecular techniques

### Fluorescence *in situ* hybridization (FISH)

Despite challenges and limitations, molecular testing does potentially provide additional information with only minimal sample input. Cytology smears, touch preps and prepared slides, including biliary brushings and pancreatic lesions sampled by EUS-FNA, could all potentially be sent for fluorescence *in situ* hybridization (FISH). As this technique relies on the binding of specific probes to chromosomal targets, the presence of neoplastic nuclei is required. FISH can even be performed on slides that have undergone routine examination with other stains. When working from formalin-fixed paraffin-embedded blocks of tissue, FISH can be performed on either whole nuclei by shaving 50 μm scrolls from the formalin-fixed paraffin-embedded block or on standard 4 μm unstained slides. The major limitations of FISH are that there is a limit to the number of probes that can be examined on any given slide and that the target aberration must be known. While some laboratories send biliary brushings for FISH analysis, this approach has not yet achieved widespread use.

### Polymerase chain reaction (PCR) and sequencing

Cell blocks prepared by the cytology laboratory and formalin-fixed paraffin-embedded tissue are amenable to polymerase chain reaction (PCR), again presuming that the mutations of interest are known. Some large laboratories offer a multiplex-PCR, capillary electrophoresis-based assay that can simultaneously check for recurrent, or "hotspot," point mutations in a panel of known oncogenes, some of which are known to be recurrent in pancreatic carcinomas. Whole genome sequencing, including next generation sequencing (NGS), has been used by some academic laboratories to examine both well-known and newly elucidated molecular alterations in a variety of diseases, particularly in oncology and congenital conditions. In fact, whole exome sequencing has been used to explore the complex genetic landscape of pancreatic cancers and has identified new avenues for research (24). NGS may soon be more widely available for clinical use and could more thoroughly characterize pancreatic and biliary pathology.

## Mutations of pancreatic neoplasms

### Precursors to pancreatic adenocarcinoma

Pancreatic adenocarcinoma has been associated with a few well-recognized precursor lesions, namely pancreatic intraepithelial neoplasia (PanIN), intraductal papillary mucinous neoplasm (IPMN) and mucinous cystic neoplasm (MCN). The progression of normal

215

pancreatic tissue to PanIN to carcinoma has been modeled as a series of accumulated genetic alterations. These changes may be classified as early (telomere shortening and KRAS mutations), intermediate (inactivating mutations or epigenetic silencing of CDKN2A) and late (inactivating mutations of TP53 and SMAD4) (1). The genetic alterations underlying IPMN and MCN are less well understood. Like in PanIN, mutations in KRAS and TP53 have been reported in IPMN, along with mutations in BRAF and STK11/LKB1; MCNs may show KRAS and TP53 mutations in higher grade lesions (24). While accumulation of these genetic alterations may indicate carcinoma progression, mutational analysis is not routine for pancreatic adenocarcinomas in most laboratories.

### Immunohistochemistry for SMAD4

Alternatively, an immunohistochemical stain available for SMAD4 could be helpful to pathologists who regularly see pancreatic adenocarcinomas in practice (Figure 14.8a–b). The SMAD4 stain demonstrates loss of staining in a subset of pancreatic adenocarcinomas and carcinomas of the Ampulla of Vater, but shows preserved staining in adenomas. However, retention of staining does not exclude the possibility of a malignant tumor.

### KRAS, GNAS and beyond

KRAS and GNAS mutations are the two major contributors to molecular testing with regard to pancreatic and biliary neoplasia. The presence of specific mutations in these genes is a significant finding that can lend support to a pathologist's or cytopathologist's diagnosis, especially if the tissue is scant or poorly visualized. If the neoplastic cells harbor KRAS or GNAS mutations, these mutations could be detected with PCR on formalin-fixed paraffin-embedded tissue, cells obtained by FNA, or even fluid aspirated from pancreatic cysts and ducts.

The most well-known and universal of the mutated genes in pancreatic adenocarcinoma, v-ki-ras2 Kirsten rat sarcoma (KRAS), is an oncogene that is almost always altered early in the development of pancreatic carcinoma. Codons 12 and 13 are the most commonly altered. While the presence of a KRAS mutation does not necessarily indicate malignancy, it does provide evidence for a neoplastic precursor or process.

Testing for KRAS mutations is more helpful in situations of an inconclusive specimen or scant material, such as pancreatic cyst sampling, since the diagnosis of pancreatic carcinoma in biopsies or resection specimens is more straightforward. KRAS mutation testing may also be helpful for directing experimental therapies and clinical trials, particularly in patients with metastatic or recurrent disease.

Most IPMNs demonstrate alterations in KRAS, GNAS or both. Interestingly, a cyst may harbor more than one KRAS mutation and different cysts within one patient's pancreas may harbor different mutations (25). Unfortunately, these mutations are present in all stages of dysplasia and the absence of both markers does not exclude the presence of a mucinous neoplasm. In addition, a negative test for KRAS and GNAS mutations could be falsely negative in cases of

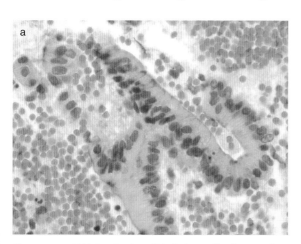
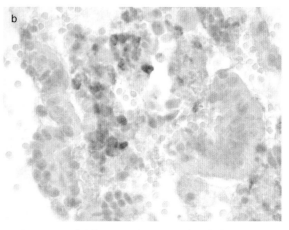

Figure 14.8 (a) H+E stain of a cellblock obtained by fine-needle aspiration, showing a well-differentiated pancreatic ductal adenocarcinoma. (b) IHC for SMAD4 showing aberrant loss of expression in the tumor cells of a well-differentiated pancreatic ductal adenocarcinoma.

insufficient cellularity. Thus, concurrent pathologic or cytologic examination is important to confirm the presence of lesional tissue.

More recently described, GNAS is an oncogene with a recurrent mutation in codon 201 that has been associated with IPMN (26). Although less frequently observed than KRAS mutations in pancreatic tumors, a mutation in GNAS distinguishes a pancreatic cyst as being an IPMN as opposed to an MCN. Furthermore, evidence suggests that secretin-stimulated pancreatic juice collected from the duodenum with GNAS mutations indicates the presence or emergence of IPMN (27). Again, testing for GNAS mutations will be most useful in inconclusive or scant cytologic specimens as part of the work-up of a pancreatic cyst or dilated pancreatic duct. GNAS and KRAS mutations can typically be tested together as part of a molecular panel, using fairly small amounts of fluid.

Although testing for KRAS and GNAS mutations are the mainstays with the most established clinical utility, other molecular alterations and corresponding tests are in the research pipeline and may eventually be used to direct patient care. Other genes that have been linked to pancreatic neoplasia include the following: ARID1A, MLL3, TGFBR1, TGFBR2, ACVR1B, RNF43, VHL and CTNNB1 (24). Serous cystadenomas may show loss of heterozygosity or loss of 3p (VHL gene), whereas solid pseudopapillary neoplasms have been closely linked to CTNNB1 mutations. Pancreatic endocrine tumors may demonstrate molecular alterations with microsatellite alternations (loss of 3p, 6pq, 10pq along with gain of 5q, 12q, 18q, 20q associated with malignant behavior). Loss of heterozygosity and polysomy have also been identified in pancreatic carcinomas.

# Pancreatic cysts

## Pancreatic cyst sampling, triage and processing

Pancreatic cysts, which may be more challenging for radiologists to distinguish as benign or malignant, lend themselves to endoscopic ultrasound-guided fine-needle aspiration (28). This method of sampling provides cyst fluid for cytological, biochemical and molecular analysis. Fresh cyst fluid should be triaged by the cytopathology laboratory and processed according to the amount of available specimen. If a small amount (<0.5 cc) of fresh pancreatic cyst fluid is obtained, priority should be given to biochemical analysis of CEA and then molecular analysis for

KRAS and GNAS mutations. An elevated CEA is associated with the presence of a mucinous cyst, one of the important questions to be answered by the pathology laboratory.

If at least 0.5 cc is obtained, 0.3 cc of the mixed sample should be sent for KRAS and GNAS analysis. Vortexing the specimen will help to ensure that any neoplastic cellular material and DNA is represented in molecular testing. The remaining fluid may be centrifuged with the supernatant sent for CEA, amylase and potential cyst fluid banking, while the cellular component may be processed for cytologic review by Cytospin.

## Pancreatic cyst fluid interpretation

### Markers of neoplasia

An elevated CEA, low amylase and the presence of a KRAS mutation together are most suggestive of a neoplastic rather than a reactive process. The presence of a GNAS mutation in a mucinous cyst supports a diagnosis of IPMN over MCN. Molecular diagnostics, in the case of KRAS and GNAS mutations, adds to biochemical and cytologic information from pancreatic cyst fluid.

### DNA yield

In addition to KRAS and GNAS testing, DNA yield from cyst fluid may be an indicator of malignancy, ranging from an optical density of 6.5 in benign cases to 16.5 in malignant cases (29). However, the ratio of neoplastic DNA compared to non-neoplastic DNA in cyst fluid may be very low, possibly below the level of detection by current methods. In this study of DNA yield, cases showing KRAS mutations with subsequent allelic loss were associated with malignancy (29).

### Commercial testing

A commercial molecular test for pancreatic cyst fluid is available for send-out testing and includes sequencing the first exon of KRAS to identify point mutations, loss of heterozygosity in a panel of tumor suppressor genes, and the determination of DNA quality and quantity (PathFinderTG, RedPath Integrated Pathology, Pittsburgh, PA) (30). The test may even be performed on extremely small amounts of fluid (200 uL). The final report uses these molecular test results to risk-stratify patients with pancreatic cysts to help guide decisions regarding surveillance versus surgery.

# Biliary brushings

## Challenges in biliary pathology

Biliary brushings obtained by endoscopic retrograde cholangiopancreaticography (ERCP) are quite challenging, due to the generally scant nature of the specimens and the morphologic overlap of certain reactive and malignant conditions. Molecular techniques do not currently play a major role in the diagnosis of carcinoma in biliary brushings, but may be helpful for negative or indeterminate results.

## Mutations of biliary neoplasia

### KRAS

KRAS mutations, present in approximately 33% of biliary intraepithelial neoplasia (BilIN) lesions, occur as an early molecular event during the progression of BilIN to intrahepatic cholangiocarcinomas, whereas p53 overexpression was identified as a late molecular event (31). Biliary brush specimens are often performed to detect whether a carcinoma of either pancreatic or biliary origin may be causing a biliary stricture. KRAS codon 12 mutational analysis of endobiliary brush cytology can be a valuable adjunct to biliary cytology in the setting of a suspicious extrahepatic biliary stenosis, especially in patients with pancreatic carcinoma (32).

## Commercial testing

Commercially available DNA probes for chromosomes 3, 7, 17 and 9p21 (UroVysion; Abbot Molecular, USA) have been demonstrated to show improved sensitivity for malignancy over routine cytology. A positive result for malignancy is when five or more cells show polysomy. However, the use of FISH with these probes should be reserved for inconclusive or negative cases after cytologic examination. The test is time-consuming, fairly labor-intensive and requires access to a fluorescence microscope. A send-out commercial test for mutations and loss of heterozygosity on biliary specimens is also available (PathFinderTG, RedPath Integrated Pathology, Pittsburgh, PA).

# Surgical resection tissue and banking

## Molecular testing in resection specimens

Surgical resection allows for determination of pathologic staging and evaluation of margins. However, resection also allows for ample tissue to be used for molecular studies. Immunohistochemistry for SMAD4 may be used to support pancreatic carcinoma

in cases where nuclear staining is lost. Other immunohistochemical markers may be used to distinguish pancreatic carcinoma from metastatic disease. However, the architecture and cytology of the tumor in histologic sections, in conjunction with clinical and radiologic information, is usually sufficient for a definitive diagnosis of carcinoma. Rarely are molecular techniques employed.

## Tissue banking

When resection specimens are received in the frozen section lab, adequate tissue for diagnosis and full histologic evaluation should be prioritized. However, should a neoplastic mass or cyst be sufficiently large ($\geq 1$ cm at the minimum, but at the discretion of the frozen section pathologist), fresh tumor may be collected and banked for research purposes or future testing. Whole genome and exome sequencing have shown that pancreatic lesions may harbor a number of mutations, and banking neoplastic tissue could allow for continued elucidation of the molecular alterations and genetic landscape of pancreatic and biliary pathology.

# Future directions

## Pathologist's role

Understanding the molecular changes underlying pancreatic and biliary pathology has the potential to personalize patient management and treatment. As pathologists, providing a morphologic diagnosis is only the beginning. With the help of ancillary tests, including molecular analysis, we can help guide the surgeon's approach, stratify a patient's risk for recurrence and prognosis, and facilitate appropriate genetic testing. There is still considerable work to be done.

## Emerging molecular tests

### FISH probes, LOH and SNPs

Emerging molecular tests include the development of FISH probe sets (TP53, p16/CDKN2A, EGFR, etc.) that may eventually be used in clinical diagnosis. The diagnostic utility of loss of heterozygosity (LOH) remains to be determined, although both pancreatic and biliary neoplasms appear to demonstrate progressive accumulated genetic alterations. IPMNs may demonstrate a LOH at 17q, affecting RNF43, a gene associated with E3 ubiquitin ligase activity (25). Furthermore, the availability of oligonucleotide arrays examining single nucleotide polymorphisms (SNPs) has obviated the need for normal tissue controls, allowing for simplified specimen collection and processing. Rare tumors, such as intraductal tubulopapillary neoplasms of the pancreas, harbor different molecular alterations compared to IPMNs. Testing for these alterations may eventually be used to aid diagnosis and guide targeted therapy.

### MicroRNAs, circulating tumor cells, circulating nucleic acids

Assays of microRNAs, which are short (20 to 25 nucleotides) RNA molecules, enable transcriptome profiling of pancreatic adenocarcinoma and other tumors. Circulating tumor cells may be captured by selecting for size, immunocapture or flow cytometry and could be examined with any of the molecular techniques requiring cells. This technique could alert providers to early metastasis and/or stratify patients based on the likelihood of metastasis. Circulating nucleic acids could become useful as a screening tool for pancreatic adenocarcinoma, since they are likely more abundant than circulating tumor cells, though they may not be specific for particular tumors. These techniques could improve the sensitivity of detecting primary carcinoma as well as recurrence, but the cost of these tests and the margin of benefit do not yet justify routine use.

### Gene expression profiling

In cases of unknown primary malignancies, gene expression profiling may be performed on fresh FNA material using RT-PCR and microarray comparison. Pancreatobiliary is one of the more common origins of an occult malignancy, and metastatic sites may be more accessible for sampling than the pancreas or extrahepatic biliary tree. Cytology lends itself to relatively easy and repeated sampling, and may be enriched for dyshesive tumor cells as compared to inflammatory and stromal cells. Sequencing pancreatic FNA specimens or corresponding surgical resections could identify genomic alterations that are actionable in terms of treating pancreatic and biliary carcinomas, particularly in cases of resistant or relapsed disease.

### Conclusion

While the use of molecular techniques demonstrates great promise, significant limitations include appropriate sampling, cost and ambiguities in the interpretation of results. The importance of a multi-modal approach, including clinical and radiologic information, biochemical cyst fluid analysis and cytologic or histologic examination, cannot be understated.

## Learning points

- The most clinically important molecular diagnostic tests in the gastrointestinal tract are APC Mutation Detection, MMR IHC and MSI Analysis, MYH mutation detection, KRAS mutation detection, BRAF mutation detection, thymidylate synthase expression, PIK3CA mutation detection, Gene Expression Signatures, HER2 amplification and KIT/PDGFRA mutation detection.
- The most clinically important molecular abnormalities in the pancreato-biliary system are KRAS mutation analysis, GNAS mutation analysis, telomere shortening, SMAD4 mutations and genetic polysomy.
- The future advancements in these areas will be dictated by further knowledge in the molecular basis of disease (molecular medicine) and by further technical advances, both in diagnostic imaging and in laboratory analysis.
- Thus, the future will require the testing of more biomarkers in each cancer type, the testing of more cancer types and the regular testing of more sample types (for instance, peripheral blood).

# References

1. Van Schaeybroeck, S., Lawler, M., Johnston, B., Salto-Tellez, M., Lee, J., Loughlin, P. et al. Colorectal Cancer. Chapter 77 in Abeloff's Clinical Oncology, 5th edn. (Philadelphia, PA: Elsevier-Saunders, 2014).

2. Hisamuddin, I. M. and Yang, V. W. Genetics of colorectal cancer. MedGenMed 2004; 6(3): 13.

3. http://surgpathcriteria.stanford.edu/gitumors/familial-adenomatous-polyposis/.

4. Subramaniam, M. M., Putti, T. C., Anuar, D., Chong, P. Y., Shah, N., Salto-Tellez, M. et al. Clonal characterization of sporadic cribriform-morular variant of papillary thyroid carcinoma by laser microdissection-based APC mutation analysis. Am J Clin Pathol 2007; 128(6): 994–1001.

5. Goodenberger, M. and Lindor, N. M. Lynch syndrome and MYH-associated polyposis: review and testing strategy. J Clin Gastroenterol 2011; 45(6): 488–500.

6. De Roock, W., Claes, B., Bernasconi, D., De Schutter, J., Biesmans, B., Fountzilas, G. et al. Effects of KRAS, BRAF, NRAS, and PIK3CA mutations on the efficacy of cetuximab plus chemotherapy in

chemotherapy-refractory metastatic colorectal cancer: a retrospective consortium analysis. *Lancet Oncol* 2010; 11(8): 753–62.

7. Kamel-Reid, S., Zhang, T., Persons, D. L., Nikiforova, M. N., Halling, K. C. and Molecular Oncology Resource Committee of the College of American Pathologists. Validation of *KRAS* testing for anti-EGFR therapeutic decisions for patients with metastatic colorectal carcinoma. *Arch Pathol Lab Med* 2012; 136(1): 26–32.

8. Sharma, S. G. and Gulley, M. L. BRAF mutation testing in colorectal cancer. *Arch Pathol Lab Med* 2010; 134(8): 1225–8.

9. Davies, H., Bignell, G. R., Cox, C., Stephens, P., Edkins, S., Clegg, S. *et al.* Mutations of the BRAF gene in human cancer. *Nature* 2002; 417(6892): 949–54.

10. Whitehall, V., Tran, K., Umapathy, A., Grieu, F., Hewitt, C., Evans, T. J. *et al.* A multicenter blinded study to evaluate KRAS mutation testing methodologies in the clinical setting. *J Mol Diagn* 2009; 11(6): 543–52.

11. Popat, S., Matakidou, A. and Houlston, R. S. Thymidylate synthase expression and prognosis in colorectal cancer: a systematic review and meta-analysis. *J Clin Oncol* 2004; 22(3): 529–36.

12. Sinicrope, F. A. and Sargent, D. J. Molecular pathways: microsatellite instability in colorectal cancer: prognostic, predictive, and therapeutic implications. *Clin Cancer Res* 2012; 18(6): 1506–12.

13. Vilar, E. and Tabernero, J. Molecular dissection of microsatellite instable colorectal cancer. *Cancer Discov* 2013; 3(5): 502–11.

14. Liao, X., Lochhead, P., Nishihara, R., Morikawa, T., Kuchiba, A., Yamauchi, M. *et al.* Aspirin use, tumor PIK3CA mutation, and colorectal-cancer survival. *New Engl J Med* 2012; 367(17): 1596–606.

15. Kelley, R. K. and Venook, A. P. Prognostic and predictive markers in stage II colon cancer: is there a role for gene expression profiling? *Clin Colorectal Cancer* 2011; 10(2): 73–80.

16. Gray, R. G., Quirke, P., Handley, K., Lopatin, M., Magill, L., Baehner, F. L. *et al.* Validation study of a quantitative multigene reverse transcriptase-polymerase chain reaction assay for assessment of recurrence risk in patients with stage II colon cancer. *J Clin Oncol* 2011; 29(35): 4611–19.

17. Kennedy, R. D., Bylesjo, M., Kerr, P., Davison, T., Black, J. M., Kay, E. W. *et al.* Development and independent validation of a prognostic assay for stage II colon cancer using formalin-fixed paraffin-embedded tissue. *J Clin Oncol* 2011; 29(35): 4620–6.

18. Bang, Y. J., Van Cutsem, E., Feyereislova, A., Chung, H. C., Shen, L., Sawaki, A. *et al.* Trastuzumab in combination with chemotherapy versus chemotherapy alone for treatment of HER2-positive advanced gastric or gastro-oesophageal junction cancer (ToGA): a phase 3, open-label, randomised controlled trial. *Lancet* 2010; 376(9742): 687–97.

19. Salto-Tellez, M., Yau, E. X., Yan, B. and Fox, S. B. Where and by whom should gastric cancer HER2/neu status be assessed? Lessons from breast cancer. *Arch Pathol Lab Med* 2011; 135(6): 693–5.

20. Tay, C. M., Ong, C. W., Lee, V. K. and Pang, B. KIT gene mutation analysis in solid tumours: biology, clinical applications and trends in diagnostic reporting. *Pathology* 2013; 45(2): 127–37.

21. Salto-Tellez, M. and Koay, E. S. Molecular diagnostic cytopathology: definitions, scope and clinical utility. *Cytopathology* 2004; 15(5): 252–5.

22. Pang, N. K., Nga, M. E., Chin, S. Y., Ismail, T. M., Lim, G. L., Soong, R. *et al.* KRAS and BRAF mutation analysis can be reliably performed on aspirated cytological specimens of metastatic colorectal carcinoma. *Cytopathology* 2011; 22(6): 358–64.

23. Pang, N. K., Chin, S. Y., Nga, M. E., Chang, A. R., Ismail, T. M., Omar, S. S. *et al.* Comparative validation of c-kit exon 11 mutation analysis on cytology samples and corresponding surgical resections of gastrointestinal stromal tumours. *Cytopathology* 2009; 20(5): 297–303.

24. Macgregor-Das, A. M. and Iacobuzio-Donahue, C. A. Molecular pathways in pancreatic carcinogenesis. *J Surg Oncol* 2013; 107(1): 8–14.

25. Matthaei, H., Norris, A. L., Tsiatis, A. C., Olino, K., Hong, S. M., dal Molin, M. *et al.* Clinicopathological characteristics and molecular analyses of multifocal intraductal papillary mucinous neoplasms of the pancreas. *Ann Surg* 2012; 255(2): 326–33.

26. Wu, J., Matthaei, H., Maitra, A., Dal Molin, M., Wood, L. D., Eshleman, J. R. *et al.* Recurrent *GNAS* mutations define an unexpected pathway for pancreatic cyst development. *Sci Transl Med* 2011; 3(92): 92ra66.

27. Kanda, M., Knight, S., Topazian, M., Syngal, S., Farrell, J., Lee, J. *et al.* Mutant GNAS detected in duodenal collections of secretin-stimulated pancreatic juice indicates the presence or emergence of pancreatic cysts. *Gut* 2013; 62(7): 1024–33.

28. Pitman, M. B. Diagnostic investigation of pancreatic cyst fluid, in Tanaka, M. (ed.), *Intraductal Papillary Mucinous*

*Neoplasm of the Pancreas* (Osaka: Springer Japan, 2013).

29. Khalid, A., McGrath, K. M., Zahid, M., Wilson, M., Brody, D., Swalsky, P. *et al.* The role of pancreatic cyst fluid molecular analysis in predicting cyst pathology. *Clin Gastroenterol Hepatol* 2005; 3(10): 967–73.

30. Melton, S. D., Genta, R. M. and Souza, R. F. Biomarkers and molecular diagnosis of gastrointestinal and pancreatic neoplasms. *Nat Rev Gastroenterol Hepatol* 2010; 7(11): 620–8.

31. Hsu, M., Sasaki, M., Igarashi, S., Sato, Y. and Nakanuma, Y. KRAS and GNAS mutations and p53 overexpression in biliary intraepithelial neoplasia and intrahepatic cholangiocarcinomas. *Cancer* 2013; 119(9): 1669–74.

32. Sturm, P. D., Rauws, E. A., Hruban, R. H., Caspers, E., Ramsoekh, T. B., Huibregtse, K. *et al.* Clinical value of K-ras codon 12 analysis and endobiliary brush cytology for the diagnosis of malignant extrahepatic bile duct stenosis. *Clin Cancer Res* 1999; 5(3): 629–35.

# Chapter 15

# Soft tissue, bone and skin tumors

Stamatios Theocharis and Jerzy Klijanienko

## Soft tissue and bone tumors – general issues

Sarcomas are rare malignant tumors arising from mesenchymal tissue at any body site. Soft tissue sarcomas comprise approximately 1% of malignant tumors, presenting more than 50 subtypes, but pleomorphic sarcoma, liposarcoma, leiomyosarcoma, synovial sarcoma and malignant peripheral nerve sheath tumor account for 75% of them (1, 2). The new World Health Organization (WHO) classification of soft tissue tumors was published in early 2013, almost 11 years after the previous edition. While the number of newly recognized entities included for the first time is fewer than that in 2002, there have instead been substantial steps forward in molecular genetic and cytogenetic characterization of this family of tumors, leading to more reproducible diagnosis, a more meaningful classification scheme and providing new insights regarding pathogenesis, which previously has been obscure in most of these lesions (3, 4). Almost 80% of sarcomas originate from soft tissues and the rest from bones. More than 10,000 new cases are diagnosed each year in the United States and they account for 0.72% of all cancers diagnosed annually, whereas they represent 7% of all cancers in children (1, 2). In Europe, quite similar data have been reported, with almost 8% of the neoplasms found in children, and half of them being less than five years of age at diagnosis (5). Between 1988 and 1997, the age-standardized incidence of soft tissue sarcomas in Europe was 9.1 per million children, with a lower range of affected patients in the western and eastern parts of the continent and a higher one in the northern. The annual incidence is 30 per million (5).

Most soft tissue sarcomas occur in adults older than 55 years and approximately 50% of bone sarcomas and 20% of soft tissue sarcomas are diagnosed under the age of 35 years. The gastrointestinal stromal tumor (GIST), regarding which frequency, incidence, prevalence and clinical aggressiveness have been underestimated, represents the most common form of soft tissue neoplasm (4). More recent data from epidemiological studies and GIST clinical trials suggest that the annual GIST incidence in the United States is at least 4,000 to 6,000 new cases (6). Some sarcomas, such as leiomyosarcoma, chondrosarcoma and GIST, are more common in adults than in children. Most high-grade bone sarcomas, including Ewing's sarcoma/peripheral neuroectodermal tumor and osteosarcoma, are much more common in children and young adults. Among children, soft tissue sarcomas are two times more common in whites than in African-Americans and Rhabdomyosarcoma is the most frequent soft tissue sarcoma (50%) at this age. Population-based data from Connecticut covering the years 1935 to 1989 have shown an increased incidence of soft tissue sarcomas in both genders, with men being more affected than women. The recent increase of acquired immune deficiency syndrome-related Kaposi's sarcoma does not explain the upward trend in soft tissue sarcoma, dating to the last few decades. A similar trend was found in a population-based study built on 5,802 cases of soft tissue sarcomas in children aged 0 to 14 years, extracted from the database of the Automated Childhood Cancer Information System (ACCIS) and registered in population-based cancer registries in Europe for the period 1978 to 1997. The incidence of soft tissue sarcomas in children increased by almost 2% per year over the period 1978 to 1997, due to the higher incidence

*Molecular Pathology: A Practical Guide for the Surgical Pathologist and Cytopathologist*, ed. John M. S. Bartlett, Abeer Shaaban and Fernando Schmitt. Published by Cambridge University Press. © Cambridge University Press, 2016.

of genitourinary rhabdomyosarcoma (3). In most soft tissue sarcoma cases, precise etiology remains unknown, although a number of associated or predisposing factors, including environmental, physical, biological and chemical factors, have been identified.

The patient's age at the first presentation should be suggestive of a given type of tissue tumor. Rhabdomyosarcoma is the most common soft tissue tumor of childhood and accounts for approximately one-half of all soft tissue sarcomas in this age group. About 65% of cases occur in children below six years of age, while it is less frequent during the early to mid-teenage years and rare in adulthood. The two most common subtypes, embryonal and alveolar, account for at least 80% of all rhabdomyosarcomas. Synovial sarcoma is at the crossroads between the pediatric and the adult age groups. Although children and adults with synovial sarcoma share a similar clinical presentation, their outcome differs, which lends to suggest that factors other than unfavorable clinical features could influence their biological behavior. Whether this difference is related to biological variables or to historically different treatment approaches for pediatric versus adult patients is a matter of debate (7). In adults, malignant fibrous histiocytoma (MFH) represents 40% and liposarcoma 25% of sarcoma cases. MFH peaks at 60 to 69 years of age (21%) with regular incidence increase between 30 and 70 years. Liposarcoma also peaks at 60 to 69 years of age (22.5%), but a high prevalence of liposarcoma is observed between 40 and 80 years. Well-differentiated liposarcoma represents the largest subgroup of malignant adipocytic neoplasms and accounts for about 40% to 45% of all liposarcoma cases. It occurs in middle-aged adults with a peak incidence in the sixth decade. Myxoid liposarcoma is a disease of young adults, with a peak incidence in the fourth and fifth decades of life. Although very rare, it is the commonest form of liposarcoma in patients younger than 20 years old, with no sex predilection. The majority of pleomorphic liposarcoma arises in elderly patients (>50 years) with an equal sex distribution. Fibrosarcoma incidence peaks at 30 to 39 years of age (24%); leiomyosarcoma peaks later at 50 to 59 years (25%).

## Sampling procedure

Up until recent years, open surgical biopsy was a standard procedure to diagnose soft tissue and bone tumors. More recently, fine-needle aspiration (FNA) or core-needle biopsy (CNB) became a diagnostic procedure. The main advantages of both FNA and CNB in the primary work-up of soft tissue lesions are that these techniques are simple, quick and cost effective. Both entail minimal tissue trauma (in contrast to open biopsy) and both are usually performed in an outpatient setting. In our experience, the combined FNA and CNB diagnosis in conjunction with clinical and radiological data has high diagnostic accuracy in the evaluation of soft tissue lesions and has been sufficient for making a treatment decision in the majority of patients with suspicion of soft tissue sarcoma admitted to our center. As FNA and CNB complement each other in the examination of soft tissue lesions (8), the double (FNA/CNB) diagnostic approach permits a combination of cellular morphology and tissue architecture and also yields tumor tissue adequate for various ancillary procedures more often than FNA or CNB alone. It is important to recognize that cell-rich and stroma-poor tumor specimens (round cell, spindle cell tumors, etc.) yield very little cellular material sufficient for all ancillary techniques application. On the contrary, cell-poor and stroma-rich specimens as from spindle cell tumors (desmoids, fibrosarcomas and dermatofibrosarcoma protuberans) yield paucicellular material and a practice of CNB is usually indicated.

## Cytologic classification of soft tissue tumors based on the principal patterns

Instead of classifying soft tissue tumors according to their histogenesis/phenotype, the cytological classification into five different patterns resulting in eight groups of entities was used for diagnosis. The five cytology-dominant patterns were individualized as spindle cell (the most frequent pattern of soft tissue tumors in adults), pleomorphic, epithelioid, myxoid and small round/ovoid cell patterns, bearing in mind that overlap between those different patterns may be present within the same specimen. For example, a rhabdoïd tumor may be classified as well as epithelioid or round cell tumor. Similarly, angiosarcoma could fit in malignant spindle cell as well as epithelioid groups and leiomyosarcoma may be classified into spindle cell, polymorphous cell, epithelioid cell and most often in myxoid groups (9, 10, 11).

Cytologic classification of soft tissue tumors is shown in Table 15.1 (12).

223

**Table 15.1** Cytologic classification of soft tissue tumors based on five cytologic patterns resulting in eight groups of various entities. Importance of molecular diagnostic markers

| Entity | Diagnostic molecular specific marker |
|---|---|
| **Low-grade spindle cell tumors of uncertain malignant potential** | |
| Fibromatoses and desmoids | No |
| Nodular fasciitis | Under investigation |
| Dermatofibrosarcoma protuberans | Yes |
| Benign fibrous histiocytoma | No |
| Solitary fibrous tumor | Yes |
| **Tumors with fibrillary stroma** | |
| Benign peripheral nerve sheath tumors | No |
| Malignant peripheral nerve sheath tumor | No |
| **Malignant spindle cell tumors** | |
| Leiomyosarcoma | No |
| Synovial sarcoma | Yes |
| Fibrosarcoma | Yes |
| Malignant fibrous histiocytoma | No |
| Malignant peripheral nerves sheath tumor | No |
| Spindle cell angiosarcoma | No |
| Kaposi sarcoma | No |
| **Myxoid tumors** | |
| Myxoid liposarcoma | Yes |
| Myxofibrosarcoma | Yes |
| Myxoid leiomyosarcoma | No |
| Myxoma and cellular myxoma | No |
| Chordoma | No |
| Extraskeletal myxoid chondrosarcoma | Yes |
| **Atypical lipomatous tumors** | |
| Well-differentiated liposarcoma | Yes |
| Spindle cell and pleomorphic lipoma | No |
| **Epithelioid tumors** | |
| Epithelioid sarcoma | Yes |
| Gastrointestinal stromal tumor | Yes |
| Epithelioid angiosarcoma | Yes |
| Granular cell tumor | No |
| Rhabdoïd tumor | Yes |
| Alveolar soft part sarcoma | Yes |
| Clear cell sarcoma | No |
| **Pleomorphic sarcomas** | |
| Pleomorphic MFH | No |
| Pleomorphic liposarcoma | No |
| Pleomorphic leiomyosarcoma and RMS | No |
| Extraskeletal osteosarcoma | No |
| Pleomorphic MPNST | No |
| **Round cell sarcomas** | |
| Embryonnal and alveolar RMS | Yes |
| Ewing's sarcoma | Yes |
| Desmoplastic small round cell tumor | Yes |
| Extraskeletal mesenchymal chondrosarcoma | Yes |
| Poorly differentiated synovial sarcoma | Yes |

## Practical notes specific for soft tissue; bone and skin tumors

Soft tissue and bone tumors present some particularities for the biopsy technique and its use for diagnosis. Following our experience, we will list briefly some particular aspects and recommendations:

- Many soft tissue malignant tumors may be deeply localized and require radiological guidance for FNA and CNB.
- Young patients should be systematically locally (Emla ®) and generally (Kalinox ®) sedated.
- We strongly recommend combined use of FNA and CNB for lesions where malignancy is suspected.
- In lesions when benignty is suspected, we recommend initial and exclusive FNA use. Rapid *on situ* evaluation (ROSE) should be practiced to confirm the benignity. The definitive diagnosis will be done on an excisional surgical specimen.
- FNA material should be used for all ancillary techniques, including molecular examinations and immunocyto/histochemistry (cell bloc).

Table 15.2 Specific chromosome translocations and gene fusions useful for diagnosis

| Entity | Chromosome translocations | Gene fusions |
|---|---|---|
| Solitary fibrous tumor | inv(12)(q13q13) | NAB2-STAT6 |
| Dermatofibrosarcoma protuberans/ giant cell fibroblastoma | r, t(17;22)(q21.33;q13.1) | COL1A1/PDGFB |
| Angiomatoid fibrous histiocytoma | t(12;16)(q13.12;p11.2) t(12;22)(q13.12;q12.2) t(2;22)(q33.3; q12.2) | FUS, EWSR1/ATF1 EWSR1/CREB1 |
| Synovial sarcoma | t(X;18)(p11.22;q11.2) | SS18/SSX1, SSX2, SSX4 |
| Infantile fibrosarcoma | t(12;15)(p13.2;q25.3) | ETV6/NTRK3 |
| Low-grade fibromyxoid sarcoma | t(7;16)(q33;p11.2) t(11;16)(p11.2;p11.2) | FUS/CREB3L2, CREB3L1 |
| Myxoid/round cell liposarcoma | t(12;16)(q13.3;p11.2) t(12;22)(q13.3;q12.2) | FUS, EWSR1/DDIT3 |
| Atypical lipoma/well-differentiated liposarcoma | t(12q14-q15) | MDM2, CDK4 |
| GIST | | KIT |
| Clear cell sarcoma | t(12;22)(q13.12;q12.2) t(2;22)(q33.3;q12.2) | EWSR1/ATF1, CREB1 |
| Alveolar soft tissue sarcoma | der(17)t(X;17)(p11.23;q25.3) | ASPSCR1/TFE3 |
| Ewing's sarcoma/ peripheral neuroectodermal tumor | t(11;22)(q24.3;q12.2) t(21;22)(q22.2;q12.2) t(7;22)(p21.2;q12.2) t(2;22)(q35;q12.2) | EWSR1/FLI1, ERG, ETV1, FEV, BCOR-CCNB3 |
| Alveolar rhabdomyosarcoma | t(2;13)(q36.1;q14.11) t(1;13)(p36.13;q14.11) | PAX3, PAX7/FOXO1 |
| Desmoplastic small round cell tumor | t(11;22)(p13;q12.2) | EWSR1/WT1, BCOR-CCNB3 |

- FNA diagnosis should be limited to eight diagnostic groups as previously shown (Table 15.2).
- CNB material should be used exclusively for standard histologic studies and immunohistochemistry. This material should not be used for ancillary examinations.
- From a practical point of view, a group of possible fusions should be studied simultaneously. For example, in case of a round cell tumor, a search of specific fusions that characterize different entities like alveolar rhabdomyosarcoma, Ewing's sarcoma, desmoplastic small cell tumor, rhabdoïd tumor and synovial sarcoma, should be applied.

## Molecular diagnosis and classification of soft tissue tumors

The diagnosis of malignancy is usually the first objective of FNA and/or CNB. The observation of genomic alterations, even unbalanced, by karyotype or comparative genomic hybridization (CGH) analysis is not a criterion of malignancy, as several types of soft tissue benign tumors bear chromosome abnormalities. The final diagnosis will be made on the specific rearrangements observed. For example, the differential diagnosis between lipoma and well-differentiated liposarcoma may be challenging, but the latter displays a characteristic amplification of the MDM2 gene (13). As another example, low-grade

225

fibromyxoid sarcoma represents a malignant tumor with bland histologic features, but bears a characteristic t(7;16) translocation leading to a fusion FUS/CREB3L2, and its detection gives the diagnosis.

## Molecular classification

Based on their genetics, soft tissue tumors can be divided into two main groups: those with simple or relatively simple recurrent chromosome rearrangements, as translocations resulting in gene fusions, or amplifications, occurring in about 40% of sarcomas, representing about 20 different types of sarcoma (14, 15, 16, 17), and those with complex rearrangements, concerning mainly pleomorphic sarcomas (18, 19).

Typically, sarcoma-associated translocations result in fusion of transcription factors or of tyrosine kinase genes, leading to their deregulation. The identification of specific rearrangements has considerably refined the classification of soft tissue tumors, since over the past three decades these molecular markers have been taken into account in the latest WHO classifications (3, 20, 21). Based on an identical translocation, histologically distinct tumors have been grouped in a single tumor type, such as Ewing's sarcoma and peripheral neuroectodermal tumor, or myxoid and round cell liposarcoma. Conversely, tumor types sometimes difficult to distinguish on the basis of their histological features, such as solid-alveolar and poorly differentiated embryonal rhabdomyosarcoma, can be reliably characterized by the presence or absence of a specific gene fusion (PAX3, PAX7/FOXO1).

Well-differentiated liposarcoma, which may raise a difficult differential diagnosis with lipoma (22), is also a tumor with relatively simple cytogenetics, with ring chromosomes in excess carrying amplifications of the MDM2 and, less frequently, CDK4 genes, mapping to chromosome bands 12q14-q15 (17). The diagnosis is easily done by FISH on tissue sections.

About 60% of soft tissue tumors, mainly adult spindle cell and pleomorphic sarcomas, and so-called MFH, lack a specific translocation and show complex rearrangements. However, the analysis of a large number of these tumors by CGH-array has shown that about 20% of them show an amplification of MDM2 and often CDK4, and therefore are dedifferentiated liposarcoma (19, 21, 23). In these cases, an additional amplification of either JUN or MAP3K5, mapping to 1p32 and 6q23, respectively occurs

(24, 25). Genome-wide profiling is the test of choice for detecting multiple potential amplifications.

The identification of specific chromosome rearrangements has made molecular techniques helpful ancillary tools for the precise diagnosis of soft tissue tumors. In practice, the strategy of the molecular diagnosis must be adapted according to the suspected type of tumor. RT-PCR or FISH is usually used as a first-line technique for translocation detection in tumors, when fresh or frozen material is available. FISH is preferentially used for paraffin-embedded material. Array-CGH is well suited for the analysis of co-amplifications characteristic of dedifferentiated liposarcoma. Interpreted in conjunction with cytological and histological data, results of all these techniques will contribute to an accurate diagnosis, which is a prerequisite for an effective treatment of the patients, particularly for the eligibility to targeted therapies (26).

Soft tissue oncology being among the poles of excellence at Institut Curie, considerable attention and much emphasis have been focused on the routine use of FNA biopsy and genetics, in terms of diagnosis, prognosis and targeted therapies decision making regarding patients with solid tumors.

## Genetic techniques

In spite of progress in histopathological classification of soft tissue tumors in recent years, their accurate diagnosis often remains challenging because of overlapping features or poor differentiation, especially for round cell tumors and undifferentiated sarcomas. A large number of soft tissue tumor types are characterized by recurrent chromosomal translocations related to the formation of specific gene fusions. This specificity verified that cytogenetic and molecular analyses are an important part of the diagnostic process in soft tissue tumors (15, 16). CNB and FNA are well suited for these techniques (12). An advantage of FNA is that it permits the collection of a large number of tumor cells, with a low contamination of stroma, especially in round cell tumors. Techniques currently used for detecting translocations are karyotyping, in situ hybridization and RT-PCR. A subset of soft tissue tumors is not associated with specific translocations, but exhibits characteristic chromosome imbalances, losses, gains or amplifications (17, 18, 19). Profiles of these imbalances can be set up using tumor DNA hybridization on genome-wide

(a)

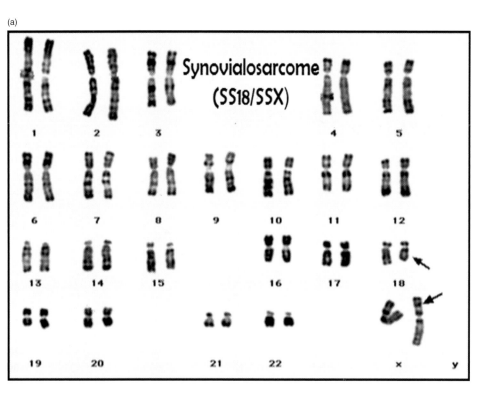

(b)

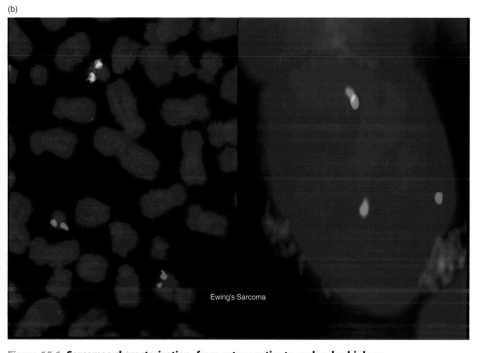

**Figure 15.1 Sarcomas characterization, from cytogenetics to molecular biology**
Sarcomas include multiple and complex tumor subtypes. Identification of specific genetic alterations, which can be used as diagnostic markers in daily practice, has always been a great challenge and has allowed to develop a panel of molecular tools dedicated to the detection to each kind of aberration. Examples of these technical evolutions integrating pathology/genetic alteration/technics are illustrated above. (a) The specific SS18/SSX translocation involved in synovialosarcoma is shown on a classical caryotype. (b) Fission of EWSR1 locus characteristic of Ewing's sarcoma can be visualized by FISH either on metaphases (left panel) or interphases.

**227**

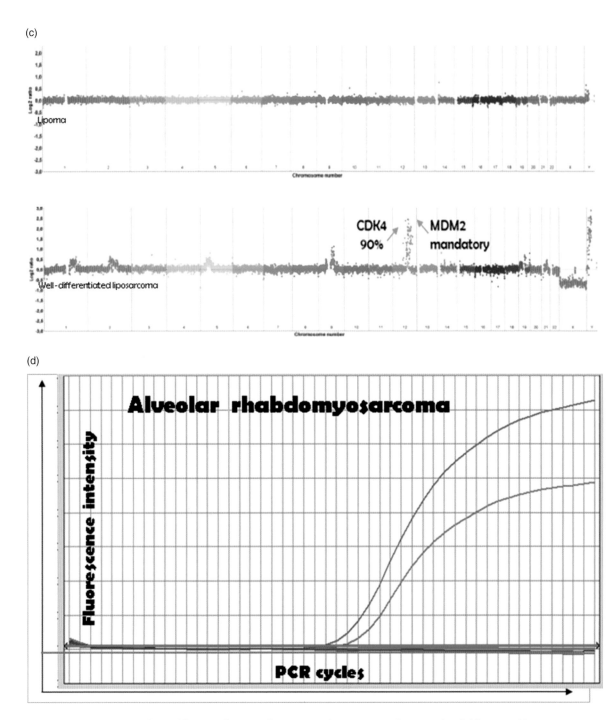

**Figure 15.1** (*cont.*) (c) Specific amplifications of CDK4 and MDM2, mandatory to assess diagnosis of well-differentiated liposarcoma vs. lipoma, are figured by aCGH. (d) PAX3/7–FKHR fusion transcript can be identified by real-time RT-QPCR and distinguish alveolar rhabdomyosarcomas.

(e)

# BCOR-CCNB3 tumor

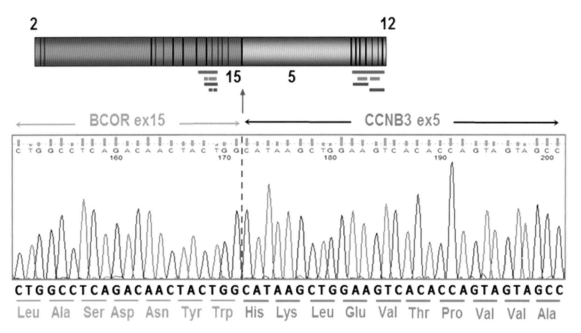

(f)

**DSRCT**

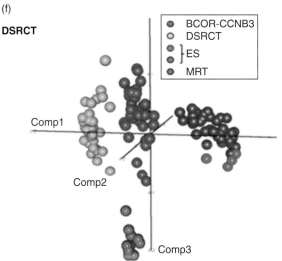

Legend:
- BCOR-CCNB3
- DSRCT
- } ES
- MRT

**Figure 15.1** *(cont.)* (e) New fusion transcripts involved in Ewing-like tumors, such as BCOR-CCNB3, can be apprehended by sequencing, and gene expression pattern analysis can clearly individualize. (f) Desmoplastcic small round cell tumors (DSRCTs), Ewing's sarcomas, BCOR-CCNB3 tumor, and malignant rhabdoïd tumor by Principal Component Analysis (PCA). We would like to thank Dr. Gaëlle Pierron from the Department of Tumour Biology, Institut Curie for the illustrations in this figure.

microarrays (CGH- or SNP-arrays) (14). Of course, other molecular assays, currently not used as first-line diagnostic tests, are used in translational research on soft tissue tumors, such as mutations and transcriptome analyses (Figure 15.1).

## Karyotyping

Karyotype analysis is the classical method for identifying chromosome rearrangements in tumors, and almost all specific translocations known in soft tissue tumors have been detected using this method.

Chromosome rearrangements known in soft tissue tumors are reported in Table 15.2. Karyotyping requires short-term culture of fresh tumor cells, after disaggregation. Round cell tumor (mainly observed in children and young adults) specimens are poorly cohesive, and are submitted to mechanical dissociation with scarpels, grown in suspension and harvested in 24 to 48 hours. Spindle cell tumor (mainly observed in adults) specimens require enzymatic disaggregation, usually by collagenase, and are grown as monolayer cultures in plastic flasks. CNB are not reliable samples for karyotyping, while FNA can yield several millions of cells in the case of round cell tumors, which are well suited for cultivation in suspension. The main interest of karyotype analysis is that it is a genome-wide technique, not requiring the knowledge of a suspected rearrangement. However, one must be aware of the fact that soft tissue tumors may not proliferate *in vitro*, and also that false-negative results can be obtained due to proliferation of inflammatory or stromal cells.

### *In situ* hybridization

This technique allows visualization of specific DNA sequences (probes) and to detection of their rearrangements on chromosomes or in interphase nuclei (27). Fluorescence *in situ* hybridization (FISH) uses probes labeled with fluorochromes, usually red and green, and chromosomes or nuclei are counterstained in blue by blue-fluorescing 4',6-diamidino-2-phenylindole (DAPI). It remains the gold standard of *in situ* hybridization techniques, even if chromogen-based methods are now emerging. The use of "break apart" dual-color probes is the most reliable strategy for detecting translocations by FISH in soft tissue tumors. The DNA sequence of the gene of interest is covered by two probes, a proximal one labeled in red, for example, and a distal one labeled in green. The two probes are separated by a gap corresponding to the region of breakpoints. A bicolor signal represents a normal gene, while a signal split in red and green spots represents a gene translocation. FISH is a very appropriate technique for the detection of amplifications. Two probes labeled with different fluorochromes are cohybridized – a locus-specific probe of the gene of interest, and a centromeric probe corresponding to the chromosome carrying the gene tested. The ratio of the copy-number of the locus-specific probe over that of the centromeric probe is calculated, and an amplification exists if this ratio is >2. Multiple copies of the amplified gene are often grouped in clusters in interphase nuclei, corresponding to the presence of homogeneously staining regions (hsr), described in metaphase chromosomes.

FISH is a very fast and sensitive technique and it has the advantage of being applicable on a variety of tumor materials: sections from frozen or paraffin-embedded CNBs, cell blocks, FNAs and cytogenetic preparations. On tissue sections, the FISH procedure preserves morphology, making it possible to focus the analysis on cells of interest, whereas lecture of cellular material allows accurate and precise "cell by cell analysis." Moreover, the bi-dimensional character of the cytological smear allows analysis of whole nuclei, which is not possible on tissue section material.

### RT-PCR

Fusion genes produce specific fusion transcripts that can be detected using the reverse transcriptase polymerase chain reaction (RT-PCR) assay (15, 16). It requires the knowledge of the potential variant fusions occurring in a given tumor type, and multiplex tests assaying several target sequences should be designed. Naturally, unknown variant fusions are missed by the test. RT-PCR can be used on frozen or paraffin-embedded material, CNBs and FNAs. Real-time RT-PCR has the advantage of a high sensitivity making it applicable on very limited amounts of material, but the result is dependent on the extracted RNA quality. Snap frozen tissue is the most reliable material for the technique, although some laboratories obtain satisfactory results from paraffin-embedded material, provided it had been adequately fixed. Attention should be paid to the risk of false positivity because of contamination in the pre-PCR step, or non-specific annealing of the primers. Amplified fragments may also be verified by sequencing. RT-PCR is a widely used test for diagnosis of fusion transcripts in soft tissue sarcoma.

### Genome-wide profiling

Some soft tissue tumor types are not characterized, at present, by specific translocations leading to gene fusions, but by non-random imbalances of chromosome segments, losses, gains or amplifications. Genome-wide profiles of these imbalances can be obtained using CGH- or SNP-arrays (28). This technique is based on hybridization of labeled tumor DNA on a whole-genome microarray (DNA chip) comprising from about $40 \times 10^3$ to more than $2 \times 10^6$ oligonucleotide probes. A resolution of 60–70

$x\ 10^3$ is, at present, sufficient for the detection of relevant copy-number changes for a diagnostic purpose in soft tissue tumors, at a reasonable cost. The tumor cell content in the sample should be more than 50%. The advantage of CGH- or SNP-arrays is the ability to obtain a high-resolution, genome-wide profile from fresh or frozen CNBs and fresh FNAs, with a resolution more than 100-fold higher than that of karyotyping, and without eventual failures related to cell culture. However, balanced rearrangements remain undetected. In is important to note that cytological FNA samples may contain a higher percentage of pure tumor cells than CNB, which usually contain stromal and inflammatory non-tumoral cells.

The microarray technology can be applied to transcriptome analysis, but this approach, while used in translational research, has not yet proven its utility in the clinical setting.

## Diagnosis using FNA or CNB and information of molecular techniques

Different tumoral entities as proposed in the previous cytological classification are presented in Table 15.2.

## Low-grade spindle cell tumors of uncertain malignant potential

Benign and malignant low-grade spindle cell soft tissue lesions include a wide variety of entities, some of which can be easily confused with high-grade malignant tumors. Over the last three to four decades, new lesions have been described and their clinicopathologic setting well identified – for example, nodular fascitis and its clinico-morphologic variants. Older lesions in the group of fibromatoses have been reclassified on the basis of better defined diagnostic criteria, immunohistochemistry and genetic profiles. The identification of the t(17;22) translocation has become a useful tool for an accurate diagnosis of dermatofibrosarcoma protuberans (DFSP) when the basic conventional cellmorphology is not totally representative of the entity. In the new WHO classification (3), solitary fibrous tumor is presenting as an entity with distinctive and specific gene fusion NAB2-STAT6, resulting in STAT6 protein over-expression that could be used as a specific immunohistochemical marker for this tumor (29).

It seems that morphological diagnoses on FNA and CNB material in low-grade spindle cell tumors should be limited to a diagnosis of "low-grade spindle cell tumor of uncertain malignant potential," to be compared to radiologic imaging information and requiring histopathologic evaluation. The diagnosis of benignity in fibromatoses and desmoids should be concluded after exclusion of DFSP and solitary fibrous tumor in accordance with radiology imaging information, molecular results and clinical presentation. DFSP is now best classified as a cutaneous fibroblastic neoplasm of intermediate malignancy. Although it can occur at any site, the trunk and proximal extremities are sites of predilection. DFSP is a slowly growing, infiltrating and locally aggressive tumor that recurs in about 50% of the affected patients. The fibrosarcomatous DFSP variety, more recently described, pursues a more aggressive clinical course, giving rise to metastatic disease. DFSP could raise difficulties in differential diagnosis with low-grade fibrosarcoma, fibromatosis and fibrohistiocytic tumors. Beside some of its histologic characteristics, its immunohistochemical profile is characteristic, showing a diffuse CD34 immunoreactivity which allows an accurate diagnosis. The distinction between different types of benign fibrous histiocytoma occasionally proves difficult, particularly with superficial biopsies. Once again, CD34 is rarely and focally expressed by benign fibrous histiocytoma. The knowledge of the clinical setting, the size and the configuration of the lesion could aid the diagnosis.

Cytogenetic analyses as well as molecular biology are useful adjuncts. The former depicts a supernumerary ring chromosome 11 and amplification sequences of chromosomes 17 and 22. The fusion transcript COL1A1-PDGF beta of the translocation t(17;22)(q21;q13) can be revealed by RT-PCR or FISH. The demonstration of similar changes in giant cell fibroblastoma allows ascertaining that this tumor is the juvenile counterpart of DFSP.

## Malignant spindle cell tumors

Among the different groups of mesenchymal malignancies, spindle cell sarcomas are well known to cause problems in differential diagnosis in terms of precising their phenotype. As emphasized above, distinguishing benign and low-grade tumors is difficult and constitutes a potential to generate false-positive and-negative results in FNA and CNB material (30, 31, 32). Due to a large group of entities with spindle cells as their main characteristic component (for example, leiomyosarcoma, synovial sarcoma, fibrosarcoma, malignant

**231**

peripheral nerve sheath tumor, Kaposi's sarcoma, angiosarcoma and malignant fibrous histiocytoma), the determination of a tumor phenotype in FNA material is both challenging and deceptive.

## Synovial sarcoma

Synovial sarcoma, both biphasic and monophasic variants, belongs to the category of spindle cell sarcomas. Obviously, poorly differentiated synovial sarcoma whose cytologic and histologic cellular composition is closer to the round cell pattern is excluded from that group. Inclusion of the biphasic variety in this group is mandatory, since a proportion of those tumors are predominantly spindle cell-rich with a minimal portion of epithelial component. The majority of synovial sarcoma recognized morphologically are of the monophasic type given better histologic identified features, the routine use of a selected panel of antibodies and the demonstration by molecular biology of both transcripts SSX-1 and SSX-2 of the translocation t(x;18) (33). On cytological grounds, synovial sarcoma has the same morphologic criteria as other members of the group.

Cytogenetic and molecular genetics findings have already been emphasized. It is particularly useful for monophasic fibrous and poorly differentiated synovial sarcoma. Some disagreement exists in terms of correlation between histologic subtype and the gene breakpoint. Fusion transcript SSX-2 has been associated with monophasic fibrous synovial sarcoma and SSX-1 with the biphasic variety and criteria that are of importance to distinguish from solitary fibrous tumors. TLE1 is a nuclear protein that functions as a transcription repressor of Wnt/Beta catenin signaling. It is a potentially useful marker of synovial sarcoma by multiple expression microarray study. It has been constantly identified as an excellent discriminator of synovial sarcoma (34).

To improve the diagnostic criteria, ancillary studies of aspirated tumor cells are helpful (35, 36, 37). It is now well established that cytogenetic analysis is a novel and objective tool for the diagnosis of soft tissue tumors and is more sensitive than conventional histologic and/or cytologic morphology, immunohistochemistry or electron microscopic analysis. It has been demonstrated (38) that the karyotypes' analysis in cytological material obtained from sarcomas is an accurate method of diagnosis. Cytogenetic studies have also revealed a specific chromosomal translocation t(X;18)(p11.2;q11.2), with a prevalence of 85% in

synovial sarcoma (39). In this context, it has been proposed that cytologic smears exhibiting a morphology suggestive of synovial sarcoma combined with a cytology-based cytogenetic analysis are sufficient for a definitive diagnosis of synovial sarcoma, rendering surgical biopsy unnecessary (40). Similarly, cytology material can also be used for analysis of specific translocation using RT-PCR technique (41) or SYT-SSX gene transcript (33).

## Fibrosarcoma

Classical adult fibrosarcoma is now a very rare tumor and, as already mentioned in this chapter, has become a diagnosis of exclusion. Despite a cellular component of compact sheets of spindle cells similar to other spindle cell sarcomas, it is defined by negative findings: absence of a representative immunohistochemical profile (vimentin positive, occasional focal positivity for CD34) and, so far, neither recognizable cytogenetic nor molecular characterization. Most past adult fibrosarcomas fall into the group of monophasic synovial sarcomas; others fall into the groups of solitary fibrous tumors (which they can closely resemble), low-grade malignant peripheral nerve sheath tumors and DFSP (42).

Two recognized variants of adult fibrosarcoma are worth highlighting – the details of myxofinrosarcoma being shown later in this chapter. Low-grade fibromyxoid sarcoma is now a well-recognized nosologic entity (43) by virtue of its unique genetic and molecular characterization with the demonstration of the chimeric fusion transcript FUS/CREB3L2 resulting from the specific translocation t(7;16)(q33;p11) (44, 45). Identical molecular findings are found in hyalinizing spindle cell tumor with giant rosettes, now considered as a variant of low-grade fibromyxoid sarcoma. The latter is a more cellular than myxoid tumor – hence, on cytohistological grounds, it is to be included in the pattern of low-grade spindle cell lesions. These tumors also depict a network of curvilinear vessels also observed in other sarcomas such as myxofibrosarcoma.

The so-called sclerosing epithelioid fibrosarcoma is an unusual variant of fibrosarcoma, of which few cases were retrieved from our own material. Quite interestingly, one of the authors reported recently a small series of low-grade fibromyxoid sarcoma with emphasis on a recurrent case whose histology was characterized by a component of typical sclerosing fibrosarcoma admixed with pleomorphic areas indistinguishable from malignant fibrous histiocytoma (46). Further immunohistochemical and molecular biology investigations tend to suggest that sclerosing epitheliod fibrosarcoma and low-grade fibromyxoid sarcoma are closely related entities sharing some morphological characteristics and depicting the same translocation (47).

## Malignant fibrous histiocytoma (MFH) – storiform pattern

Once considered as the most frequent sarcoma of adult life, its fate has somewhat followed fibrosarcoma. It rather designates a spectrum of tumors, which share morphologic features that allow their inclusion in a distinct clinicopathologic setting, although being not uniform in their histogenesis and pathogenesis (48, 49). Over the recent years, better defined histologic criteria and comparative genomic analysis have resulted in the dismemberment of MFH, which is supported by findings showing, for example, similar genomic profiles. To name only but a few, leiomyosarcoma and MFH (50, 51), liposarcoma and MFH (52, 53, 54).

At the present time, the five variants of MFH have been reclassified on the basis of morphological changes and molecular genetic profile. Storiform-pleomorphic MFH are usually dedifferentiated liposarcomas or leimyosarcomas, as well as inflammatory variant. Giant cell variant belongs to the recently reclassified soft tissue malignant giant cell tumor. Myxoid and angiomatous variants need to be revisited before they could move to another precise tumor phenotype. Cytomorphology corresponds to histological subtype. Usually, tumors are composed of spindle cells showing nuclear pleomorphism. Some cases may show atypical, multinucleated cells or roundish cells.

The angiomatoid malignant fibrous histiocytoma has been reclassified and renamed as angiomatous fibrous histiocytoma. It is recognized as a well-defined nosologic entity by virtue of its morphologic, clinical and molecular characteristics. This slow-growing neoplasm affects primarily children and young adults. It occurs in the extremities and very rarely metastasizes. Unlike morphology, it is characterized by an irregular solid mass of histiocyte-like cells which are desmin positive (50% of cases), cystic areas of hemorrhage and chronic inflammation. Molecular biology studies have shown that angiomatoid fibrous histiocytoma possesses a fusion gene which incorporates either EWRS1 or FUS gene and ATF1 (55). Recently, another study confirmed that the fusion gene EWRS1-CREBI is predominant in this entity (56).

It is beyond the scope of this chapter to detail MFH and its recognized varieties since they better fit in the already discussed patterns, namely, spindle cell, pleomorphic and myxoid.

## Myxoid tumors

Several soft tissue tumors could be included in this category of pattern which exhibit variable biological behavior, ranging from harmless entities (like intramuscular myxoma) to malignant sarcoma (like extraskeletal myxoid chondrosarcoma). In this section of the chapter, the focus is on predominantly benign and malignant myxoid tumors. The main candidates are myxoid liposarcoma, myxoid malignant fibrous histiocytoma, myxoma and extraskeletal myxoid chondrosarcoma.

The value of FNA in the differential diagnosis of adult myxoid sarcoma has already been largely investigated (57) and proved to represent a valuable diagnostic tool. Myxoid sarcomas present probably the greatest challenge when attempting to accurately diagnose with cytologic methods, but the recognition of myxoid soft tissue tumor is not complicated due to the presence of a characteristic myxoid substance.

### Myxoid liposarcoma (with or without round or spindle cells)

Liposarcoma is the most frequent soft tissue sarcoma of adult life since the reclassification of malignant fibrous histiocytomas. Myxoid variant of liposarcoma is the most frequent subtype, accounting for about 50% of all liposarcomas. Although given separate designation in the literature, its round cell variant represents the less well-differentiated end of a same nosologic spectrum. This has been substantiated by the demonstration of the typical t(12;16)(q13;p11) and t(12;22)(q13;q12) chromosomal translocations in both morphological variants (58). They are also similar in terms of age and location. In comparison to well-differentiated and dedifferentiated liposarcomas, they occur in a younger age group. They arise principally in the lower extremities, thigh and popliteal area, very rarely in the abdominal cavity and retroperitoneum. Typical well-differentiated myxoid liposarcoma is a low-grade sarcoma characterized by recurrences, whereas the round cell tumors are prone to give rise to metastasis. However, it is still debated and unclear which proportion of round cells is indicative of a metastatic potential. One study has suggested the following scheme: 0% to 5% of round cells = 23% of risk; 5% to 10% of round cells = 35% of risk; and >25% of round cells = 58% of risk (59). According to Weiss and Goldblum (60), the following labels have been attributed to round cell myxoid liposarcoma, grade I with less than 10 % of round cells, grade II with 10% to 25% and the remainder grade III. Of interest, if myxoid/round cell liposarcoma metastasize to the usual sites like lung and bone, they tend also to extend to other soft tissue sites. The immunohistochemical profile of myxoid liposarcoma does not contribute significantly to the precision of diagnosis. For more difficult cases, the molecular genetic profile is very helpful (61).

### Extraskeletal myxoid chondrosarcoma

Although extraskeletal myxoid chondrosarcoma is a rare soft tissue sarcoma, much has been reported on all aspects of this neoplasm in the past 30 years. Once named "chordoid sarcoma," the designation of extraskeletal myxoid chondrosarcoma has come to be recognized despite a morphological spectrum varying from predominantly myxoid tumors to more solid ones (62). The demonstration of a recurrent t(9;22) (q22;q12) chromosome translocation resulting in the EWS/TEC protein has been well demonstrated with a prevalence of about 75% (63). Less often, a second translocation t(9;17)(q22;q11) is also present.

Extraskeletal myxoid chondrosarcoma occurs principally in the deep soft tissues of the extremities. Similar tumors are found in the bones, but do not harbor the above-described molecular genetic findings. The biologic behavior of extraskeletal myxoid chondrosarcoma is characterized by recurrence and metastasis, sometimes several years after the initial excision. There are controversies concerning its histoprognosis, some reports suggesting that tumor cellularity could be predictive of its outcome (62, 64, 65, 66). Principal entities to consider in the differential diagnosis are myxoid liposarcoma, myxoid malignant fibrous histiocytoma and, for more solid tumors, mixed tumors of epithelial origin like chondroid syringoma.

## Atypical lipomatous tumors

Entities such as spindle cell lipoma and its morphological variant pleomorphic lipoma, well-differentiated liposarcoma and atypical lipoma are included in this category. In the WHO classification of liposarcomas, well-differentiated liposarcoma is further subclassified in lipoma-like, inflammatory and sclerosing types. Dedifferentiated tumors belong also to this subgroup given their cytogenetic and molecular characteristics. It is now accepted that well-differentiated liposarcoma, atypical lipoma and atypical lipomatous tumor are different terms that describe the same entity, i.e. well-differentiated liposarcoma.

### Well-differentiated liposarcoma/atypical lipoma

The immunohistochemical profile does not contribute to the precision of the diagnosis. However, well-differentiated liposarcomas have unique and specific genetic and molecular features. They consistently show amplified sequences of 12q13-q15 (3, 20). MDM2 and CDK4 genes harbor the mutations which can be readily demonstrated by immunohistochemical methods. They are specific and constitute an example of a sarcoma with a simple genetic profile, similar to recognized translocations. This is a very powerful tool to differentiate well-differentiated liposarcoma from some forms of large infiltrating lipomas (63).

### Spindle cell and pleomorphic lipoma

Spindle cell and pleomorphic lipoma are two distinctive pathologic variants of the same nosologic entity. Clinically, they show identical settings: the majority of patients are men between 45 and 65 years of age (91% in the Armed Forces Institute of Pathology (AFIP) series), and they arise in the subcutaneous tissue in the posterior neck or shoulder. They are also described, although rarely, in unusual sites.

Knowledge of the clinical presentation of lesions is helpful. In tumors which are more difficult to classify, cytogenetical profile could be indicative: spindle cell lipoma and pleomorphic lipoma depict characteristic abnormalities exhibiting loss of 16q material and less frequently 13q. The presence of a supernumerary ring 12 chromosome and the typical t(12;22) translocation is diagnostic of dermatofibrosarcoma protuberans. Well-differentiated liposarcoma shows a different profile already discussed above (12).

## Epithelioid tumors

This is the least frequent of the fine-needle aspiration categories of patterns in soft tissue tumors. It also includes benign lesions such as granular cell tumor and granular rhabdomyoma and sarcomas of epithelioid-like appearance. The latter comprises epithelioid angiosarcoma, epithelioid leiomyoma/ leiomyosarcoma (GIST), epitheliod sarcoma, rhabdoïd tumor, metastasis from carcinomas and malignant melanoma. A few of those are well-characterized entities, for example, epithelioid sarcoma, whereas others are not. Their general morphologic pattern has already been described. Entities within this group have been partially redefined by their immunohistochemical profile, cytogenetics and molecular features.

## Epithelioid sarcoma

Epithelioid sarcoma is a relatively rare soft tissue tumor, whose classical variant occurs in the distal portions of extremities, hand and wrist. It could be easily confused with benign and malignant conditions, especially inflammatory granulomatous process, synovial sarcoma and ulcerated squamous cell carcinoma. Typically, the neoplasm principally affects adolescents and young adults with a proportion of 2:1 male:female. With progression, multiple small nodules may develop and progress along the fascias and neurovascular structures.

Recently, a mutation of the gene hSNF5/INII similar to rhabdoïd tumor has been reported (67). Nevertheless, there is still no consensus about the definite phenotype of epithelioid sarcoma. The recent description of that gene mutation raises concern.

## Gastrointestinal stromal tumor (GIST)/epithelioid leiomyosarcoma

The term of GIST (gastrointestinal stromal tumor) has come to be recognized as the right designation for a group of mesenchymal spindle cell and/or epithelioid neoplasms originating in the abdominal cavity and gastrointestinal tract. During the four to five previous decades, a number of appellations were coined such as leiomyoblastoma (benign/ malignant), epithelioid leiomyoma/leiomyosarcoma, stromal tumor and for a limited number of identical morphological neoplasms GANN (gastrointestinal autonomic nervous tumor). Previous immunohistochemical investigations tend to identify different subgroups of entities according to profiles of antibody expression, smooth muscle, nervous or none of these, of which 60% to 70% were positive for CD34.

A consensus approach outlined the key elements to define the role of KIT immunopositivity in the diagnosis of GIST (68). The vast majority of GISTs express KIT (gene KIT mutation at 4q11) and have constitutional activation of tyrosine kinase receptor KIT and BDGFRA. However, some uncertainties are to be made precise in terms of histogenesis and biological behavior.

## Rhabdoïd tumor

Originally described in the kidney and reported as "rhabdomyosarcomatous variant of Wilms' tumor," rhabdoïd tumor has come to be defined as a distinct clinicopathologic entity. Subsequent descriptions of similar tumors arising in every extrarenal anatomic site have been well documented. Indeed, most of the rhabdoïd tumors arise in the kidney in children less than 1 year of age and pursue an aggressive clinical course. It is important to better define extrarenal rhabdoïd tumor since a wide variety of carcinomas with rhabdoïd features have been described, including urothelial carcinoma, renal cell carcinoma, colorectal carcinoma, etc. Similar features are also part of melanoma, mesothelioma, lymphoma and sarcomas of various types. Besides its clinical course, rhabdoïd tumor has unique immunohistochemical and cytogenetic profiles. Aberrations of chromosomes 11 and 22 have been reported, suggesting the presence of a muted suppressor gene at this locus. The gene hSNF5/INI has been reported to be mutated and is presently a serious candidate for the development of the tumor (36, 67).

## Alveolar soft part sarcoma

Alveolar soft part sarcoma is a rare malignant tumor of unusual clinical behavior originally described in 1952 (69). Despite a number of immunohistochemical and electron microscopic studies, its exact nature and classification are uncertain, although it was recently better characterized by the documentation of a recurrent, non-reciprocal translation, der (17)t(x;17)(p11.2;q25) (70, 71). Despite a controversial histogenesis and cryptic behavior, its histopathological picture is characteristic. Most alveolar soft part sarcomas occur in adolescents and young adults with a predilection for females during the first two years of life (69). Muscles and soft tissue of the extremities are the most common sites of involvement, followed by the trunk, head and neck and the retroperitoneum. At the time of diagnosis, several patients have

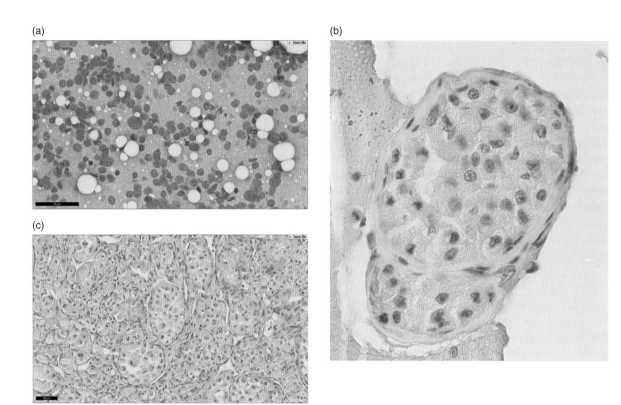

**Figure 15.2 8-year-old female with 6 cm axillary mass radiologically corresponding to an unspecific benign lesion**
(a) May-Grünwald-Giemsa (MGG) smear showing epithelioid sarcoma with roundish cells. A hypothesis of alveolar soft tissue sarcoma was made. (b) Cell bloc showing TFE3 immunohistochemical positivity which confirmed cytological diagnosis of alveolar soft tissue sarcoma. In addition, a translocation of ASPSCR1/TFE3 was also found using RT-PCR technique on cytology material. (c) Histological section of CNB performed on axillary tumor. TFE3 was also positive.

metastatic disease (72). A five-year survival rate could reach up to 80% (73) even if the ultimate prognosis is nevertheless poor (Figure 15.2).

## Clear cell sarcoma

Clear cell sarcoma of tendons and aponeuroses, formerly referred to as malignant melanoma of soft parts, is a rare malignant neoplasm derived from neural crest cells. Both females and males are affected, although women are more frequently affected. The median age of occurrence is 36 years. Most tumors occur in the extremities – the trunk, head and neck being more rarely involved. They are medium-sized neoplasms averaging 4 to 5 cm in largest diameter, well circumscribed, lobulated or multinodular. Their prognosis is poor. A large series of cases have shown a five-year survival rate of around 55% (12). A more recent study from the Japanese Oncology Group

reports an overall survival rate of 45% at five years and 36% at ten years (74).

In the past, many studies attempted to verify the nosologic classification of clear cell sarcoma and its distinction from other similar morphologic entities, particularly malignant melanoma, to which it has been closely associated. Electron microscopic and immunohistochemical investigations had shown a melanocytic differentiation for clear cell sarcoma. However, a cytogenetic hallmark of clear cell sarcoma has been demonstrated, a translocation t(12;22)(q13;q12) resulting in the chimeric EWS-ATF1 gene. Although preliminary reports tended to show that this genetic abnormality was isolated, further studies confirmed that detection of EWS-ATF1 was highly prevalent and therefore could be used as a sensitive diagnostic tool (75, 76). There is now convincing evidence that clear cell sarcoma could be separated from malignant melanoma on the basis of the molecular findings (77).

(a)

(b)

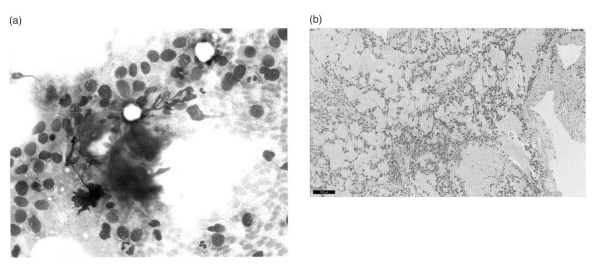

**Figure 15.3 14-year-old male with 14 cm iliaque bone mass radiologically corresponding to a Ewing's sarcoma**
(a) MGG smear showing myxoid and chondroid fragments with chondrocytes (strongly magenta on MGG stain). Moreover, numerous spindle, roundish and oval isolated cells were also detected. A cytological diagnosis of osteosarcoma with differential diagnosis of mesenchymal chondrosarcoma was made. Cellular material was prepared for molecular studies. (b) Corresponding histological sections of CNB showed small cell osteosarcoma with bone and cartilage formation. RT-PCR was performed on cytological material for research of Ewing's sarcoma (FLI1, ERG, ETV1, E1AF, FEV), alveolar rhabdomyosarcoma (PAX3, PAX7/FKHR), desmoplastic small round cell sarcoma (EWS/WT1) and synovial sarcoma (SSX1, SSX2, SSX4) and was always negative. These negative results helped in the differential diagnosis.

# Pleomorphic sarcomas

Pleomorphic sarcoma has long been considered as a wastebasket of sarcomas whose phenotype could not be determined with accuracy. Not so long ago, pathologists suscribed to the assertion that "attempts to make the diagnosis of pleomorphic sarcoma more precise is a frustrating, time-consuming and futile exercise" in terms of treatment approach and histoprognosis. The adjuncture of more recent ancillary techniques such as cytogenetics and molecular biology, added to newer immunohistochemical panels of antibodies, allow separating distinct entities within the group of pleomorphic sarcoma. Some of these studies have also shown that these distinctions were very important in view of the poor prognosis associated with particular groups of pleomorphic sarcomas, and therefore histopathological reclassification of pleomorphic sarcomas of soft tissue had clinical relevance. Candidates to include in that category are malignant fibrous histiocytoma (pleomorphic variant), liposarcoma, leiomyosarcoma, malignant peripheral nerve sheath tumor, rhabdomyosarcoma and the very rare cases of soft tissue osteosarcoma and chondrosarcoma. Previous correlative histological/cytological studies have attempted to delineate some cytological features that could, in conjunction with ancillary techniques, be helpful in making the diagnosis of pleomorphic sarcoma more precise.

Presently, most of the entities included in the subgroups of malignant fibrous histiocytoma have been reclassified, either by immunohistochemical studies or molecular genetics investigations. About 15 years ago, it was postulated that, with sufficient effort, a specific line of differentiation could be identified in the majority of pleomorphic malignant soft tissue sarcomas, including malignant fibrous histiocytoma (78). Later on, studies from the CHAMP GROUP demonstrated that due to the karyotype complexity of pleomorphic sarcomas (PLS), it seems unlikely that cytogenetic analysis could assist in the diagnosis and subclassification of PLS, including malignant fibrous histiocytoma (79). Further investigations have nevertheless shown that despite karyotypic complexities, some pleomorphic sarcomas, particularly malignant fibrous histiocytoma and liposarcoma, malignant fibrous histiocytoma and leiomyosarcoma, could share similar genomic imbalances (80, 81, 82). Tissue microarray studies tend now to identify genetic profiles among some pleomorphic sarcomas, of which pleomorphic malignant fibrous histiocytomas are candidates (Figure 15.3).

**237**

# Round cell sarcomas

Round cell sarcomas largely affect the pediatric population, while the minority of cases can be observed in adults. Indeed, in latter circumstances, in assessing small round cell tumors, it is important to rule out entities such as small cell lymphoma and primary or metastatic small cell carcinoma. Among entities included in that category of sarcomas, some of them are strongly suspected by their clinical setting – for example, mesenchymal chondrosarcoma, embryonal botryoid rhabdomyosarcoma and desmoplastic small round cell tumor. Molecular genetics play a pivotal role in the precise diagnosis, since distinctive cytogenetic and molecular abnormalities allow the distinction from one to another subtype of a given phenotype of tumor and from other round cell neoplasms. The emergence of new antibodies has widened the selected panel used to differentiate round cell neoplasms of soft tissues.

## Embryonal and alveolar rhabdomyosarcoma

Embryonal rhabdomyosarcoma and alveolar rhabdomyosarcoma belong to this category of morphologic pattern. The solid variant of alveolar rhabdomyosarcoma is often of similar morphology to embryonal rhabdomyosarcoma and both are easily confused. In such cases, molecular genetics permit to differentiate both entities, since most alveolar types have a t(2;13)(q35;q14) translocation resulting in the breakpoint within the PAX gene on chromosome 2 and the FKHR gene on chromosome 13, which is not found in embryonal rhabdomyosarcoma (83). In a minority of cases, a variant t(1;13)(p36;q14) translocation which juxtaposes the PAX7 gene with the FKHR gene is also involved in the pathogenesis of alveolar rhabdomyosarcoma (84).

Embryonal rhabdomyosarcoma accounts for about 49% of all rhabdomyosarcomas. It affects children younger than 10 years of age, sometimes adolescents and young adults. The most common sites are head and neck followed by genitourinary tract, deep soft tissues of the extremities, the pelvis and the retroperitoneum (85). In comparison with alveolar rhabdomyosarcoma, the cytogenetic abnormalities are characterized by a consistent loss of heterozygocity for closely linked loci at chromosome 11p15.5 (86). A spindle cell variant of embryonal rhabdomyosarcoma has also been characterized by virtue of its cellular component, mostly spindle cells and its

clinical setting, i.e. predilection for affecting males in paratesticular location, and appears to pursue a more favorable clinical course.

The term "botryoid" polypoid grape-like growth embryonal rhabdomyosarcoma refers to neoplasms found in mucosa-lined hollow organs, for example, the nasal cavity, nasopharynx, bile duct, urinary bladder and vagina. During the past ten years, the clinical behavior of rhabdomyosarcomas has greatly improved, particularly for the embryonal subtype, due to multidisciplinary therapeutic approach, including biopsy, surgical removal of the neoplasm and chemotherapy with or without radiotherapy.

Alveolar rhabdomyosarcoma tends to occur at a slightly older age than the embryonal type. It arises in deep soft tissues of the extremities, accounting for 50% of all rhabdomyosarcomas in this location. In contrast to embryonal rhabdomyosarcoma, its prognosis did not improve in previous decades, despite the institution of multidisciplinary therapeutic approaches.

Rhabdomyosarcoma should be differentiated from Ewing's sarcoma, rhabdoïd tumors and poorly differentiated synovial sarcoma (87, 88). Ewing's sarcoma exhibit a similar morphology with round cell tumors, but contains specific and well-characterized translocations t(11;22)(q24,q12) and t(21;22)(q22, q12), which are found with an estimated prevalence of 95%. Rhabdoïd tumors could also be confused with rhabdomyosarcoma. The presence of perinuclear cytoplasmic globular inclusions is usually more characteristic of rhabdoïd tumors. For differential diagnosis from extrarenal tumors, hypercalcemia and cytokeratin positive/desmin negative immunostaining helps in accurate tumor typing (10), although some cases with expression of desmin and myofilaments have been described (89). In poorly differentiated synovial sarcoma, smears are uniform, lack nuclear pleomorphism and are mostly composed of ovoid to rounded tumor cells with scant tapering cytoplasm (35). Branching papillary-like tumor tissue fragments with vessel stalks, acinar-like structures and comma-like nuclei are also characteristic. Cytogenetic studies have shown a specific chromosomal translocation t(X;18)(p11.2;q11.2), with an estimated prevalence of 85% in synovial sarcoma (SS) (90). Cytologic material can also be used for analysis of specific transcripts using RT-PCR technique to detect the SYT-SSX fusion transcripts whose estimated prevalence is 65% for SYT-SSX1 and 35% for SYT-SSX2 (35).

(a)

(b)

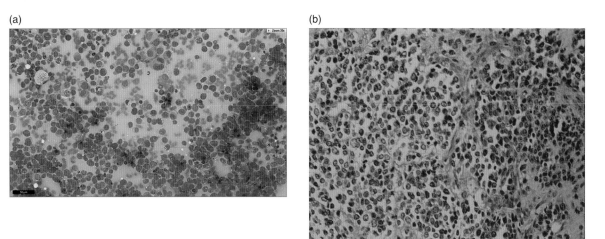

**Figure 15.4 15-year-old female with large intra-abdominal mass, radiologically corresponding to a malignant unspecific tumor**
Initial FNA on peripheral lymph node diagnosed round cell sarcoma, probably rhabdomyosarcoma, eventually desmoplastic small round cell sarcoma or rhabdoïd tumor. Malignant lymphoma was formally exluded. Moreover, FISH analysis of pleural infiltration showed t(2;13)(q35;q14) translocation. The patient was referred for intra-abdominal FNA and CNB. (a) MGG stained smears showing dense proliferation of polymorphous sarcoma cells with predominant population of round cells. Immunohistochemistry performed on cell bloc showed desmin, myogenin and alfa smooth positivity. However, RT-PCR performed on cytology material has identified PAX7/FKHR translocation. In total, a diagnosis of alveolar rhabdomyosarcoma was made. (b) CNB confirmed diagnosis of alveolar rhabdomyosarcoma using appropriate immunohistochemical and FISH analyses.

Over the last two decades, the use of immunocytochemistry to identify muscular markers substantially improves the accuracy of diagnosis (82, 83). FNA material was successfully used in the ancillary techniques to detect the characteristic t(2;13)(q35; q14) chromosomal translocation and/or the gene fusion transcripts PAX-FKHR that are detected with an estimated prevalence of 80% in alveolar rhabdomyosarcoma.

In conclusion, it is now well established that cytogenetic and RT-PCR analyses are more objective and sensitive tools than conventional histologic and/or cytologic morphology, immuno(cyto)chemistry or electron microscopic analysis for the diagnosis of soft tissue tumors (91) (Figure 15.4).

## Ewing's sarcoma

The concept of tumors of the Ewing's sarcoma spectrum has considerably evolved in recent years. It allowed the grouping in a specific category of the extraskeletal Ewing's tumor and peripheral neuroepithelioma (also reported as adult neuroblastoma and peripheral neuroepithelioma). Indeed, identification of a common cytogenetic abnormality t(11;22) (q24;q12) has been a strong argument to support the hypothesis that both neoplasms

were histogenetically linked. Additional investigations revealed variations involving 22q12 chromosome, the site of the EWS gene (90, 92).

Most patients affected are adolescents, the majority of the cohort being less than 30 years of age. They arise in the extremities for primitive neuroectodermal tumor (PNET) and paravertebral areas for Ewing's sarcoma. They are rapidly growing, deeply located large masses. Their prognosis has dramatically improved with the introduction of modern therapy, including surgery and radiation therapy/multi-agent chemotherapy. Key factors influencing prognosis are presence of metastasis at initial diagnosis, large size of the tumor, extensive necrosis and poor response to chemotherapy (Figure 15.5).

## Desmoplastic small round cell tumor

Desmoplastic small round cell tumor is the term most commonly used for this relatively rare malignant neoplasm, of which the majority of cases arise in the abdominal cavity and/or the pelvic peritoneum. Other cases occur in various anatomical sites including the parotid gland, thoracic region and central nervous system. Most patients affected are males between 15 and 35 years of age, although they have been

**239**

(a)

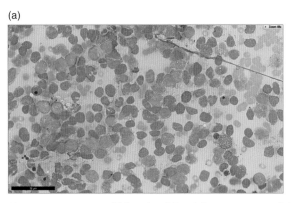

(b)

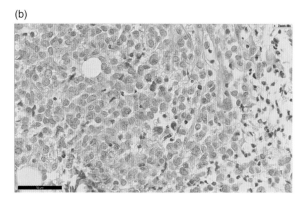

**Figure 15.5** **12-year-old female with pelvic 7 cm mass radiologically corresponding to a bone tumor**
(a) FNA showing round cell population composed of large clearer cells and smaller darker cells. Cytological diagnosis was skeletal Ewing's sarcoma. RT-PCR performed on cellular material has identified FLI1 translocation which confirmed a FNA diagnosis. (b) Corresponding histologic sections of pelvic mass showed Ewing's sarcoma. Mic2 was positive.

reported to occur in patients as young as five years and as old as 70 to 80 years. Most commonly, these are large abdominal masses with extensive peritoneal involvement. So far, it is a highly malignant polyphenotypic neoplasm of unknown histogenesis.

These tumors have a unique cytogenetic abnormality t(11;22)(p13;q12) translocation, hence they constitute a distinct nosologic and clinicopathologic entity (93, 94). The breakpoints involve the EWS gene on 22q12 and the Wilms tumor gene WT1 on 11p13 (95). WT1 is a tumor suppressor gene that encodes a transcription factor that normally inhibits promoters of growth factors such as PDGFA. The fusion transcript is detected by RT-PCR. DSRCT pursues an aggressive biologic behavior with an extremely poor prognosis (96).

### Extraskeletal mesenchymal chondrosarcoma

Extraskeletal mesenchymal chondrosarcoma is a distinct entity of relatively recent identification. It is described as a cartilaginous tumor of bimorphic appearance composed of sheets of primitive mesenchymal cells and interspersed islands of well-differentiated cartilaginous tissue. Due to its undifferentiated cell composition, it is included in the category of small cell tumors. It is a rare malignant tumor that could also occur in bone, and most commonly affects young adults and teenagers. In contrast with classical adult chondrosarcoma, principal anatomic sites are the regions of head and neck, the orbit and the meninges, followed by the extremities, especially the thigh. When occurring in the bones, different sites are involved from those related to conventional chondrosarcoma, i.e. the jaws, ribs and spine, and the tumors have a

minimal osseous participation with large tumoral extension into the surrounding soft tissues. Typical extraskeletal mesenchymal chondrosarcoma is not a difficult diagnosis in small biopsy specimens composed only of a small cell population indistinguishable from other small cell tumors. Extraskeletal mesenchymal chondrosarcoma is a very malignant neoplasm that pursues a rapid clinical course and metastasizes in a high proportion of cases. So far, extraskeletal mesenchymal chondrosarcoma was included in the category of cartilaginous tumor although the demonstration of t(11;22)(q24;q12) translocation has been documented, raising the hypothesis of a close relationship to Ewing's sarcoma/PNET tumors (97).

## Skin tumors

# Malignant melanoma of the skin

Melanoma is the sixth most common malignant neoplasm in the United States, representing the most deadly form of skin cancer and one of the most aggressive malignancies with increased incidence (98, 99). The melanoma pathogenesis is related to melanocytes' malignant transformation under environmental, genetic, molecular or unknown events. Cutaneous melanomas usually present mutations in various genes encoding for proteins of the Ras/Raf/MAPK signaling pathway, which regulates cell proliferation and also KIT gene mutations (100, 101). BRAF and NRAS mutations are more prominent in melnomas of non-chronic sunlight; damaged KIT mutations are most commonly seen in acral, mucosal and chronically sun-damaged sites (102). Although

BRAF gene mutations are the most common genetic alterations in melanoma, they are also prominent in benign nevi, so their presence cannot be used for differential diagnosis between benign and malignant melanocytic lesions (103, 104). On the other hand, the identification of such mutations, especially relating to V600E BRAF, should be predictive of the patients' response to specific BRAF inhibitors. Of similar importance is the identification of NRAS, PI3K, AKT, PTEN and c-KIT mutations in melanoma. The increasing use of BRAF and KIT inhibitors encourages the determination of mutational status for both genes in melanoma cases that could be easily and precisely applied in either FNA or CNB samples.

In melanoma diagnosis, a four-probe set targeting 6p25 (RREBi), 6p23 (MYB), IIpI3 (CCND1) and centromere 6 (CEP6) has been used to separate true melanoma cases from nevus. 11q13- and 5p15-directed probes have been also used to define the excision margins of acral lentiginous melanomas (101, 105).

# Merkel cell carcinoma

Merkel cell carcinoma (MCC) represents a rare, highly aggressive and frequently lethal neuroendocrine skin cancer. MCC primarily affects elderly and immunosuppressed individuals, and mostly occurs in sun-exposed skin areas, particularly in the head and neck (106, 107).

(a)

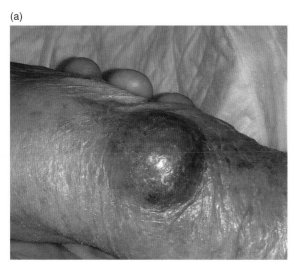

(b)

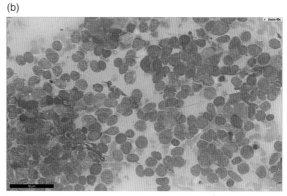

(c)

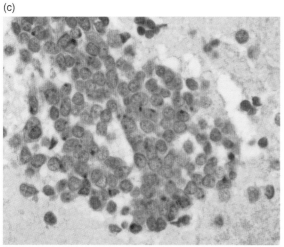

Figure 15.6 **93-year-old female with history of estrogen and progesterone receptors positive breast adenocarcinoma of ductal type**
(a) A year later she presented 3 cm wrist mass. (b) FNA showed proliferation of roundish and oval cells which were occasionally clustered. Immunohistochemistry performed on cell bloc showed estrogen, progesterone receptors and HER2-neu negativity. (c) Cytokeratin 20 was positive in para-nuclear dots which allowed the diagnosis of skin Merkel cell carcinoma and the exclusion of a breast metastasis. RT-PCR performed on cellular material has identified MCPyV (Merkel cell polyomavirus) sequences and confirmed such diagnosis.

Feng *et al.* recently identified a polyomavirus in eight out of ten MCC tumors. This virus, named Merkel cell polyoma virus (MCPyV), was also detected, but less frequently in other human tissues (108). Increasing evidence suggested a causative role of MCPyV in MCC development, although the exact tumorigenic pathway has not yet been defined.

On the other hand, recurrent chromosomal aberrations have been reported, including chromosomal loss, trisomy of chromosome 6, gene deletions and amplifications. The verification of MCPyV in tumoral samples by molecular biology techniques is a routine procedure in FNA, CBA or cell block material (Figure 15.6).

# References

1. Zahm, S. H. and Fraumeni, J. F., Jr. The epidemiology of soft tissue sarcoma. *Semin Oncol* 1997; 24(5): 504–14.

2. Jemal, A., Siegel, R., Ward, E., Murray, T., Xu, J. and Thun, M. J. Cancer statistics, 2007. *CA Cancer J Clin* 2007; 57(1): 43–66.

3. Fletcher, C. D. M., Bridge, J. A., Hogendoorn, P. C. W. and Mertens, F. (eds.), *World Health Organization Classification of Tumours of Soft Tissue and Bone*, 4th edn. (Lyon: IARC Press, 2013).

4. Fletcher, C. D. M. The evolving classification of soft tissue tumours – an update based on the new 2013 WHO classification. *Histopathology* 2014; 64(1): 2–11.

5. Pastore, G., Peris-Bonet, R., Carli, M., Martínez-García, C., Sánchez de Toledo, J. and Steliarova-Foucher, E. Childhood soft tissue sarcomas incidence and survival in European children (1978–1997): report from the Automated Childhood Cancer Information System project. *Eur J Cancer* 2006; 42(13): 2136–49.

6. Nilsson, B., Bumming, P., Meis-Kindblom, J. M., Odén, A., Dortok, A., Gustavsson, B. *et al.* Gastrointestinal stromal tumors: the incidence, prevalence, clinical course, and prognostication in the preimatinib mesylate era – a population-based study in western Sweden. *Cancer* 2005; 103(4): 821–9.

7. Sultan, I., Rodriguez-Galindo, C., Saab, R., Yasir, S., Casanova, M. and Ferrari, A. Comparing children and adults with synovial sarcoma in the Surveillance, Epidemiology, and End Results program, 1983 to 2005: an analysis of 1268 patients. *Cancer* 2009; 115(15): 3537–47.

8. Domanski, H. A., Åkerman, M., Carlén, B., Engellau, J., Gustafson, P., Jonsson, K. *et al.* Core-needle biopsy performed by the cytopathologist: a technique to complement fine-needle aspiration of soft tissue and bone lesions. *Cancer* 2005; 105(4): 229–39.

9. Layfield, L. J. *Cytopathology of Bone and Soft Tissue Tumors* (Oxford University Press, 2002).

10. Åkerman, M. and Domanski, H. A. The cytological features of soft tissue tumours in fine needle aspiration smears classified according to histotype, in Orell, S. R. (ed.), *Monographs in Clinical Cytology*. Vol. 16. *The Cytology of Soft Tissue Tumours* (Basel: Kargel, 2003), pp. 17–84.

11. Geisinger, K. and Abdul-Karim, F. W. Fine needle aspiration biopsy of soft tissue tumors, in Strauss, M. (ed.), *Enzinger and Weiss's Soft Tissue Tumors*, 5th edn. (St. Louis: Mosby, 2008), pp. 103–17.

12. Klijanienko, J. and Lagacé, R. *Soft Tissue Tumors. A Multidisciplinary, Decisional Diagnostic Approach* (Hoboken NJ: Wiley-Blackwell, 2011).

13. Dei Tos, A. P. Liposarcomas: diagnostic pitfalls and new insights. *Histopathology* 2014; 64(1): 38–52.

14. Antonescu, C. R. The role of genetic testing in soft tissue sarcoma. *Histopathology* 2006; 48(1): 13–21.

15. Lazar, A., Abruzzo, L. V., Pollock, R. E., Lee, S. and Czerniak, B. Molecular diagnosis of sarcomas: chromosomal translocations in sarcomas. *Arch Pathol Lab Med* 2006; 130(8): 1199–207.

16. Gulley, M. L. and Kaiser-Rogers, K. A. A rational approach to genetic testing for sarcoma. *Diagn Mol Pathol* 2009; 18(1): 1–10.

17. Coindre, J. M., Pédeutour, F. and Aurias, A. Well-differentiated and dedifferentiated liposarcomas. *Virchows Arch* 2010; 456(2): 167–79.

18. Dei Tos, A. P. Classification of pleomorphic sarcomas: where are we now? *Histopathology* 2006; 48(1): 51–62.

19. Guillou, L. and Aurias, A. Soft tissue sarcomas with complex genomic profiles. *Virchows Arch* 2009; 456(2): 201–17.

20. Fletcher, C. D. M., Unni, K. K. and Mertens, F. *World Health Organisation Classification of Tumours. Pathology and Genetics of Tumours of Soft Tissue and Bone* (Lyon: IARC Press, 2002).

21. Fletcher, C. D. The evolving classification of soft tissue tumours: an update based on the new WHO classification. *Histopathology* 2006; 48(1): 3–12.

22. Klijanienko, J., Caillaud, J. M. and Lagacé, R. Fine-needle aspiration in liposarcoma. Cyto-histologic correlative study including well-differentiated, myxoid, and

pleomorphic variants. *Diagn Cytopathol* 2004; 30(5): 307–12.

23. Idbaih, A., Coindre, J. M., Derré, J., Mariani, O., Terrier, P., Ranchère, D. *et al.* Myxoid malignant fibrous histiocytoma and pleomorphic liposarcoma share very similar genomic imbalances. *Lab Invest* 2005; 85(2): 176–81.

24. Mariani, O., Brennetot, C., Coindre, J. M., Gruel, N., Ganem, C., Delattre, O. *et al.* JUN oncogene amplification and overexpression block adipocytic differentiation in highly aggressive sarcomas. *Cancer Cell* 2007; 11(4): 361–74.

25. Chibon, F., Mariani, O., Derré, J., Mairal, A., Coindre, J. M., Guillou, L. *et al.* ASK1 (MAP3K5) as a potential therapeutic target in malignant fibrous histiocytomas with 12q14-q15 and 6q23 amplifications. *Gene Chromosome Canc* 2004; 40(1): 32–7.

26. Al-Zaid, T., Somaiah, N. and Lazar, A. J. Targeted therapies for sarcomas: new roles for the pathologist. *Histopathology* 2014; 64: 119–33.

27. Tanas, M. R. and Goldblum, J. R. Fluorescence in situ hybridization in the diagnosis of soft tissue neoplasms: a review. *Adv Anat Pathol* 2009; 16(6): 383–91.

28. Dutt, A. and Beroukhim, R. Single nucleotide polymorphism array analysis of cancer. *Curr Opin Oncol* 2007; 19(1): 43–9.

29. Chmielecki, J., Crago, A. M., Rosenberg, M., O'Connor, R., Walker, S. R., Ambrogio, L. *et al.* Whole-exome sequencing identifies a recurrent NAB2–STAT6 fusion in solitary fibrous tumours. *Nat Genet* 2013; 45(2): 131–2.

30. Klijanienko, J., Caillaud, J. M., Lagacé, R. and Vielh, P. Fine-needle aspiration of leiomyosarcoma. A correlative cytohistopathological study of 96 tumors in 68 patients. *Diagn Cytopathol* 2003; 28: 119–25.

31. Klijanienko, J., Caillaud, J. M., Lagacé, R. and Vielh, P. Cytohistologic correlations of 24 malignat peripheral nerve sheath tumors (MPNST) in 17 patients. The Institut Curie experience. *Diagn Cytopathol* 2002; 27: 103–8.

32. Klijanienko, J., Caillaud, J. M., Lagacé, R. and Vielh, P. Cytology in angiosarcoma including classic and epithelioid variants. Institut Curie's experience. *Diagn Cytopathol* 2003; 29: 140–5.

33. Inagaki, H., Murase, T., Otsuka, T. and Eimoto, T. Detection of SYT-SSX fusion transcript in synovial sarcoma using archival cytologic specimens. *Am J Clin Pathol* 1999; 111(4): 528–33.

34. Terry, J., Saito, T., Subramanian, S., Ruttan, C., Antonescu, C. R., Goldblum, J. R. *et al.* TLE1 as a diagnostic immunohistochemical marker for synovial sarcoma emerging from gene expression profiling studies. *Am J Surg Pathol* 2007; 31(2): 240–6.

35. Klijanienko, J., Caillaud, J. M., Lagacé, R. and Vielh, P. Cytohistologic correlations in 56 synovial sarcomas in 36 patients. The Institut Curie experience. *Diagn Cytopathol* 2002; 27(2): 96–102.

36. Srinivasan, R., Gautam, U. and Gupta, S. Synovial sarcoma: diagnosis on fine-needle aspiration by morphology and molecular analysis. *Cancer* 2009; 117(2): 128–36.

37. Liu, K., Layfield, L. J., Coogan, A. C., Ballo, M. S., Bentz, J. S. and Dodge, R. K. Diagnostic accuracy in fine-needle aspiration of soft tissue and bone lesions. Influence of clinical history and experience. *Am J Clin Pathol* 1999; 111(5): 632–40.

38. Molenaar, W. M., DeJong, B., Buist, J., Idenburg, V. J., Seruca, R., Vos, A. M. *et al.* Chromosomal analysis and the classification of soft tissue sarcomas. *Lab Invest* 1989; 60(2): 266–74.

39. Saboorian, M. H., Ashfaq, R., Vandersteenhoven, J. J. and Schneider, N. R. Cytogenetics as an adjunct in establishing a definitive diagnosis of synovial sarcoma by fine-needle aspiration. *Cancer* 1997; 81(3): 187–92.

40. Ryan, M. R., Stastny, J. F. and Wakely, P. E. The cytopathology of synovial sarcoma. A study of six cases, with emphasis on architecture and histopathologic correlation. *Cancer (Cancer Cytopathol)* 1998; 84(1): 42–9.

41. Nilsson, G., Wang, M., Wejde, J., Kanter, L., Karlén, J., Tani, E. *et al.* Reverse transcriptase polymerase chain reaction on fine needle aspirates for rapid detection of translocations in synovial sarcoma. *Acta Cytol* 1998; 42(6): 1317–24.

42. Klijanienko, J., Caillaud, J. M. and Lagacé, R. Fine-needle aspiration of primary and recurrent dermatofibrosarcoma protuberans. *Diagn Cytopathol* 2004; 30(4): 261–5.

43. Evans, H. L., Khurana, K. K., Kemp, B. L. and Ayala, A. G. Heterologous elements in the dedifferentiated component of dedifferentiated liposarcoma. *Am J Surg Pathol* 1994; 18(11): 1150–7.

44. Panagopoulos, I., Storlazzi, C. T., Fletcher, C. D., Fletcher, J. A., Nascimento, A., Domanski, H. A. *et al.* The chimeric FUS/CREB3l2 gene is specific for low-grade fibromyxoid sarcoma. *Gene Chromosome Canc* 2004; 40(3): 218–28.

45. A. Matsuyama, , M. Hisaoka, , S. Shimajiri, Hayashi, T., Imamura, T., Ishida, T. *et al.* Molecular detection of FUS-CREB3L2 fusion transcripts in low-grade fibromyxoid sarcoma using formalin-fixed, paraffin-embedded tissue specimens. *Am*

**243**

*J Surg Pathol* 2006; 30(9): 1077–84.

46. M. Périgny, , N. Dion, , C. Couture, and Lagacé, R. Low grade fibromyxoid sarcoma: a clinico-pathologic analysis of 7 cases. *Ann Pathol* 2006; 26(6): 419–25.

47. Guillou, L., Benhattar, J., Gengler, C., Gallagher, G., Ranchère-Vince, D., Collin, F. *et al.* Translocation-positive low-grade fibromyxoid sarcoma: clinicopathologic and molecular analysis of a series expanding the morphologic spectrum and suggesting potential relationship to sclerosing epithelioid fibrosarcoma: a study from the French Sarcoma Group. *Am J Surg Pathol* 2007; 31(9): 1387–402.

48. Klijanienko, J., Caillaud, J. M., Lagacé, R. and Vielh, P. Comparative fine-needle aspiration and pathologic study in malignant fibrous histiocytoma. Cytodiagnostic features of 95 tumors in 71 patients. *Diagn Cytopathol* 2003; 29(6): 320–6.

49. Klijanienko, J., Caillaud, J. M. and Lagacé, R. Fine-needle aspiration in primary and recurrent benign fibrous histiocytoma (classic, myxoid and angiomatoid variants). *Diagn Cytopathol* 2004; 31(6): 387–91.

50. J. Derré, , R. Lagacé, , A. Nicolas, Mairal, A., Chibon, F., Coindre, J. M. *et al.* Leiomyosarcomas and most malignant fibrous histiocytomas share very similar comparative genomic hybridization imbalances: an analysis of a series of 27 leiomyosarcomas. *Lab Invest* 2001; 81(2): 211–15.

51. M. Sabah, R. Cummins, M. Leader and Kay, E. Leiomyosarcoma and malignant fibrous histiocytoma share similar allelic imbalance pattern at 9p. *Virchows Arch* 2005; 446(3): 251–8.

52. Idbaih, A., Coindre, J. M., Derré, J., Mariani, O., Terrier, P.,

Ranchère, D. *et al.* Myxoid malignant fibrous histiocytoma and pleomorphic liposarcoma share very similar genomic imbalances. *Lab Invest* 2005; 85(2): 176–81.

53. Coindre, J. M., Mariani, O., Chibon, F., Mairal, A., De Saint Aubain Somerhausen, N., Favre-Guillevin, E. *et al.* Most malignant fibrous histiocytomas developed in the retroperitoneum are dedifferentiated liposarcomas: a review of 25 cases initially diagnosed as malignant fibrous histiocytoma. *Mod Pathol* 2003; 16(3): 256–62.

54. Coindre, J. M., Hostein, I., Maire, G., Derré, J., Guillou, L., Leroux, A. *et al.* Inflammatory malignant fibrous histiocytomas and dedifferentiated liposarcomas: histological review, genomic profile, and MDM2 and CDK4 status favour a single entity. *J Pathol* 2004; 203(3): 822–30.

55. Hallor, K. H., Mertens, F., Jin, Y., Meis-Kindblom, J. M., Kindblom, L. G., Behrendtz, M. *et al.* Fusion of the EWSR1 and ATF1 genes without expression of the MITF-M transcript in angiomatoid fibrous histiocytoma. *Gene Chromosome Canc* 2005; 44(1): 97–102.

56. Antonescu, C. R., Dal Cin, P., Nafa, K., Teot, L. A., Surti, U., Fletcher, C. D. *et al.* EWSR1-CREB1 is the predominant gene fusion in angiomatoid fibrous histiocytoma. *Gene Chromosome Canc* 2007; 46(12): 1051–60.

57. Kilpatrick, S. E., Ward, W. G. and Bos, G. D. The value of fine-needle aspiration biopsy in the differential diagnosis of adult myxoid sarcoma. *Cancer* 2000; 90(3): 167–77.

58. Fletcher, C. D., Akerman, M., Dal Cin, P., de Wever, I., Mandahl, N., Mertens, F. *et al.* Correlation between clinicopathological features and karyotype in lipomatous tumors: a report of 178 cases from the Chromosomes

and Morphology (CHAMP) Collaborative Study Group. *Am J Pathol* 1996; 148(2): 623–30.

59. Kilpatrick, S. E., Doyon, J., Choong, P. F., Sim, F. H. and Nascimento, A. G. The clinicopathologic spectrum of myxoid and round cell liposarcoma. A study of 95 cases. *Cancer* 1996; 77(8): 1450–8.

60. Weiss, S. W. and Goldblum, J. R. Liposarcoma, in Strauss, M. (ed.), *Enzinger and Weiss's Soft Tissue Tumors*, 5th edn. (St. Louis: Mosby, 2008), pp. 477–517.

61. Colin, P., Lagacé, R., Caillaud, J. M., Sastre-Garau, X. and Klijanienko, J. Fine-needle aspiration in myxofibrosarcoma. Experience of Institut Curie. *Diagn Cytopathol* 2010; 38(5): 343–6.

62. Dardick, I., Lagacé, R., Carlier, M. T. and Jung, R. C. Chordoid sarcoma (extraskeletal myxoid chondrosarcoma). *Virchows Arch* 1983; 399(1): 61–78.

63. Sciot, R., Dal Cin, P., Fletcher, C., Samson, I., Smith, M., De Vos, R. *et al.* t(9;22)(q22-31;q11-12) is a consistent marker of extraskeletal myxoid chondrosarcoma: evaluation of three cases. *Mod Pathol* 1995; 8(7): 765–8.

64. Huvos, A. G. Myxoid chondrosarcoma, in Mitchel, J. (ed.), *Bone Tumors. Diagnosis, Treatment and Prognosis*, 2nd edn. (Philadelphia, PA: W. B. Saunders, 1991), pp. 366–7.

65. Oliveira, A. M., Sebo, T. J., McGrory, J. E., Gaffey, T. A., Rock, M. G. and Nascimento, A. G. Extraskeletal myxoid chondrosarcoma: a clinicopathologic, immunohistochemical, and ploidy analysis of 23 cases. *Mod Pathol* 2000; 13(8): 900–8.

66. Meis-Kindblom, J. M., Bergh, P., Gunterberg, B. and Kindblom, L. J. Extraskeletal myxoid chondrosarcoma: a reappraisal of its morphologic spectrum and

prognostic factors based on 117 cases. *Am J Surg Pathol* 1999; 23(6): 636–50.

67. Hornick, J. L., Dal Cin, P. and Fletcher, C. D. Loss of INI1 expression is characteristic of both conventional and proximal-type epithelioid sarcoma. *Am J Surg Pathol* 2009; 33(4): 542–50.

68. Fletcher, C. D., Berman, J. J., Corless, C., Gorstein, F., Lasota, J., Longley, B. J. *et al.* Diagnosis of gastrointestinal stromal tumors: a consensus approach. *Hum Pathol* 2002; 33(5): 459–65.

69. Chritopherson, W. M., Foote, F. W.Jr. and Steward, F. W. Alveolar soft-part sarcoma: structurally characteristic tumors of uncertain histogenesis. *Cancer* 1952; 5(1): 100–11.

70. Ladanyi, M., Lui, M. Y., Antonescu, C. R., Krause-Boehm, A., Meindl, A., Argani, P. *et al.* The der(17)t(X;17)(p11;q25) of human alveolar soft part sarcoma fuses the TFE3 transcription factor gene ASPL, a novel gene 17q25. *Oncogene* 2001; 20(1): 48–57.

71. Sandberg, A. and Bridge, J. Updates on the cytogenetics and molecular genetics of bone and soft tissue tumors: alveolar soft part sarcoma. *Cancer Genet Cytogenet* 2002; 136(1): 1–9.

72. Portera, C. A., Jr., Ho, V., Patel, S. R., Hunt, K. K., Feig, B. W., Respondek, P. M. *et al.* Alveolar soft part sarcoma: clinical course and patterns of metastasis in 70 patients treated at a single institution. *Cancer* 2001; 91(3): 585–91.

73. Kayton, M. L., Meyers, P., Wexler, L. H., Gerald, W. L. and LaQuaglia, M. P. Clinical presentation, treatment, and outcome of alveolar soft part sarcoma in children, adolescents, and young adults. *J Pediatr Surg* 2006; 41(1): 187–93.

74. Kawai, A., Hosono, A., Nakayama, R., Matsumine, A., Matsumoto, S., Ueda, T. *et al.*

Clear cell sarcoma of tendons and aponeuroses: a study of 75 patients. *Cancer* 2007; 109(1): 109–16.

75. Antonescu, C. R., Tschernyavsky, S. J., Woodruff, J. M., Jungbluth, A. A., Brennan, M. F. and Ladanyi, M. Molecular diagnosis of clear cell sarcoma: detection of EWS-ATF1 and MITF-M transcripts and histopathological and ultrastructural analysis of 12 cases. *J Mol Diagn* 2002; 4(1): 44–52.

76. Panagopoulos, I., Mertens, F., Dêbiec-Rychter, M., Isaksson, M., Limon, J., Kardas, I. *et al.* Molecular genetic characterization of the EWS/ATF1 fusion gene in clear cell sarcoma of tendons and aponeuroses. *Int J Cancer* 2002; 99(4): 560–7.

77. Langezaal, S. M., Graadt van Roggen, J. F., Cleton-Jansen, A. M., Baelde, J. J. and Hogendoorn, P. C. Malignant melanoma is genetically distinct from clear cell sarcoma of tendons and aponeurosis (malignant melanoma of soft parts). *Br J Cancer* 2001; 84(4): 535–8.

78. Fletcher, C. D. Pleomorphic malignant fibrous histiocytoma: fact or fiction? A critical reappraisal based on 159 tumors diagnosed as pleomorphic sarcoma. *Am J Surg Pathol* 1992; 16(3): 213–28.

79. Mertens, F., Fletcher, C. D., Dal Cin, P., De Wever, I., Mandahl, N., Mitelman, F. *et al.* Cytogenetic analysis of 46 pleomorphic soft tissue sarcomas and correlation with morphologic and clinical features: a report of the CHAMP Study Group. Chromosomes and Morphology. *Gene Chromosome Canc* 1998; 22(1): 16–25.

80. Idbaih, A., Coindre, J. M., Derré, J., Mariani, O., Terrier, P., Ranchère, D. *et al.* Myxoid malignant fibrous histiocytoma and pleomorphic liposarcoma

share very similar genomic imbalances. *Lab Invest* 2005; 85(2): 176–81.

81. F. Chibon, , A. Mairal, , P. Fréneaux, Terrier, P., Coindre, J. M., Sastre, X. *et al.* The RB1 gene is the target of chromosome 13 deletions in malignant fibrous histiocytoma. *Cancer Res* 2000; 60(22): 6339–45.

82. Derré, J., Lagacé, R., Nicolas, A., Mairal, A., Chibon, F., Coindre, J. M. *et al.* Leiomyosarcomas and most malignant fibrous histiocytomas share very similar comparative genomic hybridization imbalances: an analysis of a series of 27 leiomyosarcomas. *Lab Invest* 2001; 81(2): 211–15.

83. Turc-Carel, C., Lizard-Nacol, S., Justrabo, E., Favrot, M., Philip, T. and Tabone, E. Consistent chromosomal translocation in alveolar rhabdomyosarcoma. *Cancer Genet Cytogenet* 1986; 19(3–4): 361–2.

84. Barr, F. G. Gene fusions involving PAX and FOX family members in alveolar rhabdomyosarcoma. *Oncogene* 2001; 20(40): 5736–46.

85. Klijanienko, J., Caillaud, J. M., Orbach, D., Brisse, H., Lagacé, R., Vielh, P. *et al.* Cyto-histological correlations in primary, recurrent and metastatic rhabdomyosarcoma: the institut Curie's experience. *Diagn Cytopathol* 2007; 35(8): 482–7.

86. C. Besnard-Guérin, , I. Newsham, , R. Winqvist and Cavenee, W. K. A common region of loss of heterozygosity in Wilms' tumor and rhabdomyosarcoma distal to be D11S988 locus on chromosome 11p15. *Hum Genet* 1996; 97(2): 163–70.

87. Klijanienko, J., Couturier, J., Bourdeaut, F., Fréneaux, P., Ballet, S., Brisse, H. *et al.* Fine-needle aspiration as a diagnostic technique in 50 cases of primary Ewing sarcoma/peripheral neuroectodermal tumor (ES/PNET). Institut Curie's

experience. *Diagn Cytopathol* 2012; 40(1): 19–25.

88. Thomson, T., Klijanienko, J., Couturier, J., Brisse, H., Pierron, G., Freneaux, P. *et al.* Fine needle aspiration in rhabdoïd tumor. Institut Curie's experience, *Cancer Cytopathol* 2011; 119(1): 49–57.

89. Fisher, H.P., Thomsen, H., Altmannsberger, M. and Bertram, U. Malignant rhabdoïd tumour of the kidney expressing neurofilament proteins. Immunohistochemical findings and histogenetic aspects. *Pathol Res Pract* 1989; 184: 541–7.

90. Peter, M., Gilbert, E. and Delattre, O. A multiplex real-time PCR assay for the detection of gene fusions observed in solid tumors. *Lab Invest* 2001; 81(6): 905–12.

91. Weiss, S. W. and Goldblum, J. R. Rhabdomyosarcoma, in Strauss, M. (ed.), *Enzinger and Weiss's Soft Tissue Tumors*, 5th edn. (St. Louis: Mosby, 2008), pp. 595–633.

92. Fisher, C. The diversity of soft tissue tumors with EWSR1 gene rearrangements: a review. *Histopathology* 2014; 64(1): 134–50.

93. Biegel, J. A., Conard, K. and Brooks, J. J. Translocation (11;22) (p13;q12): primary change in intra-abdominal desmoplastic small round cell tumor. *Gene Chromosome Canc* 1993; 7(2): 119–21.

94. Sawyer, J. R., Tryka, A. F. and Lewis, J. M. A novel reciprocal

chromosome translocation t (11;22)(p13;q12) in an intraabdominal desmoplastic small round-cell tumor. *Am J Surg Pathol* 1992; 16(4): 411–16.

95. Ladanyi, M. and Gerald, W. Fusion of the EWS and WT1 genes in the desmoplastic small round cell tumor. *Cancer Res* 1994; 54(11): 2837–40.

96. Klijanienko, J., Colin, P., Couturier, J., Lagacé, R., Fréneaux, P., Pierron, G. *et al.* Fine-needle aspiration in desmoplastic small round cell tumor: a report of 10 new tumors in 8 patients with clinicopathological and molecular correlations with review of the literature. *Cancer Cytopathol* 2014; 122(5): 386–93.

97. Sciot, R., Dal Cin, P., Fletcher, C., Samson, I., Smith, M., De Vos, R. *et al.* t(9;22)(q22–31;q11–12) is a consistent marker of extraskeletal myxoid chondrosarcoma: evaluation of three cases. *Mod Pathol* 1995; 8(7): 765–8.

98. Gerami, P., Gannon, B. and Murphy, M. J. Melanocytic neoplasms I: molecular diagnosis, in Murphy, M. J. (ed.), *Molecular Diagnostics in Dermatology and Dermatopathology* (New York: Springer, 2011), pp. 73–103.

99. Tsao, H., Atkins, M. B. and Sober, A. J. Management of cutaneous melanoma. *New Engl J Med* 2004; 351(10): 998–1012.

100. Sullivan, R. J. and Flaherty, K. MAP kinase signaling and

inhibition in melanoma. *Oncogene* 2013; 32(19): 2373–9.

101. Solus, J. F. and Kraft, S. Ras, RAF, and MAP kinase in melanoma. *Adv Anat Pathol* 2013; 20(4): 217–26.

102. Curtin, J. A., Fridlyand, J., Kageshita, T., Patel, H. N., Busam, K. J., Kutzner, H. *et al.* Distinct sets of genetic alterations in melanoma. *New Engl J Med* 2005; 353(20): 2135–47.

103. Hocker, T. and Tsao, H. Ultraviolet radiation and melanoma: a systematic review and analysis of reported sequence variants. *Hum Mutat* 2007; 28(6): 578–88.

104. Grossmann, A. H., Grossman, K. F. and Wallander, M. L. Molecular testing in malignant melanoma. *Diagn Cytopathol* 2012; 40(6): 503–10.

105. Elaba, Z., Phelps, A. and Murphy, M. J. Molecular diagnostic strategies: a role in the practice of dermatology. *Int J Dermatol* 2012; 51(11): 1292–302.

106. Kuwamoto, S. Recent advances in the biology of Merkel cell carcinoma. *Hum Pathol* 2011; 42(8): 1063–77.

107. Houben, R., Schrama, D. and Becker, J. Molecular pathogenesis of Merkel cell carcinoma. *Exp Dermatol* 2009; 18(3): 193–8.

108. Feng, H., Shuda, M., Chang, Y. and Moore, P. S. Clonal integration of a polyomavirus in human Merkel cell carcinoma. *Science* 2008; 319(5866): 1096–100.

# Chapter 16

# Cardio-thoracic tumors

Umberto Malapelle, Claudio Bellevicine, Elena Vigliar
and Giancarlo Troncone

## Lung cancer

### Background

Advances in predictive biomarker testing and in molecular targeted therapy of lung cancer have in the past few years driven a major change in the histological and cytological practice, calling the pathologist to closely interact with pulmonologists, oncologists and molecular biologists to optimize patient care. Several clinical trials demonstrated that tyrosine kinase inhibitor (TKI) therapy is better than conventional chemotherapy, when patients harbor epidermal growth factor receptor (EGFR) mutations (1). Similarly, the patients whose lung cancer contains anaplastic lymphoma kinase (ALK) fusion genes consistently respond to ALK inhibitors (2). These and other advances have led to the recognition that the diagnosis of lung adenocarcinoma requires a multidisciplinary approach and to the proposal of a new classification (3); even more recently the College of American Pathologists (CAP), the International Association for the Study of Lung Cancer (IASLC) and the Association for Molecular Pathology (AMP) set out to create standardized international guidelines for lung cancer biomarker testing (4).

Today, the pathologist plays different roles in lung cancer biomarker testing (Table 16.1). The pathologists may perform the molecular testing in-house, supervising the activity of his/her laboratory. Currently, however, a greater number of pathologists refer to outside molecular pathology laboratories. In any case, the pathologist is responsible for the pre-analytical phases of testing; he/she reviews a representative tissue section or a smear to determine the cellularity and purity (mucin and necrosis may inhibit amplification) of the tumor sample being submitted

for biomarker testing, also suggesting which molecular tests are more pertinent for a given cancer based on the association of specific mutation with specific histological types and subtypes. Since various mutational assays have different analytic sensitivities, the pathologist should enrich for tumor content to a level that is acceptable for the assay being used. It is noteworthy that the determination of the rate of neoplastic cells is very much "observer-dependent" and pathologists should take care not to underestimate the percentage of non-tumor cells (5). Once the results of molecular analysis are received, the pathologists may compare the mutation signals with the extent of tumor cells in the tested specimen, carefully evaluating the quality processes employed to ensure confidence in the results. One of the basic requirements to enable the practicing pathologist to perform

**Table 16.1** Pathologist's role in biomarker testing

1. Test request
   a. Reflex (regardless of a specific clinician's request in early neoplastic stages)
   b. Histological driven (based on the association between a specific mutation and a specific morphology)

2. Pre-analytical phases of testing
   a. Selection of tumor area
   b. Tumor cell enrichment
   c. Selection of reference laboratory

3. Post-analytical phases of testing
   a. Evaluation of mutation signal respect to tumor content
   b. Evaluation of quality processes
   c. Integration of the test results into the pathology report

*Molecular Pathology: A Practical Guide for the Surgical Pathologist and Cytopathologist*, ed. John M. S. Bartlett, Abeer Shaaban and Fernando Schmitt. Published by Cambridge University Press. © Cambridge University Press, 2016.

all of these tasks is educational; this chapter aims to provide the essential concepts of lung molecular pathology, whose understanding is necessary to properly handle and manage surgical pathology and cytopathology specimens for molecular testing.

## Clinical issues

### General considerations

The relevance of biomarker testing in the field of molecular lung pathology cannot be overemphasized, since this neoplasm is the number one cause of cancer death in the global population. Indeed, in the United States, deaths from lung cancer are more than the combined total of deaths from the next three most common causes of cancer deaths (colon, breast and prostate cancer). Tobacco smoking is by far the major risk factor for lung cancer; in fact, the majority of cases, approximately 85% of the lung cancer in men and 47% of the lung cancer in women, are caused by tobacco smoking. Thus, a significant number of lung cancers also develop in those who have never smoked, with distinct clinical (more frequent in female), pathological (mostly adenocarcinoma) and molecular characteristics.

Despite significant improvements in its diagnosis and treatment, lung cancer still has a poor prognosis. In patients with early-stage disease, the most effective treatment is surgery. However, 30% to 60% of patients with localized disease develop recurrence and the five-year survival rate is 50%. Furthermore, no effective screening techniques have been identified yet; most of the patients present with locally advanced or metastatic disease and they are not eligible for surgical resection. Conventional therapy for advanced-stage non-small cell lung carcinoma (NSCLC) is doublet chemotherapy that includes cisplatin or carboplatin and in selected cases patients are also treated by radiotherapy. The response to this first-line treatment is followed by disease progression. The patients may be given second-line therapy, or feasibly more lines of therapy, in an effort to control their disease. Ultimately, practically all of these patients die from lung cancer, as reflected in the figures cited above.

### Clinical information

At the time of the initial diagnosis of lung cancer, until clinical staging is not completed, it is unknown whether surgery will follow (5); thus, the pathologist must bear in mind that the first biopsy or cytological sample may be the only one available to perform the molecular studies and he/she should avoid the ancillary studies that may not be essential to establish the pathologic diagnosis (4). Communication between the members of the multidisciplinary team (MDT) should enable the pathologist to receive information on the clinical suspicion of the lesion sampled (primary tumor vs. metastasis), on previous relevant surgical, oncological, radiotherapeutic treatments and on the smoking history (never, ex (pack years, years since quitting), current smoker (pack years, years of smoking)) (3). Some patients may not be candidates for targeted therapy for clinical reasons, even if a treatable molecular alteration was found, and a good communication between the clinical care team and the testing laboratory is needed to ensure that testing is performed for patients whose management will be impacted by the test result (3, 4).

### Sampling

The current increased diagnostic demands dictate that the use of material obtained for pathological evaluation and molecular analysis should be optimized in order to reduce the need for additional invasive sampling procedures for the patient. While the requirements have increased, sample size (small bronchial biopsies, cytology specimens) has decreased. The optimal methodology for diagnostic sampling of intra-thoracic tumor at either the primary or a metastatic site of lung lesions is reviewed elsewhere (6). As a general rule, the best strategy to increase the yield of a diagnostic procedure is to combine several techniques. Thus, broncoscopic biopsy should be combined with bronchial brush in central lesions, and with transbronchial needle aspiration (TBNA) in suspected submucosal infiltration. Ultrasound-guided (EUS, EBUS) procedures and the upcoming use of a navigation system may assist in the selection of the most appropriate point of sampling. Complex procedures combining diagnosis and staging and requiring the sampling of multiple lymph node stations need to be performed within the time frame of the local anaesthesia, that is, around 30 minutes. In this setting, Rapid On-Site Examination (ROSE) – a quick cytological examination for the presence of tumor cells by the cytopathologist – is crucial to ensure that the obtained material is sufficient and properly preserved – not only for the identification of malignancy, but also for biomarker testing (7).

# Pathological strategy
## Advances in understanding of lung cancer

Remarkable advances in the understanding of lung cancer have recently been made on a molecular basis, raising hope that a genotype-driven targeted treatment approach to lung cancer, schematized in Table 16.2, will improve the survival and quality of life of patients with lung neoplasia. Most lung adenocarcinomas arise in the lung periphery from the brochioloalveolar epithelium, the so-called terminal respiratory unit (TRU). Atypical adenomatous hyperplasia (AAH) is a recognized precursor lesion in the TRU, a pre-invasive stage of epithelial dysplasia, which can progress to invasive disease through a stage of adenocarcinoma *in situ* (AIS) (3). Some of the molecular events associated with this process are now recognized. Common to all lung cancer appears to be: activation, up-regulation and expression of oncogenes which promote tumor growth and progression; and the loss of activity of genes which have the opposite effect by abrogating oncogenic action, the so-called tumor suppressor genes (TSG). The discovery in 2004 that activating somatic mutations in the tyrosine kinase (TK) domain of the epidermal growth factor receptor (EGFR) gene make the tumor sensitive to tyrosine kinase inhibitors (TKIs) treatment has probably represented the most significant breakthrough in the field of molecular oncology in the past decade (3). Three years later, in 2007, Soda

**Table 16.2** Genotype-driven targeted treatment approach to lung cancer

| Targeted gene | Drugs | Biomarker | Assay | Clinical features | Histology |
|---|---|---|---|---|---|
| EGFR | Gefitinib, Erlotinib, Afatinib, Dacomitinib | EGFR gene mutation/ deletions/insertion | PCR-based assay IHC by mutation-specific antibody | Female, Asian, non-smokers | Low-grade, papillary and lepidic pattern |
| ALK | Crizotinib | ALK gene fusions | FISH RT-PCR IHC | Young age, non-smokers | Solid, cribiform, mucinous with signet-ring cells |
| ROS1 | Crizotinib | ROS1 gene fusions | FISH IHC | Young, non-smoker | Similar to those of ALK rearrangements |
| BRAF | Verumafenib dabrafenib | BRAF gene mutation | PCR-based assay IHC by mutation-specific antibody | Smokers, advanced stage | Micropapillary, high histological grade |
| RET | Isunitinib sorafenib, vandetanib cabozantinib | RET gene rearrangements | FISH RT-PCR | Young, non-smokers | Similar to those of ALK rearrangements |
| MEK1 | Selumetinib | MEK mutation KRAS mutation | PCR-based assay | Smokers* | Intestinal-like (TTF1-; CDX2+)* |
| HER2 | Afatinib; neratinib; dacomitinib | HER2 gene mutation (insertion) HER2 gene amplification | PCR-based assay | Non-smokers Histology: low-grade, lepidic pattern | |
| MET | Onartuzumab; rilotumumab; cabozantinib; tivantinib; crizotinib | MET gene amplification MET gene mutation HGF overexpression | FISH IHC PCR-based assay | Poor prognostic factor | Inversely correlated with the lepidic subtype |

* Clinical and histological features related to KRAS mutant NSCLC.

and co-workers reported that anaplastic lymphoma kinase (ALK) rearrangement positive patients can be effectively treated with a novel ALK inhibitor (3).

These evidences have strongly supported the so-called "oncogene addiction" theory, which dominates current views of the role of oncogenic mutations in carcinogenesis and cancer treatment. Basic and clinical research has revealed that some genetic lesions are not only necessary for the initial development or progression of a specific tumor, but are also required for the maintenance of that tumor's survival. Such "driver" mutations sustain tumors, but simultaneously can serve as cancer-specific targets of vulnerability to be exploited therapeutically, with fewer of the side effects seen with cytotoxic chemotherapy.

## Subtyping of NSCLC is crucial

The pathologist's practice, including the handling and management of surgical pathology and cytopathology specimens, has undergone a major change (5). Until recently, patient management was still based on the traditional distinction between small cell carcinoma (SCLC) and NSCLC, this latter constituting approximately 85% of all lung cancers and traditionally divided into three major cell types: adenocarcinoma (approximately 50%); squamous cell carcinoma (approximately 35%); and large cell carcinoma (approximately 15%, although this is a decreasing cell type category). Until recently, subtyping of NSCLC received little attention because the treatment strategy was similar. Today, knowledge of the specific NSCLC subtype is essential prior to prescribing a number of important new drugs to treat NSCLC, including both cytotoxic chemotherapeutic and molecular targeted agents (3). As an example, the anti-folate agent pemetrexed is differentially effective in different forms of NSCLC. This drug competitively binds the thymidilate synthase (TS) – an enzyme involved in the DNA synthetic pathway. TS levels are higher in SCLC and squamous cell carcinomas than in adenocarcinomas. This is the most likely explanation for the improved anti-tumor activity of pemetrexed in adenocarcinomas than in SCLC and squamous cell carcinomas, where the drug may fail to inhibit the higher levels of TS (3). Another example is given by bevacizumab, a monoclonal antibody targeted against the vascular endothelial growth factor receptor (VEGFR), which is not licensed for use in patients who have a diagnosis of squamous cell carcinoma (3). Potentially fatal hemoptysis has been reported in early clinical trials in patients with squamous cell

carcinomas, but not with adenocarcinomas, treated with bevacizumab. The increased propensity of squamous cell carcinoma to hemorrhage may be explained partially by the fact that these tumors generally arise from the large bronchi, while adenocarcinomas usually take their origin from the peripheral lung epithelium. The potential of central tumors to invade major vessels, with blood supply from the bronchial arteries, could lead to large vessel hemorrhage at systemic pressure if treatment results in tumor necrosis. Finally, NSCLC subtyping is crucial to select patients for EGFR and ALK testing, as the prevalence of EGFR mutation and ALK rearrangements is negligible in lung cancers without an adenocarcinoma component (4). All these evidences imply that, at least for the complete resection specimens, NSCLC not otherwise specified (NOS) is no longer considered appropriate as a diagnostic term and as an operational category for clinical management (3). In the small tissue sample setting, the term NSCLC-NOS should be used as little as possible, relying on the aid of immunohistochemistry, to detect the line of differentiation in difficult cases (3).

## Revised classification for adenocarcinoma

The diagnostic criteria of the most recent World Health Organization (WHO) Thoracic Tumor Classification of 2004 were mostly based on a simpler approach based on hematoxylin and eosin (H&E) examination (3). The only applications of ancillary techniques were histochemical stains to demonstrate the presence of luminal and intracytoplasmic mucin droplets and immunohistochemistry for the demonstration of neuroendocrine differentiation in large cell neuroendocrine carcinoma. Attempts to apply this classification to small biopsy or cytology samples lead to inaccuracy and inconsistency of diagnosis. In 2011, a panel of lung cancer specialists representing the International Association for the Study of Lung Cancer (IASLC), the American Thoracic Society (ATS) and the European Respiratory Society (ERS) published proposals for a new multidisciplinary classification of lung adenocarcinoma (3). This new classification, expected to be formally adopted by WHO in a few years, combines histology with clinical, molecular, radiologic and surgical issues, with the intent to provide clinically relevant terminology. Important aspects of this proposal are the concepts of adenocarcinoma-in situ (formerly bronchioloalveolar carcinoma (BAC)) and minimally invasive adenocarcinoma and the recommendations on classifying resected

**Table 16.3** International Association for the Study of Lung Cancer (IASLC), American Thoracic Society (ATS) and European Respiratory Society (ERS), Classification of lung adenocarcinoma in resection specimens

**Pre-invasive lesions**

Atypical adenomatous hyperplasia

Adenocarcinoma *in situ* (≤3 cm formerly bronchioloalveolar carcinoma)

Non-mucinous

Mucinous

Mixed mucinous/non-mucinous

**Minimally invasive adenocarcinoma (≤3 cm lepidic predominant tumor with ≤5 mm invasion)**

Non-mucinous

Mucinous

Mixed mucinous/non-mucinous

**Invasive adenocarcinoma**

Lepidic predominant (formerly non-mucinous bronchioloalveolar carcinoma, with >5 mm invasion)

Acinar predominant

Papillary predominant

Micropapillary predominant

Solid predominant with mucin production

**Variants of invasive adenocarcinoma**

Invasive mucinous adenocarcinoma (formerly mucinous bronchioloalveolar carcinoma)

Colloid

Fetal (low and high grade)

Enteric

adenocarcinoma by the predominant tumor pattern in the lesion (Table 16.3). The predominance of certain patterns, such as micropapillary or solid pattern poorly differentiated in the lesion, portends a poorer prognosis for surgically resected tumors, while a predominance of lepidic pattern (former BAC) is associated with a relatively good prognosis (3).

## The modern work-up of lung adenocarcinoma

The IASLC/ATS/ERS-recommended adenocarcinoma work-up includes three steps: identification of malignancy; immunohistochemistry (IHC) refinement where needed; and molecular pathology (Figure 16.1)

(3). The first step is the identification of carcinoma, as opposed to other rarer malignancies, pre-invasive or reactive changes (hyperplasia and dysplasia) and non-neoplastic pathological processes (inflammation, benign tumors, etc.). If carcinoma is identified, the default diagnosis is primary lung cancer, and reflex IHC to differentiate primary from secondary tumor manifestations in the lung without further clinical information should not be performed (6). However, the pathologist must always be alert to the possibility of metastatic disease and an adequate clinical history is essential to indicate if there is any suspicion or possibility that the lung tumor under investigation could be metastatic disease. After diagnosing the tumor as primary lung carcinoma, the next step is to determine whether the tumor represents SCLC or NSCLC. Standard morphology is in most cases effective, reliable and accurate for the recognition of SCLC. Within the NSCLC group, most pathologists can easily identify well- or moderately differentiated squamous cell carcinomas or adenocarcinomas, but specific diagnoses are more difficult with poorly differentiated tumors. As an example, so-called "squamoid" features are common in many poorly differentiated cases, even in adenocarcinomas, but the only features diagnostic of squamous cell carcinoma are keratin formation and/or intercellular bridges (3, 6). Since diagnostic criteria are more dependent on architecture than on individual cellular features, only IHC can effectively reveal the line of differentiation of small biopsy samples (bronchoscopic, needle, core biopsies and cytology). Undifferentiated cells, from a tumor that is differentiated as squamous or adenocarcinoma in other parts not sampled, may express lineage markers associated with the differentiation type and the percentage of unclassifiable NSCLC can be limited using IHC.

Although large panels of markers including up to eight immunostains have been proposed, only a few antibodies (Table 16.4) are really needed to differentiate SCLC from NSCLC and in subtyping NSCLC (6). TTF-1 is the single best marker for adenocarcinoma, also providing the added value of serving as a pneumocyte marker that can help confirm a primary lung origin. TTF-1 is not expressed in squamous cell carcinomas of the lung, although TTF-1 positivity can be observed in the hyperplastic type II pneumocytes that are sometimes seen entrapped within the tumor. Commercially available antibodies to TTF-1 may show different results. The clone 8G7G3/1 is more specific for adenocarcinoma than the clone SPT24,

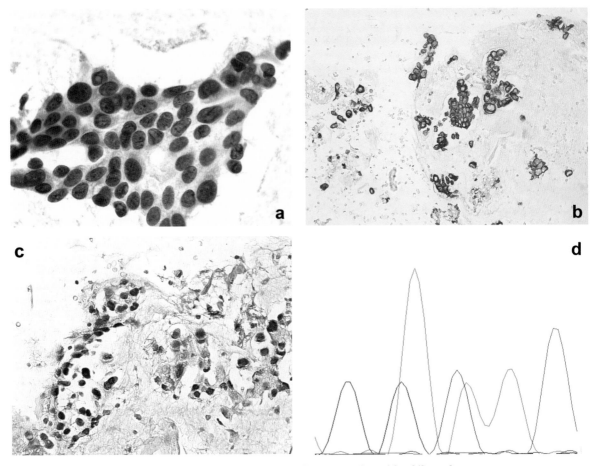

**Figure 16.1 Endoscopic-ultrasound (EUS) guided FNA in a patient presenting with a hilar pulmonary tumor mass abutting in the mediastinum**
The Papanicolaou stained smear showed sheets of unevenly spaced atypical nuclei displaying irregular contours, grooves and occasional intranuclear inclusions. These features were diagnostic of NSCLC, favoring adenocarcinoma. Immunohistochemistry performed on cell-block material showed cytoplasmatic CK7 (b) and nuclear TTF1 (c) positive staining, confirming adenocarcinoma. EGFR exon 19 deletion (15 bp) was evident on the sequencing electropherogram (d).

which stains a proportion of squamous cell carcinomas as well as a few colonic metastatic adenocarcinomas (6). Both clones besides epithelial thyroid cells may stain adenocarcinomas of the endometrium and of the breast. TTF-1 is also frequently expressed in SCLC, whereas the other adenocarcinoma marker Napsin A is negative in SCLC. Napsin A may have a sensitivity higher than TTF-1 in poorly differentiated adenocarcinomas. Chromogranin A is the most specific marker of neuroendocrine differentiation and the dot-like puntiform staining pattern is very helpful in confirming SCLC.

p63 is a reliable marker for squamous histology (6). However, p63 also stains a subset of adenocarcinoma. Several studies have found that, when co-existent,

TTF1 expression should take preference over p63 expression (3). p63 may also stain a subset of SCLC. More recently, the p40 antibody, which reacts only with the p63 truncated dominant-negative isoform, seems to have a higher specificity than conventional p63 in correctly identifying squamous cell carcinoma while not staining adenocarcinoma, even when p63 positive, and SCLC (6). As a general rule, napsin expression excludes squamous cell carcinoma and neuroendocrine tumors including small cell carcinoma; p40 expression excludes small cell carcinoma and adenocarcinoma and TTF-1 expression excludes squamous cell carcinoma (6) (Table 16.4).

It is possible to limit immunophenotyping of NSCLC to only one adenocarcinoma marker (TTF1)

Table 16.4 Immunostaining in differential diagnosis of lung cancer

| IHC markers | Squamous cell carcinoma vs. adenocarcinoma | |
|---|---|---|
| p63 | +++ (100%) | + (20–30%) |
| p40 (ΔNp63) | +++ (100%) | – |
| TTF-1 | – | ++ (80%)[i] |
| Napsin | – | ++ (80%)[ii] |
| | Squamous cell carcinoma vs. small cell carcinoma | |
| p63 | +++ (100%) | + (20%) |
| p40 (ΔNp63) | +++ (100%) | – |
| CK 34βE12 | +++ (100%) | – |
| TTF-1 | – | ++ (73–83%)[iii] |
| Chromogranin | – | +/– (dot-like)± |
| Synaptophysin | – | ++/+ (granular) ± |
| CD56 | – | +++ (membrane) ± |
| | Adenocarcinoma vs. small cell carcinoma | |
| Napsin | ++ (80%) | – |
| Chromogranin | – | +/– (dot-like)± |
| Synaptophysin | – | ++/+ (granular) ± |
| CD56 | – | +++ (membrane) ± |

(i) TTF1 negative adenocarcinomas almost never harbor mutated EGFR.
(ii) Napsin may be more sensitive than TTF1 in poorly differentiated ADC.
(iii) TTF1 expression in SCLC depends on clone used; extrapulmonary SCC may express TTF1 positivity in up
    to 36% of cases, especially in those of uterine cervix origin.
± Chromogranin and synapthophysin expression may be lost in SCLC, but most of these tumors are positive
    for CD56.

and one squamous marker (p63 or p40) when the tissue needs to be maximized for molecular testing (3). In selected cases, especially in the case of poorly cellular cytological specimens, antibody cocktails can be prepared by mixing two "different-by-lineage" antibodies to a single slide, combining a nuclear and a cytoplasmatic marker (for example, TTF-1 plus desmocollin-3 or p63 plus Napsin A) (6). Some carcinoma cases are completely unreactive to any of the currently available markers, having a "null" immuno-profile. In these cases, microRNAs – in particular the hsa-miR-205 and the hsa-let-7 family expression, which are differentially expressed in lung squamous cell carcinomas and adenocarcinomas – can be used to classify NSCLCs with a high degree of sensitivity and specificity.

Technicians should adequately section the block in order to secure the primary diagnosis, preserving as much tissue as possible for possible subsequent IHC or molecular testing. Cutting the block only once yielding sections both to establish the diagnosis and for genomic studies would be ideal to save as much tumor tissue as possible for molecular testing (5). To preserve the quality of epitopes and DNA, spare cut sections should be properly stored for future use in a thick protective coat or sealed and stored at 4°C or by special tapes ("Tissue Protector"; Pathology Institute Corp., Toyama, Japan). The principal steps of the pre-analytical mutational testing workflow are schematized in Figure 16.2.

# EGFR testing

## EGFR gene alterations

Although many additional molecular markers have been proposed, the current reality of molecular

253

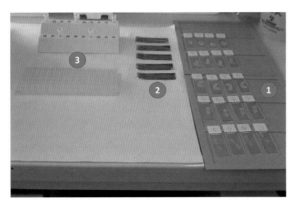

**Figure 16.2 Principal components of the pre-analytical mutational testing workflow**
Formalin-fixed paraffin-embedded sections are placed on uncharged slides and de-waxed (1). The thickness is around 10 μm, thus intact cell nuclei are likely to be contained in such sections; these are serially cut including pre and post 5 μm ematoxylin and eosin stained slides. The referral pathologist ensures for tumor adequacy selecting the neoplastic area prior to manual macrodissection. Performed by using sterile razor blades (2), the obtained material is harvested in Eppendorf tubes (3).

testing of NSCLC includes the assessment of EGFR and ALK gene alterations. These tests are the primary subject of the CAP/IASLC/AMP guidelines (4). Multiple other predictive biomarkers, to be discussed later, are mentioned in the guidelines as forthcoming. The simplest algorithm is to test for EGFR mutations first by a rapid EGFR mutation screening test and then to proceed to ALK testing if the EGFR results are wild-type. An alternative algorithm, potentially more cost effective, would begin with KRAS analysis, which represents 25% to 30% of lung adenocarcinomas. The tumors without KRAS mutations would then be EGFR and ALK tested.

Mutation at the TK domain of EGFR leads to increased proliferation, angiogenesis, metastasis and decreased apoptosis (7). Mutant EGFR is targeted by the small TKIs. The first generation of EGFR TKIs approved for treatment of advanced-stage lung cancer includes gefitinib (Iressa; AstraZeneca, London, United Kingdom) and erlotinib (Tarceva; Genentech, South San Francisco, California, and OSI Pharmaceuticals, Long Island, New York). These drugs reversibly occupy the TK ATP binding site, thereby preventing EGFR activation and downstream signaling effects. The efficacy of this treatment, as monotherapy in the first line setting, is restricted to those NSCLC patients (10% of Caucasians and 35% of East Asians) harboring EGFR mutations (1). Although

increased EGFR gene copy-number (polysomy or amplification) is observed in about 40% of cases, EGFR copy-number analysis (i.e. FISH or chromogenic *in situ* hybridization) is not recommended for selection of EGFR TKI therapy (4). The IPASS study, a large phase III randomized clinical trial with data on both EGFR mutation and amplification, showed that EGFR TKI treatment selection based on mutation status leads to better clinical outcomes in the first-line setting than selection based on EGFR gene copy-number (1). Subsequent randomized clinical trials led on patients with high stage NSCLC further established the relation between activating EGFR mutations and longer progression-free survival (4). However, no study reported improvement in overall survival, possibly because of the crossover design of these studies in which most of the patients with EGFR-mutated tumors treated initially with chemotherapy crossed over to the EGFR TKI treatment arm, confusing the analysis of overall survival data (4).

## EGFR mutation testing: which patients?

EGFR mutations are more common in women and in patients who have never smoked tobacco (7). These clinical characteristics, however, can be of value for population studies, but they are insufficiently specific to select individual patients (4). Nomograms combining several variables to define patients who have a very low probability of EGFR mutations have been developed, but still need validation. Most mutant tumors are adenocarcinomas and the CAP/IASLC/AMP guidelines do not recommend testing "pure" SqCC and SCLC (4). However, carcinoma with mixed histology (for example, adenosquamous, mixed adeno/small cell) may harbor mutations in EGFR and, if so, respond to treatment. Therefore, on specimens obtained by an incomplete sampling of the tumor (biopsy and cytology), in which the possibility of an adenocarcinoma component cannot be excluded, the opportunity of testing even cases diagnosed either as SqCC or as SCLC should be evaluated on a case-by-case basis, and clinical criteria such as young age and lack of smoking history should be taken into account (4).

## EGFR mutations testing: which samples?

According to the concept that key driver mutations are well preserved during tumor progression, the mutation patterns between primary and metastatic sites and between primary and recurrent neoplasms are similar (4). When an earlier primary lesion is available and suitable for analysis, there is no need to sample a metastasis before initiation of TKI therapy (4). A detailed study by Yatabe *et al.*, in which 50 tumors were divided into three parts and five into 100 parts, showed that testing of multiple different areas within a single tumor is not necessary (8). Similarly, mutations detected on a single cytological smear may be representative of the entire tumor and, therefore, they can predict the response to treatment (9).

When an EGFR mutation is identified by direct sequencing, both mutant and wild-type alleles are seen on the sequencing electropherograms. In some instances, even if the tumor has not been microdissected, the mutant allele may appear to be in great excess of the wild-type allele leading to mutant allele-specific imbalance (MASI), due to EGFR copy-number increase. As shown in Figure 16.3, MASI is distributed unevenly throughout the tumors, a phenomenon described as pseudo-heterogeneity (8).

## EGFR testing: which mutations?

Approximately 90% of mutations are either exon 19 short in-frame deletions resulting in the loss of four to six amino acids (E746 to S752) or a single-nucleotide substitution (L858R) in exon 21. The evidence linking these mutations to TKI benefit is extensively documented. Less common point mutations may occur throughout exons 18 to 21, while in-frame duplications and/or insertions occur mostly in exon 20. Response data are accumulating also for these less common mutations and the CAP/IASLC/AMP consensus opinion is that clinical EGFR mutation testing should be able to detect all individual mutations that have been reported with a frequency of at least 1% of EGFR-mutated lung adenocarcinomas (4). Thus, assays for EGFR exon 19 deletions should be designed to detect not just the common 15-bp and 18-bp deletions, but also the less common 9-, 12-, 24- and 27-bp deletions, as well as the uncommon 15-bp and 18-bp insertions (4). EGFR exon 18 should be analyzed for E709 and G719 mutations; exon 20 for S768, T790M

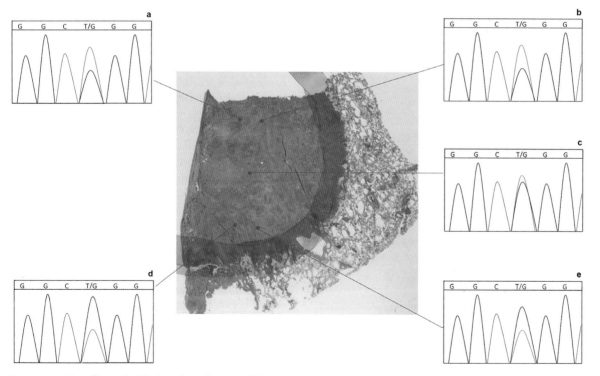

**Figure 16.3 Paraffin-embedded section of resected lung adenocarcinoma harboring the G>T transversion L858R EGFR mutation detected by Sanger sequencing**
The ratios between the mutant (black) and the wild (red) peaks were different depending on the tumor area (a–e) that had been laser microdissected due to EGFR mutant allele-specific imbalance (MASI).

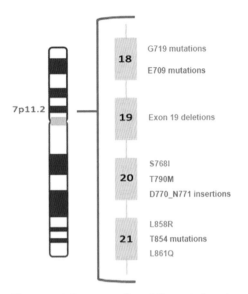

**Figure 16.4 Representation of the mutations in exons 18–21 of the EGFR gene to be detected according to the CAP/IASLC/AMP guidelines**
EGFR mutations in these exons are associated with sensitivity (green) or resistance (red) to EGFR TKI. Assays for EGFR exon 19 deletions should be designed to detect not just the common 15-bp and 18-bp deletions, but also the less common 9-, 12-, 24- and 27-bp deletions, as well as the uncommon 15-bp and 18-bp insertions. EGFR exon 18 should be analyzed for E709 and G719 mutations; exon 20 for S768, T790M and insertions; and exon 21 for L858R, T854 and L861Q mutations.

and insertions; and exon 21 for L858R, T854 and L861Q mutations (Figure 16.4).

## EGFR mutation assays: validation procedures

Any laboratory should validate its EGFR testing strategy, including both laboratory-developed tests and FDA-approved commercial assays, before clinical implementation (4). As an example of the validation process, the steps taken to assess the performance features of the fragment length assay (Figure 16.5) are detailed elsewhere (10). Any different specimen type, including frozen, fresh and fixed (comprising each fixative to be used) samples, should be separately validated. The most important performance characteristics are specificity and sensitivity. True mutations should be distinguished from sequencing artifacts; low amounts of template DNA, as in the case of DNA obtained from microdissected sections, and formalin fixation can cause random polymerase errors in nucleotide incorporation, usually being C-T or G-A transitions (4). DNA treatment with Escherichia coli

uracil N-glycosylase before amplification and genotyping on shorter amplicons may be a way to avoid artifactual mutations.

Validation experiments with no template controls and very-low-concentration wild-type specimens should ensure the analytic specificity of the method and the reliable distinction between true-positive and false-positive results. Mutational artifacts can be distinguished from true mutations by bidirectional sequencing and by confirmatory sequencing of independent PCR products (7). The detection of "novel" mutations is to be considered carefully and should be confirmed by replicate assays on new DNA extracts to rule out art factual mutations due to formalin fixation. The analytic sensitivity is the lowest concentration (or absolute cell count) of tumor cells in which a mutation is detected with 100% precision in replicates repeated both within run and between runs (4). Because of variation in EGFR copy-number, analytical sensitivity should be assessed not only on cell lines, but also on a few clinical specimens evaluating the reproducibility of the whole analytic process, including the pre-analytical assessment of tumor cell percentage and of tumor enrichment (4). The internal quality insurance process should include the continuous monitoring of the percentage of EGFR-positive cases in order to confirm whether the results match those obtained in the larger series. The number of annual EGFR tests considered optimal for guaranteeing the technical sufficiency of a laboratory is arbitrarily set at 50 (6).

Once established, testing quality should be maintained during production. To ensure the reliability of EGFR testing, external quality assessment (EQA) programmes that mirror the daily diagnostic situation have been conducted in North America and in several European countries (4). Usually, proficiency testing is performed by sending a similar sample (set) simultaneously to the participating laboratories. The participants are requested to perform mutational analysis, using their usual method, and to submit results within 10 working days to the organizing body. Because the correct mutation call rate decreases in proportion to the decreasing percentage of tumor cells in a specimen, quality assurance programs should include samples with a low tumor content. To this aim, artificial paraffin blocks consisting of mutation-positive colorectal cancer cells diluted in a background of mutation phase are useful. However, this approach does not take account of test variables

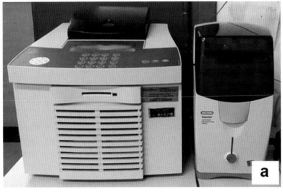

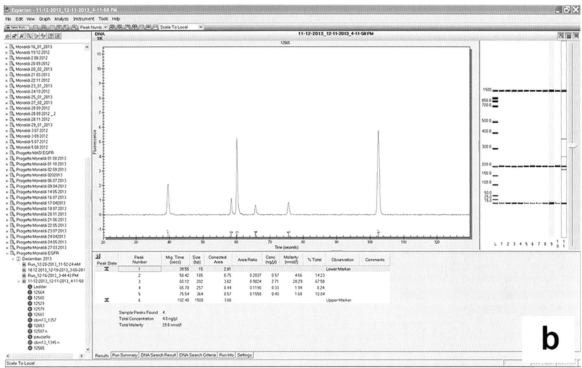

**Figure 16.5 EGFR testing by fragment length analysis**
This method detects the exon 19 alterations easily. The extracted DNA is amplified (a, left). The PCR products are separated by microfluidic technology on a chip, by an Experion electrophoresis instrument (BIORAD, Milan, Italy). The deleted allele generates in the electropherogram an additional peak, which may be detected by the use of dye molecules intercalated into DNA detected by laser-induced fluorescence with high-resolution capacity, avoiding the need for fluorescently labeled primers. The limit of mutant allele detection of this technique is 10%.

linked to the pre-analytical phase, that is, specimen fixation, dehydration, clearing and embedding.

## EGFR mutation assays: method choice

The CAP/IASLC/AMP guidelines do not recommend any individual method(s) to the exclusion of others, but laboratories may use any validated (see section above, entitled "EGFR mutation assays: validation procedures") EGFR testing method with sufficient performance characteristics (4). In practice, laboratories can opt to use commercially available kits or develop their own tests. Testing kits have the advantages of being previously validated, ready for use and quality controlled. Recently, erlotinib has been approved by the FDA for the first-line treatment of patients with EGFR activating mutation-positive NSCLC detected by the approved cobas® EGFR Mutation Test (11). Similarly, the second-generation irreversible EGFR TKI afatinib recently gained FDA approval as first-line therapy for EGFR mutation-positive NSCLC in conjunction with Qiagen's therascreen RGQ polymerase chain reaction (PCR) diagnostic test (11). In Europe, the EMA took a different approach, since the exact mutation methodology was not specified. Consequently, community testing for EGFR was developed in 2009, with many laboratories using different techniques, including laboratory-developed tests. These latter are less expensive than commercially available kits, but take time to develop and validate and may have limited quality control (7).

The Sanger method with fluorescence-tagged dideoxy terminators is the classical reference methodology (7). The analytical sensitivity of this method requires a minimum tumor content of approximately 30%. Surgical resection samples usually fulfill this requirement and in this setting the Sanger method provides good results that are representative of the whole tumor (Figure 16.6). However, even after tumor cell enrichment by macro-dissection, many routine specimens have insufficient tumor cellularity for this analytic sensitivity (7). Thus, laboratories that

exclusively validated this Sanger method would have to reject many specimens as inadequate for testing. Therefore, in addition to the Sanger method, the CAP/IASLC/AMP guidelines suggest to validate a more sensitive technique, which should be able to detect mutations in specimens with as few as 10% cancer cells, to be employed when the tumor content of the tested sample is scant (4).

Conversely, the use of ultrasensitive molecular assays based on a mutated allele-enriching strategy, such as locked nucleic acid or peptide nucleic acid clamps, co-amplification at lower denaturation temperature PCR, or enzymatic digestion of wild-type sequences, which are able to detect mutations in specimens with less than 1% of cancer cells, is controversial (12). They may be useful either for clinical samples containing an extremely low proportion of tumor cells or as a tool to overcome the need of tumor cell enrichment; however, the risk of possibly artifactual mutations is high and the detection of a very small mutated subclone has uncertain clinical significance with regard to predicting response to targeted therapy (12).

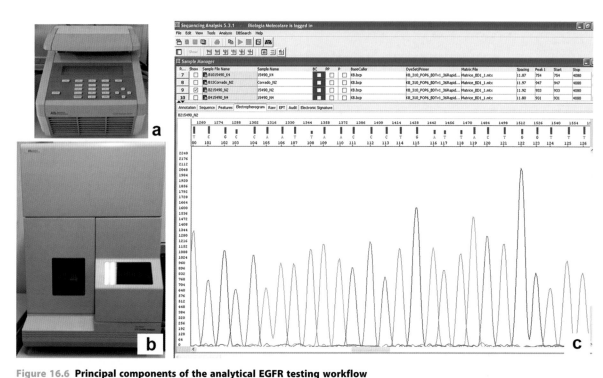

**Figure 16.6 Principal components of the analytical EGFR testing workflow**
In high cellular samples (>30% neoplastic cells), the extracted DNA is amplified (a) and the PCR products are direct sequenced (b). The sequencing electropherogram is then aligned and visually analyzed on a dedicated software (c). This latter offers the advantage of detecting all mutations, but is time-consuming and it has low sensitivity.

In this context, next generation sequencing (NGS) technologies, also known as massive parallel sequencing since they allow the parallel analysis of a very large number of DNA molecules, are significantly advancing molecular diagnostics by enabling the design of highly multiplexed assays (13). Reports on the use of NGS for the analysis of lung carcinoma cytological samples are still very few, but results are very encouraging. Remarkably, Buttitta *et al.* have shown that in principle NGS can identify EGFR mutated alleles in bronchoalveolar lavages and in the pleural fluid of samples where tumor cells were very few or even altogether absent after microscopic evaluation (14).

## EGFR mutational assays and time around testing

The time around testing (TAT) of EGFR mutational analysis has relevant clinical implications. The test is required for patients with stage IV lung cancer either at the time of diagnosis for patients presenting with advanced-stage disease or at the time of recurrence or progression in patients who originally presented with lower-stage disease, but were not previously tested (4). Since EGFR wild-type tumors respond better to conventional chemotherapy than to EGFR TKI, oncologists cannot administer EGFR TKI as first-line therapy without evidence of a sensitizing EGFR mutation (1). On the other hand, patients with EGFR mutations show superior outcomes when the targeted TKI therapies are administered as first-line agents (4). The CAP/IASLC/AMP guidelines encourage trying to incorporate EGFR screening into routine patient management, with a testing TAT of five days, but strongly recommend that EGFR results should be available within two weeks (ten working days) of receiving the specimen in the testing laboratory. In fact, a longer time may lead to administration of TKIs as second-line agents, which is less efficient. Laboratories may consider offering two assays: a rapid assay for the most common mutations, which can be reported within five days, and a more comprehensive follow-up assay to detect the remaining mutations, which may take ten days to report.

The CAP/IASLC/AMP guidelines also suggest laboratory departments to establish processes to ensure that specimens that have a final histopathologic diagnosis are sent to outside molecular pathology laboratories within three working days of receiving requests and to intramural molecular pathology laboratories within 24 hours (4). The presence within the molecular pathology laboratory of both a pathologist, who is highly trained in selecting the best specimen while considering the specific methods used by that particular laboratory, and a dedicated technician may allow expeditious histological processing of samples for molecular testing (5). Pathology departments may also consider the cost-effectiveness of a testing policy based on the reflex (upfront) testing of specimens in early-stage disease, regardless of a specific clinician's request. In fact, despite treatment during early stage, a large percentage of these patients will nevertheless have relapse, with disease progressing to an advanced stage, and they will eventually require molecular testing. Reflex testing may also not be practical, in terms of laboratory resourcing or for reimbursement reasons. However, the "upfront" procedure can enable the use of EGFR status as a prognostic factor and to select early-stage patients for TKI adjuvant therapy. Several studies are investigating the use of first-generation EGFR TKIs as adjuvant therapy in early-stage lung cancers, including the RADIANT and SELECT trials.

## EGFR mutation testing is feasible on cytology

As recently as 2009, a consensus statement from the European Epidermal Growth Factor Receptor (EGFR) Workshop Group recommended the performance of mutation testing on tissue biopsy samples rather than on cytological specimens (15). Since then, investigation was intensively carried out to eliminate the diffuse perception that cytological material was only sufficient to provide a generic diagnosis of non-small cell lung carcinoma (NSCLC). To this end, retrospective studies were designed to test EGFR mutation on a sizeable number of parallel cytological and histological samples obtained from the same patients (Table 16.5). The degree of concordance between cyto and histo was very high but not absolute, ranging between 91.6% and 100%. Even more recently, several institutions reported their prospective clinical experiences on routinely collected cytological specimens. In general, the methodologies were sufficiently robust to test satisfactorily most of the routine cases; even limited cytological materials yielding extremely small amounts of DNA were reliably tested. Different techniques, including direct sequencing and real-time PCR (RT-PCR) based methods, applied to different sample types, including exfoliative and aspirative samples, and preparations, such as direct smears, cell blocks (CB) and monolayer preparations, yielded data

Table 16.5 Summary of studies that analyzed EGFR mutational status in paired histological and cytological samples

| First author (ref) | Type of cytological sample | Paired samples (n=) | EGFR detection methods | Concordant/total(%) |
|---|---|---|---|---|
| Lozano (16) | Direct smears | 20 | Direct sequencing | 100% |
| Bozzetti (17) | Direct smears or needle washing | 9 | Direct sequencing | 100% |
| Bruno (18) | Direct smears | 50 | Direct sequencing | 100% |
| Chowdhuri (19) | Cell block | 12 | LCM and direct sequencing or pyrosequencing | 100% |
| Goto (20) | Cell pellet from bronchial brushing | 30 | PNA-LNA PCR clamp or ARMS-Scorpion | 96.6%[i] |
| Mitiushkina (21) | Direct smears | 72 | Exon 19 fragment length assay Exon 21 allele-specific real-time | 68/72 94.4% |
| Sun (22) | Direct smears and/or cell blocks | 60 | Pyrosequencing | 55/60 91.7%[ii] |
| Khode (23) | Direct smears from the same site of the histology | 37 | Pyrosequencing | 36/37 97% |
| Khode (23) | Direct smears from a different site | 23 | Pyrosequencing | 19/23 82% |

Notes:
(i) 29/30 cases were evaluated; one test failure in histology sample.
(ii) Discordant cases included two sputum specimens and three pleural effusions.

comparable to those obtained on larger tumor biopsies in terms of frequency and distribution of EGFR mutations according to sex, histology and prior smoking history. In 2013, the international guidelines for lung cancer biomarker testing issued by CAP/IASLC/AMP considered cytological samples suitable for EGFR testing (4). The key point is that the essential information should be shared among histopathologists, cytologists and molecular pathologists. This improves the precision of the diagnosis and avoids a waste of material for redundant molecular analyses.

### EGFR mutation testing and cytological preparations

Different cytopreparation types, such as direct smears, cell blocks and liquid-based cytology samples, have advantages and drawbacks (Table 16.6) (7). Due to the lack of legal regulation, the primary cytopathologist is often reluctant "to sacrifice" the morphology of malignant cells for DNA extraction and the smear sent to the centralized laboratories is not always the "good one" and is often paucicellular (9). Laser capture microdissection (LCM) enables selective cancer cell dissection (Figure 16.7). Only 25 cancer cells are needed to yield adequate DNA to reliably detect EGFR mutations and our recent data showed that EGFR mutations detected on a paucicellular smear by a centralized laboratory can predict TKI treatment response as equally well as mutations identified on histology samples (9). However, LCM requires specific training and it is very time-consuming. In the near future, computer-aided LCM will semi-automate the microdissection process, allowing a more rapid retrieval of tumor cells, saving the pathologist's time and effort. The DNA obtained from stained smears is of better quality than that extracted from cell blocks. However, cell blocks are valuable when the aspirated material, clotted after the prolonged echo-endoscopic bronchial (EBUS) or digestive (EUS) procedures, cannot be smeared. When the cytopathologist or cytotechnologist cannot provide ROSE of sample

Table 16.6 Advantages and disadvantages of different cytopreparations for EGFR mutation testing

|  | Direct smears | Cell blocks | Liquid-based cytology |
|---|---|---|---|
| Advantages | High-quality DNA<br>Selection of malignant cells<br>ROSE | Diagnostic smears preserved<br>TTF1 positive cells can be selected<br>Guidelines recommended<br>Useful for EBUS and EUS | High-quality DNA<br>Eliminates the need for slide preparation by clinicians<br>Material maximized<br>Fast method on CytoLyt derived DNA |
| Disadvantages | Delay due to coverslip removal<br>LCM may be needed<br>Lack of regulation | Poor DNA quality<br>ROSE unfeasible | ROSE unfeasible |

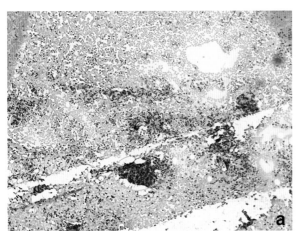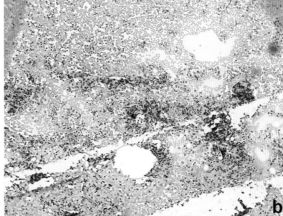

Figure 16.7 NSCLC Papanicolaou-stained smear containing few neoplastic groups whose manual selection was difficult due to the rich inflammatory background (a). Laser-capture microdissection enables the selective removal of the neoplastic cells for DNA extraction and molecular testing (b, yellow circle).

adequacy, liquid-based cytology makes the processing of material easier and eliminates the need for slide preparation by clinicians (24).

Malignant pleural effusion (MPE) is a frequent complication of advanced lung adenocarcinoma, growing at the periphery of the lung and invading the pleural cavity. The release of tumor-derived DNA into the pleural fluid through the apoptosis or necrosis of disseminated tumor cells makes MPE an easily reached source of material, as mutations can be detected in soluble DNA (7). However, since the composition of MPE includes normal, inflammatory and reactive mesothelial cells, highly sensitive molecular methods, including next generation sequencing (NGS), may be needed (14).

## EGFR mutational assays by immunohistochemistry

Immunohistochemistry (IHC) evaluation of total EGFR expression may only predict response to cetuximab (Merck Serono, Darmstadt, Germany). High EGFR expression (score of 200 or more) using the Dako pharmDx Kit (Glostrup, Denmark) correlated with increased overall survival for patients with advanced NSCLC who were receiving first-line platinum-based chemotherapy plus cetuximab, compared to chemotherapy alone, for lung squamous cell carcinomas and adenocarcinomas (4).

Conversely, EGFR total IHC does not correlate with the presence of EGFR mutations and does not carry reliable predictive information relative to the TKI treatment response (4). Instead, commercially

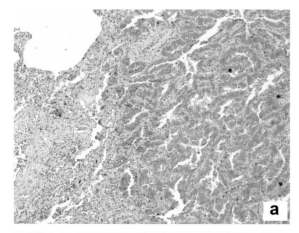

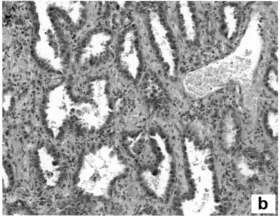

Figure 16.8 Paraffin-embedded section of two cases of resected lung adenocarcinoma harboring the E746_A750del (a) and the L858R (b) EGFR gene alterations detected by commercially available mutation-specific rabbit monoclonal antibodies. Both cases showed intense (score 3+) staining. The IHC evidences were confirmed by molecular evidences of EGFR mutation.

available mutation-specific rabbit monoclonal antibody raised against the most common mutated forms of EGFR, namely, the 15-bp/5-amino-acid deletion (E746_A750del) in exon 19 and the L858R point mutation in exon 21, are promising tools for a simple, rapid and inexpensive detection of EGFR mutation (Figure 16.8). Mutant antibodies have high specificity with elevated positive predictive value; in fact, the cases showing intense (3+) mutant antibody staining always have molecular evidence of EGFR mutation. However, the sensitivity of mutated EGFR mutant IHC is low, as each EGFR mutant antibody only targets a single specific mutation. For example, the 6B6 clone strongly reacts to EGFR proteins carrying the E746_A750del, whereas the immunoreaction is

variable or absent in tumors affected by the less common 9-, 12-, 18-24- and 27-bp deletions. Thus, in routine practice, the only useful application of these antibodies is reserved to those cases that, featuring an extremely low number or proportion of tumor cells, are not suitable for DNA-based molecular analysis. For example, in malignant effusions and in CNS liquor specimens, the EGFR mutant antibodies detected *in situ* EGFR mutations even with a few neoplastic cells. The mutant antibodies represent an attractive research tool useful to provide information on the relationship between the level of mutant protein, which is influenced by the MASI phenomenon, and the response to treatment.

## Primary and acquired resistance to EGFR TKI

Most (70%) of the patients harboring sensitizing EGFR mutations have significant clinical and radiographic responses to TKIs. However, almost all patients relapse or progress, a phenomenon termed "acquired resistance" (AR). The most common mechanism is the emergence of a subclone of resistant cells carrying a secondary EGFR TK domain mutation. The most frequent (50%) of these resistance mutations is the T790M, which occurs in cis on the same allele as the original activating mutations and increases the affinity of the receptor for ATP, thereby reducing the TKI activity. While sensitizing EGFR mutations are present in every tumor cell, the clone carrying the T790M mutation is being selected under the TKI administration pressure and progressively expands. To reliably detect the T790M, the CAP/IASLC/AMP guidelines suggest implementing mutational assays sensitive enough to detect 5% of mutant cells. Interestingly, sensitive molecular assays detected pre-treatment the T790M mutation in the 2% to 4% in TKI-naive tumors when this mutation co-existed with a sensiziting mutation. Patients carrying pre-treatment T790M mutation have a shorter EGFR TKIs response and a shorter PFS. Interestingly, recently, it was suggested that the drug-sensitive and drug-resistant EGFR-T790M mutant cells show a slower growth. Other "secondary" resistance mutations include the much rarer L747S, D761Y and T854A mutations.

Second-generation EGFR TKIs are being intensively evaluated as further lines of treatment when AR resistance onsets. Afatinib (BIBW2992; Boehringer Ingelheim, Ingelheim, Germany) is a second-generation TKI, which irreversibly binds with a higher affinity to

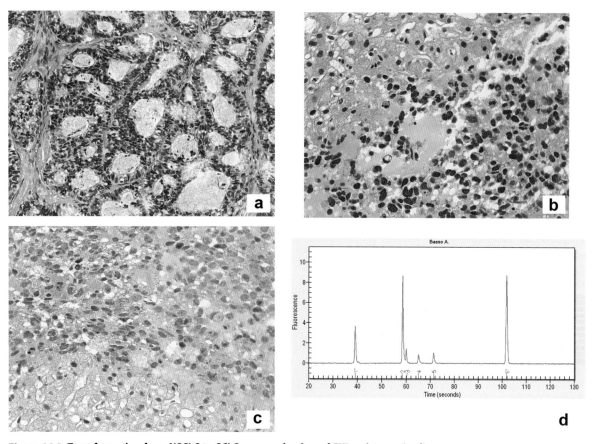

**Figure 16.9 Transformation from NSCLC to SCLC as a mechanism of TKI resistance (a–d)**
Advanced-stage lung adenocarcinoma (a, 20x) harboring EGFR exon 19 deletion. The tumor responded to TKI administration. After nine months, the disease progressed with multiple liver metastasis. These latter were core-biopsied and the histology revealed a typical small cell carcinoma morphology (b, 20x), also confirmed by positivity for neuroendocrine markers (c, Synaptophysin, 20x). In d, the fragment length assay documenting the persistence of the exon 19 deletion in the progressive disease is shown.

EGFR, even when the T790M occurs (11). Clinical evidence suggests that, in contrast to chemotherapy, anti-EGFR drugs should not be discontinued when a patient with a previously responsive EGFR tumor shows signs of progression. However, serial biopsies revealed that genetic mechanisms of resistance were lost in the absence of the continued selective pressure of EGFR inhibitor treatment, and such cancers were sensitive to a second round of treatment with EGFR inhibitors (11).

A less common mechanism of EGFR TKI resistance is the amplification of another receptor tyrosine kinase. MET amplification, which drives the ERBB3-dependent activation of the PI3K pathway, has been shown in up to 20% of AR cases with or without T790M mutations. The presence of minor clones of MET-amplified cells in TKI tumors has also been

shown. More recently, PTEN loss and ERBB2 amplification have also been linked with acquired resistance to EGFR TKIs. Histological transformation from NSCLC to SCLC at the time of TKI resistance may also occur. In these cases, the original EGFR mutation is maintained and when the pre- and post-treatment tissues are subjected to neuroendocrine immunohistochemical analyses, including staining for synaptophysin and chromogranin, only the post-treatment specimens are positive for neuroendocrine markers (Figure 16.9) (4).

## EML4-ALK testing

The identification of the gene rearrangements involving the ALK gene in lung adenocarcinoma first came through a screen for transforming cDNAs; these were

263

isolated from a tumor occurring in a 62-year-old Japanese male with a low smoking history and with EGFR and KRAS wild-type status (2). The rearrangement involved a pericentric inversion on the short arm of chromosome 2, which created a fusion gene encoding the amino-terminal portion of echinoderm microtubule-associated protein-like 4 (EML4) and the intracellular juxtamembrane region of ALK. This rearrangement had transforming potential, inducing tumor in the nude mice (2).

The EML4-ALK fusion is present in approximately 3% to 6% of adenocarcinomas, depending on the population studied and the detection methods used (2); over ten EML4-ALK variants have been identified in lung cancer, as well as other fusion partners such as TFG and KIF5B. All variants are highly sensitive to treatment by the oral ALK inhibitor crizotinib (Xalkori; Pfizer, New York, New York). (2) In addition to ALK, crizotinib inhibits ROS1, MET and RON. The treatment by crizotinib gave a response rate of around 60% and progression-free survival of around ten months, leading to accelerated approval by the FDA in August 2011 (2). Crizotinib is well tolerated, and treatment-related adverse events such as nausea, vision disorder, vomiting and diarrhea are limited. A proportion of ALK-positive patients with NSCLC (in most studies <10%) have intrinsic resistance to crizotinib treatment, while mechanisms of acquired resistance include ALK kinase domain mutations (2).

### The CAP/IASLC/AMP guidelines for ALK testing

Currently, several methods are available to identify ALK rearrangements, including IHC with different ALK-specific antibodies, quantitative real-time polymerase chain reaction (qRT-PCR) and fluorescent in situ hybridization (FISH). Molecular testing is necessary to determine ALK status and the CAP/IASLC/AMP guidelines are very similar to those issued for EGFR testing (4). Briefly, patient selection cannot be based on associated clinical characteristics; the never/light smoking history and the younger age are not shared by all carriers, who are occasionally older patients with a smoking history. Similarly, associated histological features that include solid signet-ring cell and mucinous cribriform patterns are not exclusive and any histological subtypes of adenocarcinoma can carry ALK re-arrangements (4). ALK fusions are very infrequent in squamous cell carcinomas and testing is

not recommended in lung cancers that lack any adenocarcinoma component. To determine EGFR and ALK status for initial treatment selection, primary tumors or metastatic lesions are equally suitable for testing. Reflex ALK testing of tumors at diagnosis from patients presenting with stage I, II or III disease is encouraged, but the decision to do so should be made locally by each laboratory, in collaboration with its oncology team (4).

### ALK testing by fluorescence *in situ* hybridization (FISH)

ALK testing can be carried out by in-house-developed FISH tests. These are cheap, but require extensive and rigorous validation before clinical implementation; as a matter of fact, most health centers have adopted the FDA-approved commercial break-apart kit (Abbott Molecular Probes, Abbott Park, Illinois), used as a "companion diagnostic" in clinical trials of crizotinib (4). Hybridization is carried out by a probe set including a SpectrumOrange-labeled on the telomeric 3' side of ALK and a SpectrumGreen-labeled on the centromeric 5' side. The wild-type status appears as a fused yellow signal, as both probes on the ALK gene (red and green) are close together, generating a fusion signal. Conversely, ALK rearrangement generates distinct and separated orange and green signals. However, these two split signals are still closely "paired" within the same chromosome and their correct interpretation is difficult (Figure 16.10) (2). Cells are considered ALK FISH positive when at least one set of red and green signals has a distance between the signal borders of ≥2 diameters of the largest of the two signals. A single red signal without a corresponding green signal is due to small deletions of 5' end of the ALK gene (2). Conversely, a single green signal without a corresponding red signal is considered negative. Similarly, an increased copy-number of non-rearranged ALK genes with fused signals corresponds to polysomy of chromosome 2 or ALK amplification is negative for rearrangement (2).

In clinical practice, a total of 50 nuclei should be scored selecting those with sufficient hybridization quality, in a consecutive manner, and with the microscope focus adjusted to each nucleus in order to correctly identify all of the signals present in the nucleus of the cells. A sample is considered negative if fewer than five cells (<10%) are positive and positive if more than 25 cells (>50%) are positive (4). A sample is considered equivocal if 5 to 25 cells

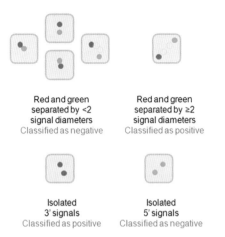

Red and green
separated by <2
signal diameters
Classified as negative

Red and green
separated by ≥2
signal diameters
Classified as positive

Isolated
3' signals
Classified as positive

Isolated
5' signals
Classified as negative

**Figure 16.10** Signal patterns in NSCLC nuclei hybridized with ALK break-apart FISH.

(10% to 50%) are positive. In this case, a second reader should evaluate the slide. If the average of the two readings contains at least 15% positive cells, the sample is considered ALK FISH positive. It is noteworthy that this interpretation algorithm is only designed and validated for histopathological use on intact formalin-fixed paraffin-embedded (FFPE) tissue biopsies or resection specimens. If cytological material is to be used, laboratories must take further steps to validate their testing methodology.

Special care is required to interpret the results and to avoid false-negative and positive results; a marked "background noise" is frequent in the adjacent non-tumor area, whereas not all cells within a positive tumor display the positive signal patterns for an ALK rearrangement (2). This heterogeneity is apparent more than real and due to technique rather than biology (25). To ensure reliable scoring, the number of fields to count should be in excess of four. Thus, a dedicated pathologist should perform the analysis him- or herself; alternatively, the pathologist could supervise other persons, who should be well trained and experienced in histo- and cytomorphology. In any case, the pathologist keeps the responsibility to validate, review and sign off the interpretation (2).

## ALK testing by qRT-PCR

As stated by CAP/IASLC/AMP guidelines, the RT-PCR is not a recommended alternative to FISH for selecting patients for ALK inhibitor therapy (4). Although in some instances qRT-PCR is very sensitive in defining both ALK fusion partner and fusion variants, this RNA-based assay method has a high failure rate in routine FFPE pathology material and carries the not negligible risk of false-negative results, owing to variability in the EML4-ALK fusion structure and the existence of other ALK fusion partners (2). To date, there have been at least 13 molecular variants of EML4-ALK reported, representing chimeric transcripts fusing EML4 exons 2, 6, 13, 14, 15, 17, 18 or 20 to ALK exon 20 or immediately upstream within intron 19 of ALK (2). Fusion of ALK to TFG and KIF5B has rarely been reported, and the possibility that other variant fusions occur cannot be ruled out. To overcome the RT-PCR limit, it would be necessary to design multi-targeted RT-PCR assays or to employ multiple pairs of primers in separate or sequential reactions to analyze the different EML4-ALK variants. However, this is technically complex, requiring a large amount of RNA, which is not always available (4).

## ALK testing by IHC

IHC-mediated identification of lung adenocarcinomas with over-expression of ALK may be a more robust, simpler, quicker and cheaper alternative to FISH-based identification of ALK rearrangements, offering the advantage of directly assessing the crizotinib protein target. However, suboptimal fixation may lead to false-negative results and be a source of intra-sample staining heterogeneity (2). Moreover, since the protein concentrations in ALK rearranged NSCLC are relatively low, standard detection methodology, as used in the identification of ALK rearranged anaplastic lymphomas, is inadequate and detection systems with a substantial degree of signal amplification, such as Novolink, (Leica/Novocastra), Advance (Dako) or Ventana i-view are required (2). The choice of antibody is also important. Currently, there are three primary antibodies commonly referred to in the published literature: ALK1 (Dako), clone 5A4 (Novocastra, Leica, but also available pre-diluted from Abcam) and D5F3 (Cell Signalling Technology) (2). The use of the two latter antibodies has resulted in both a very high negative predictive value (all IHC-negative cases are also FISH-negative) and high positive predictive values (90% to 100%

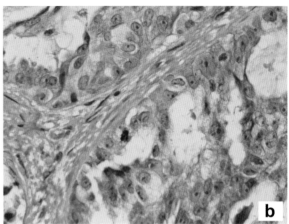

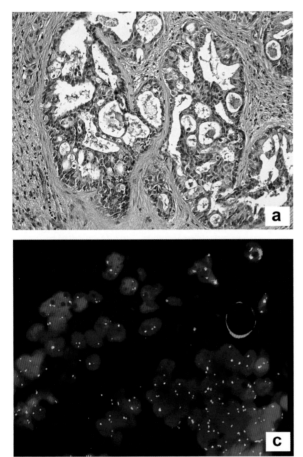

**Figure 16.11** Paraffin-embedded section of resected lung adenocarcinoma showing association between the ALK gene fusion and a specific morphology. Note in (a) the ADC cribiform pattern showing a diffuse, granular cytoplasmic positivity for anti-ALK D5F3 clone (b). The ALK rearrangement was confirmed by FISH (c).

probability of being FISH positive when IHC is strongly positive).

There is no clear consensus on how to score ALK IHC staining (2, 4). In NSCLC, ALK-rearranged staining pattern is cytoplasmic (Figure 16.11). It may have a granular character, and in some cases there may be membrane accentuation. The use of successive microscope objectives with related spatial resolutions as a physical aid in establishing intensity may lead to more uniformity in intensity scoring. Strong staining (3+) is clearly visible using a ×2 or ×4 objective, moderate staining (2+) requires a ×10 or ×20 objective to be clearly seen, while weak staining (1+) cannot be seen until a ×40 objective is used. Recent evidences suggest that in the near future (3+) staining will not require FISH confirmation (2).

## Emerging molecular markers in adenocarcinoma

In lung adenocarcinomas, besides EGFR and ALK, there are multiple other potentially actionable targets with corresponding predictive biomarkers (Table 16.2). The main genes with known or potential "driver" mutation status currently include HER2, ROS1, MET, RET, MEK1 and BRAF (11). Together with EGFR and ALK, these mutations account for around 20% of NSCLCs (11). Most of the key "driver" mutations in NSCLC have thus far been found in genes encoding signaling proteins, such as protein kinases. By transferring phosphate groups from ATP to specific target proteins, these signaling proteins are critical regulators of cellular proliferation and survival. The identification of these oncogenic drivers has led to the design of rationally targeted therapies that have produced superior clinical outcomes in tumors harboring these mutations. "Driver" mutations are also found in GTPases, such as the RAS oncogenes, which are intracellular enzymes that typically function downstream from protein kinases to propagate cell growth, proliferation and survival signals. However, the RAS oncogenes (KRAS and NRAS) are not actionable yet, as we are not aware of any molecules in clinical development that directly inhibit RAS (11).

## HER2

The epidermal growth factor receptor 2 (HER2/neu) does not have any known specific ligand and it is activated by forming heterodimers with other EGFR family members, preferentially with either EGFR or HER3. HER2/neu mutations are rare (18). They occur in approximately 2% to 4% of lung ADCs of never-smoking women with predominant lepidic pattern, nearly always being mutually exclusive with EGFR and KRAS mutation. Usually, the genetic alteration is a 12-bp insertion causing duplication of amino acids YVMA at codon 775 in exon 20 (26). Recent data suggested the potential efficacy of HER2-targeted drugs in the mutant population and routine clinical genotyping of lung ADC will soon include HER2. However, no association between HER2 mutation and HER2 overexpression was shown and whether patients with these mutations truly benefit from anti-HER2 strategies remains to be demonstrated. It is noteworthy that HER2 amplification was identified as a mechanism of acquired resistance to EGFR-TKI therapy. NSCLC patients with HER2 amplification and activating EGFR mutation may respond better to afatinib, which inhibits both HER2 and EGFR activities.

## ROS1

ROS1 is an insulin receptor family TK whose ligands have not been identified. Chromosomal rearrangements involving the ROS1 and the immediately adjacent FIG genes were first reported in glioblastomas. However, in lung adenocarcinoma, the ROS1 fusion partners may include several other genes; in all fusion events the ROS1 kinase domain is retained and overexpressed and ROS1 alteration is mutually exclusive with EGFR, KRAS and ALK (27). The frequency of ROS1-translocated ADC is 2% and their clinical and histological features are similar to those of ALK-rearranged adenocarcinoma (27). They occur in young never-smoker patients with a microscopic solid growth pattern, with mucinous/cribriform features and psammomatous calcification. Similary to ALK-rearranged adenocarcinoma, tumors harboring ROS1 rearrangements respond to the multi-targeted small molecule tyrosine kinase inhibitor crizotinib, whose approval for treatment of ROS1+ adenocarcinomas is generally expected in the not-too-distant future. The methodology to detect ROS1 fusion events includes several commercially available break-apart FISH kits. In addition, IHC screening for ROS1 translocation has promising performance data, including 100% sensitivity and 92% specificity (27).

## MET

The mesenchymal-epidermal transition (MET) receptor tyrosine kinase has a central role in the cancer cell's survival. This kinase is also called hepatocyte growth factor receptor, because it binds with high affinity to the ligand hepatocyte growth factor (HGF) (11). Dysregulation of the MET/HGF pathway can occur via several mechanisms such as MET and HGF overexpression, MET gene amplification or mutation. MET amplification occurs in 3% of cases and has a negative prognostic significance. In up to 20% of EGFR mutant tumors with acquired resistance to EGFR, MET amplification has emerged as one of the critical events. Few data are available on the role of MET mutations. They may be rare and their significance is unknown. MET has been shown to be inhibited by the small molecule tyrosine kinase inhibitor crizotinib and there are pre-clinical evidences that crizotinib can be used in the treatment of HGF-induced resistance to gefitinib in EGFR mutant lung cancer. Several HGF and MET inhibitors are in clinical development, including small molecule MET inhibitors (for example, cabozantinib), antagonistic antibodies against MET (for example, onartuzumab) and neutralizing antibodies against HGF (for example, rilotumumab). IHC staining of more than 50% of tumor cells by the Ventana CONFIRM anti-Total c-MET [SP44] rabbit monoclonal antibody is predictive of response to onartuzumab (MetMAb) (11).

## RET

Activating fusions involving the RET receptor tyrosine kinase were first reported in lung adenocarcinoma in 2012. In lung cancer, RET fusions are detected collectively in approximately 1% of NSCLCs. 5′-fusion partners include NCOA4, CCDC6 and KIF5B. Clinical characteristics associated with

RET fusions include never-smoking status, adenocarcinoma histology with a mucinous cribriform pattern and younger age at diagnosis. Importantly, such mutations are rarely, if ever, found in tumors that harbor mutations in other drivers, that is EGFR, KRAS, HER2 and ALK.

Pre-clinical studies have suggested that lung cancers harboring RET fusions should be sensitive to inhibition with RET TKIs, including sunitinib, sorafenib and vandetanib. In particular, vandetanib inhibits both RET and EGFR. In a recent report, a patient with RET-fusion-positive lung adenocarcinoma responded to vandetanib with decrease in tumor size after one week of treatment. Although data are available only for a single patient, the identification of a RET-fusion-positive lung adenocarcinoma patient with response on vandetanib treatment suggests that RET fusions indeed represent another clinically actionable driver mutation in lung cancer. Recently, it was shown that it is possibile to use RNA purified from cytological specimens to detect the RET/KIF5B gene fusion by the MassARRAY Analyzer (Sequenom Inc, San Diego, California) – an innovative technology that uses mass spectrometry to determine the sequence of rearranged genes (28).

## MEK1

MEK1 (also known as MAPK1) is a serine-threonine kinase that has an important function as a downstream target of RAS activation. MEK1 activates MAPK2 and MAPK3 downstream of BRAF (14). Rare cases of somatic mutations of MEK1 have been reported in NSCLC with 2 of 107 lung ADC found to have an activating mutation in exon 2 that did not involve the kinase domain. The mutations were exclusive of other driver mutations and were associated with gain of function *in vitro* (11).

## BRAF

BRAF is a crucial component of the Ras/mitogen-activated protein kinase (MAPK) signaling pathway; BRAF is downstream of KRAS, and directly phosphorylates MEK, which in turn phosphorylates ERK. The pathway culminates in the transcription of genes that favor proliferation and survival. The most common BRAF mutation known in lung adenocarcinoma is a valine to glutamate substitution at codon 600 (V600E). BRAF mutations are found in approximately 4% of lung adenocarcinomas (29). BRAF mutations are also mutually exclusive of EGFR, KRAS and EML4/ALK,

and are found in a relatively high proportion of smokers (29). BRAF inhibitors as vemurafenib or dabrafenib are clinically superior to conventional chemotherapy. The onset of the KRAS G12D mutation, not present in the pre-treatment tumor biopsy, is a mechanism of resistance to vemurafenib or to dabrafenib and of disease progression. V600E-mutated tumors may display an aggressive histotype characterized by micropapillary features in 80% of patients and it is significantly associated with the female sex, representing a negative prognostic factor (29). The non-V600E mutations lack prognostic significance. The usefulness of immunohistochemistry (IHC) as a new approach for the detection of BRAF V600E in cancer patients has been recently reported.

## KRAS

KRAS mutation is the most common molecular change in NSCLC, occurring in approximately 30% of ADC, 5% of SQCC and 8% of adenosquamous carcinoma. In lung adenocarcinomas, KRAS mutations mostly occur in patients with a history of tobacco smoking. KRAS mutations often associate with mucinous and intestinal-like (CDX2+, TTF1-) tumor differentiation (Figure 16.12). Most mutations are codon 12 TGT and GTT transversions. Similarly to EGFR alterations, KRAS mutations are also early events that drive tumorigenesis; thus, intratumoral heterogeneity of KRAS mutation is a rare event and primary and corresponding metastases share the same mutational status.

At this time, testing for KRAS mutation does not add any clinically useful information and the only cost-effective application is to test for KRAS mutation as a first-line "screening" as a strong negative predictor for identifying an additional aberration in either EGFR or ALK. No approved therapeutic agents are available that target KRAS. The data linking KRAS to the response to platinum-based adjuvant chemotherapy are uncertain and the same holds for KRAS prognostic significance, as evidence associating the mutation with a more aggressive clinical course is not consistent. When a KRAS mutation is identified by direct sequencing, both mutant and wild-type alleles are seen on the sequencing electropherograms (30). In some instances, even if the tumor has not been microdissected, the mutant allele may appear to be in great excess of the wild-type allele. The mutant allele may become dominant when deletion of the wild-type allele and/or chromosome hyperploidy or

268

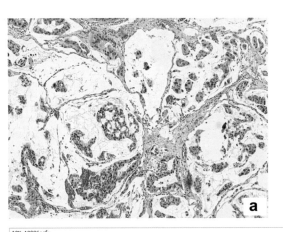

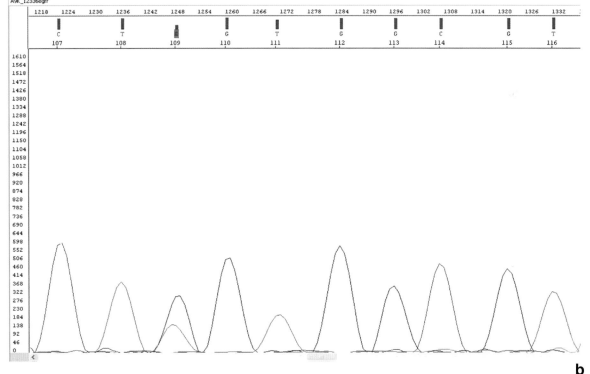

Figure 16.12 Paraffin-embedded section of resected lung adenocarcinoma showing association between the KRAS gene mutation and a specific morphology. Lung adenocarcinoma with mucinous features (a) harboring G12C KRAS mutation (b).

KRAS amplification leads to mutant allele-specific imbalance (MASI) (30). KRAS MASI correlates with a worse overall survival (OS) rate (30).

The Ras/RAF/MEK/ERK pathway is frequently deregulated in cancer; the approval of inhibitors that target this pathway downstream of RAS will make KRAS mutational analysis increasingly important. Selumetinib is an oral inhibitor of mitogen-activated protein kinase kinases (MEK) 1 and 2, which is particularly active in tumors with KRAS mutation. Preliminary data showed that in patients with advanced KRAS-mutant NSCLC, combining selumetinib with docetaxel may improve progression-free survival. A small but distinct subset of lung cancers (approximately 1%) harbor NRAS mutations. Pre-clinical models, including NRAS-mutant lung cancer cell lines, suggest that MEK inhibitors, such as selumetinib and trametinib, may be active against these tumors. Although NRAS mutations are more common in current/former smokers, the smoking-related G:C > T:A transversions are significantly less frequent in NRAS-mutated lung tumors than KRAS-mutant non-small cell lung cancer (31).

## Molecular testing in non-adenocarcinoma
### Squamous cell carcinoma

The recognition of squamous differentiation in NSCLC is crucial. Cytotoxic agents such as gemcitabine and taxanes have a better performance in SQCC than in ADC. On the other hand, the anti-angiogenic bevacizumab is potentially harmful in SQCC. While a significant proportion of patients affected by lung ADC may benefit from tailored therapy, drugs that specifically target molecular mechanisms of SQCC are not yet in clinical use. In the near future, however, thanks to recent studies that are unraveling the genetics of SQCC, new effective therapeutic targets will be available.

The PI3K signal transduction pathway is central to cell survival, metabolism, motility and angiogenesis. Significant alterations involving the PI3K pathway were identified in 47% of SQCCs by the Cancer Genome Atlas project. Pathway activation in lung carcinogenesis occurs through a variety of mechanisms, including activating mutations in PI3KCA or AKT1, as well as PIK3CA amplification, or loss of negative regulation by the tumor suppressor gene PTEN. These pathway alterations are more common in SQCC than in ADCs. PIK3CA mutations occurring in exons 9 and 20 range from 3% to 6% of SQCLCs, whereas PIK3CA amplification was observed in about 40% of SQCLC patients of Asian ethnicity. AKT1 mutation, resulting in its constitutive activation, has been reported in up to 7% of SQCC, but it has not yet been described in ADC. The PTEN activity, which negatively regulates the PI3K-AKT-mTOR pathway, may be lost by methylation and/or mutation. Low levels of PTEN expression by IHC are frequent (24%), in part due to gene methylation silencing. Furthermore, the PTEN mutation rate of 10.2% is not negligible in SQCC. Inhibitors of the PI3K pathway may represent potential treatment agents.

The discoidin domain receptor (DDR) is a TK that regulates cell adhesion, proliferation and extracellular remodeling. DDR mutations occuring in 3.2% of

SQCC may represent a useful biomarker for treatment with dasatinib, a multikinase inhibitor; other DDR2 inhibitors include nilotinib and imatinib.

The transmembrane tyrosine kinase fibroblast growth factor receptor (FGFR) is amplified in up to 20% of SQCC. Its selective inhibitors (AZD4547, BGJ398) are currently tested in clinical trials, following the evidence of tumor regression in mouse xenograft models. Amplification and over-expression of SOX2 may occur in SQCC, but, unfortunately, SOX2 amplification is not currently targetable. Interestingly, SOX2 drives the expression of differentation squamous cell markers such as p63.

Besides mutations of driver oncogenes, genetic alteration may influence the response of individual patients to chemotherapeutic drug treatment. For example, the regulation of the cellular abundance of the cytoprotective NFE2L2 agent is important. The CUL3-KEAP1 ubiquitin E3 ligase complex promotes the proteasomal degradation of NFE2L2. KEAP1 and NFE2L2 mutations have been implicated in the resistance of tumor cells against chemotherapeutic drugs.

### Small cell lung cancer

Although the genomic landscape of SCLC is being intensively investigated, currently still little is known about the underlying molecular events. Systematic genomic studies in SCLC are challenging because these tumors are usually diagnosed at unresectable stages on cytological specimens or biopsies. Thus, the lack of suitable fresh or frozen tumor specimens for genomic characterization hampers the investigations aimed to identify novel therapeutically relevant genomic alterations. SCLC is characterized by an exceptionally high number of genes carrying somatic mutations, whose clinical significances are currently being investigated. Among the oncosuppressor genes, inactivating mutations of TP53 (75% to 90%) and of RB1 (60% to 90%) are very frequent, while alterations of driver oncogenes include FGFR1, SOX2 and the RLF-MYCL1 fusion product.

The amplification of FGFR1 that occurs in 6% of SCLC may be targeted by selective FGFR inhibitors. SOX2 is a critical factor in the maintenance of pluripotency and self-renewal of stem cells; SOX2 amplification (copy-number >4) has been detected in approximately a quarter of SCLC. The inhibition of SOX2 using short hairpin RNA (shRNA) decreases the proliferation of SOX2-amplified SCLC cell lines.

This finding supports the possible role of SOX2 as a SCLC driver gene.

Gene fusions are a frequent event in SCLC, involving more than 40 different targets. RLF and MYCL1 undergo gene fusion in 9% of SCLC. Small interfering RNA-mediated targeting of MYCL1 in fusion-positive cell lines effectively reduced the proliferation of these cells, suggesting a functional role for MYCL1 in SCLC.

## Reporting the molecular pathology test

The set of data to be included in the EGFR/ALK testing clinical report is well indicated by different guidelines (4, 6). The report should be clear enough to enable the oncologists to easily understand the test outcome in relation to treatment selection and to convey the most relevant information to their patients. For example, an overall statement of the cancer's likelihood to respond to or resist EGFR TKI therapy can be of great practical value. On the other hand, the report should also include the technical information relative to the test methodology, including the DNA extraction method, the spectrum of the mutations tested and the analytic sensitivity of the method, expressed as the lower limit of detection of the mutant alleles in relation to the sample (percentage of tumor cells) being analyzed. The reasons for the rejection of an insufficient specimen or those related to assay failure should be clearly stated (4).

The format of the molecular report may be different. The data can be conveyed as a stand-alone molecular pathology report or as part of a larger surgical pathology or cytopathology report in which molecular data are integrated with histologic examination and other tests performed on the same specimen (25). The length of the report should not be more than one page. The pre-clinical section should clearly state the patient name, the date of birth, a brief patient history (tumor stage, smoking status, histological diagnosis) the date of sample arrival, the sample type and its number. The result section should be divided into two different parts, reflecting both the role of the pathologist (selection of the correct part of the sample for DNA analysis and interpretation of the test outcome) and that of the molecular biologist (responsibility for DNA extraction, molecular testing and reporting). The microscopy part should include the percentage of total nuclei that are malignant and, when relevant, the degree of necrosis or note on processing

or fixation. The result of the mutational analysis should state the names of any clinically significant mutations identified, in formal Human Genome Variation Society (HGVS) nomenclature (4). For FISH tests, colloquial nomenclature can be used, since the nomenclature of the International System for Human Cytogenetic Nomenclature (ISCN) is difficult for the non-specialist to understand (4).

## Malignant mesothelioma

Malignant mesothelioma (MM) is a locally aggressive tumor arising from pleural or peritoneal cavities; it can also develop from the serosa surfaces of the pericardium or the tunica vaginalis. Up to 80% of all cases are pleural in origin. In most of the cases, MM is associated with occupational asbestos exposure, and the latency period may be over 20 years. There are no specific signs and symptoms; consequently, MM is usually diagnosed at the advanced stage of the disease. The prognosis is poor, with a median survival of 9 to 12 months after diagnosis. MM is highly refractory to conventional chemotherapies strategies; currently, a combination of cisplatin and multi-targeted antifolate agent pemetrexed as first-line standard regimen has achieved a median survival time longer than cisplatin alone (32). The understanding of the molecular landscape of MM has been challenging due to its rarity. However, several recent genomic analyses have described comprehensive lists of genetic, epigenetic and signaling alterations in MM. Genetic analyses showed that three oncosuppressor genes (CDKN2A/ARF locus, NF2 and BAP1) are most frequently mutated in MM, and can be a potential target for the treatments (32, 33).

## CDKN2A/ARF locus

About 70% to 80% of MM specimens showed deletion in this locus located at chromosome 9p21.3; CDKN2A encodes p16INK4a, whereas ARF encodes p14ARF. p16INK4a controls the cell cycle via the cyclin-dependent kinase (CDK)4/cyclin D-retinoblastoma protein (pRB) pathway, whereas p14ARF regulates p53. Lack of p14 ARF increases MDM2 activity, which facilitates p53 degradation; lack of p16 leads to the enhanced activities of CDK4 and 6 and induces the phosphorylation of pRb. Thus, the homozygous deletion of CDKN2A/ARF locus leads to the loss of the functions of both p53 and pRb tumor suppressors (32, 33, 34). Because the targeted deletion region is often large, other genes located in the same gene cluster are also co-deleted; for example, the CDKN2B gene, adjacent to CDKN2A, is co-deleted in MM, but at a lower frequency (34).

## NF2

The neurofibromatosis type 2 (NF2) gene encodes for merlin, a tumor suppressor protein. NF2 inactivation is frequent, with rates ranging from 20 to 60% of MM. Various mechanisms of inactivation have been described, including homozygous deletions, nonsense and missense mutations (34). Merlin is regulated by extracellular signaling and modulates multiple signal transduction cascades, including the Hippo pathway and the mammalian target of rapamycin (mTOR) pathway. Under-phosphorylated merlin regulates cell growth inactivating YAP1, a transcriptional co-activator of the Hippo cascade (33, 34). The Merlin-Hippo signaling pathway has been shown to be frequently inactivated in MM cells and the resulting YAP1 activation induces transcription of multiple cancer-promoting genes, including cyclin D1 and connective tissue growth factor (33, 34). Merlin also has an inactivating role on the integrin-dependent mTORC1 signaling pathway in MM cells. mTORC1 inhibitor, rapamycin and its analogs, evelorimus and temsirolimus, showed enhanced cell death in association with cisplatin on MM cell lines (33).

## BRCA1-associated protein-1 (BAP1)

In MM, BAP1, localized on chromosome 3p21.1, is an important oncosuppressor harboring somatic mutations in about 10% of cases (32, 33). BAP1 belongs to the classes of de-ubiquitinating enzymes and it encodes a nuclear ubiquitin C-terminal hydrolase. BAP1 is implicated in DNA damage response, cell cycle regulation and histone modifications and its inactivation induces the perturbation of global gene expression profiling (33).

## Epigenetic alteration

Numerous oncosuppressor genes have been shown to be down-regulated in MM cells by epigenetic mechanisms such as DNA methylation of their transcriptional promoters. The global epigenetic profile differs between MM and normal pleura; MM also exhibits distinct methylation patterns from lung adenocarcinoma, showing that MM had a relatively infrequent number of genes with hypermethylation compared with lung cancer (33, 34). Genes involved include E-cadherin, fragile histidine triad, retinoic acid receptor-β and the Wnt inhibitory factor 1 (33).

Membrane receptor tyrosine kinases (RTKs) have been examined as a molecular target for therapy in MM patients (32, 33). MM expresses a high level of the epidermal growth factor receptor (EGFR) and the vascular endothelial growth factor (VEGF) (33, 34). Nevertheless, the tyrosine kinase inhibitor, erlotinib, and the antibody for VEGF, bevacizumab, showed no survival benefits in phase II clinical trial (32).

## Thymic carcinoma

Thymic carcinoma (TC) is a rare mediastinal aggressive malignant tumor, which in many patients is detected at an inoperable advanced stage with a poor response to multimodal chemoradiotherapy. A few biomarkers and a limited number of possible targeted treatments have been proposed; their clinical value, however, still needs careful validation. This mostly applies to the HER family members and their ligand proteins. EGFR gene mutation and amplification are uncommon. Similarly, HER2 amplification is a rare event, while other molecular alterations – including EGFR and HER2 increased gene copy-numbers and protein over-expression – may occur. In this setting, even in the absence of EGFR mutation, multi-target TKIs such as sunitinib or sorafinib can be effective in patients with metastatic thymic carcinoma. It is noteworthy that mutations involving c-KIT occur in 10% of TCs and the poorly differentiated thymic squamous cell carcinoma over-expressing CD117 should be tested for c-KIT mutations, evaluating exons 9, 11, 13, 14 and 17. Patients harboring a c-KIT mutant tumor may respond to targeted therapy with different TKI, such as imatinib, sorafenib and dasatinib. PDGFR-α mutations have not been detected in thymic carcinoma. KRAS mutations may rarely occur in TC and they may be associated with increased gene copy-number. In TC, the level of IGF1R expression is significantly higher than that in thymoma and the possibility to target IGF-1R with an anti-IGF-1R antibody has recently been shown in preclinical models.

## Cardiac tumors

Primary cardiac tumors are rare, being 50 times less frequent than tumors metastatic to the heart.

Approximately 75% of primary cardiac tumors are benign, and 50% of these benign tumors are represented by myxomas. Other primary benign tumors include lipomas, fibromas, hemangiomas, teratomas and rhabdomyomas, whereas primary malignant tumors of the heart are predominantly sarcomas. Due to their rarity, there are few studies on the molecular mechanisms of cardiac tumor; in particular, cardiac neoplasms occurring in a syndromic fashion are those better studied (35).

About 90% of cardiac myxomas (CM) are sporadic, while 5% to 10% of cases show a familial inheritance as part of the Carney complex (CNC). The sporadic variety occurs later than the familiar one affecting middle-aged women. Sporadic mixomas mostly arise from the left atrium as a single tumor and without associated conditions. Conversely, the familial variety is multicentric in one-third of the cases, and associated with extra-cardiac abnormalities. A great deal of investigation has been dedicated to unraveling the molecular basis of CM arising in CNC. Cytogenetic analysis has revealed two major loci of susceptibility genes in CNC. The CNC1 susceptibility gene is the PPKAR1A gene, which acts as a tumor suppressor gene, and this may harbor a number of different mutations leading to a premature stop codon. Recently, missense mutation (Arg674Gln) in another CNC gene, perinatal isoform of the myosin heavy chain gene MYH8, located at 17p12–31, has been identified. Although the exact mechanism of CM development is not known, it is proposed that mutation in MYH8 promotes the survival of multipotent progenitor cells in the mature heart and provides a substrate for secondary tumorigenic events. A small subset of families with CNC syndrome shows amplification in the CNC2 gene, located on 2p16, without PRKAR1A mutation. These subjects have a negative family history, are present later in life and usually do not develop myxomas. In contrast, no single gene mutation has been identified for sporadic CM, although structural rearrangement in PRKAR1A has been identified in one-third of cases (36).

Cardiac rhabdomyomas are the most common fetal heart tumor and represent a prenatal marker for Tuberous sclerosis complex (TSC), a rare autosomal dominant disease. TSC is caused by a mutation of TSC1 and TSC2, two tumor-suppressor genes located on chromosomes 9q34 and 16p13. TSC1 and TSC2 mutations may also occur in non-familial rhabdomyomas. Inhibition of the mTOR pathway has been proposed as a therapeutic option for the hamartomatous lesions of TSC (37).

Cardiac fibromas are typically solitary, intramural tumors and may be asymptomatic or may result in arrhythmias or cardiac failure depending on their location and size. Cardiac fibromas may occur as a part of Gorlin syndrome, which includes a variety of benign and malignant neoplasms. PTCH1, localized in chromosome 9q22.3, is the gene involved in the pathogenesis of Gorlin syndrome. In fact, conventional cytogenetic analysis of both syndromic and non-syndromic cardiac fibromas revealed a clonal deletion of the long arm of one chromosome 9 homologue which includes the PTCH1 gene locus (38).

## Learning points

- The use of DNA-based molecular tests to stratify lung cancer patients for targeted therapies is mandatory in routine clinical practice.
- Clinical trial-based evidence fully supports the value of EGFR and ALK as predictive markers and a number of emerging biomarkers is currently being evaluated.
- A remarkable degree of consensus has been reached on which patients and when and how they should be tested for EGFR and ALK alterations, as detailed in the CAP/IASLC/AMP guidelines.
- Thanks to a combined morphological, clinical and molecular understanding of lung cancer, the pathologist's role in biomarker testing is pivotal.

## References

1. Mok, T. S., Wu, Y. L., Thongprasert, S., Yang, C. H., Chu, D. T., Saijo, N. et al. Gefitinib or carboplatin-paclitaxel in pulmonary adenocarcinoma. *New Engl J Med* 2009; 361(10): 947–57. PubMed PMID: 19692680.

2. Thunnissen, E., Bubendorf, L., Dietel, M., Elmberger, G., Kerr, K., Lopez-Rios, F. et al. EML4-ALK testing in non-small cell carcinomas of the lung: a review with recommendations. *Virchows Arch* 2012; 461(3): 245–57. PubMed PMID: 22825000. Pubmed Central PMCID: PMC3432214. Epub: 2012/07/25. eng.

3. Travis, W. D., Brambilla, E., Noguchi, M., Nicholson, A. G., Geisinger, K. R., Yatabe, Y. et al.

International association for the study of lung cancer/American Thoracic Society/European Respiratory Society international multidisciplinary classification of lung adenocarcinoma. *J Thorac Oncol* 2011; 6(2): 244–85. PubMed PMID: 21252716.

4. Lindeman, N. I., Cagle, P. T., Beasley, M. B., Chitale, D. A., Dacic, S., Giaccone, G. *et al.* Molecular testing guideline for selection of lung cancer patients for EGFR and ALK tyrosine kinase inhibitors: guideline from the College of American Pathologists, International Association for the Study of Lung Cancer, and Association for Molecular Pathology. *Arch Pathol Lab Med* 2013; 137(6): 828–60. PubMed PMID: 23551194. Epub: 2013/04/05.eng.

5. Aisner, D. L. and Marshall, C. B. Molecular pathology of non-small cell lung cancer: a practical guide. *Am J Clin Pathol* 2012; 138(3): 332–46. PubMed PMID: 22912349. Epub: 2012/08/23.eng.

6. Thunnissen, E., Kerr, K. M., Herth, F. J., Lantuejoul, S., Papotti, M., Rintoul, R. C. *et al.* The challenge of NSCLC diagnosis and predictive analysis on small samples. Practical approach of a working group. *Lung Cancer* 2012; 76(1):1–18. PubMed PMID: 22138001. Epub: 2011/12/06.eng.

7. Malapelle, U., Bellevicine, C., Zeppa, P., Palombini, L. and Troncone, G. Cytology-based gene mutation tests to predict response to anti-epidermal growth factor receptor therapy: a review. *Diagn Cytopathol* 2011; 39(9): 703–10. PubMed PMID: 21837660.

8. Yatabe, Y., Matsuo, K. and Mitsudomi, T. Heterogeneous distribution of EGFR mutations is extremely rare in lung adenocarcinoma. *J Clin Oncol* 2011; 29(22): 2972–7. PubMed PMID: 21730270.

9. Malapelle, U., Bellevicine, C., de Luca, C., Salatiello, M., de Stefano, A., Rocco, D. *et al.* EGFR mutations detected on cytology samples by a centralized laboratory reliably predict response to Gefitinib in non small cell lung cancer patients. *Cancer Cytopathol* 2013; 121(10): 552–60.

10. Malapelle, U., Russo, S., Pepe, F., Sgariglia, R., De Luca, C., Bellevicine, C. *et al.* EGFR mutation detection by microfluidic technology: a validation study. *J Clin Pathol* 2013; 66(11): 982–4. PubMed PMID: 23794480. Epub: 2013/06/25.eng.

11. Shames, D. S. and Wistuba, I. I. The evolving genomic classification of lung cancer. *J Pathol* 2013; 232(2): 121–33. PubMed PMID: 24114583. Epub: 2013/10/12.eng.

12. Han, H. S., Lim, S. N., An, J. Y., Lee, K. M., Choe, K. H., Lee, K. H. *et al.* Detection of EGFR mutation status in lung adenocarcinoma specimens with different proportions of tumor cells using two methods of differential sensitivity. *J Thorac Oncol* 2012; 7(2): 355–64. PubMed PMID: 22157369.

13. Chin, E. L., da Silva, C. and Hegde, M. Assessment of clinical analytical sensitivity and specificity of next-generation sequencing for detection of simple and complex mutations. *BMC Genet* 2013; 14: 6. PubMed PMID: 23418865. Epub: 2013/02/20.eng.

14. Buttitta, F., Felicioni, L., Del Grammastro, M., Filice, G., Di Lorito, A., Malatesta, S. *et al.* Effective assessment of EGFR mutation status in bronchoalveolar lavage and pleural fluids by next-generation sequencing. *Clin Cancer Res* 2013; 19(3): 691–8. PubMed PMID: 23243218.

15. Pirker, R., Herth, F. J., Kerr, K. M., Filipits, M., Taron, M., Gandara, D. *et al.* Consensus for EGFR mutation testing in non-small cell lung cancer: results from a European workshop. *J Thorac Oncol* 2010; 5(10): 1706–13. PubMed PMID: 20871269.

16. Lozano, M. D., Zulueta, J. J., Echeveste, J. I., Gurpide, A., Seijo, L. M., Martin-Algarra, S. *et al.* Assessment of epidermal growth factor receptor and K-ras mutation status in cytological stained smears of non-small cell lung cancer patients: correlation with clinical outcomes. *Oncologist* 2011; 16(6): 877–85. PubMed PMID: 21572125.

17. Bozzetti, C., Negri, F. V., Azzoni, C., Naldi, N., Nizzoli, R., Bortesi, B. *et al.* Epidermal growth factor receptor and Kras gene expression: reliability of mutational analysis on cytological samples. *Diagn Cytopathol* 2013; 41(7): 595–8. PubMed PMID: 22833420. Epub: 2012/07/27.eng.

18. Bruno, P., Mariotta, S., Ricci, A., Duranti, E., Scozzi, D., Noto, A. *et al.* Reliability of direct sequencing of EGFR: comparison between cytological and histological samples from the same patient. *Anticancer Res* 2011; 31(12): 4207–10. PubMed PMID: 22199282. Epub: 2011/12/27.eng.

19. Chowdhuri, S. R., Xi, L., Pham, T. H., Hanson, J., Rodriguez-Canales, J., Berman, A. *et al.* EGFR and KRAS mutation analysis in cytologic samples of lung adenocarcinoma enabled by laser capture microdissection. *Mod Pathol* 2012; 25(4): 548–55. PubMed PMID: 22157931.

20. Goto, K., Satouchi, M., Ishii, G., Nishio, K., Hagiwara, K., Mitsudomi, T. *et al.* An evaluation study of EGFR mutation tests utilized for non-small-cell lung cancer in the diagnostic setting. *Ann Oncol* 2012; 23(11): 2914–19. PubMed PMID: 22776705. Epub: 2012/07/11.eng.

21. Mitiushkina, N. V., Iyevleva, A. G., Poltoratskiy, A. N., Ivantsov,

A. O., Togo, A. V., Polyakov, I. S. *et al.* Detection of EGFR mutations and EML4-ALK rearrangements in lung adenocarcinomas using archived cytological slides. *Cancer Cytopathol* 2013; 121(7): 370–6. PubMed PMID: 23408463. Epub: 2013/02/15.eng.

22. Sun, P. L., Jin, Y., Kim, H., Lee, C. T., Jheon, S. and Chung, J. H. High concordance of EGFR mutation status between histologic and corresponding cytologic specimens of lung adenocarcinomas. *Cancer Cytopathol* 2013; 121(6): 311–19.

23. Khode, R., Larsen, D. A., Culbreath, B. C., Parrish, S., Walker, K. L., Sayage-Rabie, L. *et al.* Comparative study of epidermal growth factor receptor mutation analysis on cytology smears and surgical pathology specimens from primary and metastatic lung carcinomas. *Cancer Cytopathol* 2013; 121(7): 361–9. PubMed PMID: 23364874. Epub 2013/02/01.eng.

24. Malapelle, U., de Rosa, N., Rocco, D., Bellevicine, C., Crispino, C., Illiano, A. *et al.* EGFR and KRAS mutations detection on lung cancer liquid-based cytology: a pilot study. *J Clin Pathol* 2012; 65(1): 87–91. PubMed PMID: 21945923.

25. Thunnissen, E., Bovee, J. V., Bruinsma, H., van den Brule, A. J., Dinjens, W., Heideman, D. A. *et al.* EGFR and KRAS quality assurance schemes in pathology: generating normative data for molecular predictive marker analysis in targeted therapy. *J Clin Pathol* 2011; 64(10): 884–92. PubMed PMID: 21947301. Epub: 2011/09/29.eng.

26. Mazieres, J., Peters, S., Lepage, B., Cortot, A. B., Barlesi, F., Beau-Faller, M. *et al.* Lung cancer that harbors an HER2 mutation:

epidemiologic characteristics and therapeutic perspectives. *J Clin Oncol* 2013; 31(16): 1997–2003. PubMed PMID: 23610105. Epub: 2013/04/24.eng.

27. Davies, K. D., Le, A. T., Theodoro, M. F., Skokan, M. C., Aisner, D. L., Berge, E. M. *et al.* Identifying and targeting ROS1 gene fusions in non-small cell lung cancer. *Clin Cancer Res* 2012; 18(17): 4570–9. PubMed PMID: 22919003. Pubmed Central PMCID: PMC3703205. Epub: 2012/08/25. eng.

28. Borrelli, N., Giannini, R., Proietti, A., Ali, G., Pelliccioni, S., Niccoli, C. *et al.* KIF5B/RET fusion gene analysis in a selected series of cytological specimens of EGFR, KRAS and EML4-ALK wild-type adenocarcinomas of the lung. *Lung Cancer* 2013; 81(3): 377–81. PubMed PMID: 23891510. Epub: 2013/07/31.eng.

29. Cardarella, S., Ogino, A., Nishino, M., Butaney, M., Shen, J., Lydon, C. *et al.* Clinical, pathologic, and biologic features associated with BRAF mutations in non-small cell lung cancer. *Clin Cancer Res* 2013; 19(16): 4532–40. PubMed PMID: 23833300. Pubmed Central PMCID: PMC3762878. Epub: 2013/07/09.eng.

30. Chiosea, S. I., Sherer, C. K., Jelic, T. and Dacic, S. KRAS mutant allele-specific imbalance in lung adenocarcinoma. *Mod Pathol*; 24(12): 1571–7. PubMed PMID: 21743433.

31. Ohashi, K., Sequist, L. V., Arcila, M. E., Lovly, C. M., Chen, X., Rudin, C. M. *et al.* Characteristics of lung cancers harboring NRAS mutations. *Clin Cancer Res* 2013; 19(9): 2584–91. PubMed PMID: 23515407. Pubmed Central PMCID: PMC3643999. Epub: 2013/03/22.eng.

32. Tada, Y., Shimada, H., Hiroshima, K. and Tagawa, M.

A potential therapeutic strategy for malignant mesothelioma with gene medicine. *BioMed Res Int* 2013; 2013: article ID 572609. PubMed PMID: 23484132. Pubmed Central PMCID: PMC3581274. Epub: 2013/03/14. eng.

33. Sekido, Y. Molecular pathogenesis of malignant mesothelioma. *Carcinogenesis* 2013; 34(7): 1413–19. PubMed PMID: 23677068. Epub: 2013/05/17.eng.

34. Jean, D., Daubriac, J., Le Pimpec-Barthes, F., Galateau-Salle, F. and Jaurand, M. C. Molecular changes in mesothelioma with an impact on prognosis and treatment. *Arch Pathol Lab Med* 2012; 136(3): 277–93. PubMed PMID: 22372904. Epub: 2012/03/01.eng.

35. Elbardissi, A. W., Dearani, J. A., Daly, R. C., Mullany, C. J., Orszulak, T. A., Puga, F. J. *et al.* Survival after resection of primary cardiac tumors: a 48-year experience. *Circulation* 2008; 118 (14 Suppl.): S7–15. PubMed PMID: 18824772.

36. Singhal, P., Luk, A., Rao, V. and Butany, J. Molecular basis of cardiac myxomas. *Int J Mol Sci* 2014; 15(1): 1315–37. PubMed PMID: 24447924.en.

37. Lee, K. A., Won, H.-S., Shim, J.-Y., Lee, P. R. and Kim, A. Molecular genetic, cardiac and neurodevelopmental findings in cases of prenatally diagnosed rhabdomyoma associated with tuberous sclerosis complex. *Ultrasound in Obstet Gynecol* 2013; 41: 306–11. PubMed PMID: 22791573.

38. Scanlan, D., Radio, S. J., Nelson, M., Zhou, M., Streblow, R., Prasad, V. *et al.* Loss of the PTCH1 gene locus in cardiac fibroma. *Cardiovasc Pathol* 2008; 17(2): 93–7. PubMed PMID: 18329553. Pubmed Central PMCID: 2342874.

# Tumors of the endocrine system

Sylvia L. Asa and Ozgur Mete

## Introduction to endocrine pathology

Endocrine tumors are an interesting group of neoplasms that have unusual molecular features. They range from very common disorders, such as pituitary tumors that are found in approximately 20% of the population (1) and clinically insignificant papillary thyroid microcarcinomas that are found in up to 24% of patients at surgery and 36% of individuals at autopsy (2), to rare but aggressive lesions that are rapidly lethal, such as anaplastic thyroid cancers and adrenal cortical carcinoma. In between are a host of neuroendocrine tumors whose behaviors are difficult to predict. The molecular changes that are characteristic of these tumors are also highly heterogeneous. This chapter will review the progress that has been made in understanding the molecular and epigenetic alterations that mediate neoplastic transformation and progression of these disorders.

## Pituitary

The pituitary is a site of common neoplastic transformation but very uncommon malignant neoplasia. Incidental pituitary tumors are found in approximately 20% of the population (1); some of these are slowly growing, hormonally inactive lesions that are incidental findings, others may be slowly growing but hormonally active, causing extensive morbidity due to hormone excess as in acromegaly or Cushing disease. Malignancy, defined by cerebrospinal and/or systemic metastatic spread, is exceptionally rare (3), but aggressive growth and invasion is a feature of a significant number of these tumors (4).

A minority of pituitary tumors are manifestations of a number of familial syndromes that are attributable to germline mutations in tumor suppressor genes. These syndromes are inherited as autosomal dominant tumor syndromes with variable penetrance. Their molecular basis has become well defined in the past 20 years.

Patients with *Multiple Endocrine Neoplasia (MEN)-1*, characterized by tumors of the pituitary, parathyroid and pancreas as well as other less common lesions, have germline inactivating mutations in the gene on chromosome 11q13 that encodes menin (5). When there is loss of heterozygosity (LOH) inactivating the normal allele in the pituitary, patients develop adenomas that most often produce prolactin and/or GH (6). Menin is not lost by mutation or LOH in sporadic pituitary adenomas (7) and is not down-regulated in most sporadic tumors (8). *MEN4* is a very rare related disorder due to germline mutation and inactivation of the CDKN1B gene that encodes p27Kip1 (9; 10); these patients also develop pituitary adenomas that may secrete GH and/or prolactin or may secrete ACTH to cause Cushing disease (11). The CDKN2C/p18INK4c gene has also been implicated in a few families that have a syndrome resembling MEN1 (12). *Isolated familial somatotropinoma (IFS)* and *familial isolated pituitary adenoma (FIPA)* are inherited syndromes of pituitary adenoma development due to germline mutations in the aryl hydrocarbon receptor interacting protein (AIP) gene (13; 14). Patients in these kindreds develop large pituitary adenomas at a young age. GH-producing adenomas are the most frequent and many of the young patients develop gigantism, but members of these kindreds also develop prolactinomas, nonfunctioning pituitary adenomas or Cushing disease. *Carney complex (CNC)* is characterized by development of a number of endocrine tumors, including pituitary adenomas, as well as myxomas (mainly

*Molecular Pathology: A Practical Guide for the Surgical Pathologist and Cytopathologist*, ed. John M. S. Bartlett, Abeer Shaaban and Fernando Schmitt. Published by Cambridge University Press. © Cambridge University Press, 2016.

cardiac) and nevi or melanocytic macules that can affect mucosal surfaces. The pituitary adenomas in this syndrome are also mainly associated with gigantism or acromegaly (15). Most of the families with this syndrome have germline mutations in the PRKAR1Aα gene that encodes the PKA regulatory subunit 1Aα (16). Mutations in SDH subunits are implicated in the development of familial paragangliomas and/or pheochromocytomas and in some cases of Carney-Stratakis syndrome; one recent report of an aggressive GH-producing tumor associated with this disorder showed mutation and LOH in the pituitary (17); however, sporadic tumors do not harbor such mutations (18).

Mutations in the far more common *sporadic pituitary adenomas* are rare. Among the first mutations identified in endocrine tumors were activating mutations in GNAS, encoding the Guanine nucleotide-binding protein (G-protein) stimulatory alpha subunit (Gsα). These "gsp" mutations result in constitutive activation of adenylate cyclase, causing increased intracellular cyclic adenosine monophosphate (cAMP) levels (19; 20) that lead to hormonally active but usually benign tumors. In the pituitary, they are found mainly in the most common variant of somatotroph adenomas of the pituitary causing acromegaly – the densely granulated type. These mutations are occasionally seen as mosaic germline events that then give rise to the *McCune-Albright syndrome*. The second most common variant of somatotroph adenoma, the sparsely granulated type, has been reported to harbor occasional inactivating mutations in the GH receptor, resulting in a different alteration in signaling pathways (21). These divergent mutations explain the differential sensitivity of the two types of somatotroph adenomas to somatostatin analogues and have a critical clinical role; the high cAMP induced by gsp mutations in densely granulated tumors is amenable to cAMP inhibition induced by somatostatin, whereas sparsely granulated adenomas do not respond as well, yet are safely targeted by the GHR antagonist Pegvisomant through its actions outside the pituitary (22).

Whole-exome sequencing of a series of clinically non-functioning adenomas has identified 24 mutations in independent genes, including platelet-derived growth factor D (PDGFD), N-myc down-regulated gene family member 4 (NDRG4) and Zipper sterile-α-motif kinase (ZAK) (23). However, these were non-recurrent events, suggesting that mechanisms other than somatic mutation underlie sporadic non-functioning pituitary adenomas. There are exceptionally rare reports of mutation of p53 (24 ;25) or RAS (26) in pituitary adenomas. RAS mutations have been reported in the metastases of rare pituitary carcinomas, but not the primary tumors (27; 28), and there is evidence of unusual clonal evolution in malignant deposits (29), with alterations in Rb and p53 in occasional lesions (30; 31). A single BRAF mutation has been reported (32).

*Hormonal regulatory pathways* are implicated in the growth of pituitary tumors. Excess GRH or CRH stimulation may play a role in somatotroph and corticotroph adenomas, respectively (33; 34). Mutation in the glucocorticoid receptor has been implicated in pituitary corticotroph adenoma development (35). Excess estrogen (36) or loss of dopaminergic inhibition may play a role in lactotroph proliferation (37), but there are no reports of any mutational basis for alterations in these pathways to account for transformation. Target organ insufficiency has been associated with the development of thyrotroph and gonadotroph adenomas (38; 39). An unusual alternatively spliced variant of the thyroid hormone receptor TRβ2 with a 135-bp deletion in the ligand-binding domain was found in one case of thyrotroph adenoma (40), accounting for lack of feedback inhibition by thyroid hormone.

*Growth factor dysregulation* is also seen in pituitary tumors. Altered expression levels have been described in the transforming growth factor β (TGF-β) family members, inhibins and activins, as well as follistatin in gonadotroph adenomas (41; 42). A truncated type I serine/threonine kinase activin receptor ActRIB (Alk4) isoform that fails to transduce activin-induced growth arrest signaling was identified in a series of gonadotroph tumors (43). Alterations in expression of FGFs and FGFRs appear to be significant in pituitary tumors; FGFs are over-expressed (44), FGFR2, which has tumor suppressor activity in the pituitary (45), is down-regulated (46; 47) and FGFR4 is up-regulated (46). A truncated ligand-independent isoform identified as ptd-FGFR4 (48) derived by alternate splicing (49) alters cell adhesion (50).

*Epigenetic dysregulation* is a common theme in pituitary adenomas. In addition to the alterations in hormones and growth factors described above, targets include Rb (51–53), p53, CDKIs (54–56), GADD45γ (57; 58), MEG3 (59), pituitary tumor apoptosis gene

(PTAG) (60), and the folate receptor in non-functioning adenomas (61). Expression profiling of pituitary tumors compared with normal pituitary tissue has identified up-regulation of cell proliferation markers such as PTTG (62; 63), ASK, CCNB1, AURKB and CENPE (63); alterations in SFRP1, TLE2, PITX2, NOTCH3 and DLK1 in the Wnt and Notch pathways were found in non-functional pituitary adenomas (64), and alterations in cell adhesion molecules ADAMTS6, CRMP1 and DCAMKL3 (adhesion) (63) and MMP-9 (65) as well as IGFBP5, MYO5A, FLT3 and NFE2L1 (66). Compared with hormonally active tumors, hormonally inactive adenomas exhibit global DNA hypermethylation, most significantly in the promoter region of the potassium voltage-gated channel KCNAB2, suggesting a role for the ion-channel activity signal pathway (67).

The mechanism of epigenetic silencing is not entirely clear. The DNA methyltransferase (DNMT) enzyme family is dysregulated; in contrast to DNMT1 and DNMT3a, DNMT3b is expressed at relatively higher levels in neoplastic pituitary cells through histone modification, and it is implicated in the silencing of pRb, p21 and p27 (68). Other mechanisms likely involve Ikaros, a transcription factor that mediates pituitary cell growth in development (69; 70) and hormone function (71). Ikaros expression is altered in adenomas (72); there is expression of a dominant negative isoform IK6 that enhances cholesterol uptake (73), decreases anti-apoptotic action (74) and mediates response to hypoxia in pituitary cells (75). High mobility group (HMG) proteins containing AT-hook domains (HMGA) are also involved in DNA binding and chromatin remodeling; they have been implicated in pituitary tumorigenesis (76; 77) through interactions with pRB/E2F1 (78) and up-regulation of cyclin B2 (79). Amplification and over-expression of HMGA2 has been reported in a small number of prolactinomas (80) and over-expression of HMGA1 has also been identified (79; 81). The altered expression of HMGA2 in primary tumors without amplification of this gene may be due to altered microRNA expression, particularly of let-7 (82). Other miRNAs that may play a role in these tumors include miR-34b, miR-326, miR-432, miR-548c-3p, miR-570 and miR-603, which are down-regulated in GH adenomas and target genes such as high mobility group A1 (HMGA1), HMGA2 and E2F1 (83).

*Germline polymorphisms* alter pituitary tumor behavior. A germline FGFR4 SNP substitutes arginine (R) for glycine (G) in the transmembrane domain resulting in FGFR4-R388 that increases growth due to Src activation and mitochondrial pS-STAT3 and decreases pY-STAT3. This change in signaling not only alters cell proliferation, but also hormone function. It relieves GH inhibition, encouraging mammosomatotroph cells to produce more GH than PRL and in patients with acromegaly, pituitary tumor size correlates with hormone excess in the presence of the FGFR4-R388, but not the FGFR4-G388 allele (84). FGFR4-R388 also enhances glucocorticoid receptor phosphorylation and nuclear translocation. Patients who are homozygous for the R388 allele are more likely to develop silent corticotroph macroadenomas, whereas those homozygous for FGFR4-G388 are more likely to have small, hormonally active microadenomas causing florid Cushing disease (85).

## Thyroid

The thyroid follicular epithelium exhibits a spectrum of proliferative lesions that range from benign multifocal clonal and polyclonal nodules, to the most aggressive anaplastic thyroid carcinoma. In between are benign functioning adenomas, indolent papillary microcarcinomas, proliferative but well-differentiated papillary and follicular carcinomas, and intermediate grade poorly differentiated carcinomas (86). In addition to this, the thyroid is a site for the development of tumors of parafollicular C cells, neuroendocrine endothelial cells that produce chromogranin, calcitonin and CEA and represent one relatively aggressive type of the group of neuroendocrine tumors of the dispersed neuroendocrine system.

The role of environmental carcinogens in neoplasia was clearly proven by the epidemics of thyroid cancer of follicular cell derivation following exposure to radioactive iodine during atomic bomb development and testing at Hanford, the Nevada Test Site and the Marshall Islands and in Japan after the Second World War (87). Further progress illustrating the impact of exposure dose and patient age was provided by the Chernobyl accident in 1986 when it became apparent that younger patients were more susceptible (88). Outside of these examples, the vast majority of these neoplasms are apparently sporadic and there is no evidence of nuclear exposure as a causative agent and the pathogenesis of these common lesions remains unknown. There is evidence of familial predisposition to follicular cell neoplasia in some cases

(89). Importantly, the elucidation of the genetic alterations underlying thyroid C cell neoplasia provided the first example of a familial cancer syndrome due to inheritance of an activated oncogene (90), thereby allowing almost 100% prediction of disease.

The entity known *as follicular nodular disease* (or *sporadic nodular goiter* when clinically significant) is the most common cause of thyroid nodules, but to date, the genetic, environmental or hormonal factors underlying this disorder are unknown. Once thought to be inflammatory (91; 92), now they are considered neoplastic since the nodules are often monoclonal (93–95).

Nodules classified as "papillary hyperplastic nodule" are actually clonal lesions that are better called "follicular adenoma with papillary architecture," since the term "papillary adenoma" has fallen out of favour, even though it is more precise (96; 97) (Figure 17.1). These lesions harbor activating mutations of the TSH receptor (TSHR) or Gsα that mediates TSH-receptor signaling (98–103), resulting in constitutive activation of adenylate cyclase, elevated levels of intracellular cAMP and increased thyroid hormone synthesis and secretion. They are usually associated with clinical or subclinical hyperthyroidism, and are "warm" or "hot" on radioactive iodine scan (104). These lesions often arise in the setting of multinodular goiter where they represent one form of neoplasia within multifocal clonal proliferations of variable morphology and molecular alterations; in this setting, the disorder is known as "Plummer's disease." Patients with McCune Albright syndrome have mosaic germline mutations and may have multiple such lesions. Patients with Carney complex, due to mutations in the PRKAR1A gene, may also develop papillary thyroid adenomas.

*Classical papillary thyroid carcinomas* with any papillary architecture, including mixed papillary and follicular tumors, stromal fibrosis and psammoma bodies, have a high incidence of the BRAFV660E mutation (Figure 17.2). Those without BRAF mutations often harbor gene rearrangements involving the RET proto-oncogene (RET-PTC), TRK, PAX8-PPARγ, ALK or AKAP9-BRAF (86; 105–107). The mutations and rearrangements are largely mutually exclusive and non-overlapping. There is geographic and temporal variation in the relative incidence of these molecular alterations (86; 106; 107). Some rearrangments, such as ETV6-NTRK3, are features of radiation-induced papillary carcinomas, but are not found in sporadic tumors (108). BRAF mutation has been suggested to predict more aggressive prognosis (109), but this is not an independent predictor and morphologic subclassification is a better predictor of lymph node metastasis and extrathyroidal extension (110).

Two variants of papillary carcinoma are associated with germline mutations that predispose to other neoplasia. The cribriform-morular variant is found almost exclusively in patients with familial polyposis coli due to germline mutations of the APC gene (111–113); rare reports indicate the possibility of sporadic mutation in CTNNB1 in tumors with this morphology (114) (Figure 17.3). A case of a "villous" variant associated with Marfan syndrome implicates mutations in the FBN1 gene that encodes fibrillin-1, which results in altered TGF-β signaling (115).

*Follicular adenomas, follicular carcinomas* and *follicular variant papillary thyroid carcinomas* with pure follicular growth patterns are characterized by a high frequency of RAS mutations (105; 106; 116–124) (Figure 17.4). Unusual BRAF mutations such as the K601E variant also occur in follicular variant papillary carcinomas (119). The Cancer Genome Atlas (TCGA) analysis has also recently uncovered mutations in EIF1AX, PPM1D and CHEK2, as well as rearrangements involving MET, LTK, ALK, FGFR2 and THADA (125). The molecular

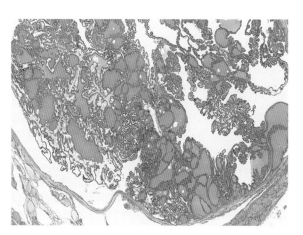

**Figure 17.1 Papillary adenoma**
Nodules classified as "papillary hyperplastic nodule" are actually clonal lesions that are better called "follicular adenoma with papillary architecture" or "papillary adenoma." These lesions harbor activating mutations of the TSH receptor (TSHR) or Gsα that mediates TSH-receptor signaling, are often associated with clinical or subclinical hyperthyroidism, and are "warm" or "hot" on radioactive iodine scan.

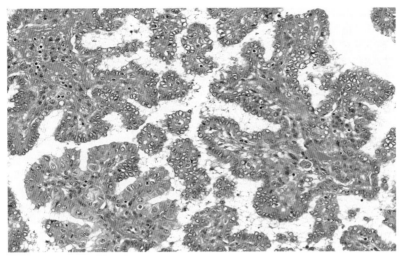

**Figure 17.2** **Papillary thyroid carcinoma with classic architecture** Tall cell, columnar cell, hobnail cell, classical and Warthin-like variants of papillary thyroid carcinomas often harbor BRAFV600E mutation. A classical variant papillary thyroid carcinoma is illustrated in this photomicrograph, together with BRAFV600E mutation status on amplification-refractory mutation system (ARMS) PCR.

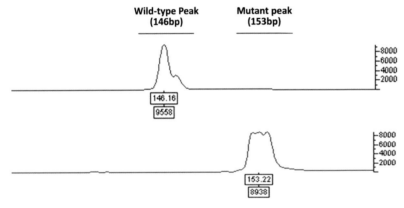

similarities between follicular carcinoma and follicular variant papillary carcinoma, and the distinct differences between them and classical papillary carcinoma, suggest that reclassification of these tumors to remove them from the papillary thyroid carcinoma category is warranted (126).

The *hyalinizing trabecular tumor* (127–129) was initially called "hyalinizing trabecular adenoma" (130) or "paraganglioma-like adenoma of thyroid" (131); however, reports of metastatic spread led to recognition of malignant potential (132–134). These tumors resemble papillary carcinoma and harbor ret/PTC rearrangements (135; 136) – therefore, many authors consider them to be variants of papillary thyroid carcinoma (3; 137; 138).

*Poorly differentiated thyroid cancer* represents a tumor that exhibits a behavior intermediate between well-differentiated and anaplastic or undifferentiated

carcinoma (139). These tumors most often arise within differentiated thyroid carcinomas and likely represent progression with additional genetic events. They harbor mutations of BRAF and RAS, as well as additional CTNNB1 and PIK3CA mutations (140–143). Rare GNAS mutations are also identified in some series (144).

*Anaplastic or undifferentiated thyroid carcinoma* is one of the most aggressive and rapidly lethal malignancies; fortunately, it only represents less than 2% of thyroid cancers (145). These tumors are characterized by frequent p53 mutations in addition to BRAF, RAS or PIK3CA alterations (86; 106), and diffuse p53 immunoreactivity is frequently identified, consistent with this additional molecular driver.

*Medullary thyroid carcinoma* is derived from a completely distinct cell type and has no differentiation features of follicular epithelium. These lesions

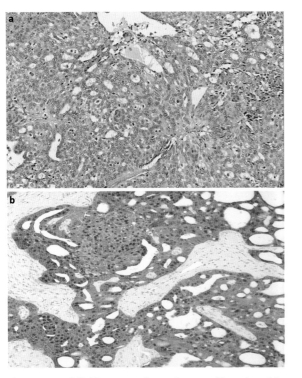

**Figure 17.3 Cribriform-morular variant papillary thyroid carcinoma**
In addition to diagnostic nuclear features of papillary thyroid carcinoma, a complex cribriform architecture and the formation of squamoid morulae (a), nuclear and cytoplasmic localization of beta-catenin (b) is regarded as a characteristic of these rare neoplasms.

result from proliferation of the calcitonin-producing C cells that are scattered in the thyroid, normally at the junction of the upper third and lower two-thirds of each lateral lobe. These tumors may be sporadic or hereditary. When hereditary but isolated, they give rise to a syndrome known as familial medullary carcinoma (FMTC). When associated with pheochromocytomas and parathyroid proliferations, they represent a component of MEN2A, and where associated with those lesions as well as mucosal ganglioneuromas and a Marfanoid habitus, the syndrome is known as MEN2B. These genetic syndromes are all due to germline-activating mutations of the RET proto-oncogene; mutations are usually present in exons 10 and 11 in FMTC or MEN2A and at codon 918 in MEN2B (90; 146); the entire list of mutations and the genotype-phenotype correlations are available at www.arup.utah.edu/database/MEN2/MEN2_welcome.php and their clinical implications are reviewed in the most recent treatment guidelines

from the American Thyroid Association (ATA) (147). Inheritance of this activated oncogene predicts thyroid cancer development with almost 100% certainty (148–150); therefore, it is recommended that affected members of kindreds undergo prophylactic thyroidectomy in childhood (151). Patients develop C cell hyperplasia as a precursor lesion; this represents an interesting misnomer, since these are all neoplastic proliferations of transformed cells rather than a polyclonal reactive process that can be seen in other settings (152). Sporadic medullary thyroid carcinomas harbor somatic RET mutations, most often in codon 918, or activating mutations of RAS genes (153).

## Parathyroid

The vast majority of parathyroid tumors are sporadic. However, a minority occur in patients with inherited genetic diseases, including MEN1, MEN2 or MEN4 syndromes, or hyperparathyroidism-jaw tumor (HPT-JT) syndrome. In inherited disease, the pathology is often multifocal (3).

*Parathyroid adenomas* are the most common parathyroid neoplasms; they are usually solitary and benign monoclonal proliferations (154; 155). A common genetic feature of sporadic tumors is intragenic deletion involving the MEN1 gene on chromosome 11q13 (155; 156). A subset of these tumors harbor a PRAD1 gene rearrangement that places the coding region of either the cyclin D1 gene or the INT2 gene encoding a fibroblast growth factor under transcriptional control of the parathyroid hormone gene promoter (157; 158), resulting in up-regulation of cyclin D1 or FGFs that drive cell proliferation.

*Parathyroid hyperplasia* accounts for 10% to 15% of primary hyperparathyroidism. This entity encompasses two different molecular profiles. Secondary hyperparathyroidism is usually characterized by diffuse hypercellularity that is polyclonal. In contrast, patients with familial syndromes including MEN1 or MEN2 have multiglandular disease that is called "hyperplasia," but actually represents multiple monoclonal adenomas; the former exhibit mutation and LOH of the MEN1 gene and the latter have germline-activating mutations of the RET proto-oncogene. Patients with secondary hyperplasia that is truly reactive can also develop autonomous clonal proliferations that accumulate additional genetic alterations and can rarely even become malignant (3).

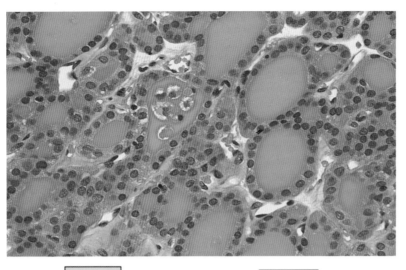

**Figure 17.4 Papillary thyroid carcinoma with pure follicular architecture**
The diagnosis of follicular variant papillary carcinoma should be restricted to follicular epithelial proliferations that exhibit 100% follicular architecture, together with nuclear features of papillary carcinoma. These lesions often harbor RAS mutations. Sanger sequence electrophoregram illustrates the presence of KRAS mutation in codon 12 (KRAS G12S).

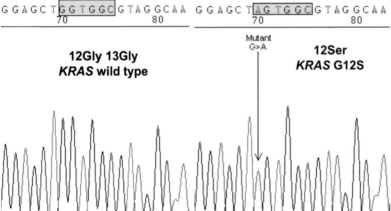

*Parathyroid carcinoma* is rare and only a small proportion of patients develop metastatic disease (159; 160). A number of genetic events are thought to underlie malignant transformation. Most of the events described represent epigenetic alterations that silence tumor suppressors such as Rb (161), p27 (162) or p53 (163), or allow over-expression of growth-enhancing proteins such as galectin-3 (164) and bcl-2 (165); the molecular changes responsible for these alterations are not known and there is no evidence of mutation in the respective genes, but all would account for increased cell proliferation and the high Ki67 labeling index found in these tumors (166).

The hyperparathyroidism-jaw tumor syndrome is a familial disorder with predisposition to the development of parathyroid carcinoma; these patients have germline mutations in the tumor suppressor HRPT2 gene (also known as CDC73) which encodes the protein parafibromin. Somatic HRPT2 mutations are found in a high proportion of sporadic parathyroid carcinomas (167; 168), resulting in global loss of parafibromin by immunohistochemistry (Figure 17.5).

## Adrenal cortex

*Adrenal cortical adenomas* are usually sporadic tumors that may or may not be clinically hormonally active; those that secrete hormones in excess can cause Cushing syndrome with glucocorticoid excess or Conn syndrome with hyperaldosteronism. Comparative genomic hybridization studies have demonstrated genetic alterations in 30% to 60% of adrenal adenomas; losses on chromosomes 1p, 11q, 17p,22p and 22q, and gains on chromosomes 4 and 5, 12 and 19 have been identified (169). Changes in

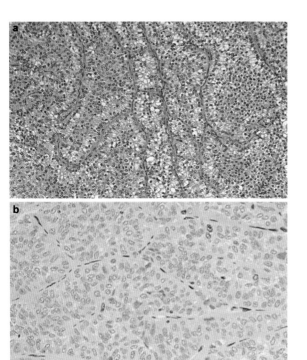

**Figure 17.5 Parathyroid carcinoma**
A parathyroid carcinoma (a) showing loss of nuclear parafibromin expression (b) is illustrated in this photomicrograph. Somatic HRPT2 mutations are found in a high proportion of sporadic parathyroid carcinomas, resulting in global loss of parafibromin by immunohistochemistry, as illustrated in this case. Please note that stromal cells and endothelial cells are positive.

chromosomes 3, 9 and X may be early events in tumors that progress to malignancy (170).

Adrenal cortical adenomas causing Cushing syndrome harbor somatic mutations in PRKACA, which encodes the catalytic subunit of cyclic AMP-dependent protein kinase (protein kinase A [PKA]) in about 37% of patients (171). ACTH receptor mutations have been reported (172), but the pathogenetic importance of these remains unclear. A different entity that mimics adrenal cortical adenoma causing adrenal glucocorticoid excess is ACTH-independent macronodular adrenal hyperplasia (AIMAH); the pathophysiology of this entity is heterogeneous, but generally involves aberrant adrenal expression and function of one or several G-protein-coupled receptors as well as germline ARMC5 mutations that promote cell proliferation and abnormal regulation of steroidogenesis (173). When the receptors are related to metabolism, the entity can be related to food intake, and when related to gonadotropins, it has been associated with pregnancy (174).

Sporadic adenomas associated with Conn syndrome and primary aldosteronism have mutations in the KCNJ5 potassium channel selectivity filter or in ATP1A1 and ATP2B3 encoding Na/K ATPases (175–177). In addition to KCJN5, ATP1A1 and ATP2B3 mutations, calcium channel mutations (CACNA1D), and aberrant wnt/beta-catenin signaling are also characteristics of aldosterone-producing adrenal cortical adenomas (178–180).

These lesions may be associated with familial disease. Patients with *MEN I* who have germline inactivating mutations of menin frequently develop small, non-functioning benign adrenal cortical adenomas (181). Those with *Carney complex* due to germline mutations in the PRKAR1Aα gene (16; 182) develop an unusual form of nodular cortical disease known as primary pigmented nodular adrenocortical disease (PPNAD). Adenomas are also more common than in the general population in patients with *familial hyperaldosteronism* and those with *congenital adrenal hyperplasia*, a group of autosomal recessive diseases due to mutations or translocations of genes encoding steroidogenic enzymes, leading to decreased negative feedback and resultant pituitary hyperstimulation (183). Cushing syndrome can occur in patients with the *McCune-Albright syndrome* and the pathology is an interesting mix of diffuse and nodular hyperplasia with adenoma formation and intervening atrophy, consistent with the mosaic pattern of the **GNAS** mutation that should cause some areas to proliferate, but the intervening non-affected tissue would undergo involution due to glucocorticoid feedback on the pituitary and ACTH suppression (184).

MicroRNA expression reveals distinct patterns in adrenal cortical adenomas that produce aldosterone and those that produce glucocorticoids; non-functioning adenomas are not distinguished in these studies. Fourteen miRNAs were common among the three adenoma subtypes (185).

*Adrenal cortical carcinoma* is a feature of several hereditary cancer syndromes: Li-Fraumeni due to germline mutation of TP53 (186; 187), Beckwith-Wiedemann associated with dysregulation of a group of growth-controlling genes on 11p15.5 – including paternal disomy of the IGF-II gene (188; 189), Lynch syndrome (190) and FAP syndrome (Familial Adenomatous Polyposis) (191). Rare cases of malignancy have also been reported in association with MEN1 (192) and Carney complex (193; 194) which are more commonly associated with benign

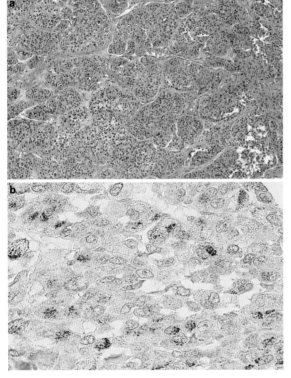

**Figure 17.6 Adrenal cortical carcinoma**
Sporadic adrenal cortical carcinomas exhibit a high frequency of rearrangements of the chromosomal locus 11 p15.5 associated with IGF-II over-expression. In this photomicrograph, an adrenal cortical carcinoma (a) showing paranuclear IGF-II expression (b) is illustrated.

A recent exome sequencing and SNP array analysis confirmed alterations in CTNNB1, TP53, CDKN2A, RB1 and MEN1 that were expected from the previous literature and also identified new mutations. ZNRF3, encoding a cell surface E3 ubiquitin ligase implicated in the beta-catenin pathway, was altered in 21% of tumors. Less frequent mutations were found in DAXX, TERT and MED12. This study defined two distinct molecular subgroups with prognostic implications, one poor outcome group characterized by numerous mutations and DNA methylation alterations, and a good prognosis group with deregulation of two microRNA clusters (203).

## Pheochromocytomas and paragangliomas

Paragangliomas are neoplasms of neuroendocrine cells of the sympathetic or parasympathetic ganglia. When they develop in the largest sympathetic ganglion, the adrenal medulla, they are known as pheochromocytomas. Although initially thought to be 10% familial and 10% multifocal, studies over the last decade have shown that approximately 35% of pheochromocytomas/paragangliomas are associated with germline mutations that predispose to these tumors (204). While the genetic data are being updated frequently, the most recent data suggest at least 15 susceptibility genes (NF-1, RET, VHL, HIF2a/EPAS1, TMEM127, KIF1Bbeta, MAX, PHD1, PHD2/EGLN1, FH, SDHA, SDHB, SDHC, SDHD, SDHAF2) involved in the pathogenesis of these neoplasms. Approximately 14% of sporadic tumors demonstrate somatic mutations in the same genes (205).

These tumors have been divided into two clusters based on the pathway alterations involved. Cluster 1 tumors have a hypoxic transcriptional signature due to mutations in SDH genes (1A) or the VHL gene (1B) or HIF2α. Cluster 2 tumors have enhanced kinase receptor signaling involving RET, NF1, TMEM127 or MAX genes (206–208). The mutations are also associated with different functional properties (209).

Mutations in the VHL gene in *von Hippel-Lindau* disease result in pheochromocytomas as well as sympathetic and parasympathetic paragangliomas. Different mutations are associated with variable constellations of the components of this disorder: hemangioblastomas, retinal angiomas, clear cell renal carcinoma, pheochromocytoma, pancreatic tumors,

lesions. The possibility of a multigenic effect was suggested by the association with a variant p53 gene in one instance (193).

Sporadic carcinomas exhibit a high frequency of somatic mutations of TP53 (195; 196) and rearrangements of the chromosomal locus 11 p15.5 associated with IGF-II hyperexpression (197; 198) (Figure 17.6). Others exhibit mutations of beta-catenin (199). LOH has been reported at 17p13, at 11q13, the site of the MEN1 gene, at 17q22–24, the site of PRKAR1A, and at 18p11, the site of the MC2-R gene (169; 170).

A microarray study using 10,000 genes (200) confirmed IGF-II as important in carcinoma and identified new candidate genes, including fibroblast growth factor receptor 1, osteopontin and 11β-hydroxylase (CYP11B1). Alterations in the expression of steroidogenic enzymes, cAMP signaling components and the IGF-II system were predictive of malignancy and, in malignant tumors, of recurrence (201; 202).

epididymal cystadenomas, and cysts of the kidney and pancreas. Type 1 mutations are not usually associated with pheochromocytomas or paragangliomas; patients with Type 2A, B or C mutations develop these tumors with differences in other associated manifestations.

The *succinate dehydrogenase (SDH) complex* is a mitochondrial enzyme complex composed of four subunits encoded by the SDHA, SDHB, SDHC and SDHD genes. SDHAF2 encodes the SDHAF2 protein which is responsible for flavination of SDHA. This complex regulates HIFα. Mutations in any of the SDH genes results in inactivation of the SDH complex, accumulation of succinate and reactive oxygen free radicals, stabilization of HIFα and activation of hypoxia-dependent pathways. Mutations in all four SDH genes and in SDHAF2 are associated with the development of pheochromocytoma and/or paraganglioma.

SDHA mutations are associated with adrenal and extra-adrenal lesions, including head and neck paragangliomas. SDHB-related tumors most commonly develop in extra-adrenal locations and have the highest rate of malignancy (210; 211) (Figure 17.7); patients with SDHB mutations also develop renal cell carcinoma, gastrointestinal stromal tumors, breast cancer and papillary thyroid cancer (212–214). SDHC and SDHD mutations are associated with head and neck paragangliomas that are not usually associated with catecholamine secretion (209; 215); a functional cardiac paraganglioma with a SDHC mutation has been reported (216). The SDHD gene exhibits maternal imprinting; therefore, disease is seen only with paternal transmission (217). Other mutations associated with SDH-related familial pheochromocytomas and paragangliomas include SDHAF2, which encodes the SDHAF2 protein responsible for flavination of SDHA, part of the SDHx complex (218; 219) that is a rare cause of multiple head and neck paragangliomas.

Activating mutations of the RET proto-oncogene in MEN2 lead to the development primarily of adrenal pheochromocytomas (220). These are usually benign, often bilateral and frequently associated with adrenal medullary hyperplasia. Clinically, they are characterized by hypersecretion of epinephrine (209). In contrast to medullary thyroid carcinoma, which is part of the MEN syndrome, there is no known specific genotype-phenotype correlation related to pheochromocytoma.

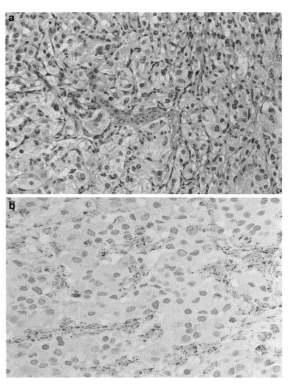

**Figure 17.7 Paraganglioma**
Approximately 35% of pheochromocytomas/paragangliomas are associated with germline mutations that predispose to these tumors. SDH-related bladder paraganglioma is illustrated (a). The tumor is negative for SDHB immunohistochemistry (b). Please note that the internal control (endothelial cells) is positive.

*Von Recklinghausen's disease* is due to inactivating mutations of the neurofibromatosis type 1 (NF-1) gene, resulting in loss of inhibition of the RAS and mTOR kinase pathways. Patients develop cutaneous or plexiform neurofibromas and other nerve sheath tumors, optic nerve gliomas, sphenoid bone dysplasia, pseudoarthrosis; café-au-lait spots and inguinal or axillary freckles and iris hamartomas (Lisch nodules). Patients with this disorder have a higher incidence of medullary thyroid carcinoma, parathyroid tumors, neuroendocrine tumors of the gut and lung, and pheochromocytomas (221). The latter, while rare, preferentially secrete epinephrine and have been reported to be malignant on occasion.

TMEM127, which encodes the TMEM-127 protein that is of unknown function (222; 223) and the MAX gene, a tumor suppressor involved in the MYC/MAX/MXD1 complex that is thought to regulate cell proliferation, differentiation and apoptosis by repressing MYC expression (224; 225); the latter two entities are mainly associated with adrenal pheochromocytomas. MAX mutations may be more frequently metastatic than other hereditary pheochromocytomas/paragangliomas, except those with SDHB/SDHD mutations. Gain-of-function mutations of HIF2α/EPAS1 (226) and mutations in the PHD2/EGLN1 gene, a prolyl hydroxylase that hydroxylates HIFα, mediating response to hypoxia (227) have been reported in rare patients with polycythemia and pheochromocytomas/paragangliomas. Using whole-exome sequencing, germline mutations in the FH gene encoding fumarate hydratase were identified recently in pheochromocytomas and paragangliomas with an increased risk of malignancy (228). Sporadic tumors have been reported to harbor mutations in the HRAS gene (229), but little else is known about the molecular alterations underlying their development.

## Tumors of the dispersed neuroendocrine system

Neuroendocrine tumors (NETs) are a heterogenous group of neoplasms arising from neuroendocrine cells of the diffuse endocrine system. These tumors can be seen in a variety of anatomic locations, and although their morphologic features and hormonal activities can be similar, their pathogenesis appears to vary with the site.

*Pulmonary NETs* are histologically divided into well-differentiated pulmonary neuroendocrine carcinoma with low-grade features (typical carcinoid tumor), well-differentiated pulmonary neuroendocrine carcinoma with intermediate grade features (atypical carcinoid tumor), and poorly differentiated (high-grade) pulmonary neuroendocrine carcinomas. High-grade neuroendocrine carcinomas are further divided into large cell and small cell subtypes. The tumorigenesis of pulmonary NETs is very complex. High-grade pulmonary neuroendocrine neoplasms often result from accumulation of cigarette smoking-related genetic and epigenetic alterations (230). No precursor lesions have been identified for high-grade neuroendocrine carcinomas, whereas precursor lesions for peripherally located low and intermediate grade well-differentiated pulmonary neuroendocrine tumors and tumorlets (microinvasive neuroendocrine tumors or microcarcinoids, <5mm) (Figure 17.8) are known as "diffuse idiopathic pulmonary neuroendocrine cell

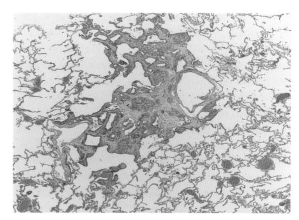

**Figure 17.8 Pulmonary neuroendocrine cell proliferations** The majority of pulmonary neuroendocrine tumors are sporadic; approximately 2% of MEN1 patients can present with multifocal well-differentiated pulmonary neuroendocrine neoplasms. This photomicrograph illustrates one of several tumorlets (microinvasive neuroendocrine tumors, <5mm) arising in a patient with MEN1 syndrome.

hyperplasia" (DIPNECH) (152). Centrally located well-differentiated pulmonary NETs are also not typically associated with precursor lesions.

The majority of pulmonary NETs are sporadic; approximately 2% of MEN1 patients can present with multifocal well-differentiated pulmonary neuroendocrine carcinomas (152). Although low-grade tumors exhibit a high frequency of LOH at 11q13, MEN1 mutations are consistently absent in sporadic pulmonary NETs (230). Instead, pulmonary NETs exhibit alterations in three important pathways, including the p53, Rb and Fas pathways, together with amplification of MYC genes, LOH at chromosomes 3p, 11q13 and 9p21, and mutations of NTRK genes (230–238). The molecular and prognostic features of high-grade pulmonary neuroendocrine carcinomas are different from well-differentiated pulmonary NETs. Low-grade (typical carcinoid tumors) and intermediate-grade (atypical carcinoid tumors) pulmonary NETs show low somatic mutation rate compared with high-grade tumors. LOH at chromosomes 3p and 9p21 and down-regulation of Fas (CD95) are common alterations in pulmonary NETs, with increasing incidence in high-grade neuroendocrine carcinomas (231; 232). High-grade neuroendocrine carcinomas of the lung are associated with inactivating mutations of TP53, RB, PTEN, CDKN2A, SLIT2, COBL and EPHA7 genes, together with amplification of MYC, MAD1L1 and FGFR1 (233; 234; 238–240).

Unlike well-differentiated NETs and small cell neuroendocrine carcinomas of the lung, NTRK gene mutations are identified exclusively in large cell pulmonary NETs (237).

Epigenetic changes are characteristic of pulmonary NETs. Methylation of the RASSF1A gene is identified in 45%, 71%, and 80% of low, intermediate and high-grade pulmonary neuroendocrine carcinomas, respectively, RAR-beta gene promoter methylation is frequent in small cell pulmonary neuroendocrine carcinoma, and inactivation of chromatin remodeling genes (MEN1 and SW1/SNF complex) is common (235; 236). Pulmonary NETs arising in different parts of the lung may have different cellular origins and/or molecular mechanisms of carcinogenesis (152; 230). High-grade pulmonary neuroendocrine carcinomas are different from both low and intermediate grade pulmonary NETs with regard to precursor lesions and molecular carcinogenesis.

*Thymic NETs* exhibit the same histologic spectrum as pulmonary NETs. These neoplasms are rare; thus, little is known about the molecular features of thymic NETs. Similar to pulmonary NETs, most are sporadic; approximately 2% of MEN1 patients present with thymic NETs arising in the background of neuroendocrine cell hyperplasia. While data on the molecular changes in sporadic tumors are scant, a small cohort of MEN1-related thymic NETs showed absence of LOH at the MEN1 locus at 11q13 and losses in the 1p region, suggesting the possibility of another tumor suppressor gene on 1p in addition to MEN1 mutations (241). Chromosomal imbalances increase with the grade of the tumor (242). Gains of 8q24 (MYC gene locus) are the most frequent alteration and one of the overlapping features between well-differentiated and poorly differentiated thymic NETs (242). cDNA profiling showed a remarkable over-expression of p21-activated kinase 3 (PAK3) and activation of the JNK pathway in well-differentiated thymic NETs associated with ectopic ACTH secretion (243). Hypomethylation of the POMC promoter in thymic carcinoids was also correlated with POMC over-expression and the ectopic ACTH syndrome (244).

*Pancreatic NETs* can be either sporadic or familial. The initial well-recognized familial syndromes associated with pancreatic NETs include MEN1 syndrome (MEN1 gene), VHL disease (VHL gene), Neurofibromatosis type 1 (NF1 gene) and tuberous sclerosis (TSC1 and TSC2 genes) (245). Recently, pancreatic NETs have also been linked to extra-colonic manifestations of Lynch syndrome (MMR genes), together with MEN4 syndrome (246; 247). Patients with MEN-4 syndrome harbor mutations in the cyclin-dependent kinase inhibitor gene (CDKN1B/p27Kip1) and present with MEN1 related states, including pancreatic NETs. Among these inherited syndromes, MEN1 syndrome is by far the most common familial syndrome associated with pancreatic NETs. In contrast to sporadic pancreatic NETs, MEN1-related pancreatic NETs are often diagnosed at an earlier age and are considered to be the most important cause of mortality in these patients. Multifocality is often associated with familial endocrine syndromes. From a morphological perspective, tuberous sclerosis- and NF-1-related pancreatic NETs cannot be distinguished from sporadic pancreatic NETs. However, those arising in the setting of MEN1 and VHL syndromes often exhibit characteristic associated findings such as peliosis of the non-tumorous islets, islet dysplasia, microadenoma or microadenomatosis, and ductulo-insular complexes (nesidioblastosis) (152). The genotype-phenotype correlations from MEN4 and Lynch syndromes are limited.

While multiple glucagon-expressing pancreatic NETs is often linked to MEN1 syndrome, a novel rare genetic disorder unassociated with MEN1, VHL or p27 mutations – *glucagon cell adenomatosis (Mahvash disease)* – has been defined (248; 249). To date, six cases have been reported; this disease is characterized by a single large pancreatic NET arising in the background of A or alpha (glucagon) cell hyperplasia of the islets leading to multiple glucagon-expressing microadenomas with occasional PP-cells (248; 250). This entity appears to be an example of a hyperplasia-neoplasia sequence that is seen in many endocrine system neoplasms (152). This entity was associated with germline inactivating mutations in the glucagon receptor (GR) gene (248); however, some patients harbor wild-type GR status (250).

The vast majority of pancreatic NETs are sporadic. Numerous studies have identified chromosomal gains or losses in sporadic pancreatic NETs. Allelic losses are commonly encountered at chromosomes loci 1p, 1q, 3p, 11p, 11q and 22q (245; 251). One of the most consistent findings in sporadic pancreatic NETs is LOH at chromosome 11q13 at the site of the MEN1 gene and up to 44% of sporadic pancreatic NETs harbor somatic inactivating MEN1 gene mutations. LOH on chromosome 3p is identified in one-third of pancreatic NETs, but no somatic mutations of the VHL gene (3p25-p26) are identified in sporadic pancreatic NETs (252).

Exomic sequencing identified that the most frequently mutated genes in pancreatic NETs involve proteins implicated in chromatin remodeling: 44% had somatic inactivating mutations in the MEN1 gene, and 43% had mutations in genes encoding the transcription/chromatin remodeling complex consisting of DAXX (death-domain-associated protein) and ATRX (α thalassemia/mental retardation syndrome X-linked) (253). Clinically, these mutations were associated with better prognosis than those with alterations in the mTOR pathway in 14% of tumors (253); however, a recent study failed to confirm these findings (254). The mTOR pathway changes explain the clinical response of some tumors to treatment with everolimus; however, there are data suggesting that the same common FGFR4 polymorphism that affects pituitary tumors, the FGFR4-G388R polymorphism, alters the clinical response (255).

DPC4/SMAD4 mutations have been reported in up to 20% of sporadic tumors (251). Mutations of TP53 and RB genes are more common in high-grade neuroendocrine carcinomas (256).

Epigenetic changes are also important in this area; the most commonly methylated genes in sporadic pancreatic NETs include RASSF/RASSF1A, MGMT, MLH1 and CDKN2A/p16 genes (257–259).

*Neuroendocrine tumors of the gastrointestinal tract* develop in multiple sites. Mutations in the genes implicated in other tumors do not seem to contribute to their pathogenesis. The most frequent alterations can be summarized as follows: (1) mutations in MEN1, NF-1, Reg1α (Reg) and CDKN1B/p27 genes; (2) LOH involving 11q13 (MEN1), 3p21.3, 18q22 (Smad4), 17p13 (p53) and the X chromosome; and (3) epigenetic silencing through promoter methylation of RASSF1A tumor suppressor gene (251).

Three types of *gastric NETs* have been described (260). Type I gastric NETs are associated with auto-immune chronic atrophic gastritis (A-CAG), and predominantly involve the corpus-fundus region; these have been considered to be reactive and potentially hyperplastic, but HUMARA clonality assays indicate that 87.5% of lesions as small as 0.5mm are monoclonal in the setting of A-CAG (261). Type II gastric NETs are associated with MEN1

and Zollinger-Ellison syndrome (MEN1-ZES). While germline mutation of the MEN1 gene is a signature of type II gastric NETs, LOH of 11q13 (MEN1) has also been reported in 48% of type I gastric NETs. Type III gastric NETs are sporadic neoplasms unassociated with MEN1 or A-CAG (152).

LOH at 3p21.3 and RASSF1A methylation has been exclusively reported in foregut (stomach, duodenum, pancreas) NETs, and these findings were absent in midgut (ileum and appendix) and hindgut NETs (260). A similar trend is also identified with MEN1 mutations and LOH of 11q13 and for the malignant behavior associated with allelic losses on chromosome X (262). In addition, the mutation of Reg1α gene is found in enterochomaffin-like cell (ECL) tumors in the setting of hypergastrinemia (263).

Colorectal NETs are uncommon in patients with MEN1 syndrome. Patients with MEN1 syndrome often have multiple small gastrin-producing G cell and somatostatin-producing D cell NETs in the small instestine (152). Patients with neurofibromatosis type 1 (NF-1, von Recklinghausen's disease) are also at risk of developing ampullary or periampullary NETs (152). Involvement of the duodenum is rare in VHL-related NET (264).

Genetic analyses of sporadic *appendiceal NETs* and *large intestinal NETs* are limited (265). Chromosomal gains, losses or both have been described in *small intestinal NETs*. While genetic alterations of intestinal NETs are still largely unknown; previous studies showed loss of chromosome 18 (251). Recently, LOH of the APC gene has been demonstrated in 15% of enterochromaffin cell ileal NETs (266). Methylation of RASSF1A and CTNNB1 genes has been reported to play an important role in the progression and metastasis of these tumors (267). Whole exome-genome sequencing studies have highlighted therapeutically relevant alterations affecting SRC, TGF-β pathway (through alterations in SMAD genes), aurora kinase A, epidermal growth factor receptor (EGFR), heat shock protein 90 and platelet-derived growth factor receptor (PDGFR), amplification of AKT1 or AKT2, and other alterations of PI3K/Akt/mTOR signaling genes in small bowel NETs (268). Moreover, 8% of small intestinal NETs harbor somatic CDKN1B mutation, suggesting cell cycle inhibitors as new treatment options for these neoplasms (269). A recent study revealed that of nine miRNAs, five (miR-96, -182, -183, -196a and -200a) were up-regulated during tumor progression, whereas four (miR-31, -129–5p, -133a and -215) were down-regulated in small intestinal NETs (270).

## Conclusions

This chapter reviewed the progress that has been made in understanding the molecular and epigenetic alterations that mediate neoplastic transformation and progression of endocrine tumors. The authors would like to recognize the advances; however, many questions remain to be answered. The molecular features of endocrine tumors are heterogeneous and depend on the anatomic location, as well as the tumor type. An important aspect of endocrine tumorigenesis is the role of epigenetic dysregulation, which often dictates the hormonal and proliferative behavior of these neoplasms.

## Learning points

- Thyroid tumors have a well-characterized molecular landscape the features of which are largely mutually exclusive and non-overlapping mutations or rearrangements in differentiated carcinomas, with evidence of cumulative events leading to progression and dedifferentiation.
- Familial genetic alterations underlie a number of tumors and preneoplastic conditions in neuroendocrine cells.
- Sporadic neuroendocrine tumors have a paucity of genetic alterations described to date.
- Epigenetic factors are implicated in the development, hormonal activity and progression of sporadic neuroendocrine neoplasms.

# References

1. Ezzat, S., Asa, S. L., Couldwell, W. T., Barr, C. E., Dodge, W. E., Vance, M. L. *et al.* The prevalence of pituitary adenomas: a systematic review. *Cancer* 2004; 101(3): 613–619.

2. Fink, A., Tomlinson, G., Freeman, J. L., Rosen, I. B. and Asa, S. L. Occult micropapillary carcinoma associated with benign follicular thyroid disease and unrelated thyroid neoplasms. *Mod Pathol* 1996; 9(8): 816–820.

3. DeLellis, R. A., Lloyd, R. V., Heitz, P. U. and Eng, C. (eds.), *Pathology and Genetics of Tumours of Endocrine Organs* (Lyon: IARC Press, 2004).

4. Asa, S. L. *Tumors of the Pituitary Gland. AFIP Atlas of Tumor Pathology*. Silverberg, S. G. (ed.), Series 4, Fascicle 15 (Silver Spring, MD: ARP Press, 2011).

5. Chandrasekharappa, S. C., Guru, S. C., Manickam, P., Olufemi, S. E., Collins, F. S., Emmert-Buck, M. R. *et al.* Positional cloning of the gene for multiple endocrine neoplasia-type 1. *Science* 1997; 276(5311): 404–407.

6. Trouillas, J., Labat-Moleur, F., Sturm, N., Kujas, M., Heymann, M.-F., Figarella-Branger, D. *et al.* Pituitary tumors and hyperplasia in multiple endocrine neoplasia type 1 syndrome (MEN1): a case-control study in a series of 77 patients versus 2509 non-MEN1 patients. *Am J Surg Pathol* 2008; 32(4): 534–543.

7. Zhuang, Z., Ezzat, S., Vortmeyer, A. O., Weil, R., Oldfield, E. H., Park, W. S. *et al.* Mutations of the MEN1 tumor suppressor gene in pituitary tumors. *Cancer Res* 1997; 57(24): 5446–5451.

8. Asa, S. L., Somers, K. and Ezzat, S. The MEN-1 gene is rarely down-regulated in pituitary adenomas. *J Clin Endocrinol Metab* 1998; 83(9): 3210–3212.

9. Pellegata, N. S., Quintanilla-Martinez, L., Siggelkow, H., Samson, E., Bink, K., Hofler, H. *et al.* Germ-line mutations in p27Kip1 cause a multiple endocrine neoplasia syndrome in rats and humans. *Proc Natl Acad Sci USA* 2006; 103(42): 15558–15563.

10. Lee, M. and Pellegata, N. S. Multiple endocrine neoplasia type 4. *Front Horm Res* 2013; 41: 63–78.

11. Georgitsi, M., Raitila, A., Karhu, A., van der Luijt, R. B., Aalfs, C. M., Sane, T. *et al.* Germline CDKN1B/p27Kip1 mutation in multiple endocrine neoplasia. *J Clin Endocrinol Metab* 2007; 92(8): 3321–3325.

12. Agarwal, S. K., Mateo, C. M. and Marx, S. J. Rare germline mutations in cyclin-dependent kinase inhibitor genes in multiple endocrine neoplasia type 1 and related states. *J Clin Endocrinol Metab* 2009; 94(5): 1826–1834.

13. Martucci, F., Trivellin, G. and Korbonits, M. Familial isolated pituitary adenomas: an emerging clinical entity. *J Endocrinol Invest* 2012; 35(11): 1003–1014.

14. Beckers, A., Aaltonen, L. A., Daly, A. F. and Karhu, A. Familial isolated pituitary adenomas (FIPA) and the pituitary adenoma predisposition due to mutations in the aryl hydrocarbon receptor interacting protein (AIP) gene. *Endocr Rev* 2013; 34(2): 239–277.

15. Carney, J. A., Gordon, H., Carpenter, P. C., Shenoy, B. V. and Go, V. L. The complex of myxomas, spotty pigmentation, and endocrine overactivity. *Medicine (Baltimore)* 1985; 64(4): 270–283.

16. Kirschner, L. S., Carney, J. A., Pack, S. D., Taymans, S. E., Giatzakis, C., Cho, Y. S. *et al.* Mutations of the gene encoding the protein kinase A type I-alpha

regulatory subunit in patients with the Carney complex. *Nat Genet* 2000; 26(1): 89–92.

17. Xekouki, P. and Stratakis, C. A. Succinate dehydrogenase (SDHx) mutations in pituitary tumors: could this be a new role for mitochondrial complex II and/or Krebs cycle defects? *Endocr Relat Cancer* 2012; 19(6): C33–C40.

18. Papathomas, T. G., Gaal, J., Corssmit, E. P., Oudijk, L., Korpershoek, E., Heimdal, K. *et al.* Non-pheochromocytoma (PCC)/paraganglioma (PGL) tumors in patients with succinate dehydrogenase-related PCC-PGL syndromes: a clinicopathological and molecular analysis. *Eur J Endocrinol* 2014; 170(1): 1–12.

19. Vallar, L., Spada, A. and Giannattasio, G. Altered $G_s$ and adenylate cyclase activity in human GH-secreting pituitary adenomas. *Nature* 1987; 330: 566–568.

20. Landis, C. A., Masters, S. B., Spada, A., Pace, A. M., Bourne, H. R. and Vallar, L. GTPase inhibiting mutations activate the alpha-chain of Gs ans stimulate adenylate cyclase in human pituitary tumors. *Nature* 1989; 340: 692–696.

21. Asa, S. L., DiGiovanni, R., Jiang, J., Ward, M. L., Loesch, K., Yamada, S. *et al.* A growth hormone receptor mutation impairs growth hormone autofeedback signaling in pituitary tumors. *Cancer Res* 2007; 67(15): 7505–7511.

22. Bhayana, S., Booth, G. L., Asa, S. L., Kovacs, K. and Ezzat, S. The implication of somatotroph adenoma phenotype to somatostatin analog responsiveness in acromegaly. *J Clin Endocrinol Metab* 2005; 90(11): 6290–6295.

23. Newey, P. J., Nesbit, M. A., Rimmer, A. J., Head, R. A., Gorvin, C. M., Attar, M. *et al.* Whole-exome sequencing studies of nonfunctioning pituitary adenomas. *J Clin Endocrinol Metab* 2013; 98(4): E796–800.

24. Levy, A., Hall, L., Yeundall, W. A. and Lightman, S. L. p53 gene mutations in pituitary adenomas: rare events. *Clin Endocrinol (Oxf)* 1994; 41: 809–814.

25. Kawashima, S. T., Usui, T., Sano, T., Iogawa, H., Hagiwara, H., Tamanaha, T. *et al.* P53 gene mutation in an atypical corticotroph adenoma with Cushing's disease. *Clin Endocrinol (Oxf)* 2009; 70(4): 656–657.

26. Karga, H. J., Alexander, J. M., Hedley-Whyte, E. T., Klibanski, A. and Jameson, J. L. Ras mutations in human pituitary tumors. *J Clin Endocrinol Metab* 1992; 74(4): 914–919.

27. Pei, L., Melmed, S., Scheithauer, B., Kovacs, K. and Prager, D. H-ras mutations in human pituitary carcinoma metastases. *J Clin Endocrinol Metab* 1994; 78: 842–846.

28. Cai, W. Y., Alexander, J. M., Hedley-Whyte, E. T., Scheithauer, B. W., Jameson, J. L., Zervas, N. T. *et al.* Ras mutations in human prolactinomas and pituitary carcinomas. *J Clin Endocrinol Metab* 1994; 78(1): 89–93.

29. Zahedi, A., Booth, G. L., Smyth, H. S., Farrell, W. E., Clayton, R. N., Asa, S. L. *et al.* Distinct clonal composition of primary and metastatic adrencorticotrophic hormone-producing pituitary carcinoma. *Clin Endocrinol (Oxf)* 2001; 55(4): 549–556.

30. Hinton, D. R., Hahn, J. A., Weiss, M. H. and Couldwell, W. T. Loss of Rb expression in an ACTH-secreting pituitary carcinoma. *Cancer Lett* 1998; 126(2): 209–214.

31. Tanizaki, Y., Jin, L., Scheithauer, B. W., Kovacs, K., Roncaroli, F. and Lloyd, R. V. P53 gene mutations in pituitary carcinomas. *Endocr Pathol* 2007; 18(4): 217–222.

32. De Martino, I., Fedele, M., Palmieri, D., Visone, R., Cappabianca, P., Wierinckx, A. *et al.* B-RAF mutations are a rare event in pituitary adenomas. *J Endocrinol Invest* 2007; 30(1): RC1–RC3.

33. Asa, S. L., Scheithauer, B. W., Bilbao, J. M., Horvath, E., Ryan, N., Kovacs, K. *et al.* A case for hypothalamic acromegaly: a clinicopathological study of six patients with hypothalamic gangliocytomas producing growth hormone-releasing factor. *J Clin Endocrinol Metab* 1984; 58(5): 796–803.

34. Stenzel-Poore, M. P., Cameron, V. A., Vaughan, J., Sawchenko, P. E. and Vale, W. Development of Cushing's syndrome in corticotropin-releasing factor transgenic mice. *Endocrinology* 1992; 130(6): 3378–3386.

35. Karl, M., Lamberts, S. W. J., Koper, J. W., Katz, D. A., Huizenga, N. E. and Kino, T. *et al.* Cushing's disease preceded by generalized glucocorticoid resistance: clinical consequences of a novel dominant-negative glucocorticoid receptor mutation. *Proc Assoc Am Physicians* 1996; 108(4): 296–307.

36. Lloyd, R. V. Estrogen-induced hyperplasia and neoplasia in the rat anterior pituitary gland. An immunohistochemical study. *Am J Pathol* 1983; 113(2): 198–206.

37. Schuff, K. G., Hentges, S. T., Kelly, M. A., Binart, N., Kelly, P. A., Iuvone, M. P. *et al.* Lack of prolactin receptor signaling in mice results in lactotroph proliferation and prolactinomas by dopamine-dependent and-independent mechanisms. *J Clin Invest* 2002; 110(7): 973–981.

38. Scheithauer, B. W., Kovacs, K. and Randall, R. V. The pituitary gland in untreated Addison's disease. A histologic and immunocytologic study of 18

adenohypophyses. *Arch Pathol Lab Med* 1983; 107(9): 484–487.

39. Scheithauer, B. W., Kovacs, K., Randall, R. V. and Ryan, N. Pituitary gland in hypothyroidism. Histologic and immunocytologic study. *Arch Pathol Lab Med* 1985; 109(6): 499–504.

40. Ando, S., Sarlis, N. J., Krishnan, J., Feng, X., Refetoff, S., Zhang, M. Q. *et al.* Aberrant alternative splicing of thyroid hormone receptor in a TSH-secreting pituitary tumor is a mechanism for hormone resistance. *Mol Endocrinol* 2001; 15(9): 1529–1538.

41. Haddad, G., Penabad, J. L., Bashey, H. M., Asa, S. L., Gennarelli, T. A., Cirullo, R. *et al.* Expression of activin/inhibin subunit messenger ribonucleic acids by gonadotroph adenomas. *J Clin Endocrinol Metab* 1994; 79: 1399–1403.

42. Penabad, J. L., Bashey, H. M., Asa, S. L., Haddad, G., Davis, K. D., Herbst, A. B. *et al.* Decreased follistatin gene expression in gonadotroph adenomas. *J Clin Endocrinol Metab* 1996; 81: 3397–3403.

43. Danila, D. C., Inder, W. J., Zhang, X., Alexander, J. M., Swearingen, B., Hedley-Whyte, E. T. *et al.* Activin effects on neoplastic proliferation of human pituitary tumors. *J Clin Endocrinol Metab* 2000; 85(3): 1009–1015.

44. Ezzat, S., Smyth, H. S., Ramyar, L. and Asa, S. L. Heterogeneous *in vivo* and *in vitro* expression of basic fibroblast growth factor by human pituitary adenomas. *J Clin Endocrinol Metab* 1995; 80: 878–884.

45. Zhu, X., Asa, S. L. and Ezzat, S. Fibroblast growth factor 2 and estrogen control the balance of histone 3 modifications targeting MAGE-A3 in pituitary neoplasia. *Clin Cancer Res* 2008; 14(7): 1984–1996.

46. Abbass, S. A. A., Asa, S. L. and Ezzat, S. Altered expression of fibroblast growth factor receptors in human pituitary adenomas. *J Clin Endocrinol Metab* 1997; 82: 1160–1166.

47. Zhu, X., Lee, K., Asa, S. L. and Ezzat, S. Epigenetic silencing through DNA and histone methylation of fibroblast growth factor receptor 2 in neoplastic pituitary cells. *Am J Pathol* 2007; 170(5): 1618–1628.

48. Ezzat, S., Zheng, L., Zhu, X. F., Wu, G. E. and Asa, S. L. Targeted expression of a human pituitary tumor-derived isoform of FGF receptor-4 recapitulates pituitary tumorigenesis. *J Clin Invest* 2002; 109(1): 69–78.

49. Yu, S., Asa, S. L., Weigel, R. J. and Ezzat, S. Pituitary tumor AP-2alpha recognizes a cryptic promoter in intron 4 of fibroblast growth factor receptor 4. *J Biol Chem* 2003; 278(22): 19597–19602.

50. Ezzat, S., Zheng, L., Winer, D. and Asa, S. L. Targeting N-cadherin through fibroblast growth factor receptor-4: distinct pathogenetic and therapeutic implications. *Mol Endocrinol* 2006; 20(11): 2965–2975.

51. Pei, L., Melmed, S., Scheithauer, B., Kovacs, K., Benedict, W. F. and Prager, D. Frequent loss of heterozygosity at the retinoblastoma susceptibility gene (RB) locus in aggressive pituitary tumors: evidence for a chromosome 13 tumor suppressor gene other than *RB. Cancer Res* 1995; 55(8): 1613–1616.

52. Woloschak, M., Roberts, J. L. and Post, K. D. Loss of heterozygosity at the retinoblastoma locus in human pituitary tumors. *Cancer* 1994; 74(2): 693–696.

53. Woloschak, M., Yu, A., Xiao, J. and Post, K. D. Abundance and state of phosphorylation of the retinoblastoma gene product in human pituitary tumors. *Int J Cancer* 1996; 67(1): 16–19.

54. Woloschak, M., Yu, A., Xiao, J. and Post, K. Frequent loss of the P16$^{INK4a}$ gene product in human pituitary tumors. *Cancer Res* 1996; 56(11): 2493–2496.

55. Woloschak, M., Yu, A. and Post, K. D. Frequent inactivation of the p16 gene in human pituitary tumors by gene methylation. *Mol Carcinog* 1997; 19(4): 221–224.

56. Dahia, P. L., Aguiar, R. C., Honegger, J., Fahlbush, R., Jordan, S., Lowe, D. G. *et al.* Mutation and expression analysis of the p27/kip1 gene in corticotrophin-secreting tumours. *Oncogene* 1998; 16(1): 69–76.

57. Zhang, X., Sun, H., Danila, D. C., Johnson, S. R., Zhou, Y., Swearingen, B. *et al.* Loss of expression of GADD45 gamma, a growth inhibitory gene, in human pituitary adenomas: implications for tumorigenesis. *J Clin Endocrinol Metab* 2002; 87(3): 1262–1267.

58. Bahar, A., Bicknell, J. E., Simpson, D. J., Clayton, R. N. and Farrell, W. E. Loss of expression of the growth inhibitory gene GADD45gamma, in human pituitary adenomas, is associated with CpG island methylation. *Oncogene* 2004; 23(4): 936–944.

59. Zhao, J., Dahle, D., Zhou, Y., Zhang, X. and Klibanski, A. Hypermethylation of the promoter region is associated with the loss of MEG3 gene expression in human pituitary tumors. *J Clin Endocrinol Metab* 2005; 90(4): 2179–2186.

60. Bahar, A., Simpson, D. J., Cutty, S. J., Bicknell, J. E., Hoban, P. R., Holley, S. *et al.* Isolation and characterization of a novel pituitary tumor apoptosis gene. *Mol Endocrinol* 2004; 18(7): 1827–1839.

61. Evans, C. O., Reddy, P., Brat, D. J., O'Neill, E. B., Craige, B., Stevens, V. L. *et al.* Differential expression

**291**

of folate receptor in pituitary adenomas. *Cancer Res* 2003; 63(14): 4218–4224.

62. Pei, L. and Melmed, S. Isolation and characterization of a pituitary tumor-transforming gene (PTTG). *Mol Endocrinol* 1997; 11: 433–441.

63. Wierinckx, A., Auger, C., Devauchelle, P., Reynaud, A., Chevallier, P., Jan, M. *et al.* A diagnostic marker set for invasion, proliferation, and aggressiveness of prolactin pituitary tumors. *Endocr Relat Cancer* 2007; 14(3): 887–900.

64. Moreno, C. S., Evans, C. O., Zhan, X., Okor, M., Desiderio, D. M. and Oyesiku, N. M. Novel molecular signaling and classification of human clinically nonfunctional pituitary adenomas identified by gene expression profiling and proteomic analyses. *Cancer Res* 2005; 65(22): 10214–10222.

65. Hussaini, I. M., Trotter, C., Zhao, Y., Abdel-Fattah, R., Amos, S., Xiao, A. *et al.* Matrix metalloproteinase-9 is differentially expressed in nonfunctioning invasive and noninvasive pituitary adenomas and increases invasion in human pituitary adenoma cell line. *Am J Pathol* 2007; 170(1): 356–365.

66. Galland, F., Lacroix, L., Saulnier, P., Dessen, P., Meduri, G., Bernier, M. *et al.* Differential gene expression profiles of invasive and non-invasive non-functioning pituitary adenomas based on microarray analysis. *Endocr Relat Cancer* 2010; 17(2): 361–371.

67. Ling, C., Pease, M., Shi, L., Punj, V., Shiroishi, M. S., Commins, D. *et al.* A pilot genome-scale profiling of DNA methylation in sporadic pituitary macroadenomas: association with tumor invasion and histopathological subtype. *PLoS ONE* 2014; 9(4): e96178.

68. Zhu, X., Mao, X., Hurren, R., Schimmer, A. D., Ezzat, S. and Asa, S. L. Deoxyribonucleic acid methyltransferase 3B promotes epigenetic silencing through histone 3 chromatin modifications in pituitary cells. *J Clin Endocrinol Metab* 2008; 93(9): 3610–3617.

69. Ezzat, S., Mader, R., Yu, S., Ning, T., Poussier, P. and Asa, S. L. Ikaros integrates endocrine and immune system development. *J Clin Invest* 2005; 115(4): 1021–1029.

70. Ezzat, S., Mader, R., Fischer, S., Yu, S., Ackerley, C. and Asa, S. L. An essential role for the hematopoietic transcription factor Ikaros in hypothalamic-pituitary-mediated somatic growth. *Proc Natl Acad Sci USA* 2006; 103(7): 2214–2219.

71. Ezzat, S., Yu, S. and Asa, S. L. The zinc finger Ikaros transcription factor regulates pituitary growth hormone and prolactin gene expression through distinct effects on chromatin accessibility. *Mol Endocrinol* 2005; 19(4): 1004–1011.

72. Ezzat, S., Yu, S. and Asa, S. L. Ikaros isoforms in human pituitary tumors: distinct localization, histone acetylation, and activation of the 5' fibroblast growth factor receptor-4 promoter. *Am J Pathol* 2003; 163(3): 1177–1184.

73. Loeper, S., Asa, S. L. and Ezzat, S. Ikaros modulates cholesterol uptake: a link between tumor suppression and differentiation. *Cancer Res* 2008; 68(10): 3715–3723.

74. Ezzat, S., Zhu, X., Loeper, S., Fischer, S. and Asa, S. L. Tumor-derived Ikaros 6 acetylates the Bcl-XL promoter to up-regulate a survival signal in pituitary cells. *Mol Endocrinol* 2006; 20(11): 2976–2986.

75. Dorman, K., Shen, Z., Yang, C., Ezzat, S. and Asa, S. L. CtBP1 interacts with ikaros and modulates pituitary tumor cell survival and response to hypoxia. *Mol Endocrinol* 2012; 26(3): 447–457.

76. Fedele, M., Battista, S., Kenyon, L., Baldassarre, G., Fidanza, V., Klein-Szanto, A. J. *et al.* Overexpression of the HMGA2 gene in transgenic mice leads to the onset of pituitary adenomas. *Oncogene* 2002; 21(20): 3190–3198.

77. Fedele, M., Pentimalli, F., Baldassarre, G., Battista, S., Klein-Szanto, A. J. P., Kenyon, L. *et al.* Transgenic mice overexpressing the wild-type form of the HMGA1 gene develop mixed growth hormone/prolactin cell pituitary adenomas and natural killer cell lymphomas. *Oncogene* 2005; 24(21): 3427–3435.

78. Fedele, M., Visone, R., De Martino, I., Troncone, G., Palmieri, D., Battista, S. *et al.* HMGA2 induces pituitary tumorigenesis by enhancing E2F1 activity. *Cancer Cell* 2006; 9(6): 459–471.

79. De Martino, I., Visone, R., Wierinckx, A., Palmieri, D., Ferraro, A., Cappabianca, P. *et al.* HMGA proteins up-regulate CCNB2 gene in mouse and human pituitary adenomas. *Cancer Res* 2009; 69(5): 1844–1850.

80. Finelli, P., Pierantoni, G. M., Giardino, D., Losa, M., Rodeschini, O., Fedele, M. *et al.* The High Mobility Group A2 gene is amplified and overexpressed in human prolactinomas. *Cancer Res* 2002; 62(8): 2398–2405.

81. Evans, C. O., Moreno, C. S., Zhan, X., McCabe, M. T., Vertino, P. M., Desiderio, D. M. *et al.* Molecular pathogenesis of human prolactinomas identified by gene expression profiling, RT-qPCR, and proteomic analyses. *Pituitary* 2008; 11(3): 231–245.

82. Qian, Z. R., Asa, S. L., Siomi, H., Siomi, M. C., Yoshimoto, K., Yamada, S. *et al.* Overexpression of HMGA2 relates to reduction of the let-7 and its relationship to clinicopathological features in pituitary adenomas. *Mod Pathol* 2009; 22(3): 431–441.

83. D'Angelo, D., Palmieri, D., Mussnich, P., Roche, M., Wierinckx, A., Raverot, G. *et al.* Altered microRNA expression profile in human pituitary GH adenomas: down-regulation of miRNA targeting HMGA1, HMGA2, and E2F1. *J Clin Endocrinol Metab* 2012; 97(7): E1128–1138.

84. Tateno, T., Asa, S. L., Zheng, L., Mayr, T., Ullrich, A. and Ezzat, S. The FGFR4-G388R polymorphism promotes mitochondrial STAT3 serine phosphorylation to facilitate pituitary growth hormone cell tumorigenesis. *PLoS Genet* 2011; 7(12): e1002400.

85. Nakano-Tateno, T., Tateno, T., Hlaing, M. M., Zheng, L., Yoshimoto, K., Yamada, S. *et al.* FGFR4 polymorphic variants modulate phenotypic features of Cushing disease. *Mol Endocrinol* 2014; 28(4): 525–533.

86. Kondo, T., Ezzat, S. and Asa, S. L. Pathogenetic mechanisms in thyroid follicular-cell neoplasia. *Nat Rev Cancer* 2006; 6(4): 292–306.

87. Robbins, J. and Schneider, A. B. Thyroid cancer following exposure to radioactive iodine. *Rev Endocr Metab Disord* 2000; 1(3): 197–203.

88. Williams, D. Radiation carcinogenesis: lessons from Chernobyl. *Oncogene* 2008; 27(Suppl 2): S9–18.

89. Khan, A., Smellie, J., Nutting, C., Harrington, K. and Newbold, K. Familial nonmedullary thyroid cancer: a review of the genetics. *Thyroid* 2010; 20(7): 795–801.

90. Mulligan, L. M., Kwok, J. B. J., Healey, C. S., Elsdon, M. J., Eng, C., Gardner, E. *et al.* Germ-line mutations of the RET proto-oncogene in multiple endocrine neoplasia type 2A. *Nature* 1993; 363(6428): 458–460.

91. Drexhage, H. A., Bottazzo, G. F., Bitensky, L., Chayen, J. and Doniach, D. Evidence for thyroid growth-stimulating immunoglobulin in some goitrous thyroid diseases. *Lancet* 1980; 2: 287–292.

92. Van der Gaag, R. D., Drexhage, H. A., Wiersinga, W. M., Brown, R. S., Docter, R., Bottazzo, G. F. *et al.* Further studies on thyroid growth-stimulating immunoglobulins in euthyroid nonendemic goiter. *J Clin Endocrinol Metab* 1985; 60(5): 972–979.

93. Apel, R. L., Ezzat, S., Bapat, B. V., Pan, N., LiVolsi, V. A. and Asa, S. L. Clonality of thyroid nodules in sporadic goiter. *Diag Mol Pathol* 1995; 4: 113–121.

94. Aeschimann, S., Kopp, P. A., Kimura, E. T., Zbaeren, J., Tobler, A., Fey, M. F. *et al.* Morphological and functional polymorphism within clonal thyroid nodules. *J Clin Endocrinol Metab* 1993; 77: 846–851.

95. Kopp, P., Kimura, E. T., Aeschimann, S., Oestreicher, M., Tobler, A., Fey, M. F. *et al.* Polyclonal and monoclonal thyroid nodules coexist within human multinodular goiters. *J Clin Endocrinol Metab* 1994; 79: 134–139.

96. Boerner, S. L. and Asa, S. L. *Biopsy Interpretation of the Thyroid* (Philadelphia, PA: Lippincott Williams & Wilkins, 2009).

97. Mete, O. and Asa, S. L. Pitfalls in the diagnosis of follicular epithelial proliferations of the thyroid. *Adv Anat Pathol* 2012; 19(6): 363–373.

98. Parma, J., Duprez, L., van Sande, J., Cochaux, P., Gervy, C., Mockel, J. *et al.* Somatic mutations in the thyrotropin recptor gene cause hyperfunctioning thyroid adenomas. *Nature* 1993; 365: 649–651.

99. van Sande, J., Parma, J., Tonacchera, M., Swillens, S., Dumont, J. and Vassart, G. Genetic basis of endocrine disease. Somatic and germline mutations of the TSH receptor gene in thyroid disease. *J Clin Endocrinol Metab* 1995; 80: 2577–2585.

100. Holzapfel, H. P., Fuhrer, D., Wonerow, P., Weinland, G., Scherbaum, W. A. and Paschke, R. Identification of constitutively activating somatic thyrotropin receptor mutations in a subset of toxic multinodular goiters. *J Clin Endocrinol Metab* 1997; 82(12): 4229–4233.

101. Parma, J., Duprez, L., Van Sandem, H., Hermans, J., Rocmans, P., Van Vliet, G. *et al.* Diversity and prevalence of somatic mutations in the thyrotropin receptor and Gs alpha genes as a cause of toxic thryoid adenomas. *J Clin Endocrinol Metab* 1997; 82(8): 2695–2701.

102. Krohn, D., Fuhrer, D., Holzapfel, H. and Paschke, R. Clonal origin of toxic thyroid nodules with constitutively activating thyrotropin receptor mutations. *J Clin Endocrinol Metab* 1998; 83: 180–184.

103. Krohn, K., Fuhrer, D., Bayer, Y., Eszlinger, M., Brauer, V., Neumann, S. *et al.* Molecular pathogenesis of euthyroid and toxic multinodular goiter. *Endocr Rev* 2005; 26(4): 504–524.

104. Bahn, R. S., Burch, H. B., Cooper, D. S., Garber, J. R., Greenlee, M. C., Klein, I. *et al.* Hyperthyroidism and other causes of thyrotoxicosis: management guidelines of the American Thyroid Association and American Association of Clinical Endocrinologists. *Endocr Pract* 2011; 17(3): 456–520.

105. Nikiforova, M. N. and Nikiforov, Y. E. Molecular diagnostics and predictors in thyroid cancer. *Thyroid* 2009; 19(12): 1351–1361.

106. Nikiforov, Y. E. and Nikiforova, M. N. Molecular genetics and diagnosis of thyroid cancer. *Nat Rev Endocrinol* 2011; 7(10): 569–580.

107. Hamatani, K., Mukai, M., Takahashi, K., Hayashi, Y., Nakachi, K. and Kusunoki, Y. Rearranged anaplastic lymphoma kinase (ALK) gene in adult-onset papillary thyroid cancer amongst atomic bomb survivors. *Thyroid* 2012; 22(11): 1153–1159.

108. Leeman-Neill, R. J., Kelly, L. M., Liu, P., Brenner, A. V., Little, M. P., Bogdanova, T. I. et al. ETV6-NTRK3 is a common chromosomal rearrangement in radiation-associated thyroid cancer. *Cancer* 2014; 120(6): 799–807.

109. Xing, M. Prognostic utility of BRAF mutation in papillary thyroid cancer. *Mol Cell Endocrinol* 2010; 321(1): 86–93.

110. Cheng, S., Serra, S., Mercado, M., Ezzat, S. and Asa, S. L. A high-throughput proteomic approach provides distinct signatures for thyroid cancer behavior. *Clin Cancer Res* 2011; 17(8): 2385–2394.

111. Cameselle-Teijeiro, J. and Chan, J. K. Cribiform-morular variant of papillary carcinoma: a distinct variant representing the sporadic counterpart of familial adenomatous polyposis-associated with thyroid carcinoma. *Mod Pathol* 1999; 12(4): 400–411.

112. Xu, B., Yoshimoto, K., Miyauchi, A., Kuma, S., Mizusawa, N., Hirokawa, M. et al. Cribiform-morular variant of papillary thyroid carcinoma: a pathological and molecular genetic study with evidence of frequent somatic mutations in exon 3 of the beta-catenin gene. *J Pathol* 2003; 199(1): 58–67.

113. Kuma, S., Hirokawa, M., Xu, B., Miyauchi, A., Kukudo, K. and Sano, T. Cribriform-morular variant of papillary thyroid carcinoma. Report of a case showing morules with peculiar nuclear clearing. *Acta Cytol* 2004; 48(3): 431–436.

114. Ito, Y., Miyauchi, A., Ishikawa, H., Hirokawa, M., Kudo, T., Tomoda, C. et al. Our experience of treatment of cribriform morular variant of papillary thyroid carcinoma; difference in clinicopathological features of FAP-associated and sporadic patients. *Endocr J* 2011; 58(8): 685–689.

115. Winer, D. A., Winer, S., Rotstein, L., Asa, S. L. and Mete, O. Villous papillary thyroid carcinoma: a variant associated with marfan syndrome. *Endocr Pathol* 2012; 23(4): 254–259.

116. Nikiforova, M. N., Kimura, E. T., Gandhi, M., Biddinger, P. W., Knauf, J. A., Basolo, F. et al. BRAF mutations in thyroid tumors are restricted to papillary carcinomas and anaplastic or poorly differentiated carcinomas arising from papillary carcinomas. *J Clin Endocrinol Metab* 2003; 88(11): 5399–5404.

117. Zhu, Z., Gandhi, M., Nikiforova, M. N., Fischer, A. H. and Nikiforov, Y. E. Molecular profile and clinical-pathologic features of the follicular variant of papillary thyroid carcinoma. An unusually high prevalence of ras mutations. *Am J Clin Pathol* 2003; 120(1): 71–77.

118. Trovisco, V., Vieira De Castro, I., Soares, P., Máximo, V., Silva, P., Magalhães, J. et al. BRAF mutations are associated with some histological types of papillary thyroid carcinoma. *J Pathol* 2004; 202(2): 247–251.

119. Trovisco, V., Soares, P., Preto, A., de Castro, I. V., Lima, J., Castro, P. et al. Type and prevalence of BRAF mutations are closely associated with papillary thyroid carcinoma histotype and patients' age but not with tumour aggressiveness. *Virchows Arch* 2005; 446(6): 589–595.

120. Adeniran, A. J., Zhu, Z., Gandhi, M., Steward, D. L., Fidler, J. P., Giordano, T. J. et al. Correlation between genetic alterations and microscopic features, clinical manifestations, and prognostic characteristics of thyroid papillary carcinomas. *Am J Surg Pathol* 2006; 30(2): 216–222.

121. Sobrinho-Simoes, M., Maximo, V., Rocha, A. S., Trovisco, V., Castro, P., Preto, A. et al. Intragenic mutations in thyroid cancer. *Endocrinol Metab Clin North Am* 2008; 37(2): 333–362, viii.

122. Fukahori, M., Yoshida, A., Hayashi, H., Yoshihara, M., Matsukuma, S., Sakuma, Y. et al. The associations between RAS mutations and clinical characteristics in follicular thyroid tumors: new insights from a single center and a large patient cohort. *Thyroid* 2012; 22(7): 683–689.

123. Gupta, N., Dasyam, A. K., Carty, S. E., Nikiforova, M. N., Ohori, N. P., Armstrong, M. et al. RAS mutations in thyroid FNA specimens are highly predictive of predominantly low-risk follicular-pattern cancers. *J Clin Endocrinol Metab* 2013; 98(5): E914–922.

124. Virk, R. K., Van Dyke, A. L., Finkelstein, A., Prasad, A., Gibson, J., Hui, P. et al. BRAFV600E mutation in papillary thyroid microcarcinoma: a genotype-phenotype correlation. *Mod Pathol* 2013; 26(1): 62–70.

125. The Cancer Genome Atlas Research Network. Integrated genomic characterization of papillary thyroid carcinoma. *Cell* 2014; 159(3): 676–690.

126. Asa, S. L. and Mete, O. Thyroid neoplasms of follicular cell derivation: a simplified approach.

*Semin Diagn Pathol* 2013; 30(3): 178–185.

127. Zipkin, P. Hyalinahniliche collagene kugeln als produkte epitelialer zellen in malignen strumen. *Virchows Arch* 1905; 182: 374–406.

128. Masson, P. Cancers thyroidiens a polarite alternative. *Bull Cancer* 1922; 11: 350–355.

129. Ward, J. V., Murray, D., Horvath, E., Kovacs, K. and Bauman, A. Hyaline cell tumor of the thyroid with massive accumulation of cytoplasmic microfilaments. *Lab Invest* 1982; 46(Abstract 88A).

130. Carney, J. A., Ryan, J. and Goellner, J. R. Hyalinizing trabecular adenoma of the thyroid gland. *Am J Surg Pathol* 1987; 11: 583–591.

131. Bronner, M. P., LiVolsi, V. A. and Jennings, T. A. PLAT: paraganglioma-like adenomas of the thyroid. *Surg Pathol* 1988; 1: 383–389.

132. Sambade, C., Franssila, K., Cameselle-Teijeiro, J., Nesland, J. and Sobrinho-Simoes, M. Hyalinizing trabecular adenoma: a misnomer for a peculiar tumor of the thyroid gland. *Endocr Pathol* 1991; 2: 83–91.

133. Molberg, K. and Albores-Saavedra, J. Hyalinizing trabecular carcinoma of the thyroid gland. *Hum Pathol* 1994; 25(2): 192–197.

134. McCluggage, W. G. and Sloan, J. M. Hyalinizing trabecular carcinoma of the thyroid gland. *Histopathology* 1996; 28(4): 357–362.

135. Cheung, C. C., Boerner, S. L., MacMillan, C. M., Ramyar, L. and Asa, S. L. Hyalinizing trabecular tumor of the thyroid: a variant of papillary carcinoma proved by molecular genetics. *Am J Surg Pathol* 2000; 24(12): 1622–1626.

136. Papotti, M., Volante, M., Giuliano, A., Fassina, A., Fusco, A., Bussolati, G. et al. RET/PTC activation in hyalinizing trabecular tumors of the thyroid. *Am J Surg Pathol* 2000; 24(12): 1615–1621.

137. Li, M., Carcangiu, M. L. and Rosai, J. Abnormal intracellular and extracellular distribution of base membrane material in papillary carcinoma and hyalinizing trabecular tumors of the thyroid: implication for deregulation secretory pathways. *Hum Pathol* 1997; 28: 1366–1372.

138. Boerner, S. L. and Asa, S. L. Hyalinizing trabecular tumor of the thyroid gland: much ado about nothing? *Am J Clin Pathol* 2004; 122(4): 495–496.

139. Carcangiu, M. L., Zampi, G. and Rosai, J. Poorly differentiated ("insular") thyroid carcinoma. A reinterpretation of Langhans' "wuchernde Struma." *Am J Surg Pathol* 1984; 8(9): 655–668.

140. Garcia-Rostan, G., Camp, R. L., Herrero, A., Carcangiu, M. L., Rimm, D. L. and Tallini, G. Beta-catenin dysregulation in thyroid neoplasms: down-regulation, aberrant nuclear expression, and CTNNB1 exon 3 mutations are markers for aggressive tumor phenotypes and poor prognosis. *Am J Pathol* 2001; 158(3): 987–996.

141. Garcia-Rostan, G., Zhao, H., Camp, R. L., Pollan, M., Herrero, A., Pardo, J. et al. ras mutations are associated with aggressive tumor phenotypes and poor prognosis in thyroid cancer. *J Clin Oncol* 2003; 21(17): 3226–3235.

142. Costa, A. M., Herrero, A., Fresno, M. F., Heymann, J., Alvarez, J. A., Cameselle-Teijeiro, J. et al. BRAF mutation associated with other genetic events identifies a subset of aggressive papillary thyroid carcinoma. *Clin Endocrinol (Oxf)* 2008; 68(4): 618–634.

143. Volante, M., Rapa, I., Gandhi, M., Bussolati, G., Giachino, D., Papotti, M. et al. RAS mutations are the predominant molecular alteration in poorly differentiated thyroid carcinomas and bear prognostic impact. *J Clin Endocrinol Metab* 2009; 94(12): 4735–4741.

144. Nikiforova, M. N., Wald, A. I., Roy, S., Durso, M. B. and Nikiforov, Y. E. Targeted next-generation sequencing panel (ThyroSeq) for detection of mutations in thyroid cancer. *J Clin Endocrinol Metab* 2013; 98(11): E1852–1860.

145. Smallridge, R. C., Ain, K. B., Asa, S. L., Bible, K. C., Brierley, J. D., Burman, K. D. et al. American Thyroid Association guidelines for management of patients with anaplastic thyroid cancer. *Thyroid* 2012; 22(11): 1104–1139.

146. Hofstra, R. M. W., Landsvater, R. M., Ceccherini, I., Stulp, R. P., Stelwagen, T., Luo, Y. et al. A mutation in the RET proto-oncogene associated with multiple endocrine neoplasia type 2B and sporadic medullary thyroid carcinoma. *Nature* 1994; 367: 375–376.

147. Wells, S. A., Jr., Asa, S. L., Dralle, H., Elisei, R., Evans, D. B., Gagel, R. F. et al. Revised American Thyroid Association guidelines for the management of medullary thyroid carcinoma. *Thyroid*; in press.

148. Marsh, D. J., Robinson, B. G., Andrew, S., Richardson, A. L., Pojer, R., Schnitzler, M. et al. A rapid screening method for the detection of mutations in the RET proto-oncogene in multiple endocrine neoplasia type 2A and familial medullary thyroid carcinoma families. *Genomics* 1994; 23: 477–479.

149. Castellone, M. D. and Santoro, M. Dysregulated RET signaling in thyroid cancer. *Endocrinol Metab Clin North Am* 2008; 37(2): 363–74, viii.

150. Jimenez, C., Hu, M. I. and Gagel, R. F. Management of medullary thyroid carcinoma. *Endocrinol*

*Metab Clin North Am* 2008; 37(2): 481–496.

151. Kloos, R. T., Eng, C., Evans, D. B., Francis, G. L., Gagel, R. F., Gharib, H. *et al.* Medullary thyroid cancer: management guidelines of the American Thyroid Association. *Thyroid* 2009; 19(6): 565–612.

152. Mete, O. and Asa, S. L. Precursor lesions of endocrine system neoplasms. *Pathol* 2013; 45(3): 316–330.

153. Agrawal, N., Jiao, Y., Sausen, M., Leary, R., Bettegowda, C., Roberts, N. J. *et al.* Exomic sequencing of medullary thyroid cancer reveals dominant and mutually exclusive oncogenic mutations in RET and RAS. *J Clin Endocrinol Metab* 2013; 98(2): E364–369.

154. Arnold, A., Staunton, C. E., Kim, H. G., Gaz, R. D. and Kronenberg, H. M. Monoclonality and abnormal parathyroid hormone genes in parathyroid adenomas. *New Engl J Med* 1988; 318(11): 658–662.

155. Arnold, A. and Kim, H. G. Clonal loss of one chromosome 11 in a parathyroid adenoma. *J Clin Endocrinol Metab* 1989; 69(3): 496–499.

156. Alvelos, M. I., Vinagre, J., Fonseca, E., Barbosa, E., Teixeira-Gomes, J., Sobrinho-Simoes, M. *et al.* MEN1 intragenic deletions may represent the most prevalent somatic event in sporadic primary hyperparathyroidism. *Eur J Endocrinol* 2013; 168(2): 119–128.

157. Arnold, A., Kim, H. G., Gaz, R. D., Eddy, R. L., Fukushima, Y., Byers, M. G. *et al.* Molecular cloning and chromosomal mapping of DNA rearranged with the parathyroid hormone gene in a parathyroid adenoma. *J Clin Invest* 1989; 83(6): 2034–2040.

158. Arnold, A. Molecular mechanisms of parathyroid neoplasia. *Endocrinol Metab Clin North Am* 1994; 23(1): 93–107.

159. Schulte, K. M. and Talat, N. Diagnosis and management of parathyroid cancer. *Nat Rev Endocrinol* 2012; 8(10): 612–622.

160. Erovic, B. M., Goldstein, D. P., Kim, D., Mete, O., Brierley, J., Tsang, R. *et al.* Parathyroid cancer: outcome analysis of 16 patients treated at the Princess Margaret Hospital. *Head Neck* 2013; 35(1): 35–39.

161. Cryns, V. L., Thor, A., Zu, H.-J., Hu, S.-X., Wierman, M. E., Vickery, A. L., Jr. *et al.* Loss of the retinoblastoma tumor-suppressor gene in parathyroid carcinoma. *New Engl J Med* 1994; 330: 757–761.

162. Erickson, L. A., Jin, L., Wollan, P., Thompson, G. B., van Heerden, J. A. and Lloyd, R. V. Parathyroid hyperplasia, adenomas, and carcinomas: differential expression of p27Kip1 protein. *Am J Surg Pathol* 1999; 23(3): 288–295.

163. Cryns, V. L., Rubio, M.-P., Thor, A. D., Louis, D. N. and Arnold, A. p53 abnormalities in human parathyroid carcinoma. *J Clin Endocrinol Metab* 1994; 78: 1320–1324.

164. Bergero, N., De Pompa, R., Sacerdote, C., Gasparri, G., Volante, M., Bussolati, G. *et al.* Galectin-3 expression in parathyroid carcinoma: immunohistochemical study of 26 cases. *Hum Pathol* 2005; 36(8): 908–914.

165. Erovic, B. M., Harris, L., Jamali, M., Goldstein, D. P., Irish, J. C., Asa, S. L. *et al.* Biomarkers of parathyroid carcinoma. *Endocr Pathol* 2012; 23(4): 221–231.

166. Abbona, G. C., Papotti, M., Gasparri, G. and Bussolati, G. Proliferative activity in parathyroid tumors as detected by Ki-67 immunostaining. *Hum Pathol* 1995; 26(2): 135–138.

167. Shattuck, T. M., Valimaki, S., Obara, T., Gaz, R. D., Clark, O. H., Shoback, D. *et al.* Somatic and germ-line mutations of the HRPT2 gene in sporadic parathyroid carcinoma. *New Engl J Med* 2003; 349(18): 1722–1729.

168. Gill, A. J., Clarkson, A., Gimm, O., Keil, J., Dralle, H., Howell, V. M. *et al.* Loss of nuclear expression of parafibromin distinguishes parathyroid carcinomas and hyperparathyroidism-jaw tumor (HPT-JT) syndrome-related adenomas from sporadic parathyroid adenomas and hyperplasias. *Am J Surg Pathol* 2006; 30(9): 1140–1149.

169. Sidhu, S., Marsh, D. J., Theodosopoulos, G., Philips, J., Bambach, C. P., Campbell, P. *et al.* Comparative genomic hybridization analysis of adrenocortical tumors. *J Clin Endocrinol Metab* 2002; 87(7): 3467–3474.

170. Russell, A. J., Sibbald, J., Haak, H., Keith, W. N. and McNicol, A. M. Increasing genome instability in adrenocortical carcinoma progression with involvement of chromosomes 3, 9 and X at the adenoma stage. *Br J Cancer* 1999; 81(4): 684–689.

171. Beuschlein, F., Fassnacht, M., Assie, G., Calebiro, D., Stratakis, C. A., Osswald, A. *et al.* Constitutive activation of PKA catalytic subunit in adrenal Cushing's syndrome. *New Engl J Med* 2014; 370(11): 1019–1028.

172. Latronico, A. C. Role of ACTH receptor in adrenocortical tumor formation. *Braz J Med Biol Res* 2000; 33(10): 1249–1252.

173. Assié, G., Libé, R., Espiard, S., Rizk-Rabin, M., Guimier, A. Luscap, W. *et al.* ARMC5 mutations in macronodular adrenal hyperplasia with Cushing's syndrome. *N Engl J Med* 2013; 369(22): 2105–2114.

174. Chui, M. H., Ozbey, N. C., Ezzat, S., Kapran, Y., Erbil, Y. and Asa, S. L. Case report: adrenal LH/hCG receptor overexpression

and gene amplification causing pregnancy-induced Cushing's syndrome. *Endocr Pathol* 2009; 20(4): 256–261.

175. Funder, J. W. The genetic basis of primary aldosteronism. *Curr Hypertens Rep* 2012; 14(2): 120–124.

176. Beuschlein, F., Boulkroun, S., Osswald, A., Wieland, T., Nielsen, H. N., Lichtenauer, U. D. *et al.* Somatic mutations in ATP1A1 and ATP2B3 lead to aldosterone-producing adenomas and secondary hypertension. *Nat Genet* 2013; 45(4): 440–442.

177. Williams, T. A., Monticone, S., Schack, V. R., Stindl, J., Burrello, J., Buffolo, F. *et al.* Somatic ATP1A1, ATP2B3, and KCNJ5 mutations in aldosterone-producing adenomas. *Hypertension* 2014; 63(1): 188–195.

178. Azizan, E. A., Poulsen, H., Tuluc, P., Zhou, J., Clausen, M. V., Lieb, A. *et al.* Somatic mutations in ATP1A1 and CACNA1D underlie a common subtype of adrenal hypertension. *Nat Genet* 2013; 45(9): 1055–1060.

179. Scholl, U. I., Goh, G., Stolting, G., de Oliveira, R. C., Choi, M., Overton, J. D. *et al.* Somatic and germline CACNA1D calcium channel mutations in aldosterone-producing adenomas and primary aldosteronism. *Nat Genet* 2013; 45(9): 1050–1054.

180. Berthon, A., Drelon, C., Ragazzon, B., Tissier, F., Amar, L., Samson-Couterie, B. *et al.* WNT/beta-catenin signalling is activated in aldosterone-producing adenomas and controls aldosterone production. *Hum Mol Genet* 2014; 23(4): 889–905.

181. Waldmann, J., Bartsch, D. K., Kann, P. H., Fendrich, V., Rothmund, M. and Langer, P. Adrenal involvement in multiple endocrine neoplasia type 1: results of 7 years prospective screening.

*Langenbecks Arch Surg* 2007; 392(4): 437–443.

182. Groussin, L., Cazabat, L., Rene-Corail, F., Jullian, E. and Bertherat, J. Adrenal pathophysiology: lessons from the Carney complex. *Horm Res* 2005; 64(3): 132–139.

183. Libe, R. and Bertherat, J. Molecular genetics of adrenocortical tumours, from familial to sporadic diseases. *Eur J Endocrinol* 2005; 153(4): 477–487.

184. Carney, J. A., Young, W. F. and Stratakis, C. A. Primary bimorphic adrenocortical disease: cause of hypercortisolism in McCune-Albright syndrome. *Am J Surg Pathol* 2011; 35(9): 1311–1326.

185. Velazquez-Fernandez, D., Caramuta, S., Ozata, D. M., Akcakaya, P., Xie, H., Hoog, A. *et al.* MicroRNA expression patterns associated with hyperfunctioning and non-hyperfunctioning phenotypes in adrenocortical adenomas. *Eur J Endocrinol* 2014; 170(4): 583–591.

186. Li, F. P., Fraumeni, J. F., Jr., Mulvihill, J. J., Blattner, W. A., Dreyfus, M. G., Tucker, M. A. *et al.* A cancer family syndrome in twenty-four kindreds. *Cancer Res* 1988; 48(18): 5358–5362.

187. Sameshima, Y., Tsunematsu, Y., Watanabe, S., Tsukamoto, T., Kawa-ha, K., Hirata, Y. *et al.* Detection of novel germ-line p53 mutations in diverse-cancer-prone families identified by selecting patients with childhood adrenocortical carcinoma. *J Natl Cancer Inst* 1992; 84(9): 703–707.

188. Henry, I., Jeanpierre, M., Couillin, P., Barichard, F., Serre, J. L., Journel, H. *et al.* Molecular definition of the 11p15.5 region involved in Beckwith-Wiedemann syndrome and probably in predisposition to adrenocortical carcinoma. *Hum Genet* 1989; 81(3): 273–277.

189. Choufani, S., Shuman, C. and Weksberg, R. Molecular findings in Beckwith-Wiedemann syndrome. *Am J Med Genet C Semin Med Genet* 2013; 163C(2): 131–140.

190. Raymond, V. M., Everett, J. N., Furtado, L. V., Gustafson, S. L., Jungbluth, C. R., Gruber, S. B. *et al.* Adrenocortical carcinoma is a Lynch syndrome-associated cancer. *J Clin Oncol* 2013; 31(24): 3012–3018.

191. Else, T. Association of adrenocortical carcinoma with familial cancer susceptibility syndromes. *Mol Cell Endocrinol* 2012; 351(1): 66–70.

192. Haase, M., Anlauf, M., Schott, M., Schinner, S., Kaminsky, E., Scherbaum, W. A. *et al.* A new mutation in the menin gene causes the multiple endocrine neoplasia type 1 syndrome with adrenocortical carcinoma. *Endocrine* 2011; 39(2): 153–159.

193. Morin, E., Mete, O., Wasserman, J. D., Joshua, A. M., Asa, S. L. and Ezzat, S. Carney complex with adrenal cortical carcinoma. *J Clin Endocrinol Metab* 2012; 97(2): E202–206.

194. Anselmo, J., Medeiros, S., Carneiro, V., Greene, E., Levy, I., Nesterova, M. *et al.* A large family with Carney complex caused by the S147G PRKAR1A mutation shows a unique spectrum of disease including adrenocortical cancer. *J Clin Endocrinol Metab* 2012; 97(2): 351–359.

195. Ohgaki, H., Kleihues, P. and Heitz, P. U. p53 mutations in sporadic adrenocortical tumors. *Int J Cancer* 1993; 54(3): 408–410.

196. Reincke, M., Karl, M., Travis, W. H., Mastorakos, G., Allolio, B., Linehan, H. M. *et al.* p53 mutations in human adrenocortical neoplasms: immunohistochemical and molecular studies. *J Clin Endocrinol Metab* 1994; 78(3): 790–794.

197. Ilvesmaki, V., Kahri, A. I., Miettinen, P. J. and Voutilainen, R. Insulin-like growth factors (IGFs) and their receptors in adrenal tumors: high IGF-II expression in functional adrenocortical carcinomas. *J Clin Endocrinol Metab* 1993; 77(3): 852–858.

198. Gicquel, C., Raffin-Sanson, M. L., Gaston, V., Bertagna, X., Plouin, P. F., Schlumberger, M. *et al.* Structural and functional abnormalities at 11p15 are associated with the malignant phenotype in sporadic adrenocortical tumors: study on a series of 82 tumors. *J Clin Endocrinol Metab* 1997; 82(8): 2559–2565.

199. Tissier, F., Cavard, C., Groussin, L., Perlemoine, K., Fumey, G., Hagnere, A. M. *et al.* Mutations of beta-catenin in adrenocortical tumors: activation of the Wnt signaling pathway is a frequent event in both benign and malignant adrenocortical tumors. *Cancer Res* 2005; 65(17): 7622–7627.

200. Giordano, T. J., Thomas, D. G., Kuick, R., Lizyness, M., Misek, D. E., Smith, A. L. *et al.* Distinct transcriptional profiles of adrenocortical tumors uncovered by DNA microarray analysis. *Am J Pathol* 2003; 162(2): 521–531.

201. de Fraipont, F., El Atifi, M., Cherradi, N., Le Moigne, G., Defaye, G., Houlgatte, R. *et al.* Gene expression profiling of human adrenocortical tumors using complementary deoxyribonucleic Acid microarrays identifies several candidate genes as markers of malignancy. *J Clin Endocrinol Metab* 2005; 90(3): 1819–1829.

202. Gicquel, C., Bertagna, X., Gaston, V., Coste, J., Louvel, A., Baudin, E. *et al.* Molecular markers and long-term recurrences in a large cohort of patients with sporadic adrenocortical tumors. *Cancer Res* 2001; 61(18): 6762–6767.

203. Assié, G., Letouzé, E., Fassnacht, M., Jouinot, A., Luscap, W., Barreau, O. *et al.* Integrated genomic characterization of adrenocortical carcinoma. *Nat Genet* 2014; 46(6): 607–612.

204. Amar, L., Bertherat, J., Baudin, E., Ajzenberg, C., Bressac-de Paillerets, B., Chabre, O. *et al.* Genetic testing in pheochromocytoma or functional paraganglioma. *J Clin Oncol* 2005; 23(34): 8812–8818.

205. Burnichon, N., Vescovo, L., Amar, L., Libé, R., de Reynies, A., Venisse, A. *et al.* Integrative genomic analysis reveals somatic mutations in pheochromocytoma and paraganglioma. *Hum Mol Genet* 2011; 20(20): 3974–3985.

206. Eisenhofer, G., Huynh, T. T., Pacak, K., Elkahloun, A., Morris, J. C., Bratslavsky, G. *et al.* Distinct gene expression profiles in norepinephrine- and epinephrine-producing hereditary and sporadic pheochromocytomas: activation of hypoxia-driven angiogenic pathways in von Hippel-Lindau syndrome. *Endocr Relat Cancer* 2004; 11(4): 897–911.

207. Dahia, P. L., Ross, K. N., Wright, M. E., Hayashida, C. Y., Santagata, S., Barontini, M. *et al.* A HIF1alpha regulatory loop links hypoxia and mitochondrial signals in pheochromocytomas. *PLoS Genet* 2005; 1(1): 72–80.

208. Lopez-Jimenez, E., Gomez-Lopez, G., Leandro-Garcia, L. J., Munoz, I., Schiavi, F., Montero-Conde, C. *et al.* Research resource: transcriptional profiling reveals different pseudohypoxic signatures in SDHB and VHL-related pheochromocytomas. *Mol Endocrinol* 2010; 24(12): 2382–2391.

209. Eisenhofer, G., Lenders, J. W., Timmers, H., Mannelli, M., Grebe, S. K., Hofbauer, L. C. *et al.* Measurements of plasma methoxytyramine, normetanephrine, and metanephrine as discriminators of different hereditary forms of pheochromocytoma. *Clin Chem* 2011; 57(3): 411–420.

210. Neumann, S., Schuchardt, K., Reske, A., Reske, A., Emmrich, P. and Paschke, R. Lack of correlation for sodium iodide symporter mRNA and protein expression and analysis of sodium iodide symporter promoter methylation in benign cold thyroid nodules. *Thyroid* 2004; 14(2): 99–111.

211. King, K. S., Prodanov, T., Kantorovich, V., Fojo, T., Hewitt, J. K., Zacharin, M. *et al.* Metastatic pheochromocytoma/paraganglioma related to primary tumor development in childhood or adolescence: significant link to SDHB mutations. *J Clin Oncol* 2011; 29(31): 4137–4142.

212. Ricketts, C., Woodward, E. R., Killick, P., Morris, M. R., Astuti, D., Latif, F. *et al.* Germline SDHB mutations and familial renal cell carcinoma. *J Natl Cancer Inst* 2008; 100(17): 1260–1262.

213. Pasini, B., McWhinney, S. R., Bei, T., Matyakhina, L., Stergiopoulos, S., Muchow, M. *et al.* Clinical and molecular genetics of patients with the Carney-Stratakis syndrome and germline mutations of the genes coding for the succinate dehydrogenase subunits SDHB, SDHC, and SDHD. *Eur J Hum Genet* 2008; 16(1): 79–88.

214. Lee, J., Wang, J., Torbenson, M., Lu, Y., Liu, Q. Z. and Li, S. Loss of SDHB and NF1 genes in a malignant phyllodes tumor of the breast as detected by oligo-array comparative genomic hybridization. *Cancer Genet Cytogenet* 2010; 196(2): 179–183.

215. Burnichon, N., Rohmer, V., Amar, L., Herman, P., Leboulleux, S., Darrouzet, V. *et al.* The succinate dehydrogenase genetic testing in a large prospective series

of patients with paragangliomas. *J Clin Endocrinol Metab* 2009; 94(8): 2817–2827.

216. Millar, A. C., Mete, O., Cusimano, R. J., Fremes, S. E., Keshavjee, S., Morgan, C. D. et al. Functional cardiac paraganglioma associated with a rare SDHC mutation. *Endocr Pathol* 2014; 25(3): 315–320.

217. Baysal, B. E. Mitochondrial complex II and genomic imprinting in inheritance of paraganglioma tumors. *Biochim Biophys Acta* 2013; 1827(5): 573–577.

218. Hao, H. X., Khalimonchuk, O., Schraders, M., Dephoure, N., Bayley, J. P., Kunst, H. et al. SDH5, a gene required for flavination of succinate dehydrogenase, is mutated in paraganglioma. *Science* 2009; 325(5944): 1139–1142.

219. Kunst, H. P., Rutten, M. H., de Monnink, J. P., Hoefsloot, L. H., Timmers, H. J., Marres, H. A. et al. SDHAF2 (PGL2-SDH5) and hereditary head and neck paraganglioma. *Clin Cancer Res* 2011; 17(2): 247–254.

220. Mulligan, L. M. and Ponder, B. A. J. Genetic basis of endocrine disease. Multiple endocrine neoplasia type 2. *J Clin Endocrinol Metab* 1995; 80: 1989–1995.

221. Zinnamosca, L., Petramala, L., Cotesta, D., Marinelli, C., Schina, M., Cianci, R. et al. Neurofibromatosis type 1 (NF1) and pheochromocytoma: prevalence, clinical and cardiovascular aspects. *Arch Dermatol Res* 2011; 303(5): 317–325.

222. Qin, Y., Yao, L., King, E. E., Buddavarapu, K., Lenci, R. E., Chocron, E. S. et al. Germline mutations in TMEM127 confer susceptibility to pheochromocytoma. *Nat Genet* 2010; 42(3): 229–233.

223. Yao, L., Schiavi, F., Cascon, A., Qin, Y., Inglada-Pérez, L., King, E.

E. et al. Spectrum and prevalence of FP/TMEM127 gene mutations in pheochromocytomas and paragangliomas. *JAMA* 2010; 304(23): 2611–2619.

224. Comino-Mendez, I., Gracia-Aznarez, F. J., Schiavi, F., Landa, I., Leandro-García, L. J., Letón, R. et al. Exome sequencing identifies MAX mutations as a cause of hereditary pheochromocytoma. *Nat Genet* 2011; 43(7): 663–667.

225. Peczkowska, M., Kowalska, A., Sygut, J., Waligórski, D., Malinoc, A., Janaszek-Sitkowska, H. et al. Testing new susceptibility genes in the cohort of apparently sporadic phaeochromocytoma/ paraganglioma patients with clinical characteristics of hereditary syndromes. *Clin Endocrinol (Oxf)* 2013; 79(6): 817–823.

226. Toledo, R. A., Qin, Y., Srikantan, S., Morales, N. P., Li, Q., Deng, Y. et al. In vivo and in vitro oncogenic effects of HIF2A mutations in pheochromocytomas and paragangliomas. *Endocr Relat Cancer* 2013; 20(3): 349–359.

227. Ladroue, C., Carcenac, R., Leporrier, M., Gad, S., Le Hello, C., Galateau-Salle, F. et al. PHD2 mutation and congenital erythrocytosis with paraganglioma. *New Engl J Med* 2008; 359(25): 2685–2692.

228. Castro-Vega, L. J., Buffet, A., de Cubas, A. A., Cascón, A., Menara, M., Khalifa, E. et al. Germline mutations in FH confer predisposition to malignant pheochromocytomas and paragangliomas. *Hum Mol Genet* 2014; 23(9): 2440–2446.

229. Crona, J., Delgado, V. A., Maharjan, R., Stålberg, P., Granberg, D., Hellman, P. et al. Somatic mutations in H-RAS in sporadic pheochromocytoma and paraganglioma identified by exome sequencing. *J Clin Endocrinol Metab* 2013; 98(7): E1266–1271.

230. Swarts, D. R., Ramaekers, F. C. and Speel, E. J. Molecular and cellular biology of neuroendocrine lung tumors: evidence for separate biological entities. *Biochim Biophys Acta* 2012; 1826(2): 255–271.

231. Viard-Leveugle, I., Veyrenc, S., French, L. E., Brambilla, C. and Brambilla, E. Frequent loss of Fas expression and function in human lung tumours with overexpression of FasL in small cell lung carcinoma. *J Pathol* 2003; 201(2): 268–277.

232. Onuki, N., Wistuba, I. I., Travis, W. D., Virmani, A. K., Yashima, K., Brambilla, E. et al. Genetic changes in the spectrum of neuroendocrine lung tumors. *Cancer* 1999; 85(3): 600–607.

233. Peifer, M., Fernandez-Cuesta, L., Sos, M. L., George, J., Seidel, D., Kasper, L. H. et al. Integrative genome analyses identify key somatic driver mutations of small-cell lung cancer. *Nat Genet* 2012; 44(10): 1104–1110.

234. Iwakawa, R., Takenaka, M., Kohno, T., Shimada, Y., Totoki, Y., Shibata, T. et al. Genome-wide identification of genes with amplification and/or fusion in small cell lung cancer. *Gene Chromosome Canc* 2013; 52(9): 802–816.

235. Toyooka, S., Toyooka, K. O., Maruyama, R., Virmani, A. K., Girard, L., Miyajima, K. et al. DNA methylation profiles of lung tumors. *Mol Cancer Ther* 2001; 1(1): 61–67.

236. Wistuba, I. I., Gazdar, A. F. and Minna, J. D. Molecular genetics of small cell lung carcinoma. *Semin Oncol* 2001; 28(2 Suppl 4): 3–13.

237. Marchetti, A., Felicioni, L., Pelosi, G., Del Grammastro, M., Fumagalli, C., Sciarrotta, M. et al. Frequent mutations in the neurotrophic tyrosine receptor kinase gene family in large cell neuroendocrine carcinoma of the

lung. *Hum Mutat* 2008; 29(5): 609–616.

238. Fernandez-Cuesta, L., Peifer, M., Lu, X., Sun, R., Ozretić, L., Seidel, D. *et al.* Frequent mutations in chromatin-remodelling genes in pulmonary carcinoids. *Nat Commun* 2014; 5: 3518.

239. Coe, B. P., Lee, E. H., Chi, B., *et al.* Gain of a region on 7p22.3, containing MAD1L1, is the most frequent event in small-cell lung cancer cell lines. *Gene Chromosome Canc* 2006; 45(1): 11–19.

240. Pelosi, G., Papotti, M., Rindi, G. and Scarpa, A. Unraveling Tumor Grading and Genomic Landscape in Lung Neuroendocrine Tumors. *Endocr Pathol* 2014; 25(2): 151–164.

241. Teh, B. T. Thymic carcinoids in multiple endocrine neoplasia type 1. *J Intern Med* 1998; 243(6): 501–504.

242. Strobel, P., Zettl, A., Shilo, K., Chuang, W. Y., Nicholson, A. G., Matsuno, Y. *et al.* Tumor genetics and survival of thymic neuroendocrine neoplasms: a multi-institutional clinicopathologic study. *Gene Chromosome Canc* 2014; 53(9): 738–749.

243. Liu, R. X., Wang, W. Q., Ye, L., Bi, Y. F., Fang, H., Cui, B. *et al.* p21-activated kinase 3 is overexpressed in thymic neuroendocrine tumors (carcinoids) with ectopic ACTH syndrome and participates in cell migration. *Endocrine* 2010; 38(1): 38–47.

244. Ye, L., Li, X., Kong, X., Wang, W., Bi, Y., Hu, L. *et al.* Hypomethylation in the promoter region of POMC gene correlates with ectopic overexpression in thymic carcinoids. *J Endocrinol* 2005; 185(2): 337–343.

245. Asa, S. L. Pancreatic endocrine tumors. *Mod Pathol* 2011; 24 (Suppl 2): S66–S77.

246. Thakker, R. V. Multiple endocrine neoplasia type 1 (MEN1) and type 4 (MEN4). *Mol Cell Endocrinol* 2014; 386(1–2): 2–15.

247. Karamurzin, Y., Zeng, Z., Stadler, Z. K., Zhang, L., Ouansafi, I., Al-Ahmadie, H. A. *et al.* Unusual DNA mismatch repair-deficient tumors in Lynch syndrome: a report of new cases and review of the literature. *Hum Pathol* 2012; 43(10): 1677–1687.

248. Zhou, C., Dhall, D., Nissen, N. N., Chen, C. R. and Yu, R. Homozygous P86S mutation of the human glucagon receptor is associated with hyperglucagonemia, alpha cell hyperplasia, and islet cell tumor. *Pancreas* 2009; 38(8): 941–946.

249. Henopp, T., Anlauf, M., Schmitt, A., Schlenger, R., Zalatnai, A., Couvelard, A. *et al.* Glucagon cell adenomatosis: a newly recognized disease of the endocrine pancreas. *J Clin Endocrinol Metab* 2009; 94(1): 213–217.

250. Kloppel, G., Anlauf, M., Perren, A. and Sipos, B. Hyperplasia to neoplasia sequence of duodenal and pancreatic neuroendocrine diseases and pseudohyperplasia of the PP-cells in the pancreas. *Endocr Pathol* 2014; 25(2): 181–185.

251. Oberg, K. The genetics of neuroendocrine tumors. *Semin Oncol* 2013; 40(1): 37–44.

252. Chung, D. C., Smith, A. P., Louis, D. N., Graeme-Cook, F., Warshaw, A. L. and Arnold, A. A novel pancreatic endocrine tumor suppressor gene locus on chromosome 3p with clinical prognostic implications. *J Clin Invest* 1997; 100(2): 404–410.

253. Jiao, Y., Shi, C., Edil, B. H., de Wilde, R. F., Klimstra, D. S., Maitra, A. *et al.* DAXX/ATRX, MEN1, and mTOR pathway genes are frequently altered in pancreatic neuroendocrine tumors. *Science* 2011; 331(6021): 1199–1203.

254. Marinoni, I., Kurrer, A. S., Vassella, E., Dettmer, M., Rudolph, T., Banz, V. *et al.* Loss of DAXX and ATRX are associated with chromosome instability and reduced survival of patients with pancreatic neuroendocrine tumors. *Gastroenterology* 2014; 146(2): 453–460.

255. Serra, S., Zheng, L., Hassan, M., Phan, A. T., Woodhouse, L., Yao, J. C. *et al.* The FGFR4-G388R single nucleotide polymorphism alters pancreatic neuroendocrine tumor progression and response to mTOR inhibition therapy. *Cancer Res* 2012; 72(22): 1–9.

256. Reid, M. D., Balci, S., Saka, B. and Adsay, N. V. Neuroendocrine tumors of the pancreas: current concepts and controversies. *Endocr Pathol* 2014; 25(1): 65–79.

257. Agathanggelou, A., Bieche, I., Ahmed-Choudhury, J., Nicke, B., Dammann, R., Baksh, S. *et al.* Identification of novel gene expression targets for the Ras association domain family 1 (RASSF1A) tumor suppressor gene in non-small cell lung cancer and neuroblastoma. *Cancer Res* 2003; 63(17): 5344–5351.

258. House, M. G., Herman, J. G., Guo, M. Z., Hooker, C. M., Schulick, R. D., Lillemoe, K. D. *et al.* Aberrant hypermethylation of tumor suppressor genes in pancreatic endocrine neoplasms. *Ann Surg* 2003; 238(3): 423–431.

259. Liu, L., Broaddus, R. R., Yao, J. C., Xie, S., White, J. A., Wu, T. T. *et al.* Epigenetic alterations in neuroendocrine tumors: methylation of RAS-association domain family 1, isoform A and p16 genes are associated with metastasis. *Mod Pathol* 2005; 18(12): 1632–1640.

260. Bordi, C. Neuroendocrine pathology of the stomach: the Parma contribution. *Endocr Pathol* 2014; 25(2): 171–180.

261. D'Adda, T., Candidus, S., Denk, H., Bordi, C. and Hofler, H.

Gastric neuroendocrine neoplasms: tumour clonality and malignancy-associated large X-chromosomal deletions. *J Pathol* 1999; 189(3): 394–401.

262. Pizzi, S., D'Adda, T., Azzoni, C., Rindi, G., Grigolato, P., Pasquali, C. *et al.* Malignancy-associated allelic losses on the X-chromosome in foregut but not in midgut endocrine tumours. *J Pathol* 2002; 196(4): 401–407.

263. Higham, A. D., Bishop, L. A., Dimaline, R., Blackmore, C. G., Dobbins, A. C., Varro, A. *et al.* Mutations of RegIalpha are associated with enterochromaffin-like cell tumor development in patients with hypergastrinemia. *Gastroenterology* 1999; 116(6): 1310–1318.

264. Gucer, H., Szentgyorgyi, E., Ezzat, S., Asa, S. L. and Mete, O. Inhibin-expressing clear cell neuroendocrine tumor of the ampulla: an unusual presentation of von Hippel-Lindau disease. *Virchows Arch* 2013; 463(4): 593–597.

265. Banck, M. S. and Beutler, A. S. Advances in small bowel neuroendocrine neoplasia. *Curr Opin Gastroenterol* 2014; 30(2): 163–167.

266. Bottarelli, L., Azzoni, C., Pizzi, S., D'Adda, T., Silini, E. M., Bordi, C. *et al.* Adenomatous polyposis coli gene involvement in ileal enterochromaffin cell neuroendocrine neoplasms. *Hum Pathol* 2013; 44(12): 2736–2742.

267. Zhang, H. Y., Rumilla, K. M., Jin, L., Nakamura, N., Stilling, G. A., Ruebel, K. H. *et al.* Association of DNA methylation and epigenetic inactivation of RASSF1A and beta-catenin with metastasis in small bowel carcinoid tumors. *Endocrine* 2006; 30(3): 299–306.

268. Banck, M. S., Kanwar, R., Kulkarni, A. A., Boora, G. K., Metge, F., Kipp, B. R. *et al.* The genomic landscape of small intestine neuroendocrine tumors. *J Clin Invest* 2013; 123(6): 2502–2508.

269. Francis, J. M., Kiezun, A., Ramos, A. H., Serra, S., Pedamallu, C. S., Qian, Z. R. *et al.* Somatic mutation of CDKN1B in small intestine neuroendocrine tumors. *Nat Genet* 2013; 45(12): 1483–1486.

270. Li, S. C., Essaghir, A., Martijn, C., Lloyd, R. V., Demoulin, J. B., Oberg, K. *et al.* Global microRNA profiling of well-differentiated small intestinal neuroendocrine tumors. *Mod Pathol* 2013; 26(5): 685–696.

# Chapter 18

# Hematological malignancies of the lymph nodes

Sarah E. Coupland and Pedro Farinha

## Introduction

Molecular genetic techniques have become an integral part of the diagnostic assessment for many lymphoid neoplasms. The demonstration of a clonal immunoglobulin or T-cell receptor gene rearrangement offers a useful diagnostic tool in cases where the combined morphological and immunophenotypical diagnosis remains equivocal. Molecular genetic detection of other genomic rearrangements may not only assist with the diagnosis, but can also provide important prognostic and predictive information. Many of these rearrangements can act as molecular markers for the detection of low levels of residual disease.

Molecular genetics has four major applications in the analysis of lymphoid malignancies. These are: (1) the demonstration of the clonal nature of a population of lymphoid cells; (2) the detection of pathogenetically important rearrangements; (3) the use of signature alterations for the detection of residual disease in monitoring disease response; and (4) the discovery of new potentially druggable molecular targets. Rearrangements of the immunoglobulin (IG) heavy and light chain and T-cell receptor (TCR) genes occur as part of the normal process of lymphoid differentiation. In a clonal population of cells, each cell will carry the same signature rearrangement, whereas in a polyclonal population, the rearrangements within all cells differ. Although it is important to remember that clonality and malignancy are not identical, the demonstration of a clonal IG or TCR gene rearrangement can be useful in the diagnosis of chronic lymphoid malignancies. The detection of pathogenetically important genetic alterations such as BCL2-IGH, CCND1 over-expression or TP53 mutation/deletion may have diagnostic and prognostic relevance. Both of these applications, in addition to being useful

diagnostically, can also assist with disease staging, determination of prognosis and the detection of minimal residual disease.

In 2006, next generation sequencing (NGS) technology was made commercially available and has since revolutionized the field of genomics. Whole genome sequencing (WGS) covers the entire genome, including all exons, introns and intergenic regions. This approach reveals all classes of alterations at an unprecedented resolution and provides comprehensive characterization of the cancer genome. Many significant discoveries have been reported in lymphoid cancers, some with a relevant impact on the diagnosis, prognosis and potential therapy of these neoplasms (1).

This chapter describes the molecular genetic abnormalities in chronic lymphoid malignancies of B- and T-cell origin. Emphasis is placed on the application of molecular genetic assays that are most relevant to diagnosis, prognosis and residual disease monitoring.

## Mature B-cell neoplasms

Mature B-cell neoplasms are malignancies of a monoclonal population of B-cells. The demonstration of the presence of a clonal population of B-cells can be achieved through the detection of a clonal IG rearrangement. This plays an important role in the diagnosis and assessment of residual disease. A large number of acquired genetic abnormalities occur in mature B lymphoid cell malignancies, some of which can be assessed using molecular genetic techniques.

### Immunoglobulin gene rearrangement assays

IG gene rearrangement occurs in a hierarchical manner during B-cell differentiation (2) (Figure 18.1). The IG heavy chain (IGH) locus on chromosome 14q32 is the first to rearrange, followed by

*Molecular Pathology: A Practical Guide for the Surgical Pathologist and Cytopathologist*, ed. John M. S. Bartlett, Abeer Shaaban and Fernando Schmitt. Published by Cambridge University Press. © Cambridge University Press, 2016.

rearrangement of IG Kappa chain (IGK) (chromosome 2p11). If IGK rearrangement results in a nonfunctional immunoglobulin protein, the IG Lambda (IGL) gene is rearranged (chromosome 22q11) and IGK is deleted. Therefore, B-cells may be classified as IGL+ or IGK+ based on the immunoglobulin light chain present on the surface. The variable domain of the immunoglobulin heavy and light chains arises as a result of rearrangement of V (variable), D (diversity; for IGH only) and J (joining) segments. In the case of the IGH locus, D-J rearrangement precedes V-DJ rearrangement. Immunoglobulin diversity is achieved in two main ways: by combinatorial diversity and junctional diversity. *Combinatorial diversity* results from the random selection of V, D and J segments into the rearranged gene. *Junctional diversity* results from deletion or insertion of nucleotides at boundaries between the segments (Figure 18.1). Both mechanisms take place in B-cell precursors within the bone marrow, before exposure to antigens. In this way, $>10^{12}$ different immununoglobulin molecules are possible (2).

Diversity is further enhanced by somatic hypermutation and class-switch recombination of IG genes in the germinal center of secondary lymph follicles (Figures 18.2 and 18.3). As a consequence, each mature B-cell has a unique antigen receptor molecule on its membrane and the chance that two different

cells have identical receptors is infinitesimal. Thus, identical rearrangements within a cell population cannot be derived from differently generated B-cells, but rather they determine the clonal nature of that population of cells. Assessment of the homogeneous versus heterogeneous nature of rearrangement is the fundament of clonality testing.

Southern hybridization utilizing a probe specific for the IG-JH segment of the IGH locus has been the gold standard for demonstration of a clonal population of B-cells (4). For the most part, PCR-based approaches have now replaced Southern hybridization in the diagnostic setting as they are more rapid and require smaller amounts of DNA (5, 6). As the quality of DNA required is smaller than that required for Southern analysis, DNA extracted from paraffin-embedded tissue can also be assessed (7). Furthermore, amplification by PCR can increase the sensitivity of detection compared with Southern hybridisation (6). A variety of PCR-based systems have been utilized for the demonstration of IG gene rearrangement, the majority utilizing rearrangement of the IGH locus. However, many of the early PCR systems showed significant rates of both false negativity (lack of recognition of all possible rearrangements) and false positivity (inability to accurately distinguish monoclonal from polyclonal PCR products). The limited use of primers aiming at the detection of

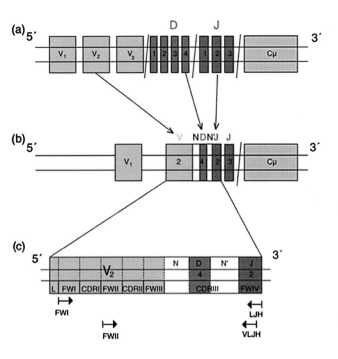

**Figure 18.1 Immunoglobulin heavy chain rearrangement and principles of polymerase chain reaction**
During B-cell development, the enormous diversity among the V regions is generated by numerous combination possibilities of different V, D and J gene segments (a) and by a random incorporation of nucleotides (known as N segments) at the VD and the DJ joints (b). The result is that each single reactive B-cell contains distinct IgH and IgL chain gene rearrangements that are specific for an individual B-cell (a molecular fingerprint). This specificity is predominantly located within the complementarity determining region (CDR) III. Using primers directed against binding sites within the variable region of the immunoglobulin heavy chain gene (c), one applies PCR to determine whether a lymphoproliferative tumor consists of neoplastic B-cells (monoclonal amplification product) or reactive ones (polyclonal amplification product).

303

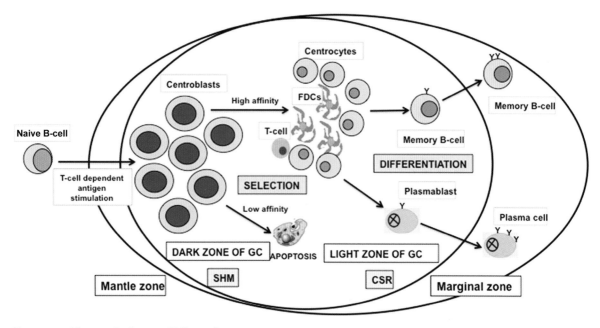

**Figure 18.2 The germinal center (GC) reaction**
Following T-cell-dependent antigen stimulation, naive B-cells migrate into secondary lymphoid tissue (e.g. tonsils, nodes or mucosa), differentiate into centroblasts and proliferate in the dark zone of the germinal centers (GCs). Within the dark zone, the centroblasts undergo somatic hypermutation (SHM), which introduces mostly single base-pair changes into the immunoglobulin variable region of the heavy- and light-chain locus, with the aim of increasing their affinity for the antigen. Centroblasts then move to the light zone, where they differentiate into centrocytes and undergo class-switch recombination (CSR). T-cells and follicular dendritic cells (FDCs) help to re-challenge the centrocytes with the antigen. Those B-cells with a low-affinity immunoglobulin-receptor are eliminated by apoptosis (approximately 90% of the B-cell population!), whereas a small subset of centrocytes with high affinity to the antigen are selected to differentiate further into either memory B-cells or plasma cells. The germinal center reaction is associated with a change in the immunophenotype of the B-cells: e.g. CBs express BCL6 in the germinal center; on exiting the germinal center, this expression is down-regulated and the cells are immunoreactive for IRF4 (also called MUM1). Therefore, in the physiological state, a B-cell does not co-express BCL6 and IRF4: this only occurs in the aberrant (i.e. neoplastic) state. Modified from ref. 3.

relatively simple gene structures, such as complete IgH V-J rearrangements, was one of the major issues.

These setbacks fueled the combined effort of multiple European centers, the BIOMED-2 consortium (currently called EuroClonality), to design probes that could cover nearly all IG targets. This assay not only offers an increased detection rate, but also allows interlaboratory standardization (8–10). Multiplex primer systems were developed to detect complete IGH VDJ rearrangements and incomplete IGH DJ rearrangements, as well as IGK and IGL rearrangements. After PCR amplification, products are analyzed by high-resolution capillary electrophoresis or polyacrylamide gel electrophoresis. A polyclonal population of cells results in multiple fluorescent peaks or a smear representing multiple PCR products (Figure 18.4). In contrast, a clonal rearrangement yields a single peak or band (Figure 18.4). Physical separation of polyclonally derived fragments from the

clonal fragment can be achieved by the formation of heteroduplex DNA molecules after denaturation and re-annealing. For some rearrangements, a nonspecific background band or peak is observed. It is therefore important to compare results with appropriate polyclonal and positive control samples and confirm that the fragment size obtained is within the expected size range. In total, eight different multiplex assays are available to assess IG gene rearrangement (8, 9).

Assessment of complete IGH VDJ rearrangement (three reactions) shows the highest detection rate, especially for pre-germinal center lymphomas (8, 9). The normal process of somatic hypermutation within the variable domain in the germinal center reduces primer-binding efficiency for IGH framework region primers. Hence, detection efficiency for post-germinal center B-cell malignancies, such as follicular lymphoma (FL), diffuse large B-cell lymphoma (DLBCL),

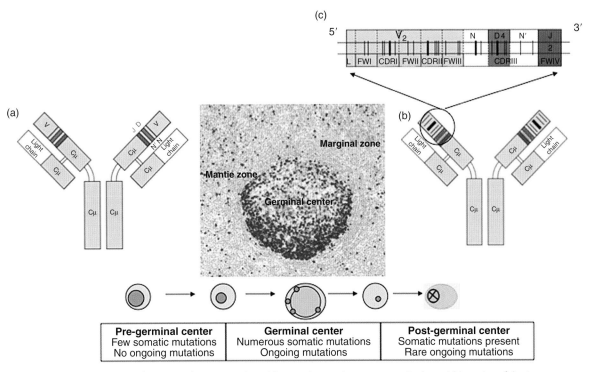

**Figure 18.3** As in Figure 18.2, the germinal center reaction with somatic mutation occurrence in the variable region of the Ig gene; principle of sequence analysis. (a) Immunoglobulin of a naive B-cell with no evidence of somatic mutations in the variable region (V) of the immunoglobulin heavy chain gene (IgH). (b) Immunoglobulin of a post-germinal B-cell with a moderate number of somatic mutations in the V of the IgH. (c) Higher "magnification" of the circled area in (b), demonstrating the somatic mutations (thin black vertical bars) in the V region of the IgH.

marginal zone lymphomas (MZL) and multiple myeloma (MM), is lower if IGH VDJ alone is assessed. The detection rate can be increased to approximately 90% to 100% for post-germinal center B-cell malignancies if incomplete IGH DJ and/or IGK rearrangements are also assessed (8, 9, 11, 12). More than ten years after their publication, the Biomed2/EuroClonality protocols have been extensively and globally validated (13, 14). Following this earlier standardization of the analytical phase of IG clonality testing, the same consortium developed a uniform reporting system, including several levels of pre- and post-analytical control that is applicable to 95% of routine cases, including formalin-fixed paraffin-embedded tissue samples.

In a clinical setting, the demonstration of a clonal IG gene rearrangement is not usually necessary for the diagnosis of all B-cell malignancies. Immunophenotypic demonstration of immunoglobulin light or heavy chain restriction of fresh or even formalin-fixed paraffin-embedded cells is more rapid and

indicates the presence of a clonal B-cell population (Figure 18.5) (2). However, molecular demonstration of clonality can be helpful in cases difficult to assess morphologically, specifically as an aid to distinguish between reactive and clonal conditions. Results should always be interpreted in conjunction with other clinical and laboratory findings as some benign reactive conditions may also demonstrate clonal IG gene rearrangement (5). Depending on the experience of the hematopathologists and the type of request, it is estimated that between 5 and 15% of cases could benefit from molecular clonality diagnostics (15).

## Chronic lymphocytic leukemia

Chronic lymphocytic leukemia (CLL) is the most common mature B-cell non-Hodgkin's lymphoma (NHL) and consists of the monoclonal proliferation of CD5+ CD23+ B-cells (Figure 18.6a). As CLL arises in a cell in which V(D)J recombination has taken place, rearrangement of IG loci may be detected by

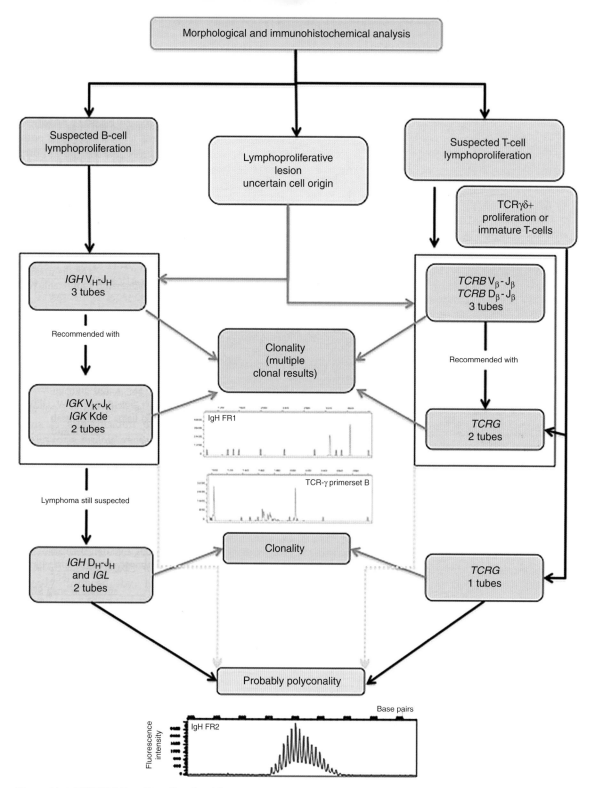

**Figure 18.4 BIOMED2/EuroClonality algorithm**

Depending on the morphological and immunohistochemical impression, DNA is extracted from the lymphoproliferative lesion and submitted for clonality analysis for immunoglobulin or TCR rearrangements. In the case of suspected B-cell neoplasms, primers for IgH are initially used, but it is recommended that this is closely followed by IgK analysis. Should it remain unclear, analysis using primers for IGH D$_H$-J$_H$ would be the next step. In those cases where a T-cell lesion is suspected, it is recommended that analyses using primers for TCRB are initially used, closely followed by those for TCRG. Primers for TCRD are used in suspected cases of neoplasms of both TCRγδ and TCRαβ expressing cells, e.g. in HSTL. Correlation of results with clinical and morphological/immunohistochemical data is always required. (Modified from Figure 1 in ref. 5.)

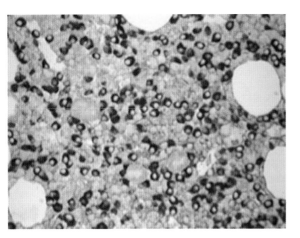

**Figure 18.5** Clear light chain restriction of Kappa in a case of multiple myeloma (PAP staining, x40 objective).

PCR (2, 8). Demonstration of clonal IG gene rearrangement is not usually necessary for the diagnosis of CLL, as clonality can usually be assessed using immunophenotypic methods. However, recurrent genomic changes are present in more than 80% of CLL cases, namely the cytogenetic imbalances, differential expression of specific genes and altered immunoglobulin mutation status, which – associated with clinical parameters – provide significant diagnostic and prognostic information (16). The current World Health Organization (WHO) guidelines recommend the assessment in the routine practice of IGH mutational status, the expression of ZAP70 (zeta-associated protein 70) and cytogenetic abnormalities, as valuable for risk stratification and therapy response (17, 18).

Analysis of the mutation status of the IGVH domain enables CLL to be divided into two groups (19). Patients with IGVH sequence showing >98% similarity to germline are termed as possessing an unmutated locus and the disease is thought to arise from a naive B-cell (20). In contrast, CLL with a mutated IGVH locus (<98% similarity) is thought to arise from a memory B-cell in which somatic hypermutation has taken place. The IGVH mutation status has clinical consequences, as patients carrying an unmutated IGVH locus demonstrate a worse overall survival rate than patients with the mutated form (21, 22). The prognostic significance of IGVH mutation status is more pronounced in patients with Binet Stage A disease (23), but still important within Binet stage B/C patients (24). The poor prognosis remains even after autologous stem cell transplantation, but can be overcome by allogeneic transplantation (25). Use of the IG VH3–21 segment alone, whether unmutated or not, appears to confer a poor prognosis (26). There is a strong but not absolute correlation between IGVH mutation status and prognostic cytogenetic abnormalities. Deletion of 11q23 and 17p13 is most commonly detected in patients with an unmutated IGVH (23). These patients suffer a particularly poor outcome irrespective of IGVH status, although the IGVH mutation status is still important in patients without a 11q23 or 17p13 deletion.

Assessment of IGVH mutation status requires DNA sequencing and subsequent analysis. As this is complex and not routinely available in all centers, surrogate markers to identify patients carrying unmutated IGVH are required. No surrogate marker has shown 100% concordance with IGVH status, but the most useful is ZAP70 up-regulation, which was identified through gene expression profiling (GEP) (27). Detection of ZAP70 protein by flow cytometry or ZAP70 mRNA by quantitative RT-PCR within B-cells shows excellent concordance with IGVH mutation status and is an indicator of poor prognosis (28). CD38 expression, despite being a prognostic marker in CLL, does not correlate with IGVH mutation status (21, 22).

Chromosomal abnormalities can be detected in up to 50% of patients with CLL and this detection rate increases to 80% with the addition of FISH (29). The consistency of these abnormalities has led to the clinical routine use of commercially available FISH panels that include probes for the detection of losses of 13q14.3, 13q34, 17p13.1, 11q22.3 and trisomy 12. FISH detection of chromosomal abnormalities of prognostic significance in CLL, such as loss of TP53 at 17p13 and loss of ATM at 11q23, both of which represent poor prognostic features, is more useful and practical than sequencing (23, 30). Functional assays to detect p53 dysfunction can also identify poor prognosis patients carrying mutations within the TP53 or ATM genes (31).

Prognostic factors such as ZAP70 expression/mutation analysis and cytogenetics are especially predictive when concordant, but none is dominant that independently predicts prognosis in discordant cases. Some investigators describe ZAP70 as the strongest risk factor, but others conclude that cytogenetics is most predictive of outcome (32–34). Yet, contrary to FISH analysis, ZAP70 testing by flow cytometry or

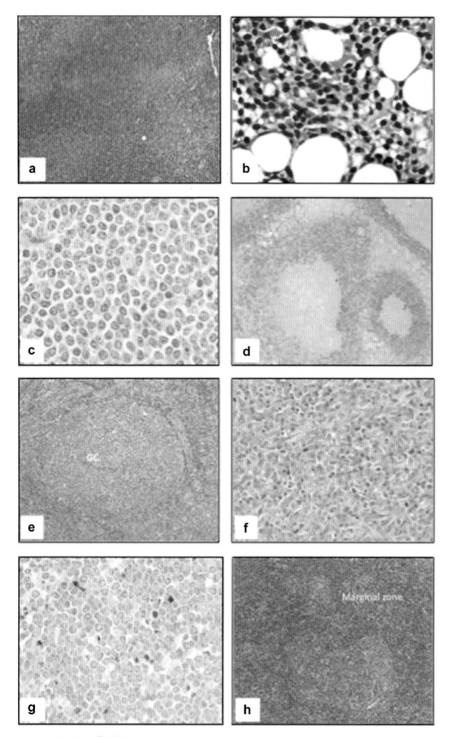

**Figure 18.6  B-cell NHL**
(a) CLL in a lymph node (H&E, x10 objective); (b) HCL in a bone marrow (H&E, x40 objective); (c) MCL in a lymph node (Giemsa, x60 objective); (d) MCL with cyclin D1 staining in the mantle zone (APAAP, x10 objective); (e) FL in a lymph node with the germinal center (GC) being filled by neoplastic cells (H&E staining, x10 objective); (f) DLBCL in a lymph node; centroblastic morphology (H&E staining, x20 objective); (g) BL in a lymph node (Giemsa, x 40 objective); (h) EMZL of the orbit with the neoplastic cells located in the marginal zone surrounding the reactive germinal center (H&E staining, x20 objective).

immunohistochemistry is not widely used due to various technical reasons.

In 2011, Puente and co-workers (35) performed NGS of four CLL cases, including two with unmutated IGH and two with mutated IGH. New recurrent mutations were found in several genes, including NOTCH1, MYD88, XPO1 and KLHL6. A large extension set was used to more firmly establish the frequency of mutations (NOTCH1 12.2%, MYD88 2.9%, XPO1 2.4%, KLHL6 1.8%). The authors showed that MYD88 and KLHL6 mutations were associated with CLL with mutated IGH, whereas NOTCH1 and XPO1 mutations were associated with CLL unmutated IGH. Fabbri *et al.* also showed NOTCH1 mutation to be associated with disease progression and poor prognosis (36). NOTCH1 mutations were present in 8.3% of CLL at diagnosis, 31% of cases in transformation, and 20.8% of cases with chemorefractoriness. This finding has potential importance as inhibitors of NOTCH signaling are available and are currently being used in some clinical trials.

Further NGS studies performed in larger cohorts of CLL patients (37–39) identified new and clinically significant SF3B1 mutations in 10% to 20% of cases. SF3B1 is a critical member of the RNA splicing machinery. This mutation is associated with treatment refractoriness and aggressive clinical behavior. It is mutually exclusive of the del17p and is associated with the presence of a del11q.

As young patients with CLL and those with poor prognosis disease are being treated aggressively with curative intent, residual disease monitoring has become an important aspect of patient management. Assessment of IGH rearrangements offers a molecular marker, which is useful to detect minimal residual disease (MRD) (40). The ideal approach is to design patient-specific oligonucleotide primers to detect low levels of disease in conjunction with sensitive detection methods such as hybridization (41) or real-time quantitative PCR (25). The value of MRD monitoring is evident from transplant recipients. Patients who have undergone autologous stem cell transplantation and have MRD detectable at 6 to 12 months post-transplant, either by the use of patient-specific or consensus primers, have a higher risk of relapse (41). Although initial data suggested that maintenance of MRD negativity ($<10^4$), once acquired, was relatively robust (41), PCR-detectable disease does eventually re-occur in the majority of patients (42). The re-appearance of PCR-detectable disease is predictive of future relapse (42). Hence, frequent monitoring of patients rather than assessment at a single time point is necessary to identify those patients likely to relapse. Similar results have been obtained for allogeneic stem cell transplant recipients. In this case, the use of very sensitive real-time PCR demonstrated complete absence of MRD approximately three months post-transplant, a situation that was not achievable in post-autograft patients, possibly reflecting a graft-versus-leukemia effect (25). Detection of minimal residual disease in CLL may also be achieved by multi-color flow cytometry (43).

## Hairy cell leukemia

Hairy cell leukemia (HCL) is a mature B-cell malignancy diagnosed on clinical features, morphology (Figure 18.6b) and phenotyping, and is generally treated with curative intent (2). IGH V(D)J recombination and usually somatic hypermutation has taken place in the neoplastic B-cell (2). As with CLL, mutations in the IGHV on hairy cells are associated with better responses to initial treatments and with prolonged survival (44). Likewise, routine cytogenetic analysis of HCL is typically not indicated, as the diagnosis can usually be made on morphologic and immunophenotypic grounds. The low proliferation of HCL renders karyotyping difficult and no prognostic genetic markers have been identified.

Response to therapy can be monitored by PCR detection of the rearranged IGH locus (45). However, in practice, flow cytometry offers similar or better sensitivity and faster analysis. In 2011, Tiacci *et al.* discovered that 100% of HCL samples analyzed had the oncogenic BRAF mutation V600E, and proposed that this is the disease's driver mutation (46). Beside the relevance of the finding in the pathobiology of this entity, it can be a significant feature for not only the diagnosis of the disease, but also as a potential therapeutic target (47).

## B-cell prolymphocytic leukemia

B-cell prolymphocytic leukemia (B-PLL) represents a malignancy of B pro-lymphocytes affecting blood, bone marrow and spleen and has a variable prognosis. Molecular genetic analysis is not routinely performed. As for CLL and other mature B lymphoid malignancies, IG genes are clonally rearranged. The majority of patients display mutated IGVH domain (48), although the prognostic importance of detecting mutation status is not clear. A number of cases of B-PLL have been reported with t(11;14) and/or over-expression of CCND1 (49). Such cases are now recognized to most likely represent a splenomegalic form of mantle cell lymphoma (MCL) (50). Therefore, detection of t(11;14) by FISH or detection of CCND1 by immunohistochemistry may distinguish B-PLL from MCL. PCR detection of t(11;14) is not helpful because of low sensitivity (see also MCL in the section directly below). Yet, recent immunophenotyping and GEP suggest that both t(11;14)-positive and-negative cases should be considered a subgroup within MCL. Both B-PLL with and without t(11;14) is highly comparable to MCL, suggesting that B-PLL is part of a spectrum, ranging from CLL-like B-PLL, leukemic MCL-like B-PLL, to nodal MCL-like B-PLL (51).

## Mantle cell lymphoma

Mantle cell lymphoma (MCL) accounts for 5% to 10% of adult NHL (Figure 18.6c). MCL arises in the primary follicle and mantle zone of lymph nodes. Hence, although IG genes are rearranged, the majority of cases do not show somatic mutations. MCL is characterized by the t(11;14) translocation that brings CCND1 (also termed PRAD1 or BCL1) upstream of an IGH JH domain (52, 53). The consequence of this rearrangement is aberrant over-expression of CCND1 (cyclin D1), which is important for G1 to S transition during the cell cycle and which can be detected in most cases using immunohistochemistry. In the setting of CCND1 negativity, immunohistochemistry for SOX11 may be informative (54).

The genomic breakpoint on chromosome 11 can lie up to 120 kb upstream of the CCND1 gene. In up to 40% of cases, the breakpoint lies within an 85-bp region termed MTC (8). However, the remainder are spread throughout a large genomic region upstream of CCND1. PCR techniques are only able to identify patients with breakpoints that lie within the MTC cluster by using a specific primer that anneals just adjacent to the cluster along with a consensus JH specific primer (8). For this reason, PCR amplification to detect the t(11;14) translocation is not a useful diagnostic test for MCL. A FISH-based approach offers a more reliable and sensitive diagnostic approach and is the genetic test of choice (55).

Given the low rate of detection by PCR, other molecular approaches for the detection of t(11;14)

have been investigated. Northern hybridization analysis of CCND1 mRNA shows high levels in patients with MCL and low or no expression in the majority of other lymphoproliferative disorders, as well as normal lymphoid tissue (56). Quantitative RT-PCR detection of CCND1 mRNA offers a useful alternative tool for the demonstration of CCND1$^+$ cases and can also be applied to formalin-fixed samples (57). CCND1 mRNA is not detected in peripheral blood from normal individuals (58) and is low or absent in most other lymphoid malignancies (57). Approximately 25% of patients with MCL demonstrate mutated IGVH genes, analogous to CLL (59, 60). This is more common in patients with nodal disease (90% of patients) than those without (44% of non-nodal cases) (60). Unlike CLL, there is no correlation between IGVH mutation status and survival in MCL (60). Certain individual IGVH genes are also more frequently rearranged in patients with MCL (59). Currently, molecular genetic analysis is not routinely performed to assess IGVH gene usage.

In those patients with a CCND1 breakpoint within the MTC, identification of an IGH-CCND1 rearrangement by PCR can be helpful to detect MRD. For patients in whom the IGH-CCND1 rearrangement cannot easily be identified by PCR, detection of IGH gene rearrangement is an alternative suitable marker of MRD (61). Achievement of molecular remission using IGH-CCND1 and/or IGH gene rearrangement was not associated with an improved survival rate in patients treated with CHOP and rituximab (R-CHOP) (62). For patients undergoing high-dose chemotherapy followed by an autograft, quantitative PCR detection of patient-specific IGH gene rearrangement may be helpful (63). In the majority of cases, PCR-detectable MCL cells are detectable in stem cell harvests (61). PCR positivity after transplantation may indicate an increased risk of relapse, but achievement of molecular remission using quantitative PCR during the first year post-transplant was associated with longer survival (63).

The blastoid variant of MCL (MCL-BV) is thought to represent transformation of classic MCL (64). MCL-BV cells have a higher mitotic index and often a complex karyotype or gross genomic imbalance. Despite this, there are no specific molecular tests to identify blastoid variants. Many genes, which control the cell cycle, are aberrantly expressed in MCL-BV, such as CDK4, CKS1, INK4A (p16), INK4B (p15) and CDKN1B (p27) (64). Inactivation of TP53 by deletion or mutation is frequent and is associated with a poorer prognosis (65).

Recent deep sequencing studies in MCL samples and cell lines identified novel genomic abnormalities with prognostic and potential therapeutic significance, namely the recurrent NOTCH1 mutations, found in 12% of a large cohort of patient MCL samples. Importantly, lymphomas that harbored a NOTCH1 mutation behaved more aggressively and were associated with an inferior overall survival rate (66).

## Follicular lymphoma

Follicular lymphoma (FL) is a neoplasm of follicle center B-cells (Figure 18.6e). Consequently, the IG genes have undergone rearrangement and somatic mutation. The hallmark of FL is the t(14;18)(q32; q21) translocation, seen in approximately 80% to 90% of patients with the disease, although it is less frequent in higher grade tumors (2, 67). The consequence of t(14;18) is the re-positioning of the BCL2 gene, located on chromosome 18, under the regulatory control of the IGH locus enhancer. BCL2 plays a key role in the inhibition of apoptosis, but also acts as a modulator of cell cycle progression. Over-expression of BCL2 prolongs cell survival both *in vitro* and *in vivo* as a consequence of inhibition of apoptosis (67). Two main breakpoint regions within the BCL2 locus have been described (8, 68). The MBR region contains two clusters (50 MBR and 30 MBR or 30 BCL2) that lie within and just downstream of exon 3. Approximately 75% of cases possess a breakpoint within the MBR region (8, 68). In approximately 15% of cases, the BCL2 breakpoint lies within the 50 mcr or mcr region (8). These regions lie 10 kb and 20 kb downstream of the 30 end of the BCL2 gene. The location of the BCL2 breakpoint does not offer prognostic information, although patients with a mcr BCL2 breakpoint tend to present with a higher grade of disease and more frequent extranodal involvement (68). The breakpoint within the IGH locus usually lies close to one of the six JH domains. Approximately 50% of patients utilize JH6, 10% to 20% use JH4 and JH5, but JH1, JH2 and JH3 are rarely if ever used (68). The type of JH domain used does not affect clinical features or survival (68).

A number of genetic methods are available for the detection of BCL2 rearrangements. These include Southern hybridization, PCR and FISH. Southern hybridization requires large amounts of high-quality DNA from diagnostic material and is therefore not the method of choice for paraffin-embedded tumor material. Standardized PCR primers have been developed that are able to detect the BCL2-IGH rearrangement in 88% of cases with a t(14;18) (8). This method utilizes a multiplex PCR amplification system incorporating a consensus JH primer and a number of different primers specific for each of the breakpoint cluster regions. The identification of the specific BCL2 breakpoint region by PCR allows the development and use of patient-specific primers for disease monitoring. The small number of t(14;18) cases in which the BCL2-IGH rearrangement is not detectable by PCR are likely to possess breakpoints between the MBR and mcr regions or, more rarely, between the MBR and 5' of the BCL2 locus. In addition to molecular genetic techniques, several FISH-based detection systems have been developed (69, 70). BCL2 protein expression can be detected by immunohistochemical methods (71), although there is not an exact correlation between the presence of a t(14;18) translocation and BCL2 expression (69, 72). Dysregulation of BCL6 is another feature of FL, and BCL6 expression can be detected in the majority of cases of FL by immunohistochemical techniques (72) or quantitative RT-PCR (73). Such expression is independent of both the presence of a 3q27 and a t(14;18) rearrangement (72). Rearrangements or mutation of BCL6 can also be detected in patients who transform to diffuse large B-cell lymphoma (DLBCL) (see the following section).

Residual FL carrying the BCL2-IGH rearrangement can be detected by molecular methods. This can be utilized for disease staging, after therapy or within autografts post purging. Original techniques utilized sensitive nested PCR approaches combined with Southern hybridization (74). Such an approach, although not necessarily quantitative, does allow the size of the PCR product to be compared with that obtained on the diagnostic sample. Quantitative PCR methods have also been developed (75) and these methods may be combined with sequencing (76) or capillary electrophoresis (77) to confirm patient-specific BCL2 rearrangement. Determination that MRD contains the same BCL2-IGH rearrangement as at diagnosis is important, as BCL2-IGH rearrangements can be detected at very low levels in the peripheral blood of normal individuals (78). It is of note that assessment of bone marrow appears to be more reliable than peripheral blood (74). Quantitative PCR analysis of bone marrow at diagnosis identifies patients with a low tumor burden ($<1$ in $10^3$ cells) who respond well to therapy and achieve a better survival rate (79).

For monitoring response to therapy, a variety of sensitive PCR-based techniques have been used to detect MRD. Patients who achieve and maintain a molecular response (PCR negative) are the most successful in terms of overall survival and relapse rate (79). PCR techniques can also be used to assess the effectiveness of purging of an autograft (40, 74). Patients infused with an autograft devoid of cells with a BCL2-IGH rearrangement, detected by nested or real-time PCR, show a better disease-free survival rate than those for whom the autograft remained PCR positive after purging (80). In post-autograft patients, detection of the BCL2-IGH rearrangement is associated with an increased risk of relapse and a worse overall survival rate (40, 74). For post-allograft patients, there are no clear data on the prognostic role for MRD monitoring.

High-grade transformation of FL to DLBCL has been correlated with acquisition of mutations within a number of genes, including BCL2 itself (81), the regulatory region of BCL6 (82), TP53 (83) and MYC (84). The BCL6 breakpoints observed in cases of high-grade FL (grade 3B according to the WHO Classification (17)) are more likely to lie within the alternative breakpoint cluster region (ABR), which lies 250 kb upstream of BCL6. The CDKN2A (p16) and CDKN2B (p15) tumor suppressor genes on chromosome 9p21 are also frequently inactivated (85, 86).

Recent NGS studies using whole-genome or whole-exome sequencing on ten transformed FL pairs followed by deep sequencing of 28 genes in an extension cohort have demonstrated the key events and evolutionary processes governing tumor initiation and transformation. It was shown that tumor evolution occurred through either a "rich" or "sparse" ancestral common progenitor clone. Further recurrent mutations were identified in linker histone, JAK-STAT ("Janus tyrosine kinase"-"signal transducers and activators of transcription") signaling, NF-κB signaling and B-cell developmental genes. Longitudinal analyses identified early driver mutations in chromatin regulator genes (CREBBP, EZH2 and KMT2D (MLL2)), whereas mutations in EBF1 and regulators of NF-κB signaling (MYD88 and TNFAIP3) were gained at transformation (87).

# Diffuse large B-cell lymphoma

Diffuse large B-cell lymphoma (DLBCL) is the most common NHL and makes up approximately 40% of NHL (Figure 18.6f) (3, 88). In terms of morphology, clinical presentation and response to treatment, it represents a heterogeneous group of diseases; molecular genetic changes underlying this heterogeneity have contributed to our understanding of these differences. In most cases, the neoplastic B-cell has undergone IG rearrangement and somatic mutation. The most common chromosomal rearrangements are t(14;18), t(3;14) and t(8;14) (Table 18.1) (67). These translocations result in the over-expression of the BCL2, BCL6 and MYC oncogenes by juxtaposition next to an IGH regulatory element (87). The presence of t(14;18) or a genomic rearrangement of the BCL2 locus, detected in 30% to 40% of DLBCL cases (72), was thought to represent transformation of FL (67). However, t(14;18) and corresponding BCL2 over-expression has been demonstrated in *de novo* DLBCL (89). Furthermore, t(14;18) is more frequent in DLBCL cases with a germinal center B-cell (GCB) phenotype and identifies a subgroup with a different expression profile (90, 91). The BCL2-IGH rearrangement may be detected by PCR, as previously described for FL. The prognostic significance of BCL2 rearrangement and expression has been a matter of some debate (92). Over-expression of BCL2 (either mRNA or protein) is probably a poor prognostic factor (89, 93), although the prognostic significance of BCL2 expression may be restricted to non-GCB group of patients (92).

Rearrangements and mutations affecting BCL6 are the most common molecular genetic change occurring in DLBCL (88). Translocations involving chromosome 3q27, the location of the BCL6 gene, are found in up to 40% of cases (94). The most common translocation partner is chromosome 14q32, which brings the BCL6 locus in juxtaposition with the IGH locus. Other chromosomal partners include chromosomes 22q11 (IGL locus) and 2p12 (IGK locus). However, translocations involving non-IG gene loci are also reported (95, 96). Translocation of BCL6 is thought to result in continued BCL6 expression and transcriptional activation of genes important for proliferation (94). The genomic breakpoints at the BCL6 locus lie within two regions. A 4 kb region termed MTC or MBR spans the first (non-coding) exon of the gene (97, 98). Most molecular detection methods have utilized Southern hybridization to identify breakpoints within this region (97, 98). However, some patients with a 3q27 translocation do not appear to possess a rearrangement of the BCL6 locus at the MTC/MBR region (97). A second breakpoint region, termed alternative breakpoint cluster region (ABR), was subsequently identified (99). This region spans 20 kb and lies approximately 250 kb upstream of BCL6 (99), but appears to be more associated with high-grade FL (see penultimate paragraph in "Follicular lymphoma," above). The use of long-range PCR to detect IG-BCL6 rearrangements has been demonstrated, but the prognostic implication of the BCL6 rearrangement is unclear, probably reflecting the heterogeneous nature of the disease (100). BCL6 mRNA over-expression can be detected using quantitative RT-PCR techniques (101). Patients displaying high BCL6 mRNA expression have a longer overall survival rate than those with low mRNA levels (101). This is supported by GEP data, which identified increased BCL6 mRNA as a good prognostic indicator within the GCB-like group (91). Increased BCL6 expression can result from several different mechanisms, including translocation to the IGH locus (t(3;14)) and point mutations within the first intron (102). Translocations and/or rearrangements of the MYC gene occur in 5% to 10% of patients and tend to involve MYC breakpoints similar to those found in sporadic Burkitt's lymphoma (103), and these have a significant clinical correlation associated with a worst clinical outcome (104, 105). PCR-based assays to detect IGH-MYC rearrangements are available, although FISH is the preferred approach (see first paragraph in "Burkitt's lymphoma," below). In a small subset of these cases, the MYC rearrangement is associated with rearrangement of BCL2, BCL6 or CCND1, the so-called "double-hit" and "triple-hit" lymphomas (105–107). Besides the molecular diagnosis by FISH, there are no clinical or morphological features that distinguish these cases. Its recognition is clinically relevant, as the standard DLBCL therapy, R-CHOP, has no impact in these lymphomas (105).

The clinical heterogeneity within DLBCL represents underlying molecular genetic differences between patients. GEP experiments have identified genetic differences responsible for such heterogeneity. According to similarities to the putative cell of origin, peripheral DLBCL can be divided into at least three different groups: (1) GC B-cell like (GCB) DLBCL, which derives from centroblasts; (2) activated B-cell like (ABC) DLBCL, which resembles features of plasmablastic B-cells committed to terminal B-cell differentiation; and (3) primary mediastinal large B-cell lymphoma, presumably arising from thymic B-cells (Table 18.1) (108). This is of clinical relevance, as patients with a GCB DLBCL had a better overall survival rate than those with an ABC-DLBCL (108). Patients can now be grouped according to the cell of origin status based on the expression status of a small number of genes, allowing prognosis to be determined at diagnosis. It must be noted that 15% to 30% of DLBCL cannot be classified neatly into any of the above GEP subgroups, including the centrally located DLBCL, i.e. PCNSL and vitreoretinal lymphomas (3, 109).

Surrogate immunohistochemical markers have been demonstrated to aid discrimination between the main DLBCL genetic subgroups, and several of these algorithms – CD10, BCL6, MUM1, B-cell lymphoma 2 (BCL2) and cyclin D2 – have been demonstrated to be predictive of survival (92). The "Hans classifier," comprising CD10, MUM1 and BCL6, can divide DLBCL into GCB-DLBCL and non-GCB-DLBCL with about 80% concordance with the GEP (92). A combination of five markers – GCTE1, CD10, BCL6, MUM1 and FOXP1 – can achieve about 90% concordance with the GEP (110).

Since the majority of DLBCL cases display a clonal IG gene rearrangement, detection of clonal IG gene rearrangement in the bone marrow at diagnosis may provide useful staging and prognostic information. The presence of a clonal IG gene rearrangement in the marrow is associated with a poorer survival, even when there is no histological evidence of bone marrow disease (111). This raises the possibility of a role for molecular staging in diffuse large B-cell lymphoma. Central nervous system (CNS) involvement by DLBCL is observed in approximately 5% of patients with the disease and usually has fatal consequences (112). Molecular detection of clonal IG gene rearrangement in the cerebrospinal fluid may identify patients for whom early treatment for CNS disease could be beneficial.

Morin et al. (113) were the first to examine DBLCL with NGS technology. They identified a recurrent and very targeted somatic mutation affecting the polycomb repressor-2 complex gene EZH2 in 22% of DLBCL, all of which were confined to the GCB subtype. EZH2 encodes a histone methyltransferase that is responsible for trimethylating Lys27 of histone H3 (H3K27) and plays an important

313

**Table 18.1** Most frequent alterations in the DLBCL subtypes

| Gene | Frequency (%) | Gene function/mechanism of transformation |
|---|---|---|
| *GCB-DLBCL subtype:* | | |
| BCL2 translocations | 30–40 | Ectopic BCL2 expression<br>Enhanced resistance to apoptosis |
| MYC translocations | 10 | Enhanced proliferation and growth, DNA replication |
| EZH2 mutations | 22 | H3K27 methyltransferase/epigenetic reprogramming |
| BCL6 mutations in BSE1 | 20 | Enhanced proliferation; impaired DNA damage responses, block in differentiation |
| MEF2B mutations | 8 | Unclear |
| *ABC-DLBCL subtype:* | | |
| BCL2 amplification | 30 | Enhanced resistance to apoptosis |
| PRDM1 (BLIMP1) mutations/deletions | 25 | Block in terminal B-cell differentiation |
| MYD88 mutations | 29 | Constitutive activation of NF-kB and JAK-STAT signaling |
| TNFAIP3 (A20) mutations/deletions | 20 | Constitutive activation of NF-kB signaling due to loss of negative regulation |
| CD79A, CD79B mutations | 20 | Constitutive activation of NF-kB and BCR signaling |
| CARD11 mutations | 9 | Constitutive activation of NF-kB signaling |
| *PMBCL:* | | |
| REL amplification | 75 | Constitutive activation of NF-kB signaling |
| JAK2 amplification | 63 | Activation of JAK-STAT pathway |
| JMJD2C amplification | 63 | Histone modification/epigenetic reprogramming |
| PDL1, PDL2 amplifications | 63 | T-cell exhaustion; reduced tumor cell immunogenicity |
| SOCS1 mutations/deletions | 45 | Enhanced JAK2 signaling due to impaired JAK2 degradation |
| STAT6 mutation | 36 | Possible activation of JAK-STAT pathway |
| CIITA translocations | 38 | Reduced tumor cell immunogenicity; Down-regulation of HLA class II |
| *Shared lesions:* | | |
| MLL2 mutations | 32 | H3K4 methyltransferase/epigenetic reprogramming |
| CREBBP/EP300 mutations/deletions | 22–40 | Epigenetic reprogramming; impaired p53 activation and BCL6 inactivation |
| BCL6 translocations | 25–40 | Enhanced proliferation; impaired DNA damage responses, block in differentiation |
| B2M mutations/deletions | 29 | Reduced tumor cell immunogenicity; down-regulation of HLA class I |
| CD58 mutations/deletions | 21 | Reduced tumor cell immunogenicity |

Note: Modified from ref. 3.

role in gene regulation. These recurrent EZH2 mutations are responsible for a gain-of-function that represents a new promising target for novel therapies, as selective EZH2 inhibitors can prevent the growth of tumor cells in DLBCL cell lines and murine xenograft models (114–116). These findings highlight the importance of NGS discoveries and their potential for rapid translation of targeted therapies into clinical practice.

Since this early study, several reports further described the mutational landscape of DLBCL using NGS techniques. Consistent with the biological distinctions that characterize DLBCLs with different cell of origin, Ngo *et al.* demonstrated recurrent somatic mutation involving MYD88 in 29% of ABC-DLBCL cases, a mutation that was virtually absent in the GCB subtype (117). MYD88 is a known adaptor protein that activates the NF-κB pathway after stimulation of toll-like receptors. The MYD88 mutations are characterized by gain-of-function, which is consistent with observations that ABC-type DLBCL is associated with constitutive activation of the NF-κB pathway. Pasqualucci *et al.* (118) expanded the list of new recurrent somatic mutations of genes involved in gene regulation, including histone and non-histone acetyltransferases CREBBP and E300 (Table 18.1). CREBBP mutations were observed in 22% of all DLBCL, with enrichment in the GCB, whereas E300 mutations were observed in 10% of all DLBCL. Morin *et al.* identified recurrent mutations in several genes affecting histone modification, especially the MLL2 gene, as a highly recurrent target for mutation, with inactivating mutations found in 32% of DLBCL cases (119). Recurrent mutations in CD58 and B2M, genes directly impacting the microenvironment and suggesting new immune-escape mechanisms in DLBCL, were also described (120). Rarer target genes of mutation but potential driver mutations in a small number of DLBCL include KRAS, BRAF and NOTCH1 (121). Finally, exclusive mutations to GCB-type DLBCL have also been identified, namely the fusion involving TBL1XR1 and TP63 present in 5% of GCB-type cases (122).

# Burkitt's lymphoma

The main pathogenetic cause of Burkitt's lymphoma (BL), a high-grade B-cell lymphoma (Figure 18.6g), is aberrant expression of MYC as a consequence of translocation between chromosome 8q32 (MYC

locus) and one of the IG genes (IGH, IGK, IGL) (123). In 80% of cases, the partner is the IGH locus resulting in the generation of the t(8;14)(q24;q32) translocation (124). In 15% of cases, MYC is aberrantly up-regulated as a consequence of juxtaposition to the IGK locus because of a t(2;8)(p12;q24) translocation. In the remaining 5% of cases, a t(8;22)(q24; q11) translocation results in expression of MYC driven by the IGL gene. Mutations of the rearranged MYC allele are also present in many patients. The consequence of these mutations is over-expression of MYC protein expressed from the mutated allele. The breakpoints within the MYC and IGH loci differ between the sporadic and endemic forms of BL (124). In endemic cases, the MYC breakpoint usually lies over 100 kb upstream of MYC and the IGH breakpoint lies within the JH domain region, resulting in control of MYC promoters by the IGH El enhancer element. In contrast, in sporadic and immunodeficient forms, the MYC breakpoint is within exon 1 or intron 1 and the IGH breakpoint usually occurs within the Sμ switch domain. Sporadic BL carrying the variant translocations t(2;8) or t(8;22) possess breakpoints downstream of MYC (123). Genomic breakpoints may be detected by Southern hybridization; however, the variability in the position of the breakpoint means that multiple hybridizations and sufficient high-quality DNA are required. The wide range of breakpoints within MYC also renders detection by conventional PCR methods difficult. PCR-based detection of rearrangements far upstream of MYC within endemic BL is not possible. However, long-range PCR methods to detect MYC-IGH rearrangements in sporadic BL have been developed (100). Good quality DNA is required for these assays, as amplification of a PCR product up to 8 kb is necessary. Furthermore, because of the variable nature of breakpoints within both the IGH and MYC loci, multiple PCR primers are required. No PCR-based methods have been developed for detection of rearrangements involving the IGL or IGK loci. In practice, in the diagnostic laboratory, FISH is a more useful approach to detect MYC rearrangements. Probes spanning the MYC locus allow FISH detection of t(8;14) as well as t(2;8) and t(8;22) through the generation of a "split" signal (124). Other molecular genetic aberrations occur in BL, including mutation of TP53 and BCL6, as well as hypermethylation of CDKN2A (p16), TP73 and DAPK1, although these aberrations are not routinely assessed (124). Besides

**315**

MYC dysregulation, BL frequently harbors mutations in ID3, TCF3 and CCND3 that activate the TCF3 pathway. Cooperation of these two pathways plays a crucial role in BL (125).

## Extranodal marginal zone B-cell lymphomas

Extranodal marginal zone B-cell lymphomas (EMZL) make up approximately 8% of non-Hodgkin's lymphomas (126) and occur at a number of extranodal sites, including stomach, intestine, lung, salivary gland and ocular adnexal tissues (Figure 18.6h) (3). EMZL are often termed "MALT" (mucosa-associated lymphoid tissue) lymphomas when involving an overlying epithelium – for example, the gastric mucosa, conjunctiva or acini of the lacrimal gland. The majority of gastric EMZL are characterized by a chronic infection by Helicobacter pylori, eradication of which can lead to tumor regression in many, but not all, cases (127). Similar associations between infectious agents and EMZL at other sites have also been observed – for example, C. jejuni, B. burgdorferi and hepatitis C virus, with EMZLs that arise in the small intestine, skin and spleen, respectively (3). The significance of C. psittaci with regard to the EMZL of the ocular adnexa remains unclear: there appears to be substantial geographic variation in its association (128).

IG genes are rearranged and have somatic mutations consistent with being derived from post-germinal center B-cells (3, 126). The most common chromosomal rearrangements in EMZL are t(11;18), t(14;18), t(3;14) and t(1;14) (Table 18.2). The t(11;18) (q21;q21) translocation results in a novel fusion protein, API2-MALT1. It is most frequently detected in lymphomas arising in the lung, stomach and intestine. All possible fusion transcripts of API2-MALT1 can be detected by one RT-PCR assay (129). However, transcript-specific PCR primer sets are required when analyzing RNA prepared from paraffin sections due to the poor quality of material that can be extracted. Detection of the API2-MALT1 fusion gene is clinically important in gastric MALT lymphoma, as it is a strong predictor of patients for whom H. pylori eradication fails to achieve tumor regression (129, 130).

The t(14;18)(q32;p21) translocation places the MALT1 gene under the control of IGH enhancer elements, resulting in MALT1 over-expression (126). The translocations t(1;14)(p22;q32) and t(1;2)(p22; p12) relocate the BCL10 locus to the IGH or IGK enhancer regions respectively, resulting in BCL10 over-expression (126). The t(3;14)(p14;q32) translocation results in deregulated expression of the forkhead transcription factor, FOXP1, by relocation of the gene to the IGH locus (131). All of these rearrangements can be detected by FISH-based assays.

Interestingly, these chromosomal aberrations in EMZL vary in frequency according to anatomical site, some occurring at the lowest frequency in the ocular adnexa (Table 18.2). In "translocation negative" ocular adnexal EMZL, it was demonstrated that the A20 gene – an essential *global* NF-κB inhibitor – was found to be inactivated either by somatic deletion and/or mutation in ocular adnexal EMZL (132, 133). The A20 deletion is most commonly heterozygous, and is mutually exclusive from the above-described MALT1 and IGH translocations. Further, it was shown that the A20 mutation/deletion is *significantly* associated with an increased expression of NF-κB target genes. These findings appear to be of clinical relevance: complete A20 inactivation is associated with a *poor lymphoma-free survival rate*, and the patients with A20 mutation/deletion required *significantly higher radiation dosages* than those without the A20 abnormalities to achieve complete remission (132, 133).

NGS has demonstrated the significance of the NOTCH signaling pathway in EMZL, particularly those arising in the spleen. The clinical relevance of alterations in NOTCH1 and NOTCH2 are yet to be ascertained (134).

## Lymphoplasmacytoid lymphoma

Lymphoplasmacytoid lymphomas (LPL) are neoplasms of small lymphocytes, lymphoplasmacytoid cells and plasma cells, and involve the bone marrow, lymph nodes and spleen. The IG gene is clonally rearranged and the majority of patients display somatic mutations within the IGVH domain (135). The t(9;14) translocation has been reported to be present in up to 50% of patients (136).

Recent WGS of bone marrow LPL cells in patients with both Waldenström's macroglobulinemia (WM) and non-IgM LPL identified a highly recurrent point mutation in MYD88, occurring in more than 90% of cases (137). The mutation is the same one described in ABC-type DLBCL (see Table 18.1), which results in a L265P amino acid substitution, with gain-of-function activity and constitutive downstream

Table 18.2 Most frequent chromosomal alterations in EMZL

| Location | Chromosomal alteration | Frequency (%) |
|---|---|---|
| Ocular adnexa | t(11;18)(q21;q21) | 10 |
| | t(14;18)(q32;q21) | 19 |
| | t(3;14)(p14.1;q32) | 14 |
| | A20 inactivation (6q23 deletion) | 20 |
| | Trisomy 3, 18 | ? |
| | 5q (ODZ2) and 9p (JMJD2C) | ? |
| Stomach | t(11;18)(q21;q21) | 22–24 |
| | t(1;14)(p22;q32) | 3 |
| | Trisomy 3, 7, 12, 18‡ | |
| Skin | t(14;18)(q32;q21) | 14 |
| | t(3;14)(p14.1;q32 | 10 |
| | Trisomy 3, 18 | |
| | 5q (ODZ2) | |
| Intestine | t(11;18)(q21;q21) | 13 |
| | t(1;14)(p22;q32) | 10 |
| | Trisomy 3, 12, 18 | |
| Lung | t(14;18)(q32;q21) | 38–53 |
| | t(1;14)(p22;q32) | 11 |
| | Trisomy 3, 12, 18 | 7 |
| Salivary gland | t(11;18)(q21;q21) | 1 |
| | t(14;18)(q32;q21) | 5 |
| | A20 inactivation | ? |
| | Trisomy 3, 7, 18 | |
| Thyroid gland | t(3;14)(p14.1;q32) | 50 |
| | A20 inactivation | ? |
| | Trisomy 3, 12 | |
| Breast | Trisomy 3, 18 | Rare |

Note: Modified from ref. 3.

activation of the NF-kB pathway. The mutation is only rarely identified in other post-germinal center B-cell neoplasms with plasmacytic differentiation, including MZL and multiple (plasma cell) myeloma (MM), suggesting it is relatively specific for LPL/WM and, thus, of potential use in the routine diagnosis of this entity (137).

## Multiple myeloma

Multiple (or plasma cell) myeloma (MM) is a clonal plasma cell malignancy derived from post-germinal center B-cells. Myeloma may be preceded by a pre-malignant stage, termed monoclonal gammopathy of

undetermined significance (MGUS (138)). Translocations involving the IGH locus on chromosome 14q32 are detected in approximately 60% of MM cases (138). The remaining cases tend to be hyperdiploid, demonstrating trisomy of a number of chromosomes (139). At the molecular level, virtually all patients with myeloma demonstrate over-expression of one or more of the cyclin D proteins (CCND1, CCND2, CCND3 (139)). The five most common translocations involving IGH are t(11;14) (CCND1), t(6;14) (CCND3), t(4;14) (MMSET and FGFR3), t(14;16) (MAF) and t(14;20) (MAFB). All of these translocations result in over-expression of a D type of cyclin, either directly by juxtaposition with the IGH locus or indirectly by over-expression of a transcription factor (139). Many of these translocations have prognostic significance, especially in conjunction with the expression level of one or more of the CCND genes. For example, both CCND1 over-expression and the presence of a t(11;14) have been associated with a better overall survival rate (139). As myeloma represents a clonal post-germinal center malignancy, IGH gene rearrangement and often somatic hypermutation has occurred in the neoplastic cell. Approximately 85% of patients possess PCR-detectable VDJ rearrangements, with 60% carrying detectable incomplete D-J rearrangements (140). In contrast to CLL, the acquisition of somatic mutations or the type of domain utilized does not correlate with prognosis (140). However, sequence identification of a patient's rearrangement does offer the ability for detection of minimal residual disease, particularly in patients undergoing transplantation. Sensitive detection of minimal residual disease before or after transplantation may be carried out by qualitative PCR using patient-specific primers (141), by semi-quantitative PCR using fluorescently labeled primers (142), by real-time quantitative PCR or by NGS (143). After transplantation, patients with residual tumor cells, as detected by PCR, have an increased risk of relapse and an increase in the level of residual disease precedes relapse by up to three to six months.

## T-cell lymphomas

There are only a few specific acquired pathogenetic abnormalities within mature T-cell neoplasms that are amenable to routine molecular diagnostic assessment. However, demonstration that a population of

317

T-cells is clonal through the use of assays that detect TCR gene rearrangement has tremendous value in the diagnostic work-up of suspected T-cell lymphoproliferative disorders. Ordered rearrangement of the T-cell receptor loci takes place during T-cell ontogeny, as the T-cells progress from the thymus to the peripheral lymphoid tissue and mature during the differentiation pathway (Figure 18.7). Such rearrangement is responsible for the very large number of different forms of the T-cell receptor that potentially can be generated. Two types of TCR molecule result from this. Most T-cells express a TCR molecule composed of α and β chains encoded by the TCRA (chromosome 14q12) and TCRB genes (chromosome 7q32), respectively. A minority of T-cells contain a γδ heterodimer encoded by the TCRG (chromosome 7p15) and TCRD genes (chromosome 14q12), respectively. The variable domain of these proteins results from rearrangement of a number of V, D (in the case of TCRB and TCRD) and J segments (*combinatorial diversity*). Antigen recognition is further diversified as a result of insertion/deletion of nucleotides at the junctions between the 2 or 3 domains (*junctional diversity*). The four TCR loci undergo gene rearrangement in a fixed order. TCRD is the first to rearrange, followed by TCRG. In γδ containing T-cells, this is followed by TCRB and TCRA rearrangement. As TCRD lies within the TCRA locus, this final rearrangement is accompanied by deletion of the TCRD locus. As T-cell malignancies represent clonal disorders, each cell within the malignant clone will carry the same type of TCR gene rearrangement. By contrast, a polyclonal population of T-cells will contain many different rearrangements as a consequence of both combinatorial and junctional diversity. The number of different domains varies among the four loci, the most complex being the TCRA locus with 70 VA domains and 61 JA domains. Detection of a clonal TCR gene rearrangement can be performed by Southern hybridization (5) by assessing the TCRB locus. This approach can detect over 90% of T-cell NHL, with a sensitivity of 1% to 5% of clonal cells. New PCR-based approaches have now replaced Southern hybridization in a diagnostic laboratory setting and offer advantages similar to those previously described for detection of IG gene rearrangement, including speed, greater sensitivity and a requirement for only small amounts of DNA.

PCR-based assays have been developed for the assessment of TCRD, TCRG and TCRB loci and these are able to detect clonal TCR gene rearrangement in almost all cases of mature T-cell malignancies (Figure 18.4) (8, 15). Assays assessing the TCRG locus are particularly useful, since the TCRG locus is rearranged in both TCRγδ and TCRαβ expressing cells. The highly complex nature of the TCRA locus precludes the development of PCR-based assays to assess TCRA rearrangement. Primer sets developed by the European BIOMED2/Euro-Clonality consortium are now in use in many laboratories worldwide (8). As for detection of IG gene rearrangements, these assays utilize multiple primers within each tube. For example, detection of TCRG gene rearrangements is achieved using two separate multiplex PCR amplifications (termed tube A and tube B). Tube A contains primers that will amplify rearrangements involving TCRG VcfI and Vc10 domains, whereas tube B will amplify rearrangements of Vc9 and Vc11 domains (8). As TCRG rearrangements may involve non-functional Vc domains, rearrangement of both alleles is common, enabling detection using both tube A and tube B. Analysis of the PCR products can be performed by high-resolution capillary electrophoresis or polyacrylamide gel electrophoresis to visualize the band or peak obtained from a clonal T-cell population. Particular caution needs to be observed while interpreting the results of TCR gene rearrangement assays. Background bands or peaks may sometimes be observed, leading to false positives. Assessment of multiple loci (for example, TCRG and TCRB) is beneficial to confirm unexpected results. The relatively limited repertoire of TCRD and TCRG V(D)J domains combined with the small percentage of TCRγδ expressing cells may lead to amplification of an apparently clonal rearrangement from normal T-cells – termed pseudoclonality. T-cells carrying certain rearrangements (for example, TCRG Vc9-Jc1.2) appear to be more frequent within the peripheral blood. The percentage of clonal T-cells in peripheral blood can also increase with age, viral infections or immunodeficiency. Hence, it should be stressed that the demonstration of a clonal population of T-cells by TCR rearrangement assays does not, by itself, indicate a T-cell malignancy, and clonality results must be interpreted within the clinical context (5). Furthermore, the identification of a clonal TCR rearrangement does not define the cell lineage of the tumor. TCR

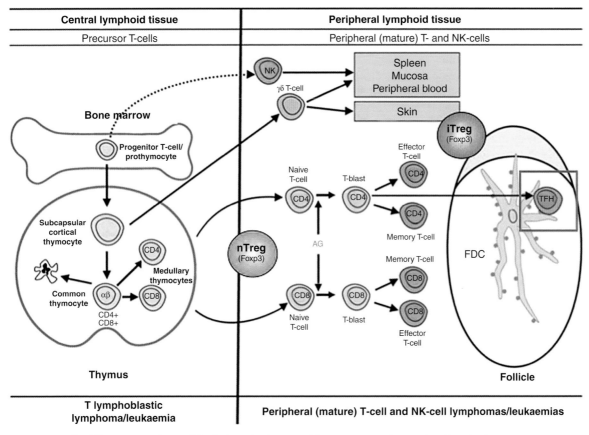

**Figure 18.7** The differentiation pathway of T-cells from the thymus and bone marrow to the peripheral lymphoid tissues.

rearrangements may be detected, albeit at low frequency, within mature B-cell NHL. In fact, approximately 10% of both mature B-cell and T-cell malignancies demonstrate rearrangement of both IG and TCR loci. In addition, non-functional TCRG rearrangements are frequently detected in TCRγδ malignancies and non-functional rearrangements of TCRB can be detected in TCRγδ lymphomas.

Recently, a NGS-based T-cell clonality assay has been developed and has in preliminary studies demonstrated itself to be suitable for routine clinical testing, either alone or as an adjunct to traditional methods (144). This requires further validation in the form of a multicenter analysis.

## T-cell prolymphocytic leukemia

T-cell prolymphocytic leukemia (T-PLL) is a rare aggressive leukemia derived from post-thymic T-cells usually expressing TCRγδ (145). Clonal rearrangement of the TCRB and TCRG loci can be detected in virtually all patients with T-PLL (146). Multiple chromosomal abnormalities are frequently detected in patients with T-PLL (147, 148). The most common of these chromosomal aberrations result in the juxtaposition of genes of the TCLI family adjacent to TCR loci, resulting in aberrant expression. These include inv(14)(q11;q32) and t(14;14)(q11;q32) rearrangements (147), which juxtapose the TCRA/D locus with at least two related genes, TCL1A and TCL1B, and t(X;14)(q28;q11) and t(X;7)(q28;q35) translocations, which juxtapose MTCP1 (a TCL1 family member) to the TCRA/D or TCRB loci, respectively (148). These rearrangements are best detected by FISH. Loss of chromosome 11q is observed in approximately 60% to 70% of patients with T-PLL (148) and this is accompanied by mutation in the remaining ATM allele (148). Mutation of the ATM gene was observed in approximately 50% of unselected TPLL patients, which probably represents an underestimate because of the large number of exons and size of the

ATM locus. Detection of 11q deletion is best achieved by FISH using a probe spanning the ATM locus, as karyotypes are often complex and mutation screening of the ATM gene is not routine.

NGS (both WGS and WES) identified novel mutations in recurrently altered genes not previously implicated in T-PLL, including EZH2, FBXW10 and CHEK2 (149, 150). Strikingly, WGS and/or WES showed largely mutually exclusive mutations affecting IL2RG, JAK1, JAK3 or STAT5B in 38 out of 50 T-PLL genomes (76.0%). Notably, gain-of-function IL2RG mutations are novel and have not been reported in any form of cancer. Further, high-frequency mutations in STAT5B have not been previously reported in T-PLL. These results for the first time provide a portrait of the mutational landscape of T-PLL and implicate deregulation of DNA repair and epigenetic modulators, as well as high-frequency mutational activation of the IL2RG-JAK1-JAK3-STAT5B axis in the pathogenesis of T-PLL. These findings offer opportunities for novel targeted therapies in this aggressive leukemia (149).

## T-cell large granular lymphocyte leukemia

T-cell LGL leukemia represents a clonal proliferation of cytotoxic T-cells and is characterized by cytopenias (151). In the vast majority of patients, the clonal nature of the T-cell compartment can be demonstrated by PCR assessment of TCRG locus and the TCRB locus. Clonal expansion of CD8+ T-cells including LGLs may be detected in normal individuals, particularly in elderly individuals. Hence, the presence of a clonal TCR gene rearrangement by itself does not necessarily indicate a T-cell malignancy.

A NGS study showed in a series of 50 CLPD-NKs and 120 T-LGL frequent recurrent STAT3 gene mutations present in approximately one-third of patients with both T and NK diseases, suggesting a similar molecular dysregulation in malignant chronic expansions of NK and CTL origin (152). Patients with mutations were characterized by symptomatic disease, history of multiple treatments, and a specific pattern of STAT3 activation and gene deregulation, including increased expression of genes activated by STAT3. Treatment with STAT3 inhibitors, both in wild-type and mutant cases, resulted in accelerated apoptosis. Importantly, STAT3 mutations may distinguish truly malignant lymphoproliferations involving T and NK cells from reactive expansions (152).

## Adult T-cell leukemia/lymphoma

Adult T-cell leukemia/lymphoma (ATLL) (Figure 18.8a–b) is a peripheral T-cell lymphoma caused by infection of the HTLV-1 virus, which is endemic in certain regions such as Japan, the Caribbean and Northern Australia (153). ATL has a poor prognosis with a mean survival time of 13 months, and is refractory to currently available combination chemotherapy. ATL is incurable because we do not have a complete understanding of its molecular basis, leading to the lack of molecular targeting. Although HTLV-1 is an apparent causative agent of ATL, several studies have demonstrated that viral gene expression is rare, except for the expression of the HTLV-1 anti-sense gene product HBZ.

Integration of the HTLV-1 virus into the host genome can be demonstrated by Southern analysis and by PCR (153). TCR genes are clonally rearranged and the demonstration of a clonal population of T-cells in the peripheral blood of healthy HTLV-1 carriers may identify patients at risk of developing ATLL. Abnormal karyotypes are frequent and certain abnormalities such as 14q are associated with a poor prognosis. Gain of chromosome 7q is associated with a good prognosis (153).

Mounting evidence has shown that ATLL does not contain the somatic mutant genes that can explain its aggressiveness. However, it is evident that ATLL cells possess multiple deregulations of genome and gene regulation, namely the molecular hallmarks of ATL, which include cell cycle dysregulation (for example, CDKN2A, p53 and chromosomal alterations), sustained signal transduction (NF-KB, JAK-STAT, mTOR/Akt, Notch, RhoA) and specific gene expression (cytokines). Since 1985, numerous excellent studies have identified signaling abnormalities in HTLV-1-associated cells, mainly induced by HTLV-1 Tax. The classical oncogenic function of Tax was first demonstrated in a study of cell cycle regulation. 'Tax" also participates in genetic damage and can activate several signaling pathways and lead to abnormal gene expression (a Tax-dependent molecular hallmark) and overproduction of several cytokines. IL-2 and its receptor are especially important for T-cell activation. IL-2 signals through its receptor are primarily delivered by two molecular families, the JAKs and STATs, whose activation leads to lymphocyte proliferation. More recent work highlights the

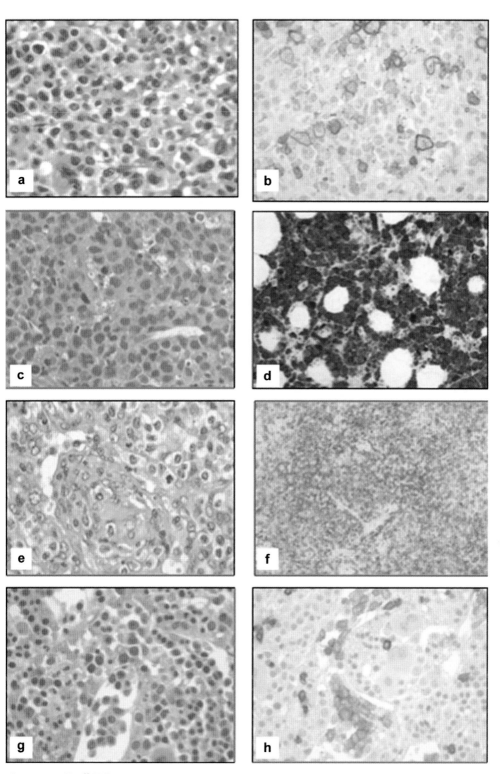

**Figure 18.8  T-cell NHL**
(a) ATLL in the bone marrow (H&E staining, x60 objective); (b) CD25 staining of the same ATLL (APAAP staining, x60 objective); (c) ALCL involving a lymph node and the surrounding adipose tissue (H&E staining, x40 objective); (d) ALK positivity of the same ALCL (PAP staining, x40 objective); (e) AITL in a lymph node (H&E staining, x40 objective); (f) PD1 positivity in the same AITL (PAP staining, x20 objective).

importance of miRNA deregulation, and epigenetic reprogramming in ATLL (153).

# Cutaneous T-cell lymphomas

Cutaneous T-cell lymphomas (CTCL), primarily Sezary syndrome and mycosis fungoides (MF), are mature T-cell malignancies with a predilection for the skin. The demonstration of clonally rearranged TCR loci is an important tool to aid the diagnosis of CTCL (154). Rearrangements of TCRG and/or TCRB genes are detectable by PCR in approximately 75% of cases of CTCL, showing good correlation with Southern hybridization (155). However, clonal rearrangement of TCRG and TCRB loci was identified within 1 out of 12 patients with benign dermatoses (155). The significance of such findings is unclear, but does emphasize the importance of interpreting TCR clonality analysis in the context of histological and other clinical assessment. Identical TCR gene rearrangements can be detected in peripheral blood and/or lymph node of patients with a CTCL. Use of gene rearrangement assays may offer staging and prognostic information, particularly for cases of MF. Patients demonstrating T-cell clonality within lymph nodes by PCR or Southern hybridization had a reduced survival rate compared with those without evidence of TCR gene rearrangement (156).

GEP studies have shown that increased signaling from the TCR can be considered a driving force of CTCL and that neoplastic T-cells can show a degree of phenotypic plasticity, as characterized by the expression of a variety of lineage markers (157). Recent NGS studies of CTCL demonstrated multiple mutations that affected several signaling pathways, such as TCRs, nuclear factor κB or JAK/STAT. Interestingly, the gene PLCG1, which is a critical mediator of TCR signaling, was found to be mutated in between 19% and 30% of samples. Immunohistochemical analysis for "nuclear factor of activated T-cells" (NFAT) showed that PLCG1-mutated cases exhibited strong NFAT nuclear immunostaining. There is potential translation of these results in routine hematopathology.

# Peripheral T-cell lymphomas

Peripheral T-cell lymphomas (PTCL) are a heterogeneous and poorly understood group of non-Hodgkin's lymphomas. PTCLs are subclassified into various subtypes, each of which are typically considered to be separate diseases based on their distinct clinical differences. Most of these subtypes are very rare; the three most common subtypes of PTCL are peripheral T-cell lymphoma not otherwise specified (PTCL-NOS), anaplastic large-cell lymphoma (ALCL), and angioimmunoblastic T-cell lymphoma (AITL), which account for approximately 70% of all PTCLs (154).

## PTCL-NOS

PTCL-NOS refers to a group of diseases that do not fit into any of the other subtypes of PTCL. PTCL-NOS is the most common PTCL subtype, constituting up to 50% of all PTCLs. The term PTCL can be confusing as it can refer to the entire spectrum of mature T-cell lymphomas, but also to the specific PTCL-NOS subtype. Although most patients with PTCL-NOS are diagnosed with their disease confined to the lymph nodes, sites outside the lymph nodes, such as the liver, bone marrow, gastrointestinal tract and skin, may also be involved. This group of PTCLs is aggressive and requires combination chemotherapy upon diagnosis (154).

Recent gene expression profiling and NG studies have revealed new findings that will have a major impact on the current classification. Iqbal et al. identified by GEP from more than 300 PTCLS two molecular subgroups characterized by high expression of either GATA3 or TBX21 trasncriptor factors and corresponding target genes (158). This difference not only is associated with different clinical prognosis, but shows biology correlation. Both transcript factors are master regulators of physiological Thelper (Th) cells, skewing Th cells towards Th2 (GATA3) and Th1 (TBX21). These findings reinforce the evidence that T-cell lineage, or a T-cell of origin, is like in DLBCL a major determinant of PTCL biology and prognosis, as both follicular helper T-cells represent the cellular origin of angioimmunoblastic lymphomas (AITL) and T regulatory phenotype with expression of FOXP3 is associated with HTLV1+ ATLL (158).

## Anaplastic large cell lymphoma

Anaplastic large cell lymphoma (ALCL) is an uncommon T-cell lymphoma characterized by CD30 positivity (159), and accounts for about 3% of all lymphomas in adults (about 15% to 20% of all PTCLs) and between 10% and 30% of all lymphomas in children. ALCL can appear in the skin or in other organs throughout the body (systemic ALCL). A significant proportion of ALCL are characterized by aberrant expression of the anaplastic lymphoma kinase (ALK) protein, termed ALK$^+$ ALCL (Figure 18.8c–d).

ALK$^+$ ALCL is characterized by specific morphological and clinical features and is usually observed in younger patients, whereas ALK$^-$ ALCL usually occurs in older patients and has a poorer prognosis (160). ALK is a receptor tyrosine kinase that is normally only expressed within the nervous system (159). Aberrant ALK expression is the consequence of a translocation between chromosome 2p33, the site of the ALK gene, with a variety of partner chromosomes. Approximately 75% of ALK$^+$ ALCL cases involve a t(2;5) translocation that gives rise to the NPM-ALK fusion protein (Figure 18.8d). Other partners for ALK include TPM3 (chromosome 1), TFG (chromosome 3), ATIC (chromosome 2) and CTCL (chromosome 17) (159). Immunohistochemistry, FISH and molecular genetic methods can all be used to analyze ALCL. Aberrant expression of ALK fusion proteins may be detected by immunohistochemical methods using anti-ALK antibodies (161). The NPM-ALK fusion gene may be detected using a two-color FISH assay, which allows interrogation of non-dividing cells. FISH utilizing a break-apart probe spanning the ALK locus also allows detection of t(2;5) and other ALK rearrangements (162). Molecular genetic methods are available for the detection of NPM-ALK for diagnostic and monitoring purposes. Genomic breakpoints lie within NPM intron 4 and ALK intron 16, allowing detection of the rearrangement by RT-PCR or by long-range PCR of genomic DNA (162). The NPM-ALK fusion transcript can be detected in patients without a detectable t(2;5) because of unsuccessful chromosome preparation or cryptic translocation (162). Both nested RT-PCR assays and real-time RT-PCR have been developed and are able to detect the fusion transcript at a sensitivity of 1 cell in $10^6$. It is worth noting, however, that low levels of NPM-ALK fusion transcripts can be detected in peripheral blood of normal individuals and reactive lymphoid tissue (162). Sensitive RT-PCR assays will be useful for monitoring of minimal residual disease. Both conventional and quantitative RT-PCR for the NPM-ALK fusion transcript have shown bone marrow involvement at diagnosis in patients for whom conventional morphology or immunophenotyping failed to do so. Such patients had a lower progression-free survival rate than those in whom marrow involvement could not be detected. This suggests that RT-PCR-based methods should be routinely performed on staging bone marrow samples at diagnosis and for disease monitoring.

Feldman and co-workers (163) used NGS as a discovery tool in ALK$^-$ ALCL, and found that the DUSP22 phosphatase on chromosome 6p25.3 formed a translocation with the fragile site FRA7H on chromosome 7q32.3. Using FISH in a series of 29 patients, 45% of these cases harbored the t(6;7) (p25.3;q32.3), showing that it is a recurrent event in ALK$^-$ ALCLs. The t(6;7)(p25.3;q32.3) was associated with down-regulation of DUSP22 and up-regulation of MIR29 microRNAs on 7q32.3, suggesting that DUSP22 may act as a tumor suppressor, whereas MIR29 may have an oncogenic function.

After describing two PTCL cases with the inversion (3)(q26q28) leading to a TBL1XR1/TP63 gene fusion that encoded a protein homologous to DNp63, a dominant-negative p63 isoform that inhibits the p53 pathway, Vasmatzis et al. surveyed 190 cases of various peripheral T-cell lymphomas for this abnormality (164). Using FISH, they identified recurrent rearrangements involving TP63 in 9.2% of PTCL-NOS and 11.8% of ALK$^-$ ALCLs (164).

Using a larger cohort of 73 ALK$^-$ ALCLs and 32 ALK$^+$ ALCLs, the same authors found that chromosomal rearrangements of DUSP22 and TP63 were identified in 30% and 8% of ALK-negative ALCLs, respectively. These rearrangements were mutually exclusive and were absent in ALK$^+$ ALCLs. Five-year overall survival rates were 85% for ALK$^+$ ALCLs, 90% for DUSP22-rearranged ALCLs, 17% for TP63-rearranged ALCLs and 42% for cases lacking all three genetic markers. Thus, ALK$^-$ ALCL is a genetically heterogeneous disease with widely disparate outcomes following standard therapy. DUSP22 and TP63 rearrangements may serve as predictive biomarkers to help guide patient management (165).

### Angioimmunoblastic T-cell lymphoma

Angioimmunoblastic T-cell lymphoma (AITL) (Figure 18.8e) is a peripheral T-cell lymphoma associated with systemic disease and has a distinctive immunoprofile, including positivity for PD1 (Figure 18.8f). It is an aggressive T-cell lymphoma that accounts for about 2% of all NHL cases (about 10% to 15% of all PTCLs). This type of lymphoma often responds to milder therapies, such as steroids, although it often progresses and requires chemotherapy and other medications. In advanced cases, bone marrow transplantation may be used.

The majority of cases demonstrate TCR gene rearrangements (166). Assessment of lymphoid clonality is complicated by the presence of both TCR and IG gene rearrangements in a subset of patients (8). These patients may have a poorer prognosis compared with those with rearrangement of TCR loci only. The EBV genome can be detected in the majority of cases (167).

Recent NGS work on AITL has demonstrated high frequencies of overlapping mutations in epigenetic modifiers and targetable mutations in a subset of cases (168). For example, TET2 was mutated in 65 (76%) AITLs, including 43 that harbored two or three TET2 mutations. DNMT3A mutations occurred in 28 (33%) AITLs. This opens the potential for druggable targets in this aggressive T-cell lymphoma.

### Hepatosplenic T-cell lymphoma

Hepatosplenic T-cell lymphoma (HSTL) is a rare systemic T-cell lymphoma with an aggressive clinical course (Figure 18.8g–h) (169). The neoplastic cells are generally of TCRγδ type, although a minority of cases are of TCRαβ type. Hence, clonal rearrangement of TCRD and TCRG loci can be detected by PCR in virtually all patients (169). Non-productive rearrangements of the TCRB locus are also observed; isochromosome 7q is frequently present (170, 171).

Compared with other T-cell lymphomas, HSTL have a distinct molecular signature irrespective of TCR cell lineage (171). Compared with PTCL-NOS and normal γδ T-cells, HSTL over-express genes encoding NK-cell-associated molecules, oncogenes (FOS and VAV3), the sphingosine-1-phosphatase receptor 5 involved in cell trafficking, and the tyrosine kinase SYK, whereas the tumor-suppressor gene AIM1 (absent in melanoma 1) was among the most commonly under-expressed. Interestingly, Syk is a protein tyrosine kinase involved in BCR signaling, and its activation is associated with cell growth and survival in B-cell lymphomas. Normal mature T lymphocytes lack Syk expression. However, the Syk protein has been reported recently as a feature common to most PTCL; this may represent a novel therapeutic target, because, in addition to its aberrant expression in many PTCLs, inhibition of Syk induces

apoptosis and blocks proliferation in T-cell lymphoma cell lines (171).

## Natural killer cell malignancies

Natural killer (NK) cell malignancies are an uncommon group of diseases with an aggressive clinical course (172, 173). The molecular pathogenesis of these disorders is incompletely understood, precluding the application of molecular genetic techniques in diagnosis and disease management. Both TCR and IG gene loci are in germline configuration. Deletion of 6q is the most frequent chromosomal change (173). The use of molecular genetic and cytogenetic techniques has also demonstrated other frequent chromosomal aberrations, such as loss of 13q and gain of 1q. The majority of cases of NK cell malignancies show EBV infection (174), which can be demonstrated by *in situ* hybridization detection of EBV-encoded RNA molecules (Figure 18.9a–d) (EBER). Furthermore, quantification of circulating EBV DNA levels offers useful prognostic information (172, 173). Higher levels of plasma EBV DNA, which can be assessed by real-time quantitative PCR, correlate with a much shorter survival rate. Furthermore, patients who do not achieve undetectable levels of plasma EBV DNA, in response to therapy, have a poorer outlook. Hence, the amount of plasma EBV DNA can be a useful marker of residual disease (172, 173).

Recent studies suggest that there is a role of JAK3 mutations in T-/NK-cell lymphomas (175, 176). JAK3 mediates diverse types of cytokine receptor signaling by interacting with the common gamma chain of IL receptors for IL-2, -4, -7, -9, -15 and -21. Recurrent mutations in JAK3 have been found in 20% to 35% of extranodal NK-/T-cell lymphoma samples (175). Most identified JAK3 mutations are missense mutations, A572V or A573V, and less frequently V722I in the pseudokinase domain. JAK3 mutations result in constitutive phosphorylation of JAK3 tyrosine 980 and activation of downstream signaling, such as phosphorylation of STAT5, STAT3, AKT and ERK (175). Activation of JAK3 signaling by these mutations enhances proliferation and invasiveness of NK-/T-cell lymphoma cell lines, which is abrogated by chemical inhibitors or siRNAs targeting mutant JAK3. It remains to be demonstrated whether these findings are of clinical or diagnostic relevance.

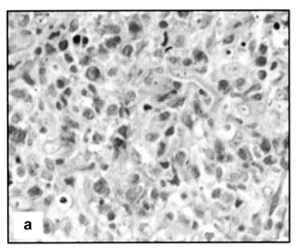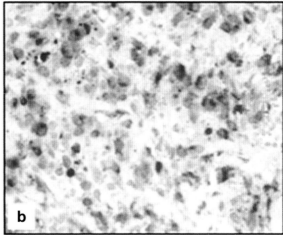

**Figure 18.9** (a) T/NK lymphoma of the orbit (H&E staining, x40 objective); (b) EBV encoded RNA molecules (EBER) positivity demonstrated using FISH (x40 objective).

# Hodgkin's lymphoma

Hodgkin's lymphoma (HL) is derived from mature B-cells and is subdivided into classical HL (cHL) (Figure 18.10) and nodular lymphocyte predominant HL (NLPHL). Accounting for 25% of all lymphomas and nearly 95% of all Hodgkin's lymphomas, patients with cHL are typically young adults. HL is unique among human B-cell lymphomas because of the scarcity of the lymphoma cells within the tumors: the Hodgkin and Reed-Sternberg (HRS) cells in cHL (Figure 18.10b) and the lymphocyte predominant (LP) cells in NLPHL. They usually account for only 0.1% to 10% of the cells in the affected tissues.

The development of laser capture microdissection techniques in the 1990s (177) firmly established the clonal B-cell identity of HRS cells (178). Since then, several studies have used cell lines, primary cHL tumor suspensions and/or microdissected HRS cells to examine genomic imbalances, copy-number alterations (179) or GEP signatures in HL (178, 180). For example, studies of microdissected HRS cells demonstrated that they derive from germinal center (GC) or post-GC B-cells because they carry somatically mutated IGVH genes. Destructive IGVH gene mutations in a fraction of cases suggest a derivation of HRS cells from GC B-cells that acquired such mutations and normally would undergo apoptosis. However, HRS cells are latently infected by EBV in about 40% of patients, and EBV is thought to be capable of rescuing pre-apoptotic germinal center B-cells from apoptosis. On the other hand, the over-expression of CFLIP and XIAP protein has also been detected in HRS cells, and it has also been proposed that they seem to be central to the resistance to apoptosis that is evident in these cells (178).

Furthermore, it was demonstrated that HRS cells are unique in the extent to which they have lost their B-cell-typical gene expression pattern. Deregulation of transcription factor networks plays a key role in this reprogramming process. In addition, HRS cells show strong constitutive activity of the transcription factor NF-κB. Multiple mechanisms are likely to contribute to this deregulated activation, including signaling through particular receptors and genetic lesions. Moreover, inactivating mutations in the TNFAIP3 tumor suppressor gene, encoding a negative regulator of NF-κB activity, were identified in about 40% of patients with classical HL (178).

Rapid strides made in NGS recently has enabled high throughput testing of larger numbers of HL cases, providing valuable information to the pathogenesis of these tumors (181, 182). A genome-wide transcriptional analysis of microdissected HRS cells compared with other B-cell lymphomas, cHL lines and normal B-cell subsets showed that HRS cells differ significantly from the usually studied cHL cell lines, that the lost B-cell identity of cHLs is not linked to the acquisition of a plasma cell-like gene expression program, and that EBV infection of HRS cells has a

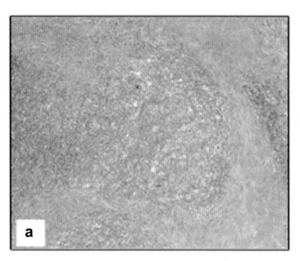
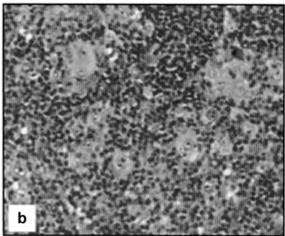

**Figure 18.10** (a) Classic HL of nodular sclerosing subtype in a lymph node (H&E staining, x20 objective); (b) higher magnification demonstrating the Hodgkin and Reed-Sternberg cells (H&E staining, x40 objective).

minor transcriptional influence on the established cHL clone. Moreover, although cHL appears to be a distinct lymphoma entity overall, HRS cells of its histologic subtypes diverged in their similarity to other related lymphomas. Unexpectedly, two molecular subgroups of cHL were identified and were associated with differential strengths of the transcription factor activity of the NOTCH1, MYC and IRF4 proto-oncogenes. Finally, HRS cells appear to display deregulated expression of several genes potentially highly relevant to lymphoma pathogenesis, including silencing of the apoptosis-inducer BIK and of INPP5D, an inhibitor of the PI3K-driven oncogenic pathway (178).

## Learning points

- Molecular genetic analysis has now become an integral part of routine diagnostic work-up and monitoring of patients with many of the mature lymphoid neoplasms. This has in large part been achieved through the efforts of the pan-European BIOMED2/EuroClonality consortium.
- The development and standardization of these molecular genetic assays has enabled them to be utilized routinely in diagnostic laboratories. However, there are still some limitations in their use and further standardization is needed. Consensus is required as to which molecular genetic tests are essential for a diagnosis, how frequently molecular analysis should be

performed to assess residual disease, what is the required sensitivity of the test and what are the most appropriate cut-off values for a positive result. Also, the role for molecular analysis in disease staging, including assessment of the CNS, needs to be addressed.

- Our knowledge of the pathogenetic mechanisms underlying mature lymphoid malignancies has progressed significantly through the development of novel molecular techniques such as GEP and more recently NGS. NGS technology has been applied to lymphoid neoplasms and has provided some early insight into the mutational landscape of several lymphoid cancers.
- A major challenge now is to determine which of these new genetic markers is important for diagnosis or prognosis and how to incorporate these novel molecular findings into clinical practice. For some of these novel genetic findings, molecular analysis may not be the most appropriate investigation. Other simpler methods such as immunophenotyping and cytogenetics may be able to provide the information regarding the expression of a gene or gene product of interest. Likewise, deep-sequencing protocols will definitively change the routine practice of hematopathology in the near future. The role of molecular genetics must, therefore, be considered together with these other test modalities, particularly when designing clinical trials and assessing novel therapies.

# References

1. Morin, R. D. and Gascoyne, R. D. Newly identified mechanisms in B-cell non-Hodgkin lymphomas uncovered by next-generation sequencing. *Semin Hematol* 2013; 50(4): 303–313.

2. Harris, N. L., Stein, H., Coupland, S. E., Hummel, M., Favera, R. D., Pasqualucci, L. *et al.* New approaches to lymphoma diagnosis. *Hematology Am Soc Hematol Educ Program* 2001; 194–220.

3. Coupland, S. E. Molecular pathology of lymphoma. *Eye (Lond)* 2013; 27(2): 180–189.

4. Rezuke, W. N., Abernathy, E. C. and Tsongalis, G. J. Molecular diagnosis of B- and T-cell lymphomas: fundamental principles and clinical applications. *Clin Chem* 1997; 43(10): 1814–1823.

5. Spagnolo, D. V., Ellis, D. W., Juneja, S., Leong, A. S., Miliauskas, J., Norris, D. L. *et al.* The role of molecular studies in lymphoma diagnosis: a review. *Pathology* 2004; 36(1): 19–44.

6. Sandberg, Y., van Gastel-Mol, E. J., Verhaaf, B., Lam, K. H., van Dongen, J. J. and Langerak, A. W. BIOMED-2 multiplex immunoglobulin/T-cell receptor polymerase chain reaction protocols can reliably replace Southern blot analysis in routine clonality diagnostic. *J Mol Diagn* 2005; 7(4): 495–503.

7. Lukowsky, A., Marchwat, M., Sterry, W. and Gellrich, S. Evaluation of B-cell clonality in archival skin biopsy samples of cutaneous B-cell lymphoma by immunoglobulin heavy chain gene polymerase chain reaction. *Leuk Lymphoma* 2006; 47(3): 487–493.

8. van Dongen, J. J., Langerak, A. W., Brüggemann, M., Evans, P. A., Hummel, M., Lavender, F. L. *et al.* Design and standardization of PCR primers and protocols for detection of clonal immunoglobulin and T-cell receptor gene recombinations in suspect lymphoproliferations: report of the BIOMED-2 Concerted Action BMH4-CT98-3936. *Leukemia* 2003; 17(12): 2257–2317.

9. Evans, P. A., Pott, Ch., Groenen, P. J., Salles, G., Davi, F., Berger, F. *et al.* Significantly improved PCR-based clonality testing in B-cell malignancies by use of multiple immunoglobulin gene targets. Report of the BIOMED-2 Concerted Action BHM4-CT98-3936. *Leukemia* 2007; 21(2): 207–214.

10. Langerak, A. W., Groenen, P. J., Brüggemann, M., Beldjord, K., Bellan, C., Bonello, L. *et al.* EuroClonality/BIOMED-2 guidelines for interpretation and reporting of Ig/TCR clonality testing in suspected lymphoproliferations. *Leukemia* 2012; 26(10): 2159–2171.

11. Halldórsdóttir, A. M., Zehnbauer, B. A. and Burack, W. R. Application of BIOMED-2 clonality assays to formalin-fixed paraffin embedded follicular lymphoma specimens: superior performance of the IGK assays compared to IGH for suboptimal specimens. *Leuk Lymphoma* 2007; 48(7): 1338–1343.

12. Payne, K., Wright, P., Grant, J. W., Huang, Y., Hamoudi, R., Bacon, C. M. *et al.* BIOMED-2 PCR assays for IGK gene rearrangements are essential for B-cell clonality analysis in follicular lymphoma. *Br J Haematol* 2011; 155(1): 84–92.

13. Liu, H., Bench, A. J., Bacon, C. M., Payne, K., Huang, Y., Scott, M. A. *et al.* A practical strategy for the routine use of BIOMED-2 PCR assays for detection of B- and T-cell clonality in diagnostic haematopathology. *Br J Haematol* 2007; 138(1): 31–43.

14. Patel, K. P., Pan, Q., Wang, Y., Maitta, R. W., Du, J., Xue, X. *et al.* Comparison of BIOMED-2 versus laboratory-developed polymerase chain reaction assays for detecting T-cell receptor-gamma gene rearrangements. *J Mol Diagn* 2010; 12(2): 226–237.

15. van Krieken, J. H., Langerak, A. W., Macintyre, E. A., Kneba, M., Hodges, E., Sanz, R. G. *et al.* Improved reliability of lymphoma diagnostics via PCR-based clonality testing: report of the BIOMED-2 Concerted Action BHM4-CT98-3936. *Leukemia* 2007; 21(2): 201–206.

16. Gribben, J. G. Molecular profiling in CLL. *Hematology Am Soc Hematol Educ Program* 2008: 444–449.

17. Swerdlow, S. H., Campo, E., Harris, N. L., Jaffe, E. S., Pileri, S. A., Stein, H. *et al. WHO Classification of Tumours of Haematopoietic and Lymphoid Tissues*, 4th edn. (Lyon: IARC Press, 2008).

18. Hauswirth, A. W. and Jäger, U. Impact of cytogenetic and molecular prognostic markers on the clinical management of chronic lymphocytic leukemia. *Haematologica* 2008; 93(1): 14–19.

19. Fais, F., Ghiotto, F., Hashimoto, S., Sellars, B., Valetto, A., Allen, S. L. *et al.* Chronic lymphocytic leukemia B cells express restricted sets of mutated and unmutated antigen receptors. *J Clin Invest* 1998; 102(8): 1515–1525.

20. Stevenson, F. K. and Caligaris-Cappio, F. Chronic lymphocytic leukemia: revelations from the B-cell receptor. *Blood* 2004; 103(12): 4389–4395.

21. Damle, R. N., Wasil, T., Fais, F., Ghiotto, F., Valetto, A., Allen, S. L. *et al.* Ig V gene mutation status and CD38 expression as novel prognostic indicators in chronic lymphocytic leukemia. *Blood* 1999; 94(6): 1840–1847.

22. Hamblin, T. J., Davis, Z., Gardiner, A., Oscier, D. G. and Stevenson, F. K. Unmutated Ig V (H) genes are associated with a

more aggressive form of chronic lymphocytic leukemia. *Blood* 1999; 94(6): 1848–1854.

23. Oscier, D. G., Gardiner, A. C., Mould, S. J., Glide, S., Davis, Z. A., Ibbotson, R. E. *et al.* Multivariate analysis of prognostic factors in CLL: clinical stage, IGVH gene mutational status, and loss or mutation of the p53 gene are independent prognostic factors. *Blood* 2002; 100(4): 1177–1184.

24. Vasconcelos, Y., Davi, F., Levy, V., Oppezzo, P., Magnac, C., Michel, A. *et al.* Binet's staging system and VH genes are independent but complementary prognostic indicators in chronic lymphocytic leukemia. *J Clin Oncol* 2003; 21(21): 3928–3932.

25. Ritgen, M., Stilgenbauer, S., von Neuhoff, N., Humpe, A., Brüggemann, M., Pott, C. *et al.* Graft-versus-leukemia activity may overcome therapeutic resistance of chronic lymphocytic leukemia with unmutated immunoglobulin variable heavy-chain gene status: implications of minimal residual disease measurement with quantitative PCR. *Blood* 2004; 104(8): 2600–2602.

26. Tobin, G. and Rosenquist, R. Prognostic usage of V(H) gene mutation status and its surrogate markers and the role of antigen selection in chronic lymphocytic leukemia. *Med Oncol* 2005; 22(3): 217–228.

27. Rosenwald, A., Alizadeh, A. A., Widhopf, G., Simon, R., Davis, R. E., Yu, X. *et al.* Relation of gene expression phenotype to immunoglobulin mutation genotype in B cell chronic lymphocytic leukemia. *J Exp Med* 2001; 194(11): 1639–1647.

28. Crespo, M., Bosch, F., Villamor, N., Bellosillo, B., Colomer, D., Rozman, M. *et al.* ZAP-70 expression as a surrogate for immunoglobulin-variable-region mutations in chronic lymphocytic

leukemia. *New Engl J Med* 2003; 348(18): 1764–1775.

29. Döhner, H., Stilgenbauer, S., Benner, A., Leupolt, E., Kröber, A., Bullinger, L. *et al.* Genomic aberrations and survival in chronic lymphocytic leukemia. *New Engl J Med* 2000; 343(26): 1910–1916.

30. Stilgenbauer, S. and Döhner, H. Campath-1H-induced complete remission of chronic lymphocytic leukemia despite p53 gene mutation and resistance to chemotherapy. *New Engl J Med* 2002; 347(6): 452–453.

31. Pettitt, A. R., Sherrington, P. D., Stewart, G., Cawley, J. C., Taylor, A. M. and Stankovic, T. *Blood* 2001; 98(3): 814–822.

32. Rassenti, L. Z., Jain, S., Keating, M. J., Wierda, W. G., Grever, M. R., Byrd, J. C. *et al.* Relative value of ZAP-70, CD38, and immunoglobulin mutation status in predicting aggressive disease in chronic lymphocytic leukemia. *Blood* 2008; 112(5): 1923–1930.

33. Shanafelt, T. D., Geyer, S. M. and Kay, N. E. Prognosis at diagnosis: integrating molecular biologic insights into clinical practice for patients with CLL. *Blood* 2004; 103(4): 1202–1210.

34. Grever, M. R., Lucas, D. M., Dewald, G. W., Neuberg, D. S., Reed, J. C., Kitada, S. *et al.* Comprehensive assessment of genetic and molecular features predicting outcome in patients with chronic lymphocytic leukemia: results from the US Intergroup Phase III Trial E2997. *J Clin Oncol* 2007; 25(7): 799–804.

35. Puente, X. S., Pinyol, M., Quesada, V., Conde, L., Ordóñez, G. R., Villamor, N. *et al.* Whole-genome sequencing identifies recurrent mutations in chronic lymphocytic leukaemia. *Nature* 2011; 475(7354): 101–105.

36. Fabbri, G., Rasi, S., Rossi, D., Trifonov, V., Khiabanian, H., Ma, J. *et al.* Analysis of the chronic

lymphocytic leukemia coding genome: role of NOTCH1 mutational activation. *J Exp Med* 2011; 208(7): 1389–1401.

37. Rossi, D., Bruscaggin, A., Spina, V., Rasi, S., Khiabanian, H., Messina, M. *et al.* Mutations of the SF3B1 splicing factor in chronic lymphocytic leukemia: association with progression and fludarabine-refractoriness. *Blood* 2011; 118(26): 6904–6908.

38. Quesada, V., Conde, L., Villamor, N., Ordóñez, G. R., Jares, P., Bassaganyas, L. *et al.* Exome sequencing identifies recurrent mutations of the splicing factor SF3B1 gene in chronic lymphocytic leukemia. *Nat Genet* 2011; 44(1): 47–52.

39. Wan, Y. and Wu, C. J. SF3B1 mutations in chronic lymphocytic leukemia. *Blood* 2013; 21(23): 4627–4634.

40. Gribben, J. G. Monitoring disease in lymphoma and CLL patients using molecular techniques. *Best Pract Res Clin Haematol* 2002; 15(1): 179–195.

41. Provan, D., Bartlett-Pandite, L., Zwicky, C., Neuberg, D., Maddocks, A., Corradini, P. *et al.* Eradication of polymerase chain reaction-detectable chronic lymphocytic leukemia cells is associated with improved outcome after bone marrow transplantation. *Blood* 1996; 88(6): 2228–2235.

42. Milligan, D. W., Fernandes, S., Dasgupta, R., Davies, F. E., Matutes, E., Fegan, C. D. *et al.* Results of the MRC pilot study show autografting for younger patients with chronic lymphocytic leukemia is safe and achieves a high percentage of molecular responses. *Blood* 2005; 105(1): 397–404.

43. Rawstron, A. C., Böttcher, S., Letestu, R., Villamor, N., Fazi, C., Kartsios, H. *et al.* Improving efficiency and sensitivity: European Research Initiative in

CLL (ERIC) update on the international harmonised approach for flow cytometric residual disease monitoring in CLL. *Leukemia* 2013; 27(1): 142–149.

44. Forconi, F., Sozzi, E., Cencini, E., Zaja, F., Intermesoli, T., Stelitano, C. et al. Hairy cell leukemias with unmutated IGHV genes define the minor subset refractory to single-agent cladribine and with more aggressive behavior. *Blood* 2009; 114(21): 4696–4702.

45. Ravandi, F., Jorgensen, J. L., O'Brien, S. M., Verstovsek, S., Koller, C. A., Faderl, S. et al. Eradication of minimal residual disease in hairy cell leukemia. *Blood* 2006; 107(12): 4658–4662.

46. Tiacci, E., Trifonov, V., Schiavoni, G., Holmes, A., Kern, W., Martelli, M. P. et al. BRAF mutations in hairy-cell leukemia. *New Engl J Med* 2011; 364(24): 2305–2315.

47. Samuel, J., Macip, S. and Dyer, M. J. Efficacy of vemurafenib in hairy-cell leukemia. *New Engl J Med* 2014; 370(3): 286–288.

48. Davi, F., Maloum, K., Michel, A., Pritsch, O., Magnac, C., Macintyre, E. et al. High frequency of somatic mutations in the VH genes expressed in prolymphocytic leukemia. *Blood* 1996; 88(10): 3953–3961.

49. Ruchlemer, R., Parry-Jones, N., Brito-Babapulle, V., Attolico, I., Wotherspoon, A. C., Matutes, E. et al. B-prolymphocytic leukaemia with t(11;14) revisited: a splenomegalic form of mantle cell lymphoma evolving with leukaemia. *Br J Haematol* 2004; 125(3): 330–336.

50. Schlette, E., Lai, R., Onciu, M., Doherty, D., Bueso-Ramos, C. and Medeiros, L. J. Leukemic mantle cell lymphoma: clinical and pathologic spectrum of twenty-three cases. *Mod Pathol* 2001; 14(11): 1133–1140.

51. van der Velden, V. H., Hoogeveen, P. G., de Ridder, D., Schindler-van der Struijk, M., van Zelm, M. C., Sanders, M. et al. B-cell prolymphocytic leukemia: a specific subgroup of mantle cell lymphoma. *Blood* 2014; 124(3): 412–19.

52. Medeiros, L. J., van Krieken, J. H., Jaffe, E. S. and Raffeld, M. Association of bcl-1 rearrangements with lymphocytic lymphoma of intermediate differentiation. *Blood* 1990; 76(10): 2086–2090.

53. Rosenberg, C. L., Wong, E., Petty, E. M., Bale, A. E., Tsujimoto, Y., Harris, N. L. et al. PRAD1, a candidate BCL1 oncogene: mapping and expression in centrocytic lymphoma. *Proc Natl Acad Sci USA* 1991; 88(21): 9638–9642.

54. Mozos, A., Royo, C., Hartmann, E., De Jong, D., Baró, C., Valera, A. et al. SOX11 expression is highly specific for mantle cell lymphoma and identifies the cyclin D1-negative subtype. *Haematologica* 2009; 94(11): 1555–1562.

55. Vaandrager, J. W., Schuuring, E., Zwikstra, E., de Boer, C. J., Kleiverda, K. K., van Krieken, J. H. et al. Direct visualization of dispersed 11q13 chromosomal translocations in mantle cell lymphoma by multicolor DNA fiber fluorescence in situ hybridization. *Blood* 1996; 88(4): 1177–1182.

56. Bosch, F., Jares, P., Campo, E., Lopez-Guillermo, A., Piris, M. A., Villamor, N. et al. PRAD-1/cyclin D1 gene overexpression in chronic lymphoproliferative disorders: a highly specific marker of mantle cell lymphoma. *Blood* 1994; 84(8): 2726–2732.

57. Aguilera, N. S., Bijwaard, K. E., Duncan, B., Krafft, A. E., Chu, W. S., Abbondanzo, S. L. et al. Differential expression of cyclin D1 in mantle cell lymphoma and other non-Hodgkin's lymphomas. *Am J Pathol* 1998; 153(6): 1969–1976.

58. Uchimaru, K., Taniguchi, T., Yoshikawa, M., Asano, S., Arnold, A., Fujita, T. et al. Detection of cyclin D1 (bcl-1, PRAD1) overexpression by a simple competitive reverse transcription-polymerase chain reaction assay in t(11;14)(q13;q32)-bearing B-cell malignancies and/or mantle cell lymphoma. *Blood* 1997; 89(3): 965–974.

59. Thorsélius, M., Walsh, S., Eriksson, I., Thunberg, U., Johnson, A., Backlin, C. et al. Somatic hypermutation and V(H) gene usage in mantle cell lymphoma. *Eur J Haematol* 2002; 68(4): 217–242.

60. Orchard, J., Garand, R., Davis, Z., Babbage, G., Sahota, S., Matutes, E. et al. A subset of t(11;14) lymphoma with mantle cell features displays mutated IgVH genes and includes patients with good prognosis, nonnodal disease. *Blood* 2003; 101(12): 4975–4981.

61. Corradini, P., Ladetto, M., Zallio, F., Astolfi, M., Rizzo, E., Sametti, S. et al. Long-term follow-up of indolent lymphoma patients treated with high-dose sequential chemotherapy and autografting: evidence that durable molecular and clinical remission frequently can be attained only in follicular subtypes. *J Clin Oncol* 2004; 22(8): 1460–1468.

62. Howard, O. M., Gribben, J. G., Neuberg, D. S., Grossbard, M., Poor, C., Janicek, M. J. et al. Rituximab and CHOP induction therapy for newly diagnosed mantle-cell lymphoma: molecular complete responses are not predictive of progression-free survival. *J Clin Oncol* 2002; 20(5): 1288–1294.

63. Pott, C., Schrader, C., Gesk, S., Harder, L., Tiemann, M., Raff, T. et al. Quantitative assessment of molecular remission after high-dose therapy with autologous stem cell transplantation predicts long-term remission in mantle cell lymphoma. *Blood* 2006; 107(6): 2271–2278.

**329**

64. Bertoni, F., Zucca, E. and Cotter, F. E. Molecular basis of mantle cell lymphoma. *Br J Haematol* 2004; 124(2): 130–140.

65. Louie, D. C., Offit, K., Jaslow, R., Parsa, N. Z., Murty, V. V., Schluger, A. *et al.* p53 overexpression as a marker of poor prognosis in mantle cell lymphomas with t(11;14)(q13;q32). *Blood* 1995; 86(8): 2892–2899.

66. Kridel, R., Meissner, B., Rogic, S., Boyle, M., Telenius, A., Woolcock, B. *et al.* Whole transcriptome sequencing reveals recurrent NOTCH1 mutations in mantle cell lymphoma. *Blood* 2012; 119(9): 1963–1971.

67. Willis, T. G. and Dyer, M. J. The role of immunoglobulin translocations in the pathogenesis of B-cell malignancies. *Blood* 2000; 96(3): 808–822.

68. Buchonnet, G., Jardin, F., Jean, N., Bertrand, P., Parmentier, F., Tison, S. *et al.* Distribution of BCL2 breakpoints in follicular lymphoma and correlation with clinical features: specific subtypes or same disease? *Leukemia* 2002; 16(9): 1852–1856.

69. Vaandrager, J. W., Schuuring, E., Raap, T., Philippo, K., Kleiverda, K. and Kluin, P. Interphase FISH detection of BCL2 rearrangement in follicular lymphoma using breakpoint-flanking probes. *Gene Chromosome Canc* 2000; 27(1): 85–94.

70. Belaud-Rotureau, M. A., Parrens, M., Carrere, N., Turmo, M., Ferrer, J., de Mascarel, A. *et al.* Interphase fluorescence in situ hybridization is more sensitive than BIOMED-2 polymerase chain reaction protocol in detecting IGH-BCL2 rearrangement in both fixed and frozen lymph node with follicular lymphoma. *Hum Pathol* 2007; 38(2): 365–372.

71. Falini, B. and Mason, D. Y. Proteins encoded by genes involved in chromosomal alterations in lymphoma and leukemia: clinical value of their detection by immunocytochemistry. *Blood* 2002; 99(2): 409–426.

72. Skinnider, B. F., Horsman, D. E., Dupuis, B. and Gascoyne, R. D. Bcl-6 and Bcl-2 protein expression in diffuse large B-cell lymphoma and follicular lymphoma: correlation with 3q27 and 18q21 chromosomal abnormalities. *Hum Pathol* 1999; 30(7): 803–808.

73. Jardin, F., Buchonnet, G., Parmentier, F., Contentin, N., Leprêtre, S., Lenain, P. *et al.* Follicle center lymphoma is associated with significantly elevated levels of BCL-6 expression among lymphoma subtypes, independent of chromosome 3q27 rearrangements. *Leukemia* 2002; 16(11): 2318–2325.

74. Gribben, J. G., Neuberg, D., Freedman, A. S., Gimmi, C. D., Pesek, K. W., Barber, M. *et al.* Detection by polymerase chain reaction of residual cells with the bcl-2 translocation is associated with increased risk of relapse after autologous bone marrow transplantation for B-cell lymphoma. *Blood* 1993; 81(12): 3449–3457.

75. Luthra, R., McBride, J. A., Cabanillas, F. and Sarris, A. Novel 5' exonuclease-based real-time PCR assay for the detection of t(14;18)(q32;q21) in patients with follicular lymphoma. *Am J Pathol* 1999; 153(1): 63–68.

76. Iqbal, S., Jenner, M. J., Summers, K. E., Davies, A. J., Matthews, J., Norton, A. *et al.* Reliable detection of clonal IgH/Bcl2 MBR rearrangement in follicular lymphoma: methodology and clinical significance *Br J Haematol* 2004; 124(3): 325–328.

77. Sanchez-Vega, B., Vega, F., Hai, S., Medeiros, L. J. and Luthra, R. Real-time t(14;18)(q32;q21) PCR assay combined with high-resolution capillary electrophoresis: a novel and rapid approach that allows accurate quantitation and size determination of bcl-2/JH fusion sequences. *Mod Pathol* 2002; 15(4): 448–453.

78. Limpens, J., Stad, R., Vos, C., de Vlaam, C., de Jong, D., van Ommen, G. J. *et al.* Lymphoma-associated translocation t(14;18) in blood B cells of normal individuals. *Blood* 1995; 85(9): 2528–2536.

79. Rambaldi, A., Lazzari, M., Manzoni, C., Carlotti, E., Arcaini, L., Baccarani, M. *et al.* Monitoring of minimal residual disease after CHOP and rituximab in previously untreated patients with follicular lymphoma. *Blood* 2002; 99(3): 856–862.

80. Galimberti, S., Guerrini, F., Morabito, F., Palumbo, G. A., Di Raimondo, F., Papineschi, F. *et al.* Quantitative molecular evaluation in autotransplant programs for follicular lymphoma: efficacy of in vivo purging by Rituximab. *Bone Marrow Transplant* 2003; 32(1): 57–63.

81. Matolcsy, A., Casali, P., Warnke, R. A. and Knowles, D. M. Morphologic transformation of follicular lymphoma is associated with somatic mutation of the translocated Bcl-2 gene. *Blood* 1996; 88(10): 3937–3944.

82. Szereday, Z., Csernus, B., Nagy, M., László, T., Warnke, R. A. and Matolcsy, A. Somatic mutation of the 5' noncoding region of the BCL-6 gene is associated with intraclonal diversity and clonal selection in histological transformation of follicular lymphoma. *Am J Pathol* 2000; 156(3): 1017–1024.

83. Lo Coco, F., Gaidano, G., Louie, D. C., Offit, K. and Chaganti, R. S. Dalla-Favera R. p53 mutations are associated with histologic transformation of follicular

lymphoma. *Blood* 1993; 82(8): 2289–2295.

84. Yano, T., Jaffe, E. S., Longo, D. L. and Raffeld, M. MYC rearrangements in histologically progressed follicular lymphomas. *Blood* 1992; 80(3): 758–767.

85. Elenitoba-Johnson, K. S., Gascoyne, R. D., Lim, M. S., Chhanabai, M., Jaffe, E. S. and Raffeld, M. Homozygous deletions at chromosome 9p21 involving p16 and p15 are associated with histologic progression in follicle center lymphoma. *Blood* 1998; 91(12): 4677–4685.

86. Pinyol, M., Cobo, F., Bea, S., Jares, P., Nayach, I., Fernandez, P. L. *et al.* p16(INK4a) gene inactivation by deletions, mutations, and hypermethylation is associated with transformed and aggressive variants of non-Hodgkin's lymphomas. *Blood* 1998; 91(8): 2977–2984.

87. Okosun, J., Bödör, C., Wang, J., Araf, S., Yang, C. Y., Pan, C. *et al.* Integrated genomic analysis identifies recurrent mutations and evolution patterns driving the initiation and progression of follicular lymphoma. *Nat Genet* 2014; 46(2): 176–178.

88. Abramson, J. S. and Shipp, M. A. Advances in the biology and therapy of diffuse large B-cell lymphoma: moving toward a molecularly targeted approach. *Blood* 2005; 106(4): 1164–1174.

89. Barrans, S. L., O'Connor, S. J., Evans, P. A., Davies, F. E., Owen, R. G., Haynes, A. P. *et al.* Rearrangement of the BCL6 locus at 3q27 is an independent poor prognostic factor in nodal diffuse large B-cell lymphoma. *Br J Haematol* 2002; 117(2): 322–332.

90. Barrans, S. L., Evans, P. A., O'Connor, S. J., Kendall, S. J., Owen, R. G., Haynes, A. P. *et al.* The t(14;18) is associated with germinal center-derived diffuse large B-cell lymphoma and is a

strong predictor of outcome. *Clin Cancer Res* 2003; 9(6): 2133–2139.

91. Rosenwald, A. and Staudt, L. M. Gene expression profiling of diffuse large B-cell lymphoma. *Leuk Lymphoma* 2003; 44(Suppl. 3): S41–47.

92. Hans, C. P., Weisenburger, D. D., Greiner, T. C., Gascoyne, R. D., Delabie, J., Ott, G. *et al.* Confirmation of the molecular classification of diffuse large B-cell lymphoma by immunohistochemistry using a tissue microarray. *Blood* 2004; 103(1): 275–282.

93. Gascoyne, R. D. Pathologic prognostic factors in diffuse aggressive non-Hodgkin's lymphoma. *Hematol Oncol Clin North Am* 1997; 11(5): 847–862.

94. Vega, F., Orduz, R. and Medeiros, L. J. Chromosomal translocations and their role in the pathogenesis of non-Hodgkin's lymphomas. *Pathology* 2002; 34(5): 397–409.

95. Akasaka, T., Ueda, C., Kurata, M., Yamabe, H., Uchiyama, T. and Ohno, H. Nonimmunoglobulin (non-Ig)/BCL6 gene fusion in diffuse large B-cell lymphoma results in worse prognosis than Ig/BCL6. *Blood* 2000; 96(8): 2907–2909.

96. Lu, Z., Tsai, A. G., Akasaka, T., Ohno, H., Jiang, Y., Melnick, A. M. *et al.* BCL6 breaks occur at different AID sequence motifs in Ig-BCL6 and non-Ig-BCL6 rearrangements. *Blood* 2013; 121(22): 4551–4554.

97. Bastard, C., Deweindt, C., Kerckaert, J. P., Lenormand, B., Rossi, A., Pezzella, F. *et al.* LAZ3 rearrangements in non-Hodgkin's lymphoma: correlation with histology, immunophenotype, karyotype, and clinical outcome in 217 patients. *Blood* 1994; 83(9): 2423–2427.

98. Lo Coco, F., Ye, B. H., Lista, F., Knowles, D. M., Offit, K., Chaganti, R. S. *et al.* Rearrangements of the BCL6 gene

in diffuse large cell non-Hodgkin's lymphoma. *Blood* 1994; 83(7): 1757–1759.

99. Butler, M. P., Iida, S., Capello, D., Rossi, D., Rao, P. H., Nallasivam, P. *et al.* Alternative translocation breakpoint cluster region 5' to BCL-6 in B-cell non-Hodgkin's lymphoma. *Cancer Res* 2002; 62(14): 4089–4094.

100. Akasaka, T., Ohno, H., Mori, T. and Okuma, M. Long distance polymerase chain reaction for detection of chromosome translocations in B-cell lymphoma/leukemia. *Leukemia* 1997; 11(Suppl. 3): 316–317.

101. Lossos, I. S., Jones, C. D., Warnke, R., Natkunam, Y., Kaizer, H., Zehnder, J. L. *et al.* Expression of a single gene, BCL-6, strongly predicts survival in patients with diffuse large B-cell lymphoma. *Blood* 2001; 98(4): 945–951.

102. Pasqualucci, L., Migliazza, A., Basso, K., Houldsworth, J., Chaganti, R. S. and Dalla-Favera, R. Mutations of the BCL6 proto-oncogene disrupt its negative autoregulation in diffuse large B-cell lymphoma. *Blood* 2003; 15(101): 2914–2923.

103. Ladanyi, M., Offit, K., Jhanwar, S. C., Filippa, D. A. and Chaganti, R. S. MYC rearrangement and translocations involving band 8q24 in diffuse large cell lymphomas. *Blood* 1991; 77(5): 1057–1063.

104. Zhou, K., Xu, D., Cao, Y., Wang, J., Yang, Y. and Huang, M. C-MYC aberrations as prognostic factors in diffuse large B-cell lymphoma: a meta-analysis of epidemiological studies. *PLoS ONE* 2014; 9(4): e95020.

105. Vaidya, R. and Witzig, T. E. Prognostic factors for diffuse large B-cell lymphoma in the R(X) CHOP era. *Ann Oncol* 2014; 25(11): 2124–2133.

106. Macpherson, N., Lesack, D., Klasa, R., Horsman, D., Connors, J. M., Barnett, M. *et al.* Small noncleaved, non-Burkitt's

**331**

(Burkitt-like) lymphoma: cytogenetics predict outcome and reflect clinical presentation. *J Clin Oncol* 1999; 17(5): 1558–1567.

107. Johnson, N. A., Savage, K. J., Ludkovski, O., Ben-Neriah, S., Woods, R., Steidl, C. et al. Lymphomas with concurrent BCL2 and MYC translocations: the critical factors associated with survival. *Blood* 2009; 114(11): 2273–2279.

108. Alizadeh, A. A., Eisen, M. B., Davis, R. E., Ma, C., Lossos, I. S., Rosenwald, A. et al. Distinct types of diffuse large B-cell lymphoma identified by gene expression profiling. *Nature* 2000; 403(6769): 503–511.

109. Deckert, M., Montesinos-Rongen, M., Brunn, A. and Siebert, R. Systems biology of primary CNS lymphoma: from genetic aberrations to modeling in mice. *Acta Neuropathol* 2014; 127(2): 175–188.

110. Choi, W. W., Weisenburger, D. D., Greiner, T. C., Piris, M. A., Banham, A. H., Delabie, J. et al. A new immunostain algorithm classifies diffuse large B-cell lymphoma into molecular subtypes with high accuracy. *Clin Cancer Res* 2009; 15(17): 5494–5502.

111. Mitterbauer-Hohendanner, G., Mannhalter, C., Winkler, K., Mitterbauer, M., Skrabs, C., Chott, A. et al. Prognostic significance of molecular staging by PCR-amplification of immunoglobulin gene rearrangements in diffuse large B-cell lymphoma (DLBCL). *Leukemia* 2004; 18(6): 1102–1107.

112. van Besien, K., Ha, C. S., Murphy, S., McLaughlin, P., Rodriguez, A., Amin, K., Forman, A., Romaguera, J. et al. Risk factors, treatment, and outcome of central nervous system recurrence in adults with intermediate-grade and immunoblastic lymphoma. *Blood* 1998; 91(4): 1178–1184.

113. Morin, R. D., Johnson, N. A., Severson, T. M., Mungall, A. J., An, J., Goya, R. et al. Somatic mutations altering EZH2 (Tyr641) in follicular and diffuse large B-cell lymphomas of germinal-center origin. *Nat Genet* 2010; 42(2): 181–185.

114. Sneeringer, C. J., Scott, M. P., Kuntz, K. W., Knutson, S. K., Pollock, R. M., Richon, V. M. et al. Coordinated activities of wild-type plus mutant EZH2 drive tumor-associated hypertrimethylation of lysine 27 on histone H3 (H3K27) in human B-cell lymphomas. *Proc Natl Acad Sci USA* 2010; 107(49): 20980–20985.

115. Qi, W., Chan, H., Teng, L., Li, L., Chuai, S., Zhang, R. et al. Selective inhibition of Ezh2 by a small molecule inhibitor blocks tumor cells proliferation. *Proc Natl Acad Sci USA* 2012; 109(52): 21360–21365.

116. McCabe, M. T., Ott, H. M., Ganji, G., Korenchuk, S., Thompson, C., Van Aller, G. S. et al. EZH2 inhibition as a therapeutic strategy for lymphoma with EZH2-activating mutations. *Nature* 2012; 492(7427): 108–112.

117. Ngo, V. N., Young, R. M., Schmitz, R., Jhavar, S., Xiao, W., Lim, K. H. et al. Oncogenically active MYD88 mutations in human lymphoma. *Nature* 2011; 470(7332): 115–119.

118. Pasqualucci, L., Dominguez-Sola, D. Chiarenza, A., Fabbri, G., Grunn, A., Trifonov, V. et al. Inactivating mutations of acetyltransferase genes in B-cell lymphoma. *Nature* 2011; 471(7337): 189–195.

119. Morin, R. D., Mendez-Lago, M., Mungall, A. J., Goya, R., Mungall, K. L., Corbett, R. D. et al. Frequent mutation of histone-modifying genes in non-Hodgkin lymphoma. *Nature* 2011; 476(7360): 298–303.

120. Pasqualucci, L., Trifonov, V., Fabbri, G., Ma, J., Rossi, D., Chiarenza, A. et al. Analysis of the coding genome of diffuse large B-cell lymphoma. *Nat Genet* 2011; 43(9): 830–837.

121. Lohr, J. G., Stojanov, P., Lawrence, M. S., Auclair, D., Chapuy, B., Sougnez, C. et al. Discovery and prioritization of somatic mutations in diffuse large B-cell lymphoma (DLBCL) by whole-exome sequencing. *Proc Natl Acad Sci USA* 2012; 109(10): 3879–3884.

122. Scott, D. W., Mungall, K. L., Ben-Neriah, S., Rogic, S., Morin, R. D., Slack, G. W. et al. TBL1XR1/TP63: a novel recurrent gene fusion in B-cell non-Hodgkin lymphoma. *Blood* 2012; 119(21): 4949–4952.

123. Magrath, I. The pathogenesis of Burkitt's lymphoma. *Adv Cancer Res* 1990; 55: 133–270.

124. Hecht, J. L. and Aster, J. C. Molecular biology of Burkitt's lymphoma. *J Clin Oncol* 2000; 18(21): 3707–3721.

125. Love, C., Sun, Z., Jima, D., Li, G., Zhang, J., Miles, R. et al. The genetic landscape of mutations in Burkitt lymphoma. *Nat Genet* 2012; 44(12): 1321–1325.

126. Farinha, P. and Gascoyne, R. D. Molecular pathogenesis of mucosa-associated lymphoid tissue lymphoma. *J Clin Oncol* 2005; 23(26): 6370–6378.

127. Wotherspoon, A. C., Diss, T. C., Pan, L. X., Schmid, C., Kerr-Muir, M. G., Lea, S. H. et al. Primary low-grade B-cell lymphoma of the conjunctiva: a mucosa-associated lymphoid tissue type lymphoma. *Histopathology* 1993; 23(5): 417–424.

128. Chanudet, E., Zhou, Y., Bacon, C. M., Wotherspoon, A. C., Müller-Hermelink, H. K., Adam, P. et al. Chlamydia psittaci is variably associated with ocular adnexal MALT lymphoma in different geographical regions. *J Pathol* 2006; 209(3): 344–351.

129. Liu, H., Ye, H., Ruskone-Fourmestraux, A., De Jong, D., Pileri, S., Thiede, C. et al. T(11;18) is a marker for all stage gastric MALT lymphomas that will not respond to H. pylori eradication. *Gastroenterology* 2002; 122(5): 1286–1294.

130. Liu, H., Ye, H., Dogan, A., Ranaldi, R., Hamoudi, R. A., Bearzi, I. et al. T(11;18)(q21;q21) is associated with advanced mucosa-associated lymphoid tissue lymphoma that expresses nuclear BCL10. *Blood* 2001; 98(4): 1182–1187.

131. Streubel, B., Vinatzer, U., Lamprecht, A., Raderer, M. and Chott, A. T(3;14)(p14.1;q32) involving IGH and FOXP1 is a novel recurrent chromosomal aberration in MALT lymphoma. *Leukemia* 2005; 19(4): 652–658.

132. Chanudet, E., Huang, Y., Ichimura, K., Dong, G., Hamoudi, R. A., Radford, J. et al. A20 is targeted by promoter methylation, deletion and inactivating mutation in MALT lymphoma. *Leukemia* 2010; 24(2): 483–487.

133. Chanudet, E., Ye, H., Ferry, J., Bacon, C. M., Adam, P., Müller-Hermelink, H. K. et al. A20 deletion is associated with copy number gain at the TNFA/B/C locus and occurs preferentially in translocation-negative MALT lymphoma of the ocular adnexa and salivary glands. *J Pathol* 2009; 217(3): 420–430.

134. Rossi, D., Ciardullo, C. and Gaidano, G. Genetic aberrations of signaling pathways in lymphomagenesis: revelations from next generation sequencing studies. *Semin Cancer Biol* 2013; 23(6): 422–430.

135. Walsh, S. H., Laurell, A., Sundström, G., Roos, G., Sundström, C. and Rosenquist, R. Lymphoplasmacytic lymphoma/ Waldenström's macroglobulinemia derives from an extensively hypermutated B cell that lacks ongoing somatic hypermutation. *Leuk Res* 2005; 29(7): 729–734.

136. Offit, K., Parsa, N. Z., Filippa, D., Jhanwar, S. C. and Chaganti, R. S. t(9;14)(p13;q32) denotes a subset of low-grade non-Hodgkin's lymphoma with plasmacytoid differentiation. *Blood* 1992; 80(10): 2594–2599.

137. Treon, S. P., Xu, L., Yang, G., Zhou, Y., Liu, X., Cao, Y. et al. MYD88 L265P somatic mutation in Waldenström's macroglobulinemia. *New Engl J Med* 2012; 367(9): 826–833.

138. Hideshima, T., Bergsagel, P. L., Kuehl, W. M. and Anderson, K. C. Advances in biology of multiple myeloma: clinical applications. *Blood* 2004; 104(3): 607–618.

139. Bergsagel, P. L. and Kuehl, W. M. Molecular pathogenesis and a consequent classification of multiple myeloma. *J Clin Oncol* 2005; 23(26): 6333–6338.

140. González, D., González, M., Alonso, M. E., López-Pérez, R., Balanzategui, A., Chillon, M. C. et al. Incomplete DJH rearrangements as a novel tumor target for minimal residual disease quantitation in multiple myeloma using real-time PCR. *Leukemia* 2003; 17(6): 1051–1057.

141. Martinelli, G., Terragna, C., Zamagni, E., Ronconi, S., Tosi, P., Lemoli, R. et al. Polymerase chain reaction-based detection of minimal residual disease in multiple myeloma patients receiving allogeneic stem cell transplantation. *Haematologica* 2000; 85(9): 930–934.

142. Novella, E., Giaretta, I., Elice, F., Madeo, D., Piccin, A., Castaman, G. et al. Fluorescent polymerase chain reaction and capillary electrophoresis for IgH rearrangement and minimal residual disease evaluation in multiple myeloma. *Haematologica* 2002; 87(11): 1157–1164.

143. Martinez-Lopez, J., Lahuerta, J. J., Pepin, F., González, M., Barrio, S., Ayala, R. et al. Prognostic value of deep sequencing method for minimal residual disease detection in multiple myeloma. *Blood* 2014; 123(20): 3073–3079.

144. Schumacher, J. A., Duncavage, E. J., Mosbruger, T. L., Szankasi, P. M. and Kelley, T. W. A comparison of deep sequencing of TCRG rearrangements vs traditional capillary electrophoresis for assessment of clonality in T-Cell lymphoproliferative disorders. *Am J Clin Pathol* 2014; 141(3): 348–359.

145. Matutes, E. T-cell prolymphocytic leukemia. *Cancer Control* 1998; 5(1): 19–24.

146. Foroni, L., Foldi, J., Matutes, E., Catovsky, D., O'Connor, N. J., Forster, A. et al. Alpha, beta and gamma T-cell receptor genes: rearrangements correlate with haematological phenotype in T cell leukaemias. *Br J Haematol* 1987; 67(3): 307–318.

147. Matutes, E., Brito-Babapulle, V., Swansbury, J., Ellis, J., Morilla, R., Dearden, C. et al. Clinical and laboratory features of 78 cases of T-prolymphocytic leukemia. *Blood* 1991; 78(12): 3269–3274.

148. Delgado, P., Starshak, P., Rao, N. and Tirado, C. A. A comprehensive update on molecular and cytogenetic abnormalities in T-cell prolymphocytic leukemia (T-pll). *J Assoc Genet Technol* 2012; 38(4): 193–198.

149. Kiel, M. J., Velusamy, T., Rolland, D., Sahasrabuddhe, A. A., Chung, F., Bailey, N. G. et al. Integrated genomic sequencing reveals mutational landscape of T-cell prolymphocytic leukemia. *Blood* 2014; 124(9): 1460–1472.

150. Bergmann, A. K., Schneppenheim, S., Seifert, M., Betts, M. J., Haake, A., Lopez, C. et al. Recurrent mutation of JAK3 in T-cell

**333**

prolymphocytic leukemia. *Gene Chromosome Canc* 2014; 53(4): 309–316.

151. Rose, M. G. and Berliner, N. T-cell large granular lymphocyte leukemia and related disorders. *Oncologist* 2004; 9(3): 247–258.

152. Jerez, A., Clemente, M. J., Makishima, H., Koskela, H., Leblanc, F., Peng Ng, K. *et al.* STAT3 mutations unify the pathogenesis of chronic lymphoproliferative disorders of NK cells and T-cell large granular lymphocyte leukemia. *Blood* 2012; 120(15): 3048–3057.

153. Yamagishi, M. and Watanabe, T. Molecular hallmarks of adult T cell leukemia. *Front Microbiol* 2012; 17(3): 334.

154. Willemze, R., Jaffe, E. S., Burg, G., Cerroni, L., Berti, E., Swerdlow, S. H. *et al.* WHO-EORTC classification for cutaneous lymphomas. *Blood* 2005; 105(10): 3768–3785.

155. Sandberg, Y., Heule, F., Lam, K., Lugtenburg, P. J., Wolvers-Tettero, I. L. M., van Dongen, J. J. *et al.* Molecular immunoglobulin/T-cell receptor clonality analysis in cutaneous lymphoproliferations. Experience with the BIOMED-2 standardized polymerase chain reaction protocol. *Haematologica* 2003; 88(6): 659–670.

156. Assaf, C., Hummel, M., Steinhoff, M., Geilen, C. C., Orawa, H., Stein, H. *et al.* Early TCR-beta and TCR-gamma PCR detection of T-cell clonality indicates minimal tumor disease in lymph nodes of cutaneous T-cell lymphoma: diagnostic and prognostic implications. *Blood* 2005; 105(2): 503–510.

157. Vaqué, J. P., Gómez-López, G., Monsálvez, V., Varela, I., Martínez, N., Pérez, C. *et al.* PLCG1 mutations in cutaneous T-cell lymphomas. *Blood* 2014; 123(13): 2034–2043.

158. Iqbal, J., Wright, G., Wang, C., Rosenwald, A., Gascoyne, R. D.,

Weisenburger, D. D. *et al.* Gene expression signatures delineate biological and prognostic subgroups in peripheral T-cell lymphoma. *Blood* 2014; 123(19): 2915–2923.

159. Stein, H., Foss, H. D., Dürkop, H., Marafioti, T., Delsol, G., Pulford, K. *et al.* CD30(+) anaplastic large cell lymphoma: a review of its histopathologic, genetic, and clinical features. *Blood* 2000; 96(12): 3681–3695.

160. Gascoyne, R. D., Aoun, P., Wu, D., Chhanabhai, M., Skinnider, B. F., Greiner, T. C. *et al.* Prognostic significance of anaplastic lymphoma kinase (ALK) protein expression in adults with anaplastic large cell lymphoma. *Blood* 1999; 93(11): 3913–3921.

161. Pulford, K., Lamant, L., Morris, S. W., Butler, L. H., Wood, K. M., Stroud, D. *et al.* Detection of anaplastic lymphoma kinase (ALK) and nucleolar protein nucleophosmin (NPM)-ALK proteins in normal and neoplastic cells with the monoclonal antibody ALK1. *Blood* 1997; 89(4): 1394–1404.

162. Kutok, J. L. and Aster, J. C. Molecular biology of anaplastic lymphoma kinase-positive anaplastic large-cell lymphoma. *J Clin Oncol* 2002; 20(17): 3691–3702.

163. Feldman, A. L., Dogan, A., Smith, D. I., Law, M. E., Ansell, S. M., Johnson, S. H. *et al.* Discovery of recurrent t(6;7)(p25.3;q32.3) translocations in ALK-negative anaplastic large cell lymphomas by massively parallel genomic sequencing. *Blood* 2011; 117(3): 915–919.

164. Vasmatzis, G., Johnson, S. H., Knudson, R. A., Ketterling, R. P., Braggio, E., Fonseca, R. *et al.* Genome-wide analysis reveals recurrent structural abnormalities of TP63 and other p53-related genes in peripheral T-cell

lymphomas. *Blood* 2012; 120(11): 2280–2289.

165. Parilla Castellar, E. R., Jaffe, E. S., Said, J. W., Swerdlow, S. H., Ketterling, R. P., Knudson, R. A. *et al.* ALK-negative anaplastic large cell lymphoma is a genetically heterogeneous disease with widely disparate clinical outcomes. *Blood* 2014; 124(9): 1473–1480.

166. Willenbrock, K., Roers, A., Seidl, C., Wacker, H. H., Küppers, R. and Hansmann, M. L. Analysis of T-cell subpopulations in T-cell non-Hodgkin's lymphoma of angioimmunoblastic lymphadenopathy with dysproteinemia type by single target gene amplification of T-cell receptor-beta gene rearrangements. *Am J Pathol* 2001; 158(5): 1851–1857.

167. Anagnostopoulos, I., Hummel, M., Finn, T., Tiemann, M., Kobjuhn, P., Dimmler, C. *et al.* Heterogeneous Epstein-Barr virus infection patterns in peripheral T-cell lymphoma of angioimmunoblastic lymphadenopathy type. *Blood* 1992; 80(7): 1804–1812.

168. Odejide, O., Weigert, O., Lane, A. A., Toscano, D., Lunning, M. A., Kopp, N. *et al.* A targeted mutational landscape of angioimmunoblastic T-cell lymphoma. *Blood* 2014; 123(9): 1293–1296.

169. Calvaruso, M., Gulino, A., Buffa, S., Guarnotta, C. and Franco, G. Challenges and new prospects in hepatosplenic γδ T-cell lymphoma. *Leuk Lymphoma* 2014; 10: 1–9.

170. Wlodarska, I., Martin-Garcia, N., Achten, R., De Wolf-Peeters, C., Pauwels, P., Tulliez, M. *et al.* Fluorescence in situ hybridization study of chromosome 7 aberrations in hepatosplenic T-cell lymphoma: isochromosome 7q as a common abnormality accumulating in forms with

features of cytologic progression. *Gene Chromosome Canc* 2002; 33(3): 243–251.

171. Travert, M., Huang, Y., de Leval, L., Martin-Garcia, N., Delfau-Larue, M. H., Berger, F. *et al.* Molecular features of hepatosplenic T-cell lymphoma unravels potential novel therapeutic targets. *Blood* 2012; 119(24): 5795–5806.

172. Kwong, K. L. Natural killer-cell malignancies: diagnosis and treatment. *Leukemia* 2005; 19(12): 2186–2194.

173. Tse, E. and Kwong, Y. L. Management of advanced NK/T-Cell lymphoma. *Curr Hematol Malig Rep* 2014; 9(3): 233–242.

174. Ruskova, A., Thula, R. and Chan, G. Aggressive Natural Killer-Cell Leukemia: report of five cases and review of the literature. *Leuk Lymphoma* 2004; 45(12): 2427–2438.

175. Koo, G. C., Tan, S. Y., Tang, T., Poon, S. L., Allen, G. E., Tan, L.

*et al.* Janus kinase 3-activating mutations identified in natural killer/T-cell lymphoma. *Cancer Discov* 2012; 2(7): 591–597.

176. Bouchekioua, A., Scourzic, L., de Wever, O., Zhang, Y., Cervera, P., Aline-Fardin, A. *et al.* JAK3 deregulation by activating mutations confers invasive growth advantage in extranodal nasal-type natural killer cell lymphoma. *Leukemia* 2014; 28(2): 338–348.

177. Emmert-Buck, M. R., Bonner, R. F., Smith, P. D., Chuaqui, R. F., Zhuang, Z., Goldstein, S. R. *et al.* Laser capture microdissection. *Science* 1996; 274(5289): 998–1001.

178. Küppers, R. New insights in the biology of Hodgkin lymphoma. *Hematology Am Soc Hematol Educ Program* 2012; 2012: 328–334.

179. Steidl, C., Diepstra, A., Lee, T., Chan, F. C., Farinha, P., Tan, K. *et al.* Gene expression profiling of microdissected Hodgkin Reed-

Sternberg cells correlates with treatment outcome in classical Hodgkin lymphoma. *Blood* 2012; 120(17): 3530–3540.

180. Liu, Y., Razak, F. R., Terpstra, M., Chan, F. C., Saber, A., Nijland, M. *et al.* The mutational landscape of Hodgkin lymphoma cell lines determined by whole exome sequencing. *Leukemia* 2014; 28(11): 2248–2251.

181. Steidl, C., Telenius, A., Shah, S. P., Farinha, P., Barclay, L., Boule, M. *et al.* Genome-wide copy number analysis of Hodgkin Reed-Sternberg cells identifies recurrent imbalances with correlations to treatment outcome. *Blood* 2010; 116(3): 418–427.

182. Tiacci, E., Döring, C., Brune, V., van Noesel, C. J., Klapper, W., Mechtersheimer, G. *et al.* Analyzing primary Hodgkin and Reed-Sternberg cells to capture the molecular and cellular pathogenesis of classical Hodgkin lymphoma. *Blood* 2012; 120(23): 4609–4620.

# Chapter 19

# Pediatric tumors

Paul Roberts, Susan Picton and Jens Stahlschmidt

## Introduction

Compared to adult incidence, pediatric malignancies are exceedingly rare. In England, Wales and Scotland, the population-based National Registry of Childhood Tumour (NRCT) records show approximately 1,500 new cases each year of malignancies in children and teenagers under the age of 15 years (1). The most common types of malignancy are leukemias (approximately 32%), followed by CNS tumors (approximately 25%) and lymphomas (approximately 10%). Other solid tumors of this age group are significantly less frequent.

Many solid tumors of infancy and childhood are characterized by a blastemal phenotype commonly referred to as "small round blue cell tumor." For diagnosis alone, the vast majority of these cases require immunolabeling and molecular techniques. This makes these tumors distinctively different from those in the adult age group, where the majority of primary diagnosis can be made on conventional H&E stain alone. Conversely, typical adult epithelial malignancies are very rare in children and confined to a limited range of organs, such as thyroid, liver and skin, to name a few.

Other differences from adult malignancies include a high proliferation index of the tumors which does not necessarily indicate a malignant behavior (for example, in infantile hemangioendotheliomas). In addition, despite a high proliferation rate, it is possible that certain tumors undergo spontaneous regression or substantial differentiation (for example, neuroblastomas).

Another feature of pediatric tumors is their marked histological heterogeneity – for example, the diagnosis of Wilms' tumor subtype requires a caution after a needle core biopsy as it may not be representative of the whole tumor.

**Table 19.1** Pediatric tumors

| | |
|---|---|
| Classical pediatric small round blue cell tumors – variable sites | Neuroblastoma<br>Ewing's sarcoma<br>Rhabdomyosarcoma<br>Non-Hodgkin's lymphoma<br>Small cell osteosarcoma<br>Mesenchymal chondrosarcoma<br>Rhabdoïd tumor<br>Desmoplastic small cell tumor<br>Germ cell tumor |
| Classical pediatric small round blue cell tumors – organ-specific sites | Wilms' tumor<br>Hepatoblastoma<br>Sialoblastoma<br>Pancreatoblastoma<br>Pleuropulmonary blastoma |

In this chapter, a selection of tumors which confront the histopathologist as a "small round blue cell tumor" are discussed and a brief overview and general approach to the diagnosis, including molecular genetic work-up, is outlined (Table 19.1).

## Processing open pediatric tumor biopsies

All pediatric tumor biopsies should be submitted fresh to the histopathology department immediately after the biopsy has been taken to triage tissue for molecular biological studies, including tissue banking and to set up karyotype cultures. Tissue banking of fresh tumor samples is essential for translational research and can be invaluable in cases of tumor recurrence for additional marker studies for targeted therapy. The results of the subsequent H&E stained

*Molecular Pathology: A Practical Guide for the Surgical Pathologist and Cytopathologist*, ed. John M. S. Bartlett, Abeer Shaaban and Fernando Schmitt. Published by Cambridge University Press. © Cambridge University Press, 2016.

section from submitted tissue must be recorded – particularly regarding the presence of tumor, the amount of normal tissues in the biopsies (for example, for the interpretation of karyotype cultures) or the presence of tumor degenerative changes and necrosis (which may predict failure or success of DNA testing, karyotype culture or the reliability of immunolabeling and/or *in situ* hybridization). It is important to have effective communication pathways between pediatric surgeons, theater staff, oncologists, the pathologist and the molecular geneticist.

## Molecular genetics

Genetic investigations in pediatric tumors can provide valuable information to aid diagnosis, subclassification, inform prognosis and guide treatment choices. There are several different technologies available for molecular testing, summarized in Table 19.2. Technology choices depend on whether a targeted, panel-based or genome-wide investigation is necessary. At the moment, the main benefit of molecular testing in pediatric tumors is a targeted approach focused on known disease-specific and prognostically important changes. As with other tumor types, it is expected that molecular testing will broaden out to encompass investigation of multiple molecular markers. At present, the main purpose of molecular testing in pediatric tumors is to assist with histopathology diagnosis. Table 19.3 shows the wide variety of non-CNS tumor-specific molecular findings on which many molecular oncology services are presently focusing their testing.

In this chapter, we focus on the following pediatric tumors with important genetic changes, some of which have therapeutic, diagnostic or prognostic significance:

- rhabdomyosarcoma;
- neuroblastoma;
- Ewing's sarcoma;
- desmoplastic small round cell tumors;
- inflammatory myofibroblastic tumor;
- dermatofibrosarcoma protuberance;
- hepatoblastoma;
- rhabdoïd tumors; and
- lipoblastoma.

# Rhabdomyosarcomas

Rhabdomyosarcomas are malignant mesenchymal tumors that derive from primitive mesenchymal stem

cells and phenotypically show features of skeletal muscle differentiation.

In the most recent WHO Classification (2013 (2)), a unifying classification scheme has been proposed. The main pediatric categories include embryonal rhabdomyosarcomas (ERMS), including the botryoid variant and alveolar rhabdomyosarcoma (ARMS), which will be discussed in this chapter. Other subtypes include the pleomorphic rhabdomyosarcoma (PRMS) (a subtype almost exclusively reported in adults) and the spindle cell sclerosing rhabdomyosarcoma (SRMS).

Rhabdomyosarcomas display various stages of primitive striated muscle differentiation on histology and immunohistochemistry. They are a relatively frequent tumor in the first 10 years of age (mean age between 3 and 5 years) and, compared to other small round blue cell tumors, also fairly frequent in the second decade of life (medulloblastomas excluded).

Rhabdomyosarcomas can occur in a variety of localizations, mainly the head and neck region, with approximately one-third occurring in the orbital region and approximately 50% in the so-called parameningeal region (tumors localized in nasopharynx, sinuses and the middle ear location). The latter tumors have a poorer prognosis, which may be partly due to their proximity to the central nervous system. These sites are also difficult areas for surgeons to achieve complete excision without significant morbidity or cosmetic problems.

Other common sites include the urogenital tract (paratesticular, urinary bladder, vagina and uterus). Thus, although derived from primitive striated muscle cells, the location is not always within the expected anatomical planes of skeletal muscle.

### Pathology

Grossly, the tumors are usually poorly defined soft tissue lesions showing focal areas of mucoid degeneration, hemorrhage or necrosis. Rhabdomyosarcomas infiltrating mucosal surfaces often show a polypoid-nodular, grape-like (botryoid) appearance. Histologically, rhabdomyosarcomas can display variable features which can render histological classification difficult.

### Embryonal rhabdomyosarcoma

Embryonal rhabdomyosarcoma (ERMS) is the most common single category of soft tissue sarcomas in children and adolescents, accounting for approximately

**Table 19.2** Technology options for molecular testing

| Technology | Pros | Cons |
| --- | --- | --- |
| G-banding | Genome-wide<br>Dosage changes and structural rearrangements<br>Shows spatial arrangements<br>Identifies different clones | Requires cell culture<br>Limited resolution (6 mb)<br>Can be poor quality<br>Normal cell overgrowth<br>Labor intensive<br>Overgrowth by certain clones |
| FISH | Targeted test<br>Rapid<br>Simple process<br>Fresh and archived tissue | Limited no. of targets<br>Multiplexing difficult |
| RT-PCR | Specific fusion transcript<br>Multiplexing of samples and transcript types | Requires RNA<br>Only answers specific question<br>Contamination by normal tissue<br>Requires positive controls – difficult for rare transcripts |
| Array CGH | Genome-wide<br>SNPs can assess LOH<br>Gives positional information<br>Fresh and archived tissue | Dosage changes only<br>May not call large amplifications<br>Needs good quality DNA<br>Need at least 10% tumor tissue<br>Low level clones missed<br>No information on different clones |
| MLPA | Targeted test<br>Multiplexing – multiple patients and up to 50 targets<br>Fresh and archived tissue | Needs good quality DNA<br>Need >15% tumor tissue<br>Results can be skewed if there are complex changes and/or multiple clones |
| Sanger sequencing | Fresh and archived tissue<br>Specific | Limited targets<br>Large dosage changes problematic<br>Needs >20% tumor DNA<br>Homozygosity for mutations can give false-negative |
| Pyrosequencing | Fresh and archived tissue<br>Analysis simple<br>Multiplexing possible | Only works with short fragment sizes |
| Next generation sequencing | Fresh and archived tissue<br>Specific<br>Multiple targets (panels) possible<br>Multiplexing of patients<br>One stop test feasible – mutations, dosage changes and rearrangements | Needs expensive equipment<br>Needs scalability – not cost effective for single cases |
| Real-time PCR | Fresh and archived tissue<br>Multiplexing of targets and patients<br>Sensitive – down to 1% tumor | Only answers specific question<br>Contamination by normal tissue<br>Requires positive controls – difficult for rare transcripts |

Table 19.3 Genetic changes in non-CNS pediatric tumors

| Histological type | Genetic change | Genes |
|---|---|---|
| Ewing's sarcoma/PNET | t(11;22)(q24;q12) | EWSR1-FLI1 |
| | t(21;22)(q22;q12) | EWSR1-ERG |
| | t(7;22)(p22;q12) | EWSR1-ETV1 |
| | t(17;22)(q12;q12) | EWSR1-E1AF |
| | t(2;22)(q33;q12) | EWSR1-FEV |
| | t(20;22)(q13;q12) | EWSR1-NFATC2 |
| | t(2;22)(q31;q12) | EWSR1-SP3 |
| | t(1;22)(p36.1;q12) | EWSR1-ZNF278 |
| | t(6;22)(p21;q12) | EWSR1-POU5F1 |
| Clear cell sarcoma of soft parts | t(12;22)(q13;q12) | EWSR1-ATF1 |
| | t(2;22)(q34;q12) | EWSR1-CREB1 |
| Desmoplastic small round cell tumor | t(11;22)(q13;q12) | EWSR1-WT1 |
| Extraskeletal myxoid chondrosarcoma | t(9;22)(q22;q12) | EWSR1-NR4A3 |
| | t(9;17)(q22;q11) | TAF15-NR4A3 |
| | t(9;15)(q22;q21) | TCF12-NR4A3 |
| | t(9;22)(q22;q15) | TFG-NR4A3 |
| Angiomatoid fibrous histiocytoma | t(2;22)(q34;q12) | EWSR1-CREB1 |
| | t(12;22)(q13;q12) | EWSR1-ATF1 |
| | t(12;16)(q13;p11) | FUS-ATF1 |
| Synovial sarcoma | t(X;18)(p11.2;q11.2) | SS18-SSX1 |
| | t(X;18)(p11.2;q11.2) | SS18-SSX2 |
| | t(X;18)(p11.2;q11.2) | SS18-SSX4 |
| Myxoid liposarcoma | t(12;16)(q13;p11) | FUS-DDIT3 |
| | t(12;22)(q13;q12) | EWSR1-DDIT3 |
| Low-grade fibromyxoid sarcoma | t(7;16)(q34;p11) | FUS-CREB3L2 |
| | t(11;16)(p11;p11) | FUS-CREB3L1 |
| Alveolar rhabdomyosarcoma | t(2;13)(q35;q14) | PAX3-FOXO1A |
| | t(1;13)(p36;q14) | PAX7-FOXO1A |
| | t(2;2)(q35;p23) | PAX3-NCOAI |
| | t(X;2)(q13;q35) | PAX3-AFX |
| | t(2;8)(q35;q13) | PAX3-NCOA2 |
| DFSP | t(17;22)(q22;q13)/r(17;22) | COL1A1-PDGFB |
| ASPS | der(17)t(X;17)(p11;q25) | ASPSCR1-TFE3 |
| Congenital fibrosarcoma / mesoblastic nephroma | t(12;15)(p13;q25) | ETV6-NTRK3 |
| Endometrial stromal sarcoma | t(7;17)(p15;q21) | JAZF1-JJAZ1 |
| | t(6;7)(p21;p15) | JAZF1-PHF1 |
| | t(6;10)(p21;p11) | EPC1-PHF1 |
| Inflammatory myofibroblastic tumor | t(1;2)(q22;p23) | TPM3-ALK |
| | t(2;19)(p23;p13) | TPM4-ALK |
| | t(2;17)(p23;q23) | CLTC-ALK |
| | t(2;2)(p23;q13) | RANBP2-ALK |
| | inv(2)(p23;q35) | ATIC-ALK |
| | t(2;4)(p23;q21) | SEC31A-ALK |
| | t(2;11)(p23;p15) | CARS-ALK |

Table 19.3 *(cont.)*

| Histological type | Genetic change | Genes |
| --- | --- | --- |
| Lipoblastoma | 8q12 rearrangements | HAS2-PLAG1<br>COLIA1-PLAG1 |
| Neuroblastoma | Double minutes/<br>homogenously staining regions<br>11q23 deletion<br>1p36 deletion<br>ALK mutation | MYCN |
| Extra-cranial malignant rhabdoïd tumor | 22q11 deletion | SMARCB1/INI1/SNF5/BAF47 |

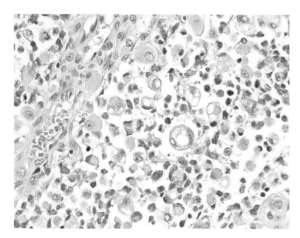

Figure 19.1 Unusual pleomorphic embryonal rhabdomyosarcoma in the periorbital region of an 11–year-old male (H&E, x400).

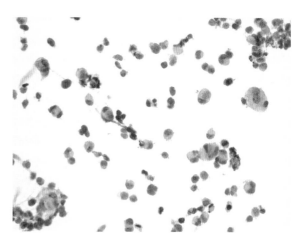

Figure 19.2 A smear preparation of the case in Figure 19.1: mono- and multinucleated cells are present. No cytoplasmic inclusions are noted (H&E, x400).

80% of all RMS. EMRS occurs predominantly in children below the age of 10 years and approximately 4% of cases affect infants. A few congenital cases have also been reported. Common sites of involvement include the head and neck region and the genitourinary urinary tract.

Histologically, the tumor cells usually form solid sheets of moderately pleomorphic small round blue cells with variable amounts of cytoplasm forming slender bipolar or unipolar (so-called tadpole or tennis racket cells) spindle cells (Figures 19.1 to 19.3). The cytoplasm is usually eosinophilic and PAS positive. Occasional cytoplasmic striations can be identified. The tumor cells can form aggregates in a loose myxoid background. In the botryoid variant, they can condense beneath a mucosal layer to form a so-called cambium layer. These lesions can protrude into a space with a polypoid, grape-like appearance. When maturing, rhabdomyoblasts may form giant cells.

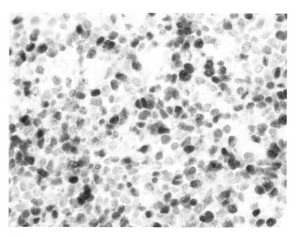

Figure 19.3 Myogenin labeling of the case in Figure 19.1, present in approximately 50% of tumor nuclei. This tumor did not show FOX01 rearrangement and was classified as an embryonal rhabdomyosarcoma with diffuse anaplasia (x400).

Treatment involves neoadjuvant chemotherapy followed by local therapy (surgery +/– radiotherapy) and further post-operative chemotherapy. Outcome for non-metastatic disease is good, at more than 70% long-term survival.

## Alveolar rhabdomyosarcomas

Alveolar rhabdomyosarcomas (ARMS) usually form clusters of discohesive, typically small round blue cells with high nuclear-cytoplasmic ratios and only minimal eosinophilic cytoplasmic differentiation. Tumor nuclei are usually hyperchromatic and have irregular outlines. Occasional Touton-type giant cells can be seen. The tumor islands show no central vascularization or reticulin fiber deposition and are at least partially separated by variable extensive fibrovascular septae. Degenerative changes create alveolar, empty spaces with lumina lined by tumor cells. Solid variants of alveolar rhabdomyosarcoma lack the fibrovascular septae and form dense sheets of undifferentiated cells with no obvious rhabdomyoblastic differentiation.

Nuclear anaplasia (including atypical mitotic figures) has been associated with a worse prognosis than tumors without anaplasia (3).

In terms of immunohistochemistry, the labeling profile reflects the myogenic properties of the tumors and commonly there is at least focal positivity for desmin and myogenin. The nuclear labeling pattern for myogenin has a high sensitivity and specificity. A high myogenin labeling index is described with a poor prognosis (4).

The principles of treatment of ARMS are similar to those of treatment of ERMS, but outcomes are significantly poorer and metastases more common.

## Triton tumor

This describes a malignant peripheral sheath tumor showing rhabdomyosarcomatous differentiation. Histologically, there is rhabdomyosarcomatous differentiation in a background of a pleomorphic spindle cell of the malignant peripheral nerve sheath tumor.

# Molecular genetics
## Alveolar rhabdomyosarcoma

The genetic hallmark of alveolar rhabdomyosarcoma (ARMS) is a PAX-FOXO1 gene rearrangement (77% of cases), most usually seen as a t(2;13)(q35;q14) (PAX3-FOXO1) translocation (55% of cases), and occasionally as a t(1;13)(p36;q14) (PAX7-FOXO1)

translocation (22% of cases) (5). Up to 10% of ARMs contain a rarer, cryptic fusion variant involving PAX3. This has been reported as a t(X;2)(q13;q35) (PAX3-AFX) translocation (6), or as translocations involving members of the nuclear receptor co-activator family of genes, either as a t(2;2)(q35;p23) (PAX3-NCOA1) or a t(2;8)(q35;q13) (PAX3-NCOA2) (7). All of the above translocations encode a chimeric protein composed of the paired box and homeodomain DNA-binding domain of a PAX gene and the transactivating domain of the partner gene.

The chimeric products of PAX-FOXO1 rearrangements are highly expressed in tumor cells and are more potent transcriptional activators than PAX or FOXO1 wild-type. PAX genes encode related members of the paired box transcription family, and FOXO1 also encodes a transcription factor. The chimeric PAX–FOXO1 fusion transcript on the der(13) encodes a novel transcription factor with altered transcriptional potential, altered transcriptional targets and altered post-translational regulation. This results in deregulated expression of downstream genes of PAX3 and possibly novel targets. Distinguishing the FOXO1 fusion partner is important, since PAX7-FOXO1A-positive tumors are reported to be locally less invasive and are more frequent in younger children (5). However, metastatic tumors presenting with PAX3-FOXO1A fusion have a less favorable outcome than those with PAX7-FOXO1A fusion, with a four-year survival rate of 8% vs. 75% for patients with PAX7-FOXO1 fusion. The transcriptional capability of PAX3-NCOA fusion is comparable to that of PAX-FOXO1 fusion. The approximate remainder of 13% of ARMS cases can be regarded as PAX fusion negative.

Oncogene amplification is a frequent finding in ARMS, seen cytogenetically as supernumerary double minutes. It is found either as amplification of the PAX-FOXO1 translocation products (Figure 19.4), most commonly seen in cases with PAX7-FOXO1 fusion, or as amplification of several other genes, most notably MYCN (8) (32% to 60% of cases), 12q13 (28% to 56% of cases) or 13q31–32 (14% to 19% of cases). Those with MYCN amplification are less likely to survive and more likely to relapse than those with no gain (9). Similarly, patients with high levels of MYCN expression also have a worse prognosis, although high levels of expression do not always correlate with high-level genomic gains. It is suggested that the association of MYCN amplification

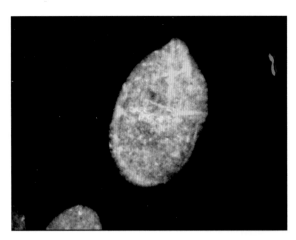

**Figure 19.4** Interphase FISH studies showing co-amplification of FOXO1 (red) and PAX3 (green).

with poor outcome in ARMS may be linked to growth promotion and repression of myoblast differentiation (10). Functional studies have demonstrated that the PAX3-FOXO1 protein cooperates with MYCN to enhance oncogenic activity, and can contribute to MYCN expression, emphasizing the importance of this relationship in tumorigenesis.

A suitable genetic testing strategy for ARMS should therefore be available to detect and discriminate fusion gene type and assess MYCN amplification status. This can be done by FISH using a break-apart FOXO1 probe, followed by specific FOXO1/PAX analysis either by FISH or RT-PCR. Assessment of MYCN amplification is best performed by FISH.

The somatic mutation rate in ARMS is low and PAX gene fusion is the dominant driver. Through its transcriptional reprogramming, it alters a host of downstream genes. Genomic analysis studies have shown a variety of target genes for PAX-FOXO1, including MYCN, IGF2, MET, CXCR4, CNR1, TFAP2B, FGFR4 and p-cadherin (11). PAX-FOXO1 cooperating factors include abrogation of the p53 pathway, IGF2 deregulation, MUCN and miR17–92 amplification, and IR1210 expression. A greater understanding of how these factors contribute and interact will enhance our understanding of ARMS tumorigenesis.

PAX-fusion negative ARMS tumors appear to mimic the clinical course of embryonal rhabdomyosarcoma (ERMS). Gene fusion status rather than histology is therefore the critical risk factor in RMS. Fusion-negative ARMS tumors accumulate a higher degree of aneuploidy and mutational burden than fusion-positive cases. The RAS pathway is mutationally activated in around 45% of fusion-negative cases, with BCOR mutations in 7.4%. Gene expression profiles of fusion-negative ARMS are also similar to those for ERMS.

## Embryonal rhabdomyosarcoma (ERMS)

Since the clinical courses of ERMS and PAX fusion-negative ARMs cases are similar and more favorable than in PAX-fusion positive ARMS tumors, patient stratification can be partly based on PAX-fusion status rather than simply just on a diagnosis of ERMS or ARMS. The genetic profile of ERMS is different from that of ARMS, although there are no genetically diagnostic markers of ERMS. Array CGH and earlier cytogenetic studies have shown that chromosomal aneuploidies are very common in ERMS, with gains of chromosome 8 particularly common (seen in 90% of patients) (12). Other common gains include chromosomes 2, 11, 12, 13, 19 and 20 (25% to 50% of cases), with losses of chromosomes 6, 9, 10, 14, 15, 16 and 18 in 50% to 95% of cases (12).

11p15.5 loss of heterozygosity or loss of imprinting is a frequent finding in ERMS, and increased expression of IGF2 appears to be important in RMS in general (13). Several recurrent mutations are described in ERMS, including p53, NRAS, KRAS, HRAS, PIK3CA, CTNNB1 and FGFR4 (11). FGFR4 is broadly over-expressed in RMS and distinguishes this from other small round cell tumors. FGFR4 antagonists could represent potential future therapeutic options.

## Neuroblastic tumors (Ewing's sarcoma and neuroblastoma family)

Neuroblastoma and Ewing's sarcoma are neuroblastic tumors, both with similar histomorphological features. The main difference is the age of presentation, which is usually below the age of 5 years in neuroblastomas, compared to the young adult and adolescent affected by Ewing's sarcoma.

## Ewing's sarcomas

Ewing's sarcomas (formerly Ewing's sarcoma/peripheral primitive neuroectodermal tumor, now considered as a single entity in the most recent WHO classification (2)) commonly present as a bony lesion or soft tissue lesion in children and young adults. The kidney is the third most common primary tumor site. Soft tissue locations include the retroperitoneum, paravertebral region, chest wall (Askin tumor) and the extremities.

## Pathology

These are usually large, fleshy tumors which can contain extensive necrosis. Bone tumors are usually eroding bone.

Histologically, they comprise relatively monotonous, evenly distributed, dense sheets of small round blue cells with round to oval nuclei. Nucleoli are usually inconspicuous. On occasions there is a variable staining intensity of the nuclear basophilia dividing these cells in pale and darker groups. Focal cytoplasmic vacuolation due to cytoplasmic glycogen and neuroectodermal rosette formation is present.

Atypical Ewing's sarcoma includes tumors with more nuclear pleomorphism, irregular nuclear membranes and prominent nucleoli. These relatively large-sized cells can cause confusion with lymphomas. In the kidney, differentiation from a blastemal Wilms' tumor component is essential; here, thorough sampling may reveal other components of Wilms' tumor.

Ewing's sarcoma shows features of neuroblastic differentiation and characteristic membranous labeling patterns with CD99 (Figures 19.5 and 19.6). The latter can also be seen in non-Hodgkin's lymphomas and leukemias and additional lymphoid markers should be included in a panel. Focal keratin labeling is also noted. Rhabdomyoblastic differentiation markers are not identified in Ewing's sarcoma.

Treatment consists of neoadjuvant chemotherapy, local therapy (surgery, radiotherapy or both) and further chemotherapy. Prognosis is related to the response to neoadjuvant chemotherapy and is assessed by the degree of tumor necrosis in the resected tumor. The chemotherapy-induced necrosis and involvement of tumor margins is essential for the planning of post-operative radiotherapy. The outlook is dependent on stage – with a good outlook for non-metastatic tumors (approximately 70% overall survival rate), an extremely poor outlook for patients with bone or bone marrow metastases and an intermediate prognosis for those with lung metastases only (approximately 30% overall survival rate) (1).

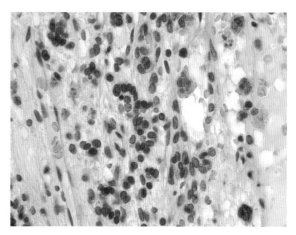

**Figure 19.5** Residual viable Ewing's sarcoma with post-chemotherapy effect (hemosiderosis) in the chest wall of a 12-year-old male (H&E, x400).

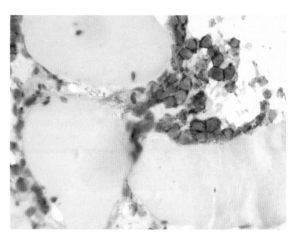

**Figure 19.6** Distinct membranous CD99 labeling of focal Ewing's sarcoma infiltrating between skeletal muscle fibers (x630).

## Molecular genetics

Ewing's sarcoma family tumors (ESFTs) are defined by translocations between the EWSR1 gene (usually exon 7) at 22q12 and members of the ETS gene family. The most frequent gene rearrangement is the t(11;22)(q24;q12), found in 85% of cases, resulting in EWSR1–FLI1 gene fusion (14). Two types of this translocation have been identified. In type 1, EWSR1 exons 1 to 7 are fused to FLI1 exons 6 to 10, while in type II exon 7 is fused to exon 5. The type 1 fusion was thought to impart a better prognosis (15), but this has been questioned. A further 10% to 15% contain other EWSR1–ETS gene rearrangements (reviewed by

Fisher (16), including t(21;22), t(2;22), t(17;22) and a t(6;22), with a small cohort showing FUS rearrangement instead of EWSR1, seen either as a t(16;21)(p11;q22) (FUS-ERG) or t(2;16)(q35;p11) (FUS-FEV) (reviewed by Romeo and Dei Tos (17)). EWSR1 translocation results in fusion of the N-terminal portion of EWSR1 to the DNA-binding domain of the partner ETS gene. In the resultant chimeric protein, the RNA-binding domain of the protein encoded by EWSR1 is replaced by the DNA-binding domain of the FLI1 gene product. The chimeric protein contributes to the malignant ESFT phenotype through altered transcriptional regulation of downstream target genes.

Because of the numerous variant translocations and fusions, molecular investigation can be negative in a morphologically typical ESFT if only the common rearrangements are screened for. A useful approach can either be assessment of an EWSR1 rearrangement using a break-apart FISH probe (Figure 19.7), followed by RT-PCR to assess the common fusion transcript types. Dual fusion FISH may also be employed to detect specific rearrangements, most usually the EWSR1-FLI1 fusion (Figure 19.8). Where no EWSR1 rearrangement is detected, assessment of a FUS rearrangement by FISH may be a useful second-line approach. CIC–DUX4 fusions, associated with t(4;19)(q35;q13) or t(10;19 (q26.3;q13), have been identified in a subset of EWSR1-negative undifferentiated small round cell sarcomas occurring mainly in extremities of young adult males (18). While genetic investigation has therefore increased diagnostic accuracy, cytogenetics does not provide absolute specificity, as evidenced by the description of exceptional cases of ARMS and polyphenotypic sarcomas with a t(11;22) (19). It is therefore important to correlate genetic results with accurate histopathology evaluation.

Another compounding problem is the wide variety of tumor types with EWSR1 rearrangement. These include Ewing-like small round cell tumors, desmoplastic small round cell tumors, myxoid liposarcoma, extraskeletal myxoid chondrosarcoma and angiomatoid fibrous histiocytoma, clear cell sarcoma of soft parts, clear cell sarcoma like tumors of the gastrointestinal tract, primary pulmonary myxoid sarcoma, extra salivary myoepithelial tumors and sporadic types of low-grade fibromyxoid sarcoma, sclerosing epithelioid fibrosarcoma and mesothelioma. EWSR1 is described as a promiscuous gene

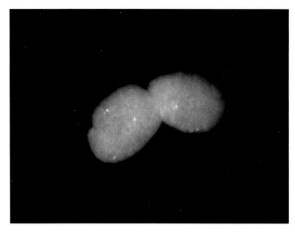

**Figure 19.7** Interphase FISH with EWSR1 break-apart probe showing EWSR1 rearrangement (red and green separated).

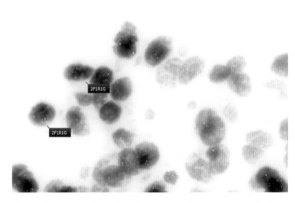

**Figure 19.8** Interphase FISH image showing EWSR1-FLI1 dual fusion (green = EWSR1, red = FLI1).

as it can fuse with multiple different partners and result in a phenotypically identical tumor, or it can partner with the same genes in morphologically and behaviorally different tumors. Where histopathology diagnosis is still uncertain, the investigation of tumor-specific fusion transcript types is the most effective means of pointing to a clearer diagnosis.

Eighty percent of ESFTs show additional secondary chromosome abnormalities at diagnosis. These include gains of chromosomes 8, 12 and 20, deletions of 1p36, 9p21, 16q21 and 17p13, 1q gain and unbalanced der(1;16) translocations (20). While the prognostic significance of some of these changes is equivocal, a complex karyotype at diagnosis appears to indicate an adverse outlook (21).

# Neuroblastoma family

Neuroblastomas are embryonal solid tumors showing remarkable heterogeneity in cellular differentiation and prognosis. They are thought to arise from immature neural crest cells and tumor sites correlate with normal tissues of the sympathetic nervous system. Neuroblastoma cells often produce neurotransmitters (measured in the urine and valuable for diagnosis and response monitoring).

## Pathology

Grossly, neuroblastomas typically display a lobulated, encapsulated and hemorrhagic cut surface and areas showing gritty calcifications.

Neuroblastomas show a wide range of histological features. These tumors are currently classified according to the INPC classification (22). Briefly, they are categorized as undifferentiated, poorly differentiated or differentiating, according to the percentage of neuroblasts in a lesion showing differentiation towards ganglion cells. Neuroblastomas are classified as stroma rich with more than 50% of Schwannian cells, or stroma poor with less than 50% of Schwannian cells. Undifferentiated neuroblastoma is the classical small round blue cell tumor for which immunohistochemistry is required to delineate its origin. In poorly differentiated neuroblastoma, associated fine acellular hair-like eosinophilic material (neuropil) is present. The neuroblastic tumor cells appear to float in a background of neuropil and hemorrhage (Figures 19.9 to 19.11). Focal Homer Wright rosette formation is described, but is only rarely present in our experience. Nuclei are typically neuroblastic with salt and pepper chromatin patterns and inconspicuous nucleoli.

The assessment of the mitotic karyorrhectic (MKI) can be used and the age-linked Shimada classification can be utilized to classify the tumors into Shimada favorable and unfavorable histology, although molecular diagnostics are increasingly

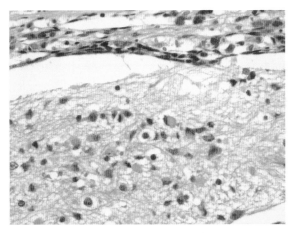

**Figure 19.10** The same case as Figure 19.9. There is extensive chemotherapy-induced necrosis. Viable tumor is still identifiable in lymphovascular spaces. Note "floating" neuropil in the background with neuroblasts showing focal ganglionic differentiation (H&E, x400).

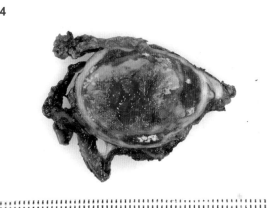

**Figure 19.9** Adrenalectomy of high-risk neuroblastoma in a 3-year-old boy. Presented with cranial and skin metastases (original histology: undifferentiated neuroblastoma) 11 weeks previously. There is extensive chemotherapy-induced degenerative change with hemorrhage. The focal chalky areas represent calcifications.

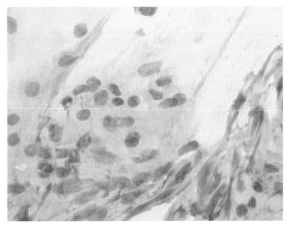

**Figure 19.11** Smear preparation of a fresh tumor biopsy in a 9-month-old girl with abdominal tumor deposits. Characteristic neuropil and neuroblastic nuclei confirm the diagnosis of neuroblastoma (H&E, x620).

becoming more useful in risk stratification. The prognosis is age dependent and in heterogenous tumors the area of most primitive differentiation, such as in ganglioneuroblastoma, nodular subtype will determine the prognosis. At the opposite end of the spectrum, a fully differentiated tumor represents a benign ganglioneuroma in which the tumor comprises mature neoplastic ganglion cells enmeshed in a spindle cell Schwannian stroma.

Immunohistochemically, S100 protein is useful for the identification of Schwannian stroma. NB84 is a useful marker of neuroblastic differentiation. Other markers such as NSE, synaptophysin and CD56 are also positive. Vimentin and CD99 are negative.

Treatment is dependent on risk factors such as age of the child, clinical stage of the tumor and molecular subtype. Chemotherapy, surgery, radiotherapy and differentiation therapy are all components of the complex treatment of childhood neuroblastoma.

## Molecular genetics

The most common focal genetic lesion in neuroblastoma is amplification of MYCN (more than ten copies for a diploid genome or >fourfold signal relative to chromosome 2), seen in 20% of all cases, and in 45% of high-risk cases, and is associated with a poor outcome. MYCN is a transcription factor that binds to DNA within promoters of an extensive network of genes and controls expression of many target genes. This in turn regulates fundamental cellular processes, including proliferation, cell growth, protein synthesis, metabolism, apoptosis and differentiation. Targets directly induced by MYCN include HMGA1,

MCM7, MDM2 and MRP1. MYCN is vital for proliferation, migration and stem cell homeostasis, while decreased levels are associated with decreased proliferation and terminal neuronal differentiation.

MYCN is one of the few genetic predictors of poor outcome, with a survival rate of 15% to 35%. It is manifest cytogenetically either as double minutes or as homogenously staining regions (hsrs). This will give an appearance of localized increased MYCN signal numbers (hsrs) confined to one area of the cell or as widespread MYCN signals covering the multiple areas or the whole cell (double minutes) (Figure 19.12). Amplification or over-expression is also reported in several other cancers, most frequently those of embryonic and/or neuroendocrine origin (reviewed in Westermark *et al.* (23)). High-risk neuroblastomas without MYCN amplification frequently display increased C-MYC expression and/or activation of MYC signaling pathways. Expression of the neurotrophin receptor TrkA is associated with good prognosis, ability to differentiate and spontaneous regression, while expression of the related TrkB receptor is correlated with poor prognosis and MYCN amplification.

The aggressive phenotype of MYCN may not only be associated with MYCN copy-number, but also with other signals that regulate MYCN expression, such as RNA-binding proteins and microRNAs.

MYCN expression signatures have been described that define high-risk patients – the majority show altered expression or stabilization of MYCN. New therapeutic targets have identified five classes of direct and indirect inhibitors of MYCN (24):

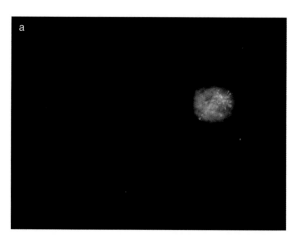
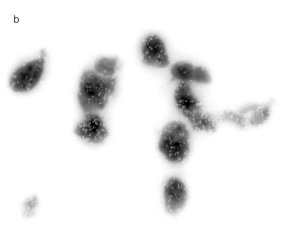

**Figure 19.12** Interphase FISH images showing MYCN amplification (MYCN = red, chromosome 2 centromere = green). (a) = hsr; (b) = double minutes.

1. targeting DNA-binding function of MYCN;
2. targeting MYCN transcription;
3. targeting synthetic lethal interactions of MYCN;
4. targeting oncogenic stabilization of MYCN; and
5. targeting expression or function of MYCN.

There are key differences in the genetic profiles of low- and high-risk neuroblastomas. Low-risk, inter-mediate-risk and stage IVS neuroblastomas have numerical gains, while high-risk neuroblastomas have intrachromosomal rearrangements. The incidence of these rearrangements increases with age at diagnosis and is strongly predictive of outcome. Together with MYCN amplification, these chromosomal aberrations may lead to deregulation of mRNAs, microRNAs and other non-coding RNAs that interfere with apoptosis, differentiation and immune surveillance.

Other established markers of poor prognosis include losses of 1p and 11q, 17q gain, losses of 3p, 4p, 9p and 14q, and gain of 1q, 2p, 7q and 11p. 11q loss is associated with older age at diagnosis, absence of MYCN amplification and more chromosomal breaks. Segmental chromosome aberrations (SCA) with or without MYCN amplification are associated with poorer outcome, with a higher risk of repalse even when associated with numerical chromosome changes (25, 26). Tumor progression is frequently associated with accumulation of segmental imbal-ances, suggesting an underlying aberration in DNA maintenance or repair.

Allelic loss of 1p36.3 is seen in 25% to 35% of neuroblastomas, is highly associated with MYCN amplification and advanced disease (27) and is found in 70% of aggressive neuroblastomas. 1p loss is inde-pendently associated with poor survival. Loss of heterozygosity (LOH) at 1p36 most likely results in loss of a tumor suppressor gene, with candidate genes CHD5, CAMTA1, CASZ1, EBE4B and APITD1 (28). 1p status is also independently predictive of event-free survival in patients with low and intermediate risk disease.

Unbalanced 11q loss is seen in 15% to 20% of neuroblastoma at diagnosis and is associated with advanced stage, older age and unfavorable histology. It is inversely associated with MYCN amplification, although a small subset shows both. Studies have shown segmental 11q LOH is independently predict-ive of inferior three-year event-free survival and overall survival rates, and suggest that MYCN amplification and 11q LOH neuroblastomas are

two different types of neuroblastoma (29). In tumors with 11q loss, segmental aneuploidy is more frequent. This may be partly explained by loss of the H2AFX gene at 11q23.3 – this plays a role in genomic stabi-lity modification and enhanced cancer susceptibility in mice. Loss of other candidate genes such as CADM1 on 11q may also be important in tumors with 11q loss.

The most frequent acquired imbalance is 17q gain (17q21-qter), seen in 70% of neuroblastomas, which results from unbalanced translocations. It is associ-ated with more aggressive/advanced disease, increased age, 1p LOH, 11q LOH and MYCN amplification, and decreased survival. It is often associated with 1p or 11q unbalanced translocation. Bown et al. (30) showed unbalanced 17q gain to be an independent predictor of poor survival, but multivariate analysis by Spitz et al. (31) indicated that 11q and MYCN status rather than 17q status are more important prognostic markers.

Detection of MYCN amplification is most usually done by interphase FISH. While other segmental imbalances can be distinguished by targeted FISH assays (Figure 19.13), given the wide variety of seg-mental imbalances and prognostic significance, it is more effective to use technologies such as MLPA or array CGH, which allow dosage assessment of mul-tiple genomic locations simultaneously.

Neuroblastomas demonstrate a low mutation rate, although recurrent changes are described in five genes – MYCN, PTPN1, ALK, ATRX and NRA (32). Activating mutations of the ALK gene are seen

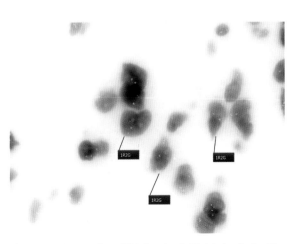

**Figure 19.13** Interphase FISH showing 1p36 deletion (red) with 1q25 control (green).

in 50% of germline neuroblastomas and 6% to 10% of sporadic cases. The most frequent ALK mutation (reviewed in Azarova *et al.* (33)), F1174L, is associated with MYCN amplification. This combination confers a worse prognosis than MYCN amplification alone, suggesting a cooperative effect on neuroblastoma formation by these two proteins. ALK is an oncogenic driver for neuroblastoma, and activation of ALK by mutation or amplification in combination with MYCN is lethal. F1174L has shown more potent transforming activity than the second most common activating mutation, R1275Q. The R1275Q mutation is found in both familial and sporadic neuroblastoma, while F1174L mutation is restricted to sporadic tumors. Both mutations are associated with constitutive phosphorylation of ALK and that of downstream targets such as ERK, STAT3 and AKT. ALK mutations are evenly distributed among the clinical stages of tumor progression. With the exception of F1174L mutations in MYC-amplified tumors, somatic ALK mutations do not appear to be associated with survival. Amplification of ALK is seen in 2% of cases, but there is presently no evidence that this has any independent correlation with aggressive disease when MYCN status is taken into account.

ALK represents a therapeutic target. Crizotinib has been clinically evaluated in adult ALCL, NSCLC and IMFT. Early studies suggest that Crizotinib inhibits proliferation of neuroblastoma cells with R1275Q-mutated ALK or amplified wild-type ALK, but not those with the FI174L mutation (34). It is likely that therapeutic suppression of the activities of MYCN and mutated ALK will become a clinical reality.

Hereditary neuroblastoma is relatively rare (2% of cases) and in this group around 90% have heritable mutations of ALK in the majority or PHOX2B (7% of cases) (35). Genetic testing should be considered where there is a family history of neuroblastoma or other disorders of neural crest origin, or for patients with evidence of multifocal primary neuroblastomas. Other mutations occasionally described in neuroblastoma include loss of function mutations and deletions of TIAM1, ARID1A and ARID1B (36).

# Desmoplastic small round cell tumor (DSRCT)

This is also known as desmoplastic small cell tumor of childhood, polyphenotypic small round cell tumor and intra-abdominal desmoplastic round cell tumor, and is a rare, highly malignant primitive mesenchymal tumor which mainly occurs in male adolescents as an intra-abdominal or retroperitoneal/pelvic mass with diffuse serosal involvement. DSRCTs are irregular gritty yellow/tan lesions with a firm fibrous cut surface (35). Histologically, the characteristic features include desmoplastic or sclerotic stroma surrounding round or angulated nests of small primitive cells with high nuclear-cytoplasmic ratios. The lesional cells are characterized by hyperchromatic nuclei. Many cells have an epithelioid appearance or may show rhabdoïd features with eosinophilic cytoplasmic inclusions. They are characterized by a polyphenotypic immunophenotype characterized by labeling with cytokeratin, EMA, desmin (usually cytoplasmic dot-like) and nuclear WT1 (clones with carboxy-terminus). Nuclear WT1 labeling for the carboxy-terminus must be seen in context, as it can be seen in other soft tissue sarcomas. Treatment involves both chemotherapy and surgery, but complete excision is rarely possible and the outlook is poor.

## Molecular genetics

DSRCTs are characterized by a t(11;22)(p13;q12) (EWSR1-WT1) translocation (36). This is not seen in any other tumor type and hence is of diagnostic importance. The resultant fusion protein is a transcription factor with a downstream effect on several genes, including PDGFRA. Recently, two intra-abdominal pediatric tumors expressing EWSR1–WT1 fusion transcript and with a morphology and immunophenotype consistent with a diagnosis of leiomyosarcoma have been reported (37). Similarly, as in ESFTs, the existence of polyphenotypic neoplasms morphologically similar to DSRCT but containing chimeric transcripts associated with the ES/PNET category (EWSR1–FLI1 and EWSR1–ERG) underlines the importance of strict correlation between conventional morphology and genetic analysis. As with ESFTs, EWSR1 break-apart FISH studies are effective as a first-line test, but follow-up studies either using EWSR1-WT1 FISH or RT-PCR are necessary given the promiscuous involvement of EWSR1 in a wide variety of different tumor types.

# Inflammatory myofibroblastic tumor (IMT)

This fibroblastic/myofibroblastic tumor with an indeterminate malignant potential has typical lymphoplasma cell-rich infiltrates associated with a

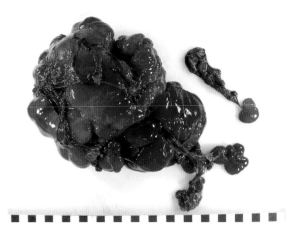

Figure 19.14 A 1400g-multinodular inflammatory myofibroblastic tumor in a 14-year-old female.

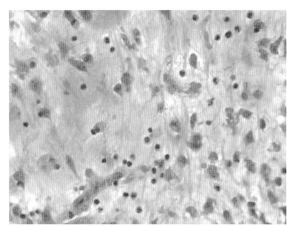

Figure 19.15 Histological features of Figure 19.14; there is a nodular fasciitis-like pattern with plumb ganglion cell-like myofibroblasts and mononuclear inflammatory cells (H&E, x400).

distinctive plump myofibroblastic and fibroblastic spindle cell component showing various stages of maturation (38). It occurs in the soft tissues and within the abdominal cavity of children and young adults.

Histologically, spindly fibroblastic myofibroblastic cells are dominant and can show three basic histological patterns: a myxoid pattern with spindle myofibroblasts in an oedematous background; a vesicular spindle cells component with variable myxoid and collagenized areas; and a fibromatosis-like pattern with a lower cellularity. Typical is the presence of lymphocytes, plasma cells and eosinophils (Figures 19.14 and 19.15).

Lesional cells label with smooth muscle antigen and focally desmin. Nuclear ALK1 labeling can be noted in approximately 50% of cases.

Treatment is ideally complete surgical excision, but this is often not possible and residual tumor requires close observation. Occasionally, medical treatment is necessary.

## Molecular genetics

ALK activation is a recurrent event in IMFS, most usually seen as an ALK gene rearrangement involving fusion with the TPM4 or TPM3 loci or other genes (39). Receptor tyrosine-kinase oncogenes are associated with striking ALK expression in the IMT myofibroblastic spindle cells. ALK expression is normally restricted to the central nervous system. High-level ALK expression, in IMTs, is notable because ALK is expressed at low or undetectable levels in non-neoplastic fibroblasts. These findings suggest that IMTs might be neoplasms in which the myofibroblastic component is transformed, in some cases, by chromosomal mechanisms targeting ALK. 2p rearrangements in IMTs create ALK fusion. Given the variety of fusion partners, an effective means of identifying ALK rearrangement is through the use of a break-apart ALK FISH probe, or via ALK expression studies.

# Dermatofibrosarcoma protuberans

This is a dermal-based fibroblastic fibrohistiocytic tumor of intermediate malignancy. It is classically characterized by a storiform growth pattern in which tumor cells are radiating around a central point, producing spokes. The tumor infiltrates diffusely into fat in a checker-board pattern. Giant cells or xanthomatous cells are usually absent. There is diffuse immunolabeling with CD34. There is no labeling with S100 protein. Treatment is surgical resection with clear margins.

## Molecular genetics

DFSP is characterized in over 90% of cases by either a t(17;22)(q22;q13) or, more commonly, a supernumerary ring (17;22) chromosome derived from the t(17;22). Translocations are more frequent in children, whereas ring chromosomes predominate in adults. The ring chromosomes usually contain chromosome 22 centromere and low-level amplification of interstitial segments of 17q23~24 and

**349**

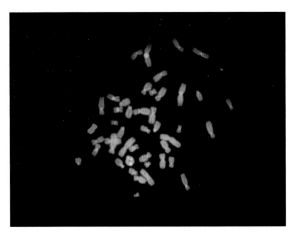

**Figure 19.16** Metaphase FISH with chromosome 17 (red) and 22 (green) whole chromosome paints showing ring (17;22).

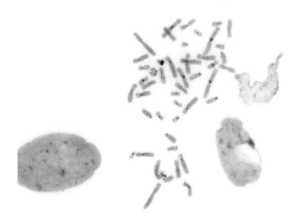

**Figure 19.17** Metaphase FISH using dual fusion COL1A1-PDGFβ probes (COL1A1 = red, PDGFβ = green).

22q11~q13 (40). Both rings and translocations have been shown to contain the same molecular rearrangements, with fusion of the COL1A1 and PDGFβ genes and the production of a chimeric autocrine factor (41). The fusion causes deregulation of the PDGFβ gene by placing it under direct control of the COL1A1 promoter, resulting in unscheduled production of PDGF, thought to be an important event in the development of DFSP. FISH studies using dual fusion probe sets are an effective means of identifying COL1A1-PDGFβ fusions. Metaphase FISH also provides a clear perspective on the appearance and composition of ring chromosomes (Figures 19.16 and 19.17).

## Hepatoblastoma

This is a malignant embryonal tumor of the liver occurring in early childhood. It resembles features of embryonal and fetal hepatocellular development (42). There is no association with infection such as hepatitis or metabolic disorders.

The tumor can arise multifocally. A pure epithelial type can be distinguished from a mixed epithelial and mesenchymal type. The epithelial component can be categorized into fetal embryonal and small cell variants. Approximately one-third of hepatoblastomas show a mesenchymal component, usually with osteoid formation. So-called teratoid hepatoblastoma are mixed tumors with an epithelial and a teratoid background characterized by primitive mesenchymal tissue containing osteoid, squamous, mucinous epithelial components, neuroglial structures and/or yolk sac elements.

The epithelial component of hepatoblastoma usually labels with glypican 3, glutamine synthetase (most intense labeling in the fetal variant), beta catenin (at least focally nuclear labeling pattern), pan-cytokeratins, Hep-Par 1 (usually present in fetal, less in the embryonal and usually absent in the small cell variants). Lack of INI1 labeling in diffuse undifferentiated small cell hepatoblastoma can identify tumors with a malignant rhabdoïd tumor-like biological behavior. INI1 labeling is retained in the other hepatoblastoma types.

Treatment is immediate surgical resection or neoadjuvant chemotherapy in order to reduce tumor size to enable complete excision followed by further chemotherapy. Very extensive tumors involving the majority of the liver may require total hepatectomy and liver transplantation.

Post-chemotherapy hepatoblastomas show advanced regressive changes with extension of the mesenchymal component. Hepatocellular carcinoma is the main differential diagnosis.

## Molecular genetics

Underlying genetic syndromes are present in around 15% of hepatoblastomas. These include familial adenomatous polyposis coli (FAP), overgrowth syndromes (i.e. Beckwith-Weidemann syndrome, Simpson–Golabi–Behmel syndrome and Sotos syndrome), trisomy 18 and Li Fraumeni (43).

Although genetic studies are of lesser importance in the diagnosis and prognostic assessment of hepatoblastoma, cytogenetic studies can be helpful where there is diagnostic uncertainty. The cytogenetic hall-mark of hepatoblastoma tumors is gain or loss of whole chromosomes – most usually gains of chromosomes 2, 8 and 20, and loss of chromosome 18. Array CGH has further characterized recurrent gains of 1q, 2q, 8q and 20q, and losses of 4q (44). Gains of chromosomes 2 and 20 are associated with less favorable disease, while 4q loss is associated with more advanced tumors and a less favorable disease (45). The first recurrent translocation described in hepatoblastoma was a der(4)t(1;4)(q12;q34) (46). Later studies showed that this was part of a family of trans-locations involving a breakpoint at 1q12 or 1q24, with various different partners (47). These translocations are always unbalanced, and result in a duplication of 1q and loss of chromosome material on the reciprocal chromosome. There are several candidate tumor suppressor genes and oncogenes in the SOR regions of 4q loss, 1q32.1 gain/amplification and 2q gain, and the precise roles of these genes in the tumorigenesis of hepatoblastoma is uncertain. 22q11 rearrangements have been described in the small cell variant, either as 22q11 translocations or SMARCB1 deletions, in a similar way to rhabdoïd tumors (48).

Mutations of several genes have been described, including APC, CTNNB1, AXIN1 and AXIN2, PIK3CA point mutation, and amplification of PIK3C2B or PLAG1 or MDM4, although these are less frequent than chromosome changes. Imprinted genes also appear to play a role – IGF2 is the most commonly up-regulated imprinted gene, and uniparental disomy and deletions of 11pter-p14.1 are frequent findings (49). Over-expression of DLK1, PEG3, PEG10, BEX1, MEG3 and NDN has also been described (43). The molecular mechanism involved in the development and progression of hepatoblastoma includes over-expression of IGF2, down-regulation of RASSF1A by promoter hypermethylation and alterations of genes in the Wnt signaling pathway, most notably a high incidence of CTNNB1 mutations (50).

RASSF1A methylation and terminal 4q deletion but not 16q deletion or 1q gain appear to be independent prognostic factors (50), and RASSF1A may be a promising molecular marker to predict treatment outcome.

# Malignant rhabdoïd tumor

Malignant rhabdoïd tumor was originally described by Beckwith and Palmer in 1978 (51), who described the new category of an aggressive pediatric renal tumor. Later, malignant rhabdoïd tumor was identified in extrarenal sites such as soft tissues, liver, genitourinary tract and in the deep soft tissues of the neck and adjacent spine. This tumor occurs mainly in young children and infants. Grossly, these invasive tumors are non-encapsulated, soft and fleshy. Histologically, typical rhabdoïd cells with eccentric nuclei and prominent nucleoli are identified. These can have round cytoplasmic inclusions. They characteristically co-express cytokeratins (CK8/18), vimentin and epithelial membrane antigen and lack nuclear INI1 labeling (52). Treatment is a combination of chemotherapy, surgery and in some cases radiotherapy, but overall the prognosis is poor.

## Molecular genetics

Germline and somatic mutations of the SMARCB1/INI1/SNF5/BAF47 gene at 22q11 are seen in the majority of cases of renal and extra renal rhabdoïd tumors and atypical teratoid/rhabdoïd tumors (ATRT) (53). SMARCB1 deletions/mutations are also a feature of other tumors, including epithelioid sarcoma, renal medullary carcinoma, undifferentiated sarcoma, choroid plexus carcinoma, schwannomatosis and a subset of hepatoblastomas (54). In patients with malignant rhabdoïd tumors, SMARCB1 appears to function as a classic tumor suppressor gene, whereby germline mutations and deletions predispose to the development of these malignancies. Inactivation of both copies of the gene leads to loss of protein expression in the nucleus. Germline mutation or deletion of SMARCB1 is seen in up to 35% of rhabdoïd tumors, while 98% of tumors show SMARCB1 loss and deletion/mutation of the other allele. It is likely that there is more than one rhabdoïd tumor locus. Tumors with whole or large chromosome 22 deletions are exclusive to rhabdoïd tumors of the brain. In contrast, the soft tissue rhabdoïd tumors are more likely to have smaller deletions in 22q11.22 than to 22q11.23. Rhabdoïd tumors are mostly diploid with few other genomic imbalances.

INI1 is expressed in all normal cells at all stages of development, with an important role in regulation of transcriptional activity of a wide variety of target genes. SMARCB1 appears to play a role in the Rb cyclin D1 pathway; however, the specific function of SMARCB1 with regard to development of human rhabdoïd tumors has not yet been elucidated. Detection of SMARCB1 loss can be done by targeted FISH studies and/or mutation analysis.

# Lipoblastomas

Lipoblastomas are well-defined benign fatty tumors mainly occurring in the trunk and extremities of young children, but can occur at other sites, including solid organs. Lipoblastomas resemble embryonal white fat.

Macroscopically, this is a well-defined yellowish to tanned tumor focally, with extensive myxoid change. The tumors measure on average less than 5cm in maximum dimension.

Histology shows a lobulated tumor composed of vascular fat with variable amounts of myxoid and mesenchymal stroma resembling early developmental fat. Focal multinucleated lipoblasts are present. In addition, there are immature spindle cells and areas resembling fibrolipoma. The lesional cells label with S100 and CD34. Treatment is surgical and recurrence after incomplete resection is observed.

## Molecular genetics

Genetic studies can be helpful in distinguishing lipoblastomas from other lipomatous tumors. Genetic changes in lipoblastoma most commonly involve gain and/or rearrangement of chromosome 8. Seventy percent of cases show rearrangement of the pleomorphic adenoma gene 1 (PLAG1) gene at 8q21.1 (55) and polysomy 8 is seen in 18% of cases with or without PLAG1 rearrangement. 8q (PLAG1) rearrangements are rare in other lipomatous tumors and thus provide a useful distinguishing feature from myxoid liposarcoma, fibrous hamartoma of infancy, hibernoma and other lipomatous tumors.

A variety of different translocation partners have been described, including 8q24, 7q22, 1p13 and 3q12 (56). To date, two fusion partners have been identified in lipoblastomas: HAS2 and COL1A2. The HAS2-PLAG1 fusion results from a t(8;8) or from an intra-chromosomal rearrangement of chromosome 8 that leads to the union of the 8q12::q24.1 bands, whereas the COL1A2-PLAG1 fusion results from a t(7;8)(q21; q12). PLAG1 is a developmentally regulated zinc finger gene involved in mitogenesis, proliferation and apoptosis and in the up-regulation of IGF2. This oncogene is believed to be responsible for the tumorigenesis of lipoblastoma through a promoter-swapping event in which the PLAG1 promoter is replaced by an active promoter from either the HAS2 or COL1A2 genes, resulting in the up-regulation of PLAG1 (57). The promoter-swapping mechanism results in over-expression of a normal PLAG1 protein. Over-expression of PLAG1 has been a crucial event in the development of several human tumors, including pleomorphic adenoma of the salivary glands, lipoblastoma, hepatoblastoma and AML. The molecular mechanism of PLAG1 activation in lipoblastoma is very similar to that in pleomorphic adenomas of the salivary gland, but the fusion partners differ in these tumors.

An alternative mechanism for the up-regulation of PLAG1 is low-level amplification of chromosome 8 with or without PLAG1 rearrangement (58). Gain of chromosome 8 results in an increase in gene dosage, which can cause up-regulation of the PLAG1 which is involved in mitogenesis, proliferation, apoptosis and IGF2 up-regulation (61). Although PLAG1 is normally expressed in fetal tissues during the prenatal period and at low levels in the postnatal period, up-regulation of PLAG1 in lipoblastoma results in the over-expression of PLAG1 protein and may lead to the abnormal differentiation of white fat tissues, resulting in tumorigenesis (59; 60).

Since distinguishing lipoblastoma from other fatty tumors (especially more aggressive cases of myxoid liposarcoma) can aid diagnosis and assessment of tumor behavior, cell culture and cytogenetic analysis is an effective method of analysis (Figure 19.18), especially given the variety of types of rearrangements and chromosome changes in this tumor type.

## Learning points

- Childhood tumors encompass a wide range of entities which can sometimes mimic each other histologically due to the shared, primitive phenotype of small round blue cells.
- The majority of pediatric tumors should be received fresh for molecular diagnosis and

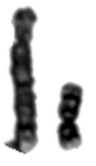

**Figure 19.18** G-banded images showing t(8;8) (left) and t(3;8) (right) as variant PLAG1 rearrangements in lipoblastoma.

treatment stratification, and tissue storage for future targeted treatment if necessary.

- Immunolabeling is essential in the diagnosis of primitive small round blue cell tumors.

- Although children can present with advanced metastatic disease, survival rates are significantly higher than in the adult population following complex multimodality treatment.

# References

1. Stiller, C. *Childhood Cancer in Britain: Incidence, Survival, Mortality*, 1st edn. (Oxford University Press, 2007).

2. Fletcher, C. D. M., Bridge, J. A., Hagendoorn, P. C. W. and Mertens, F. (eds.), *WHO Classification of Soft Tissue and Bone Tumours*, 4th edn. (Lyon: IARC, 2013).

3. Hawkins, H. K. and Camacho-Velasquez, J. V. Rhabdomyosarcoma in children. Correlation of form and prognosis in one institution's experience. *Am J Surg Pathol* 11(7): 531–542, 1987.

4. Heerema-McKenney, A., Wijnaendts, L. C., Pulliam, J. F., Lopez-Terrada, D., McKenney, J. K., Zhu, S. *et al.* Diffuse myogenin expression by immunohistochemistry is an independent marker of poor survival in pediatric rhabdomyosarcoma: a tissue microarray study of 71 primary tumors including correlation with molecular phenotype. *Am J Surg Pathol* 32(10): 1513–1522, 2008.

5. Sorensen, P. H., Lynch, J. C., Qualman, S. J., Tirabosco, R., Lim, J. F., Maurer, H. M. *et al.* PAX3-FKHR and PAX7-FKHR gene fusions are prognostic indicators in alveolar rhabdomyosarcoma: a report from the children's oncology group. *J Clin Oncol* 20(11): 2672–2679, 2002.

6. Barr, F. G., Qualman, S. J., Macris, M. H., Melnyk, N., Lawlor, E. R., Strzelecki, D. M. *et al.* Genetic heterogeneity in the alveolar rhabdomyosarcoma subset without typical gene fusions.

*Cancer Res* 62(16): 4704–4710, 2002.

7. Sumegi, J., Streblow, R., Frayer, R. W., Dal Cin, P., Rosenberg, A., Meloni-Ehrig, A. *et al.* Recurrent t(2;2) and t(2;8) translocations in rhabdomyosarcoma without the canonical PAX-FOXO1 fuse PAX3 to members of the nuclear receptor transcriptional coactivator family. *Gene Chromosome Canc* 49(3): 224–236, 2010.

8. Hachitanda, T., Toyoshima, S., Akazawa, K. and Tsuneyoshi, M. N-myc gene amplification in rhabdomyosarcoma detected by FISH: its correlation with histologic features. *Mod Pathol* 11(12): 1222–1227, 1998.

9. Williamson, D., Lu, Y.-J., Gordon, T., Sciot, R., Kelsey, A., Fisher, C. *et al.* Relationship between MYCN copy number and expression in rhabdomyosarcomas and correlation with adverse prognosis in alveolar subtype. *J Clin Oncol* 23(4): 880–888, 2005.

10. Xia, S. J. and Barr, F. G. Chromosome translocations in sarcomas and the emergence of oncogenic transcription factors. *Eur J Cancer* 41: 2513–2527, 2005.

11. Shern, J. F., Chen, L., Chmielecki, J. *et al.* Comprehensive genomic analysis of rhabdomyosarcoma reveals a landscape of alterations affecting a common genetic axis in fusion positive and fusion negative tumours. *Cancer Discov* 4(2): 216–231, 2014.

12. Paulson, V., Chandler, G., Rakheja, D., Galindo, R. L., Wilson, K., Amatruda, J. F. *et al.* High-resolution array CGH identifies common mechanisms that drive embryonal

rhabdomyosarcoma pathogenesis. *Gene Chromosome Canc* 50(6): 397–408, 2011.

13. Scrable, H., Witte, D., Shimada, H., Seemayer, T. A., Wang Wuu, S., Soukup, S. *et al.* Molecular differential pathology of rhabdomyosarcoma. *Gene Chromosome Canc* 1(1): 23–35, 1989.

14. de Alava, E. and Gerald, W. L. Molecular biology of the Ewing's sarcoma/primitive neuroectodermal tumour family. *J Clin Oncol* 18(1): 204–213, 2000.

15. de Alava, E., Kawai, A., Healy, J. H., Fligman, I., Meyers, P. A., Huvos, A. G. *et al.* EWS-FLI1 fusion transcript structure is an independent determinant of prognosis in Ewing's sarcoma. *J Clin Oncol* 16(4): 1248–1255, 1998.

16. Fisher, C. The diversity of soft tissue tumours with EWSR1 gene rearrangements: a review. *Histopathol* 64(1): 134–150, 2014.

17. Romeo, S. and Dei Tos, A. P. Soft tissue tumours associated with EWSR1 translocation. *Virchows Arch* 456(2): 219–234, 2010.

18. Salto Kawamura, M., Yamazaki, Y., Kaneko, K., Kawaguchi, N., Kanda, H., Mukai, H. *et al.* Fusion between CIC and DUX4 upregulates PEA3 family genes in Ewing-like sarcomas with t(14;19)(q35;q13) translocation. *Hum Mol Genet* 15: 2125–2137, 2005.

19. Thorner, P., Squire, J., Chilton-MacNeill, S., Marrano, P., Bayani, J., Malkin, D. *et al.* Is the EWS/FLI1 fusion transcript specific for Ewing sarcoma and peripheral neuroectodermal tumour? A report of 4 cases showing this

transcript in a wider range of tumour types. *Am J Pathol* 148(4): 1125–1138, 1996.

20. Hattinger, C. M., Potschger, U., Tarkkanen, M., Squire, J., Zielenska, M., Kiuru-Kuhlefelt, S. *et al.* Prognostic impact of chromosomal aberrations in Ewing tumours. *Br J Cancer* 86(11): 1763–1769, 2002.

21. Roberts, P. Cancer cytogenetics. *Encyclopedia of Life Sciences* (Wiley J.), www.els.net, 2008.

22. Shimada, H., Ambros, I. M., Dehner, L. P., Hata, J., Joshi, V. V., Roald, B. *et al.* The International Neuroblastoma Pathology Classification (the Shimada system) *Cancer* 86(2): 364–372, 1999.

23. Westermark, U. K., Wilhelm, M., Frenzel, A. and Arsenian Henriksson, M. The MYCN oncogene and differentiation in neuroblastoma. *Semin Cancer Biol* 21(4): 256–266, 2011.

24. Barone, G., Anderson, J., Pearson, D. J., Petrie, K. and Chesler, L. *et al.* New strategies in neuroblastoma: therapeutic targeting of MYCN and ALK. *Clin Cancer Res* 19(21): 5814–5821, 2013.

25. Janoueix-Lerosey, I., Schleiermacher, G., Michels, E., Mosseri, V., Ribeiro, A., Lequin, D. *et al.* Overall genomic pattern is a predictor of outcome in neuroblastoma. *J Clin Oncol* 27(7): 1026–1033, 2009.

26. Schleiermacher, G., Janoueix-Lerosey, I., Ribeiro, A., Klijanienko, J., Couturier, J., Pierron, G. *et al.* Accumulation of segmental alterations determines progression in neuroblastoma. *J Clin Oncol* 28(19): 3122–3130, 2010.

27. White, P. S., Thompson, P. M., Gotoh, T., Okawa, E. R., Igarashi, J., Kok, M. *et al.* Definition and characterisation of a region of 1p36.3 consistently deleted in

neuroblastoma. *Oncogene* 24(16): 2684–2694, 2005.

28. Domingo-Fernandez, R., Watters, K., Piskareva, O., Stallings, R. L. and Bray, I. The role of genetic and epigenetic alterations in neuroblastoma disease pathogenesis. *Paediatr Surg Int* 29(2): 101–119, 2013.

29. Michels, E., Vandesompele, J., De Preter, K., Hoebeeck, J., Vermeulen, J., Schramm, A. *et al.* Array CGH based classification of neuroblastoma into genomic subgroups. *Gene Chromosome Canc* 46(12): 1098–1108, 2007.

30. Bown, N., Cotterill, S., Lastowska, M., O'Neill, S., Pearson, A. D., Plantaz, D. *et al.* Gain of chromosome arm 17q and adverse outcome in patients with neuroblastoma. *New Engl J Med* 340(25): 1954–1961, 1999.

31. Spitz, R., Hero, B., Ernestus, K. and Berthold, F. Gain of distal chromosome arm 17q is not associated with poor prognosis in neuroblastoma. *Clin Cancer Res* 9(13): 4835–4840, 2003.

32. Pugh, T. J., Morozova, O., Attiyeh, E. F., Asgharzadeh, S., Wei, J. S., Auclair, D. *et al.* The genetic landscape of high risk neuroblastoma. *Nat Genet* 45(3): 279–84, 2013.

33. Azarova, A. M., Gautam, G. and George, R. E. Emerging importance of ALK in neuroblastoma. *Sem Cancer Biol* 21(4): 267–275, 2011.

34. Wood, A. C., Laudenslager, M., Haglund, E. A., Attiyeh, E. F., Pawel, B., Courtwright, J. *et al.* Inhibition of ALK mutated neuroblastomas by the selective inhibitor PF-02341066. *J Clin Oncol* 27: 10008b, 2009.

35. Mosse, Y. P., Laudenslager, M., Khazi, D., Carlisle, A. J., Winter, C. L., Rappaport, E. *et al.* Germline PHOXB2 mutation in hereditary neuroblastoma. *Am J Hum Genet* 75(4): 727–730, 2004.

36. Sausen, M., Leary, R. J., Jones, S., Wu, J., Reynolds, C. P., Liu, X. *et al.* Integrated genomic analyses identify ARID1A and ARID1B alterations in the childhood cancer neuroblastoma. *Nat Genet* 45(1): 12–17, 2013.

37. Chang, F. Desmoplastic small round cell tumours: cytologic, histologic, and immunohistochemical features. *Arch Pathol Lab Med* 130(5): 728–732, 2006.

38. Sandberg, A. A. and Bridge, J. A. Updates on the cytogenetics and molecular genetics of bone and soft tissue tumours: DSRCT. *Cancer Genet Cytogenet* 138(1): 1–10, 2002.

39. Alaggio, R., Rosolen, A., Sartori, F., Leszl, A., d'Amore, E. S., Bisogno, G. *et al.* Spindle cell tumour with EWSR1-WTI transcript and a favorable clinical course: a variant of DSRCT, a variant of leiomyosarcoma, or a new entity? Report of 2 paediatric cases. *Am J Surg Pathol* 31(3): 454–459, 2007.

40. Coffin, C. M., Hornick, J. L. and Fletcher, C. D. Inflammatory myofibroblastic tumour: comparison of clinicopathologic, histologic, and immunohistochemical features including ALK expression in atypical and aggressive cases. *J Surg Pathol* 31(4): 509–520, 2007.

41. Lawrence B, Perez-Atayde, A., Hibbard, M. K., Rubin, B. P., Dal Cin, P., Pinkus, J. L. *et al.* TPM3-ALK and TPM4-ALK oncogenes in inflammatory myofibroblastic tumours. *Am J Pathol* 157(2): 377–384, 2000.

42. Naeem, R., Lux, M. L., Huang, S.-F., Naber, S. P., Corson, J. M. and Fletcher, J. A. Ring chromosomes in DFSP are composed of interspersed sequences from chromosomes 17 and 22. *Am J Pathol* 147(6): 1553–1558, 1995.

43. Simon, M.-P., Pedeutour, F., Sirvent, N., Grosgeorge, J., Minoletti, F., Coindre, J.-M. *et al.* Deregulation of the platelet derived growth facto B-chain gene via fusion with collagen gene COL1A1 in DFSP and giant-cell fibroblastoma. *Nat Genet* 15: 95–98, 1997.

44. López-Terrada, D., Alaggio, R., de Dávila, M. T., Czauderna, P., Hiyama, E., Katzenstein, H. *et al.* Children's Oncology Group Liver Tumor Committee: towards an international pediatric liver tumor consensus classification: proceedings of the Los Angeles COG liver tumors symposium. *Mod Pathol* 27(3): 472–491, 2014.

45. Tomlinson, G. E. and Kappler, R. Genetics and epigenetics of hepatoblastoma. *Paediatr Blood Cancer* 59(5): 785–792, 2012.

46. Weber, R. G., Pietsch, T., von Schweinitz, D. and Lichter, P. Characterisation of genomic alterations in hepatoblastomas: a role for gains on chromosomes 8q and 20 as predictors of poor outcome. *Am J Pathol* 157(2): 571–578, 2000.

47. Kumon, K., Kobayashi, H., Namiki, T., Tsunematsu, Y., Miyauchi, J., Kikuta, A. *et al.* Frequent increase of DNA copy number in the 2q24 chromosomal region and its association with a poor clinical outcome in hepatoblastoma: cytogenetic and comparative genomic hybridisation analysis. *Jpn J Cancer Res* 92(8): 854–862, 2001.

48. Schneider, N., Cooley, L., Finegold, M., Douglass, E. C., Tomlinson, G. E. *et al.* Report of the first recurring chromosome translocation: der(4)t(1;4)(q12; q34). *Gene Chromosome Canc* 19(4): 291–294, 1997.

49. Tomlinson, G. E., Douglass, E. C., Pollock, B. H., Finegold, M. J. and Schneider, N. R. Cytogenetic analysis of a large series of hepatoblastoma: numerical aberrations with recurring translocations involving 1q12–21. *Gene Chromosome Canc* 44(2): 177–184, 2005.

50. Trobaugh-Lotario, A. D., Tomlinson, G. E., Finegold, M. J., Gore, L. and Feusner, J. H. Small cell undifferentiated variant of hepatoblastoma: adverse clinical and molecular features similar to rhabdoïd tumours. *Paediatr Blood Cancer* 52(3): 328–334, 2009.

51. Gray, S. G., Eriksson, T., Elkstrom, C., Holm, S., von Schweinitz, D., Kogner, P. *et al.* Altered expression of members of the IGF-axis in hepatoblastomas. *Br J Cancer* 82(9): 1561–1567, 2000.

52. Arai, Y., Honda, S., Haruta, M., Kasai, F., Fujiwara, Y., Ohshima, J. *et al.* Genome-wide analysis of allelic imbalances reveals 4q deletions as a poor prognostic factor and MDM4 amplification at 1q32.1 in hepatoblastoma. *Gene Chromosome Canc* 49(7): 596–609, 2010.

53. Beckwith, J. B. and Palmer, N. F. Histopathology and prognosis of Wilms' tumours: results from the First National Wilms' Tumour Study. *Cancer* 41 (5): 1937–1948, 1978.

54. Oda, Y. and Tsuneyoshi, M. Extrarenal rhabdoïd tumours of soft tissue: clinicopathological and molecular genetic review and distinction from other soft-tissue sarcomas with rhabdoïd features. *Pathol Int* 56(6): 287–295, 2006.

55. Biegel, J. A., Zhou, J., Rorke, L. B., Stenstrom, C., Wainwright, L. M., Fogelgren, B. *et al.* Germline and acquired mutations of INI1 in atypical teratoid rhabdoïd tumours. *Cancer Res* 59(1): 74–79, 1999.

56. Jackson, E. M., Sievert, A. J., Gai, X., Hakonarson, H., Judkins, A. R., Tooke, L. *et al.* Genomic analysis using high density SNP based oligonucleotide arrays and MLPA provides a comprehensive analysis of INI1/SMRCB1 in malignant rhabdoïd tumours. *Clin Cancer Res* 15(6): 1923–1930, 2009.

57. Bandal, P., Bjerkegagen, B. and Heim, S. Rearrangements of chromosomal region 8q11–13 in lipomatous tumours; correlation with lipoblastoma morphology. *J Pathol* 208(3): 388–394, 2006.

58. Deen, M., Ebrahim, S., Schloff, D. and Mohammed, A. N. A novel PLAG1-RAD51L1 gene fusion resulting from a t(8;14)(q12;q24) in a case of lipoblastoma. *Cancer Genetics* 206(6): 233–237, 2013.

59. Hibbard, M. K., Kozakewich, H. P., Dal Cin, P., Sciot, R., Tan, X., Xiao, S. *et al.* PLAG1 fusion oncogenes in lipoblastoma. *Cancer Res* 60(17): 4869–4872, 2000.

60. Ropke, A., Kalinski, T., Kluba, U., von Falkenhausen, U., Wieacker, P. F. and Ropke, M. PLAG1 activation in lipoblastoma coinciding with low-level amplification of a derivative chromosome 8 with a deletion del (8)(q13q21.2). *Cytogenet Genome Res* 119(1–2): 33–38, 2007.

61. Zatkova, A., Rouillard, J. M., Hartmann, W., Lamb, B. J., Kuick, R., Eckart, M. *et al.* Amplification and overexpression of the IGF2 regulator PLAG1 in hepatoblastoma. *Gene Chromosome Canc* 39(2): 126–137, 2004.

Ben Davidson

## Introduction

The serosal cavities, i.e. the peritoneal, pleural and pericardial spaces, are frequently affected by malignant tumors, and serous effusions constitute one of the most commonly seen specimen types in cytopathology. The identification of tumor cells in effusions may constitute the first evidence of cancer or be the first site of metastasis in a previously diagnosed malignancy. Cancers involving the serosal cavities are most frequently metastatic, of which the most commonly encountered ones are adenocarcinomas of breast, lung, ovarian and gastrointestinal origin. However, practically any tumor type, including other carcinomas, as well as hematological cancers, sarcomas, germ cell tumors, malignant melanomas and childhood cancers originating from embryonal tissues have been reported at this anatomic site. Primary cancers of the serosal cavities include malignant mesothelioma (MM), primary peritoneal carcinoma (PPC), primary effusion lymphoma and other, rarer entities [1].

The role of cytopathology has in recent years been minimized, debated or challenged in several organ systems, including fine-needle aspiration of the prostate and the breast and cervical cytology, in the context of core biopsies and HPV testing, respectively. Effusions, however, cannot be superseded by surgical pathology, as cytology is the only method by which one may retrieve cells from fluid. The role of effusion cytology becomes still more evident when solid lesions are not detected or when obtaining a biopsy from the latter is more difficult and costly, and/or entails much greater discomfort or risk for the patient.

Molecular techniques are assuming an ever-greater role in the diagnostic, therapeutic, predictive and prognostic setting in cancer. Effusions are often large-volume and easy to tap, and consist of viable cells that are dissociated or are arranged in small groups, making these specimens ideal for molecular analyses.

This chapter provides an overview of our current knowledge and experience with regard to the application of molecular techniques in malignant effusions. While immunohistochemistry (IHC) and electron microscopy are time-honored techniques in effusion cytology, they will not be discussed in this chapter, as they are not regarded as "molecular" in the narrower interpretation of this term. Enzyme-linked immunosorbent assay (ELISA), flow cytometry and related antibody-based techniques are similarly not discussed due to space considerations. Hematological cancers represent a diagnostic field which differs considerably from the remaining malignancies affecting the serosal cavities, and are beyond the scope of this chapter. The studies discussed in this chapter are those describing molecular assays that are currently used in effusion cytology, or that are perceived to have a potential diagnostic role in this setting.

## In situ hybridization (ISH)

Gross changes in chromosomal number and structure are effectively detected by cytogenetic analysis, a method that has been extensively applied to cancer diagnosis, including effusion cytology [2]. Cytogenetics is nevertheless a laborious and relatively slow procedure requiring culturing of cells. ISH is an effective method allowing the combination of molecular analysis and morphological assessment of specimens. It may be effectively performed on archival material, including cell blocks, and is more cost-effective and less time-consuming than traditional

*Molecular Pathology: A Practical Guide for the Surgical Pathologist and Cytopathologist*, ed. John M. S. Bartlett, Abeer Shaaban and Fernando Schmitt. Published by Cambridge University Press. © Cambridge University Press, 2016.

cytogenetics, which it has largely superseded [3]. Visualization may be achieved by colorimetric reaction (chromogenic ISH; CISH), silver (SISH) or fluorescence (FISH).

Several early studies have focused on the role of ISH in confirming or excluding malignancy in effusion specimens. Analysis of 24 reactive effusions showed absence of trisomy 7 in these specimens, suggesting this may be a marker favoring a nonneoplastic condition [4]. Cytological evaluation, cytogenetic analysis and FISH using probes for chromosomes 7, 8, 12, 18, X and Y were assessed for their diagnostic role in differentiating benign from malignant pleural effusions in a series of 26 specimens from 25 patients, of whom 14 and 11 had malignancy and benign conditions, respectively. Malignant specimens consisted of both epithelial and non-epithelial cancers. Cytology and FISH detected 8 and 6 of 14 of cases as pathologic, whereas cytogenetics was informative in 5 of 11 successfully cultured specimens. In the benign specimens, cytology and FISH were uniformly normal, whereas cytogenetic analysis detected an abnormal clone in 1 of 11 specimens [5].

Zojer and co-workers studied 57 effusions from breast carcinoma (BC) patients using FISH probes for chromosomes 7, 11, 12, 17 and 18. Aneuploidy was found in 32 of 34 (94%) effusions with positive morphological evaluation, as well as in 11 of 23 cytology-negative specimens [6]. Analysis by the same group of 25 effusions from patients diagnosed with malignant tumors of the exocrine or endocrine pancreas using FISH probes for chromosomes 7, 8, 11 and 18 showed chromosomal imbalances in all effusions, most frequently affecting chromosome 8, and MYC, residing on that chromosome, was amplified in 2 out of 10 effusions [7]. Aneuploidy of chromosome 8 was additionally found in 75% of 40 BC effusions [8]. The same group nevertheless reported on hyperdiploidy, as well as aneuploidy in small populations, in reactive mesothelial cells, applying FISH probes for chromosomes 7, 8, 11, 12, 17 and 18, calling for caution in determining cut-offs for the diagnosis of malignancy based on FISH [9]. A complementary role for this FISH assay and cytology was subsequently reported by this group in two larger series of 201 and 358 effusions, the latter including the former [10, 11].

Data supporting the use of FISH as adjunct to cytology have recently been published by other groups. Analysis of 72 malignant effusions consisting of various cancer types and 21 benign effusions showed sensitivity and specificity of 88% and 94.5%, respectively, for the combination of morphology and FISH analysis using probes for chromosomes 7, 11 and 17 [12]. Another study of 200 effusions applying FISH probes for chromosomes 7 and 17 similarly found the combination of this technique with morphology as beneficial, and FISH was particularly helpful in establishing the diagnosis of malignancy in cases with suspicious but inconclusive cytology [13].

Recent research has increasingly focused on the application of FISH to more specific entities, either as a diagnostic tool or as a basis for patient selection for targeted therapy.

HER2 is the protein product of the gene ERBB2, located at chromosome 17q, and is receptor tyrosine kinase of the epidermal growth factor receptor (EGFR) family. HER2 is over-expressed in 30% of BC, and HER2-over-expressing metastatic tumors are targeted by several drugs, including trastuzumab (Herceptin®), lapatinib (Tykerb®), pertuzumab (PERJETA™) and ado-trastuzumab emtansine [14]. Targeted therapy against HER2 is additionally used in metastatic gastric and gastro-esophageal junction carcinoma, a tumor in which HER2 gene amplification is found in 20% of cases [15]. HER2 status is routinely evaluated at the protein level using IHC or at the gene level applying CISH, SISH or FISH (Figures 20.1 and 20.2).

HER2 status results using IHC and FISH, performed on 42 cytological BC specimens, including 15 effusions, were shown to correlate well [16]. However, results between these two methods were more discrepant in another study, with some of the discordant observations attributed to chromosome 17 polyploidy [17]. HER2 status in metastatic tumors cannot be deduced from expression data in the primary carcinoma, as shown in analysis of 100 patient-matched specimens, including seven effusions, by FISH, in which nine metastases had a different HER2 status from the primary tumor [18]. In contrast, analysis of a total of 72 patient-matched primary and metastatic gastric carcinomas, the latter including 15 effusions, showed concordance levels of 98.5% and 94.9% for tumors analyzed by FISH (n=68) and IHC (n=39), respectively, suggesting that HER2 status in the primary tumor may reflect that of the corresponding metastasis [19].

Several studies have explored the role of FISH in the diagnosis of MM. MM have frequently homozygous deletion of the CDKN2A gene at chromosome 9p21, encoding the tumor suppressor proteins p14

357

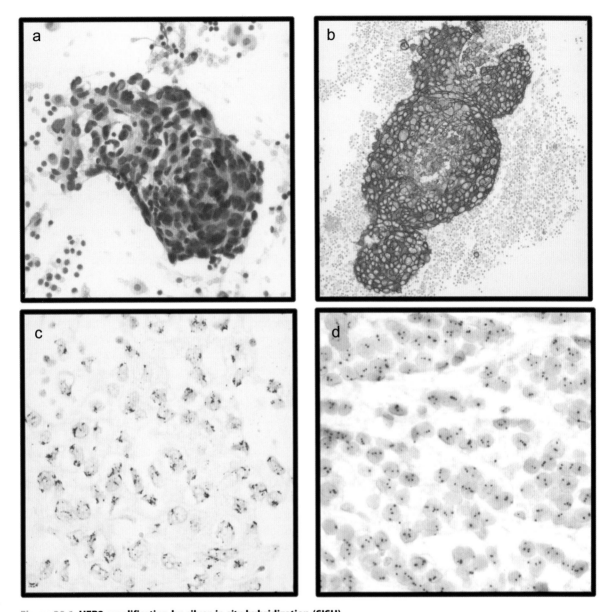

**Figure 20.1 HER2 amplification by silver *in situ* hybridization (SISH)**
(a) PAP-stained smear from a breast carcinoma pleural effusion (X200 magnification); (b) HER2 immunostaining, score = 3 (X100 magnification); (c) HER2 SISH analysis. Tumor cells have aggregates of black dots, corresponding to HER2 amplification. Chromosome 17 copy-number (red dots) does not exceed 2/cell (X400 magnification). (d) Example of needle biopsy from a primary breast carcinoma with normal HER2 status, evidenced by the presence of black: red dot ratio ≤2 (X400 magnification).

and p16. Illei *et al.* analyzed 32 effusions, of which 19, 6 and 7 were cytologically diagnosed as negative, suspicious for MM and diagnostic for MM, respectively. All six suspicious specimens and six out of seven cytologically malignant specimens had homozygous deletion of the CDKN2A gene by FISH, whereas none of the benign effusions showed this finding [20]. These results were reproduced by other investigators [21, 22]. Notably, both heterozygous and homozygous 9p21 deletions were observed in metastatic carcinomas, suggesting this finding is not specific for MM [21].

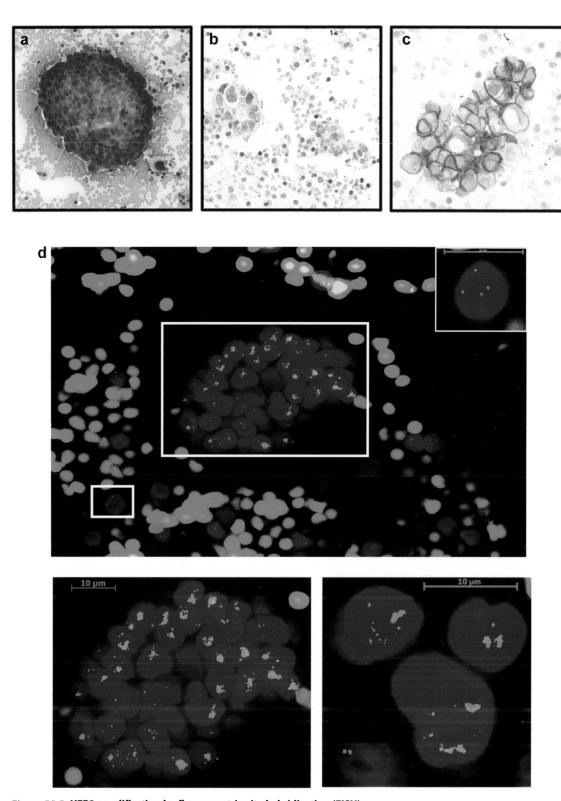

**Figure 20.2 HER2 amplification by fluorescent *in situ* hybridization (FISH)**
(a) Diff-Quik-stained smear from a breast carcinoma pleural effusion, showing a characteristic ball-shaped group of tumor cells (X200 magnification); (b) H&E-stained cell block section (X300 magnification); (c) HER2 immunostaining, score = 3 (X400 magnification); (d) HER2 FISH analysis showing amplification of this gene. A cluster of tumor cells (large frame), in which cells have HER2 copy-number >20 (pink clusters). The CEP17 centrosomal probe detects 1–2 copies (green dots) per cell. High power detail is shown in the lower panel.

Two studies applied the UroVysion™ kit, which contains centromeric probes for chromosomes 3, 7 and 17 and a probe for chromosome 9p21, to the diagnosis of effusions.

Flores-Staino et al. studied 68 effusions, including 21 MM, 29 metastatic tumors and 18 reactive specimens [23]. Deletions at 9p21 were observed in 12 of 21 MM and 3 of 29 other cancers, and were uniformly absent in benign specimens, while gains at 9p21 were observed in 2 of 21 MM, 20 of 29 non-MM cancers and 0 of 18 benign specimens. Gains in chromosomes 3, 7 and 17 were frequent in malignant tumors of both groups, and rare in benign effusions.

Savic et al. analyzed 52 MM and 28 reactive specimens. Positive FISH, defined as 10% of mesothelial cells with increased copy-number of at least one signal of at least one chromosome, and/or at least 15% of mesothelial cells with heterozygous or homozygous 9p21 deletion, was found in 41 of 52 (79%) MM and none of the benign specimens, and the most frequent aberration was 9p21 deletions. Promoter hypermethylation of the genes coding for p14, p15 or p16 was found in some of the FISH-negative MM [24].

Example of the 9p21 assay is shown in Figure 20.3.

Analysis of 17 MM and 17 benign effusions using centromeric probes for chromosomes 7 and 9 found this assay to be useful in differentiating these two conditions [25].

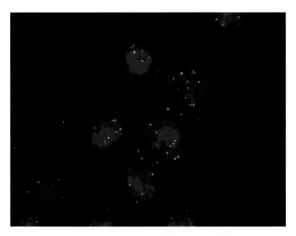

**Figure 20.3 Chromosome 9p21 deletion by FISH**
Malignant mesothelioma (MM) pleural effusion analyzed using a probe for chromosome 9p21 (UroVysion™ kit). Two large MM cells have absence of yellow dots, corresponding to homozygous chromosome 9p21 deletion. Reactive lymphocytes at the periphery have two yellow dots, denoting intact gene.
Courtesy of Professor Anders Hjerpe, Karolinska Institute, Stockholm, Sweden.

Few additional studies have applied ISH for a potentially diagnostic purpose. Frequent mRNA expression of MUC2 and MUC5AC, more strongly for the former, was observed in pseudomyoxoma peritonei specimens using a [35S]UTP-labeled probe [26]. Thyroid transcription factor-1 (TTF1) gene amplification by FISH was found in 13 of 175 primary lung carcinomas, 2 of 52 lymph node metastases and 2 of 46 malignant effusions. TTF1 mRNA and protein expression in effusions by PCR and IHC was related to longer survival, though not in multivariate analysis [27].

## Polymerase chain reaction (PCR)

PCR is one of the most widely applied methods in both the diagnostic and experimental settings, and has been utilized in a large number of studies focused on effusions.

One of the most focused-upon topics has been telomerase status as a diagnostic test for malignancy. Normal cells undergo repeated telomere shortening during senescence, which leads to cellular aging and death. Telomerase, a ribonucleoprotein complex, prevents this shortening, thereby conferring immortality to cancer cells. The role of telomerase in cancer biology has long been recognized and recent insights point to its role in stem cell biology [28].

Telomerase activity may be investigated using different assays, of which the most frequently used are the telomere repeat amplification protocol (TRAP) and the direct primer-extension activity assay [29].

In analysis of 144 effusions using the TRAP assay, 64 of 70 cytologically malignant effusions, 20 of 22 suspicious specimens and 3 of 22 benign effusions tested positive, resulting in sensitivity and specificity of 91.4% and 94.2%, respectively. The three telomerase-positive benign effusions were all from tuberculosis patients [30]. Several smaller studies, including one applying an in situ telomerase assay, generated comparable results [31–36]. ISH using probes for human telomerase mRNA component (hTERC) and telomerase reverse transcriptase (hTERT) mRNA was similarly efficient in this differential diagnosis [37]. However, two studies, of which one analyzed 291 effusions, reported relatively frequent false-positive analyses in reactive specimens [38, 39]. To date, this test has not gained recognition as a routine ancillary test in the majority of laboratories.

Several additional genes have been assessed for their diagnostic role in effusions applying PCR. Yamashita *et al.* analyzed 49 cytological specimens, including 44 effusions and 5 bile samples, for KRAS status at exons 1 and 2. KRAS point mutations were found in the effusion supernatant in eight out of nine pancreatic, two out of eight colorectal and one out of eight gastric carcinomas, including three cytology-negative specimens using single strand conformation polymorphism (SSCP) analysis, and were absent in all benign conditions [40].

Yu and co-workers applied a quantitative RT-PCR assay for the mucin genes MUC1, MUC2 and MUC5AC to 112 pleural effusion specimens, including 54 malignant effusions, the majority from lung carcinoma patients, 35 effusions from patients with benign conditions, and 23 cytology-negative effusions from patients with previous cancer diagnosis. Assay combining MUC1 and MUC5AC resulted in sensitivity and specificity at 86.1% and 91.5%, respectively. MUC2 was not valuable in this differential diagnosis [41].

In another study, an RT-PCR assay for the EGP2, also known as EPCAM, the gene which codes for epithelial glycoprotein 2, was applied to 110 peritoneal and pleural effusions, including 18 cytology-malignant and 92 benign specimens. EGP2 mRNA was found in 17 of 18 of the former and 11 of 92 of the latter group, and 6 of 11 positive effusions in the benign group were from cancer patients. The assay detected ten malignant cells added to $10^7$ benign cells [42].

The melanoma-associated antigen (MAGE) family constitutes a large group of cancer-related antigens that are under consideration as therapeutic targets [43]. A PCR assay for MAGE1 and MAGE3 and for the related genes BAGE and GAGE1–2 was applied to 44 effusions (27 effusions from women diagnosed with ovarian carcinoma (OC) and 17 specimens from patients with non-neoplastic diseases). BAGE, MAGE, MAGE3 and GAGE1–2 were detected in 17, 2, 8 and 8 malignant effusions, respectively, and with the exception of one BAGE-positive specimen, were absent from benign effusions [44].

An RT-PCR assay for prepro-gastrin releasing peptide (prepro-GRP) was reported to be specific for small cell lung carcinoma and was positive in all six tested effusions containing this tumor [45].

Fiegl and co-workers added an assay for the BC-related genes hMAM and hMAMB, coding for the BC markers mammaglobin and mammaglobin B to their above-described FISH assay for the detection of malignant cells in effusions. The hMAM and hMAMB assay was positive in 20 and 17 of 20 BC effusions, respectively. Of note, these genes were also frequently found in malignant effusions from other gynecologic carcinomas, and less frequently in gastro-intestinal carcinomas, and hMAMB was expressed in the majority of metastatic lung carcinomas [46].

Measurement of gene copy-numbers of the cell cycle marker cyclin E (size 100 bp) by quantitative PCR (qPCR) efficiently differentiated malignant (n=88) from benign (n=70) effusions [47].

Analysis of BIRC5 mRNA levels by qPCR in supernatants from 81 malignant and 31 benign pleural and peritoneal effusions showed over-expression of this mRNA, encoding for the anti-apoptotic marker Survivin, in malignant effusions, with sensitivity and diagnostic accuracy of 79% and 81.3%, respectively. Combination with CEA increased these values to 86.4% and 88.4%, respectively [48].

In another study, cell pellets from 56 malignant and 19 benign effusions were analyzed for mRNA expression of CLDN1, CLDN4, CLDN18, CEA, EPCAM, CK19, CK20, MUC1 and MUC16 using qPCR. All markers except CLDN18 and CK19 were over-expressed in malignant effusions, and the use of CLDN4, EPCAM and CK20 as adjunct to cytology resulted in an 86% detection rate [49].

Undoubtedly, the area in which PCR-based methodology has practical clinical relevance to date is in the testing of *EGFR* mutation status in advanced non-small cell lung carcinoma (NSCLC) (Figures 20.4 and 20.5). Activating mutations in EGFR are found in exons 18 to 21 of the tyrosine kinase domain in the EGFR gene and are associated with sensitivity to the tyrosine kinase inhibitors erlotinib (Tarceva®) and gefitinib (Iressa®). The most common EGFR mutations are short in-frame deletions at exon 19, located around amino acid residues 747 to 750, and point mutation L858R at exon 21. Testing for EGFR mutations can be done using different methods, including direct sequencing, denaturing high-performance liquid chromatography (dHPLC), high-resolution melting analysis (HRMA), pyro-sequencing, amplification-refractory mutation system (ARMS) PCR and PCR-restriction fragment length polymorphisms (PCR-RFLP) [50]. In a recent review, 33 studies in which EGFR mutation analysis was performed on cytological material were listed, of

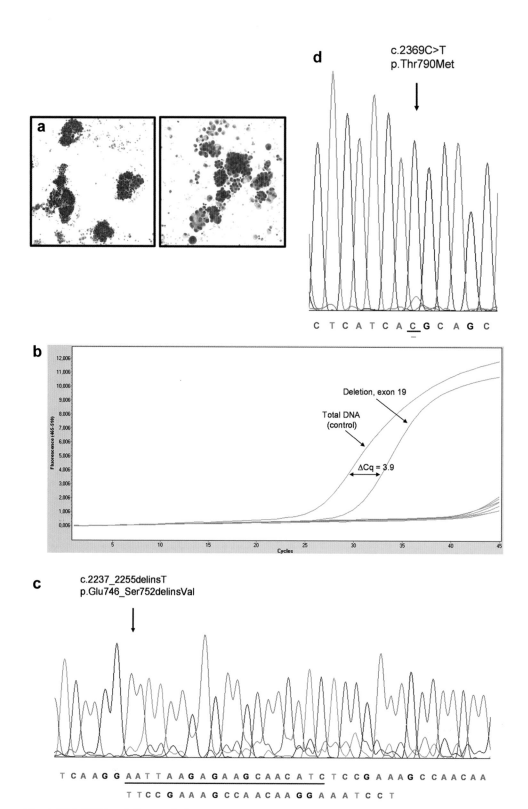

**Figure 20.4 EGFR mutation analysis**
A pleural effusion from a NSCLC patient treated with EGFR TKI. (a) Diff-Quik-stained (left) and PAP-stained (right) smears showing adenocarcinoma groups with papillary architecture. EGFR exon 19 deletion was shown by an ARMS PCR assay (therascreen EGFR PCR kit; Qiagen, Manchester, UK) (b) and identified as Glu746_Ser752delinVal (c.2237_2255delinsT) using Sanger sequencing (c). Sanger sequencing detected Thr790Met (c.2369C>T) mutation, consistent with acquired TKI resistance (d). The presence of both mutations was additionally demonstrated by an allele-specific PCR assay (Cobas® EGFR Mutation test; Roche Diagnostics, Mannheim, Germany; results not shown).

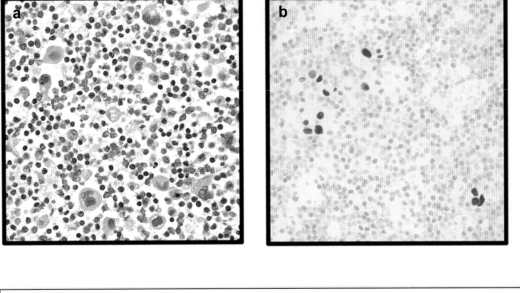

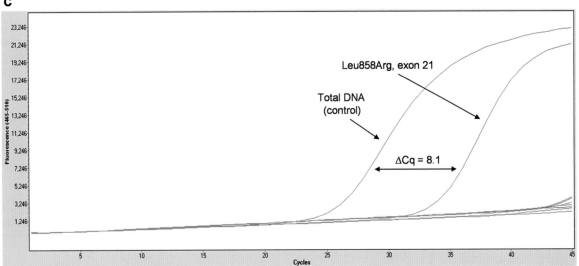

**Figure 20.5 EGFR mutation analysis**
Pleural effusion from a NSCLC patient. (a) H&E stained section showing adenocarcinoma cells, dissociated and in small groups; (b) TTF1 immunostaining showing nuclear expression in tumor cells; (c) EGFR exon 21 mutation Leu858Arg (c.2573T>G) was shown by an ARMS PCR assay (therascreen EGFR PCR kit; Qiagen, Manchester, UK). Mutated DNA, estimated from $\Delta$Cq value of 8.1 to be present in low percentage in this sample, could not be detected by Sanger sequencing, due to its limited sensitivity (~20% Mut DNA/Wt DNA; results not shown).

which approximately 50% analyzed effusion specimens, and the use of cytology specimens for this analysis resulted in satisfactory detection rates [50], an observation further reinforced in two recent papers published after the literature search for the aforementioned review [51, 52].

Another molecular finding detected in some NSCLC patients is fusion between the echinoderm microtubule-associated protein-like 4 (EML4) and the anaplastic lymphoma kinase (ALK) genes, both located on the short arm of chromosome 2, and a small inversion involving the two loci results in generation of the EML4-ALK fusion in lung cancer. The EML4-ALK tyrosine kinase undergoes constitutive dimerization, resulting in kinase activation and transforming ability, making it a therapeutic target in

363

cancer [53]. Analysis of 808 lung carcinoma specimens from 754 patients using multiplex PCR identified EML4-ALK transcripts in 36 specimens from 32 patients, including five pleural effusions [53]. In another study, in which pleural effusions from 116 patients with wild-type EGFR were studied, 39 tumors (34%) contained the *EML4-ALK* fusion gene by RT-PCR, and good agreement (85%) was seen with FISH in cases from which a cell block was available [54].

## DNA methylation

In addition to genetic changes, cancer cells exhibit altered epigenetic regulation. Epigenetic changes in tumor cells are related to DNA methylation, histone modifications, non-coding RNA and mitotic retention of gene regulatory machinery. DNA methylation mediates both transient and long-term gene silencing. Addition of methyl groups on CpG islands within gene promoters is done by three methyltransferases, DNMT1, DNMT3a and DNMT3b, and prevents binding of transcription factors and thereby gene transcription. Silenced genes are typically related to cell cycle regulation, DNA repair and survival/apoptosis. In contrast, oncogenes may be hypomethylated, with resulting transcriptional activation [55].

Benlloch *et al.* analyzed 87 pleural effusions (53 malignant, 34 benign) for the methylation status of death-associated protein kinase (DAPK), Ras association domain family 1A (RASSF1A), retinoic acid receptor-β (RARB) and p16/INK4a. Aberrant methylation was detected in 31 (58.5%) malignant effusions, the majority in one or two genes, and was absent in all benign effusions [56].

Another study applied an assay for the same four genes, as well as $O^6$-methylguanine-DNA methyltransferase (MGMT) as the fifth gene, to analysis of 47 malignant and 34 benign effusions. The number of methylation-positive specimens ranged between 3 out of 47 (MGMT) and 19 out of 47 (RARB) for malignant effusions, with MGMT, p16/INK4a and RASSF1A being the most specific assays and DAPK the least specific one. Methylation of any of the four genes other than DAPK was found in 28 malignant and seven benign effusions, corresponding to sensitivity and specificity of 59.6% and 79.4%, respectively [57].

The same five-gene panel was recently applied to the differential diagnosis of pleural MM (n=39), lung carcinoma (n=46), benign asbestos pleurisy (n=25)

and benign effusions of other etiology (n=30). The number of methylation-positive specimens ranged between 0 (MGMT) and 12 out of 39 (RASSF1A) for MM, and between 1 (MGMT) and 24 out of 46 (RARB) for lung carcinomas, with significantly higher RASSF1A, RARB and p16/INK4a methylation in the latter group. Benign asbestos pleurisy specimens had a methylation profile comparable to MM, whereas other benign specimens had infrequent methylation at all five genes [58].

Another gene evaluated for its methylation status in pleural effusion specimens is Wnt inhibitory factor 1 (WIF1). In analysis of 36 NSCLC and 35 benign effusions, WIF1 hypermethylation was detected in 25 (69.4%) malignant specimens and none of the benign effusions [59].

A different gene panel, including CHFR (checkpoint with forkhead and ring finger domains), p16/INK4a, RUNX3 (runt-related transcription factor 3), CDH1 (E-cadherin), hMLH1 (mutL homolog 1), ABCG2 (ATP-binding cassette, subfamily G, member 2) and BNIP3 (BCL2/adenovirus E1B 19 kDa interacting protein 3), was applied to 80 peritoneal effusions from gastric carcinoma patients. Cases were divided into three groups based on the depth of tumor invasion in the gastric wall and the presence of disseminated disease. CHFR, CDH1 and BNIP3 were increasingly more frequently observed in the transition from less invasive to more invasive and to disseminated disease [60].

## Loss of heterozygosity (LOH) / microsatellite instability (MSI)

Cancer cells are characterized by extensive genomic changes which include the activation of oncogenes and inactivation of tumor suppressor genes. LOH represents loss of one of the two alleles found for each gene in normal cells, and often affects tumor suppressor genes.

In MSI, the number of repeats of short sequences of DNA called microsatellites is different from the number in normal DNA. MSI represents a defect in the DNA repair system of the cell.

De Matos Granja *et al.* analyzed 41 pleural effusions from patients diagnosed with BC, including 24 malignant, 14 suspicious and 3 benign specimens for LOH at chromosomes 1p32 (MycL1), 7q31 and 17q21. LOH at 1p32 (MycL1), 7q31 and 17q21 was found in 7 of 32, 4 of 15 and 7 of 22 informative specimens, respectively, and was limited to malignant or suspicious effusions [61]. The same group reported on LOH at 16q22.1, which includes the locus of the E-cadherin gene CDH1, in 5 of 13 informative BC effusions [62].

Comparative analysis of LOH and MSI in 40 malignant and 17 tuberculous pleural effusions applying four microsatellite markers showed more frequent alterations in the former group (63% vs. 35% for all assays combined), but both sensitivity and specificity were regarded as insufficient. The same was true for FHIT and TP53 mutations [63].

In another study, cell pellets and supernatants from 14 malignant and six benign pleural effusions were studied for MSI and LOH using 12 microsatellite markers from eight chromosome regions. Analysis of the effusion supernatants was associated with 79% sensitivity and 100% specificity, and combination of this assay with cytology increased the sensitivity for detecting malignancy to 79%, compared to 57% for cytology alone [64].

Analysis of 48 pleural effusions, including 26 malignant and 22 benign effusions, the former predominantly lung carcinomas, for MSI and/or LOH using six microsatellite markers from five chromosome regions led to disappointing results, with only two malignant and one benign specimen showing genetic alterations [65].

## High-throughput analyses

Methods which enable researchers to analyze the entire genome, transcriptome, proteome and metabolome of tumor cells have been at the forefront of cancer research in recent years, with rapidly increasing platform complexity and its accompanying bioinformatics challenges. Efforts have largely been driven by the vision of personalized medicine, in which characterization of the metastatic disease, as in effusions, is of paramount importance. Some of the studies of effusions which may have direct diagnostic or clinical relevance are discussed in this section.

## Comparative genomic hybridization (CGH)

CGH is a method which compares the genome of tumor cells with that of normal tissue reference, thereby providing information regarding copynumber changes. The first study of effusion specimens applying CGH analyzed 15 cytological specimens, including 11 effusions, from patients with

OC, BC, colon carcinoma and MM. Analysis was successful in 14 out of 15 specimens, and showed a range of genetic changes in each of the tumor types investigated. Findings corresponded well with those of classic cytogenetics, when comparison was possible, and data quality was equal to or superior to data obtained from frozen biopsies, available for three patients [66].

Pirker and co-workers analyzed short-term cultures from 48 malignant melanoma specimens at different anatomic sites, including five effusions. The most frequent alterations involved gains in chromosomes 20q, 7q, 7p, 20p, 6p and 17q and losses of chromosomes 9p, 10q, 6q, 10p, 4q and 11q. Gains and amplifications at chromosomes 5p and 3q included the loci for hTERT and hTERC telomerase genes [67].

CGH analysis of 31 lung adenocarcinoma effusions showed multiple genetic alterations in tumor cells, with amplifications and deletions each involving 13 chromosomes. Loss of the 19q and 22q chromosome arms was more common than in previously reported analyses of primary carcinomas, and changes in chromosomes 3, 11 and/or X differed between males and females and between smokers and non-smokers [68].

## Gene expression microarrays

As discussed above, effusions are not infrequently the first malignant specimen obtained in a patient with no previous history of cancer. Consequently, the clinical question reverts from focusing on whether the effusion contains malignant cells to attempts to find the organ of origin. High-throughput technology offers a possibility to compare different cancers affecting the serosal cavities at the DNA, mRNA and protein levels.

The author's group performed three microarray studies using Affymetrix and Illumina platforms to differentiate between serous OC/PPC and MM, between serous OC/PPC and BC, and between BC and lung adenocarcinoma [69–71]. In each of these studies, 200 to 300 genes were found to be differentially expressed, often with cross-validation of the other studies (for example, over-expression of the folate receptor genes FOLR1 and FOLR3 in OC/PPC compared to both MM and BC; over-expression of the carbonic anhydrase family member CA12 and the trefoil factors TFF1 and TFF3 in BC compared to both OC/PPC and lung adenocarcinoma). Validation studies of larger series applying qPCR identified FOLR1, FOLR3, the retinoic acid suppressor PRAME, the Ets transcription factor family member EHF and the trafficking molecule RAB25 as markers of serous OC/PPC in the differential diagnosis from MM [72–75]. Scavanger receptor class A, member 3 (SCARA3), a molecule protecting cells from oxidative damage, was validated as an over-expressed gene in OC/PPC compared to BC [76], whereas the Ets family member SPDEF and the major histocompatibility complex (MHC)-related marker AZGP1 were over-expressed in BC compared to OC/PPC by qPCR [77]. TNXB, encoding the extracellular protein Tenascin-X, was validated as a novel MM marker at both the mRNA and protein levels [78].

The Tissue of Origin Test array® (Pathwork Diagnostics, Redwood City, CA), performed on mRNA from effusion cell blocks, was applied to 27 malignant and nine reactive effusions, the majority of the former being metastatic adenocarcinomas. There were four specimens with discordant results with regard to the clinical diagnosis, but upon re-evaluation of the cell content and immunostaining results, the test was reported as having correctly classified 16 out of 17 specimens containing more than 60% tumor cells [79].

qPCR analysis of effusion specimens based on gene panels generated through comparison of solid lung carcinoma and MM correctly classified all 13 studied specimens [80]. Microarray analysis of cell lines generated from pleural effusions identified markers differentiating MM from lung adenocarcinoma [81].

MicroRNAs (miRNAs) are short, non-coding RNAs regulating gene expression in physiological and pathological conditions. miRNAs exert their regulatory function by binding to the 3'-UTR of their target mRNA, thereby inhibiting target gene translation into proteins. Deregulated miRNA profiles have been shown in various malignancies. Circulating miRNAs are present in biological fluids such as blood, saliva, urine and ascites, and are therefore currently evaluated as potential cancer biomarkers in the diagnostic setting [82, 83].

Analysis of 13 miRNAs in 11 benign and 18 malignant effusion supernatants, the latter from patients with gastric and lung carcinoma, identified miR-24, miR-26a and miR-30d as over-expressed in the malignant specimens. Patients with malignant effusions who had higher levels of miR-152 had better response to Docetaxel [84].

In a recent study, miRNA microarrays, applied to comparative analysis of ten benign and ten lung adenocarcinoma pleural effusion supernatants, identified miR-198 as under-expressed in the malignant effusions, a finding validated by the authors in a larger case series. miR-198 performed at the same level as CEA and better than the cytokeratin fragment CYFRA in this differential diagnosis, and combination of all three markers resulted in sensitivity and specificity of 89.2% and 85%, respectively [85].

The author's group compared the miRNA content of small membrane particles secreted by cells, called exosomes, in OC supernatants, supernatants from benign reactive effusions and OC cell pellets from effusions, and identified differentially expressed miRNAs in each group [86].

## Proteomics and metabolomics

Different proteomics platforms have been evaluated in recent years in studies aimed at identifying tumor-specific markers that will help in the diagnostic and therapeutic settings. Some of these studies have analyzed five malignant effusions or less, and are therefore not discussed in this chapter. However, several larger studies have been published.

Tyan et al. studied 43 pleural effusions from patients with lung adenocarcinoma using a two-dimensional nano-high-performance liquid chromatography electrospray ionization tandem mass spectrometry (2D nano-HPLC-ESI-MS/MS) system. At higher confidence level, 124 proteins were identified, including both secreted and cellular proteins, the majority of which were molecules with a biological role in metabolism, transport, cell communication and cell growth [87].

In another study, 14 malignant pleural effusions, the majority from lung carcinoma patients, and 13 benign transudates were analyzed using two-dimensional gel electrophoresis. Protein spots with differential expression were identified by time-of-flight mass spectrometry and liquid chromatography/tandem mass spectrometry, with further target validation by ELISA and Western blots. Seven spots which were smaller in the malignant specimens were identified, including the fibrinogen β- and γ-chain precursors and pigment epithelium-derived factor [88].

Comparative analysis of serous OC peritoneal effusions and benign effusions using discovery-based proteomics, bioinformatics prioritization and targeted proteomics quantification using Selected Reaction Monitoring Mass Spectrometry (SRM-MS) identified 51 differentially expressed candidate proteins, of which some have previously been identified in analyses of OC effusion cells or supernatants, or in analyses of OC cell lines, including known OC markers such as CA 125/MUC16, mesothelin and kallikrein family members [89].

Yu *et al.* performed a pooled analysis of 13 malignant effusions from lung carcinoma patients after removal of six high-abundance plasma proteins. One-dimensional SDS-PAGE combined with nano-LC_MS/MS was used for evaluation of 482 non-redundant proteins. Four proteins, consisting of alpha-2-HSglycoprotein (AHSG), angiogenin, cystatin-C and insulin-like growth factor-binding protein 2 (IGFBP2), were validated for their diagnostic role in a larger series of malignant effusions from different cancers and benign effusions using ELISA. IGFBP2 was the most significantly over-expressed marker in malignant effusions, irrespective of cancer type [90].

Two studies using lysate array proteomics evaluated the diagnostic role of this method in differentiating OC effusions from benign reactive effusions, as well its clinical relevance in OC. In the first paper, 61 malignant and nine reactive effusions were studied for expression of 26 proteins related to cell survival, proliferation and apoptosis. Significantly higher expression of AKT, cAMP-responsive element binding protein (CREB), c-Jun-NH2-kinase (JNK), phosphorylated extracellular-regulated kinase (p-ERK) and p-CREB were found in OC effusions compared to their benign counterparts. Pre-chemotherapy OC effusions tapped at diagnosis had significantly different expression levels of several of the studied molecules compared to post-chemotherapy disease recurrence effusions, and the prognostic markers identified for each of these two groups were different [91].

In the second paper, the proteomic profiles of 51 malignant and 20 reactive effusions were studied for expression of 16 proteins mediating adhesion and intracellular signaling. The majority of studied proteins were over-expressed in OC effusions, and several, including cadherin family members, focal adhesion kinase (FAK), AKT and p-AKT, Pyk and p-Pyk, were significantly related to clinicopathologic parameters and/or survival [92].

Metabolic profiling of body fluids provides information regarding differences in the levels of endogenous metabolites across physiological and various pathological states, and may aid in monitoring cellular responses following therapeutic interventions. Metabolomics has consequently a potential role in cancer diagnosis and has been applied to the differentiation of benign from malignant ascites [93].

In a collaborative study, the author's group recently applied high-resolution magnetic resonance (MR) spectroscopy to analysis of 115 effusion supernatants, including 95 OC, 10 BC and 10 MM. OC specimens included eight paired peritoneal effusions obtained pre- and post-chemotherapy from the same patient. OC effusions had elevated levels of ketones (aceto-acetate and beta-hydroxybutyrate) and lactate compared to MM and BC, whereas the latter had more glucose, alanine and pyruvate. Post-chemotherapy OC effusions had significantly higher glucose and lipid levels compared to pre-chemotherapy patient-matched specimens [94].

## Concluding remarks

The body of data discussed in this chapter, although incomplete, provides clear evidence regarding the potential of effusion specimens in the context of complex analyses at the DNA, RNA and protein levels. Indeed, effusions have been repeatedly shown to perform at least as good as biopsy specimens in multiple assays. While analyses such as HER2 status and EGFR mutation status are required by clinicians and thus performed in multiple laboratories, the choice of other assays as diagnostic adjuncts depends on the expertise level and experience of each lab. Many of the assays discussed in this chapter appear promising, but require validation in additional series from independent institutions.

In view of their accessibility, the large volume which can often be tapped, the high state of viability of cells in these specimens and their relevance within the advanced cancer setting, the role of effusions in cancer diagnosis, prediction of treatment response and prognostication is likely to increase. A recent paper which analyzed sequential OC ascites specimens along tumor progression using deep sequencing [95] is likely to be the first of many studies in which this cutting-edge technology will be used, potentially bringing cancer therapy ever closer to truly personalized medicine.

# References

1. Davidson, B., Firat, B. P. and Michael, C. W. (eds.), *Serous Effusions* (London: Springer, 2011).

2. Sandberg, A. A. and Meloni-Ehrig, A. M. Cytogenetics and genetics of human cancer: methods and accomplishments. *Cancer Genet Cytogenet* 2010; 203(2): 102–26.

3. Reis-Filho, J. S. and de Landér Schmitt, F. C. Fluorescence in situ hybridization, comparative genomic hybridization, and other molecular biology techniques in the analysis of effusions. *Diagn Cytopathol* 2005; 33(5): 294–9.

4. Larramendy, M. L., Björkqvist, A. M., Tammilehto, L., Taavitsainen, M., Mattson, K. and Knuutila, S. Absence of trisomy 7 in nonneoplastic human ascitic and pleural fluid cells. An interphase cytogenetic study. *Cancer Genet Cytogenet* 1994; 78(1): 78–81.

5. Johnson, T. M., Kuffel, D. G. and Dewald, G. W. Detection of hyperdiploid malignant cells in pleural effusions with chromosome-specific probes and fluorescence in situ hybridization. *Mayo Clin Proc* 1996; 71(7): 643–8.

6. Zojer, N., Fiegl, M., Angerler, J., Müllauer, L., Gsur, A., Roka, S. *et al.* Interphase fluorescence in situ hybridization improves the detection of malignant cells in effusions from breast cancer patients. *Br J Cancer* 1997; 75(3): 403–7.

7. Zojer, N., Fiegl, M., Müllauer, L., Chott, A., Roka, S., Ackermann, J. *et al.* Chromosomal imbalances in primary and metastatic pancreatic carcinoma as detected by interphase cytogenetics: basic findings and clinical aspects. *Br J Cancer* 1998; 77(8): 1337–42.

8. Roka, S., Fiegl, M., Zojer, N., Filipits, M., Schuster, R., Steiner, B. *et al.* Aneuploidy of chromosome 8 as detected by interphase fluorescence in situ hybridization is a recurrent finding in primary and metastatic breast cancer. *Breast Cancer Res Treat* 1998; 48(2): 125–33.

9. Fiegl, M., Zojer, N., Kaufmann, H., Müllauer, L., Schuster, R., Huber, H. *et al.* Hyperdiploidy and apparent aneusomy in mesothelial cells from non-malignant effusions as detected by fluorescence in situ hybridization (FISH). *Cytometry* 1999; 38(1): 15–23.

10. Fiegl, M., Kaufmann, H., Zojer, N., Schuster, R., Wiener, H., Müllauer, L. *et al.* Malignant cell detection by fluorescence in situ hybridization (FISH) in effusions from patients with carcinoma. *Hum Pathol* 2000; 31(4): 448–55.

11. Fiegl, M., Massoner, A., Haun, M., Sturm, W., Kaufmann, H., Hack, R. *et al.* Sensitive detection of tumour cells in effusions by combining cytology and fluorescence in situ hybridisation (FISH). *Br J Cancer* 2004; 91(3): 558–63.

12. Han, J., Cao, S., Zhang, K., Zhao, G., Xin, Y., Dong, Q. *et al.* Fluorescence in situ hybridization as adjunct to cytology improves the diagnosis and directs estimation of prognosis of malignant pleural effusions. *J Cardiothorac Surg* 2012; 7: 121.

13. Rosolen, D. C., Kulikowski, L. D., Bottura, G., Nascimento, A. M., Acencio, M., Teixeira, L. *et al.* Efficacy of two fluorescence in situ hybridization (FISH) probes for diagnosing malignant pleural effusions. *Lung Cancer* 2013; 80(3): 284–8.

14. Gradishar, W. J. Emerging approaches for treating HER2-positive metastatic breast cancer beyond trastuzumab. *Ann Oncol* 2013; 24(10): 2492–500.

15. Pazo Cid, R. A. and Antón, A. Advanced HER2-positive gastric cancer: current and future targeted therapies. *Crit Rev Oncol Hematol* 2013; 85(3): 350–62.

16. Shabaik, A., Lin, G., Peterson, M., Hasteh, F., Tipps, A., Datnow, B. *et al.* Reliability of Her2/neu, estrogen receptor, and progesterone receptor testing by immunohistochemistry on cell block of FNA and serous effusions from patients with primary and metastatic breast carcinoma. *Diagn Cytopathol* 2011; 39(5): 328–32.

17. Schlüter, B., Gerhards, R., Strumberg, D. and Voigtmann, R. Combined detection of Her2/neu gene amplification and protein overexpression in effusions from patients with breast and ovarian cancer. *J Cancer Res Clin Oncol* 2010; 136(9): 1389–400.

18. Arihiro, K., Oda, M., Ogawa, K., Tominaga, K., Kaneko, Y., Shimizu, T. *et al.* Discordant HER2 status between primary breast carcinoma and recurrent/metastatic tumors using fluorescence in situ hybridization on cytological samples. *Jpn J Clin Oncol* 2013; 43(1): 55–62.

19. Bozzetti, C., Negri, F. V., Lagrasta, C. A., Crafa, P., Bassano, C., Tamagnini, I. *et al.* Comparison of HER2 status in primary and paired metastatic sites of gastric carcinoma. *Br J Cancer* 2011; 104(9): 1372–6.

20. Illei, P. B., Ladanyi, M., Rusch, V. W. and Zakowski, M. F. The use of CDKN2A deletion as a diagnostic marker for malignant mesothelioma in body cavity effusions. *Cancer* 2003; 99(1): 51–6.

21. Onofre, F. B., Onofre, A. S., Pomjanski, N., Buckstegge, B., Grote, H. J., Böcking, A. *et al.* 9p21 deletion in the diagnosis of malignant mesothelioma in serous effusions additional to immunocytochemistry, DNA-ICM, and AgNOR analysis. *Cancer* 2008; 114(3): 204–15.

22. Matsumoto, S., Nabeshima, K., Kamei, T., Hiroshima, K., Kawahara, K., Hata, S. et al. Morphology of 9p21 homozygous deletion-positive pleural mesothelioma cells analyzed using fluorescence in situ hybridization and virtual microscope system in effusion cytology. Cancer Cytopathol 2013; 121(8): 415–22.

23. Flores-Staino, C., Darai-Ramqvist, E., Dobra, K. and Hjerpe, A. Adaptation of a commercial fluorescent in situ hybridization test to the diagnosis of malignant cells in effusions. Lung Cancer 2010; 68(1): 39–43.

24. Savic, S., Franco, N., Grilli, B., Barascud Ade, V., Herzog, M., Bode, B. et al. Fluorescence in situ hybridization in the definitive diagnosis of malignant mesothelioma in effusion cytology. Chest 2010; 138(1): 137–44.

25. Shin, H. J., Shin, D. M., Tarco, E. and Sneige, N. Detection of numerical aberrations of chromosomes 7 and 9 in cytologic specimens of pleural malignant mesothelioma. Cancer 2003; 99(4): 233–9.

26. O'Connell, J. T., Hacker, C. M. and Barsky, S. H. MUC2 is a molecular marker for pseudomyxoma peritonei. Mod Pathol 2002; 15(9): 958–72.

27. Li, X., Wan, L., Shen, H., Geng, J., Nie, J., Wang, G. et al. Thyroid transcription factor-1 amplification and expressions in lung adenocarcinoma tissues and pleural effusions predict patient survival and prognosis. J Thorac Oncol 2012; 7(1): 76–84.

28. Günes, C. and Rudolph, K. L. The role of telomeres in stem cells and cancer. Cell 2013; 152(3): 390–3.

29. Podlevsky, J. D. and Chen, J. J. It all comes together at the ends: telomerase structure, function, and biogenesis. Mutat Res 2012; 730(1–2): 3–11.

30. Yang, C. T., Lee, M. H., Lan, R. S. and Chen, J. K. Telomerase activity in pleural effusions: diagnostic significance. J Clin Oncol 1998; 16(2): 567–73.

31. Cunningham, V. J., Markham, N., Shroyer, A. L., and Shroyer, K. R. Detection of telomerase expression in fine-needle aspirations and fluids. Diagn Cytopathol 1998; 18(6): 431–6.

32. Mu, X. C., Brien, T. P., Ross, J. S., Lowry, C. V. and McKenna, B. J. Telomerase activity in benign and malignant cytologic fluids. Cancer 1999; 87(2): 93–9.

33. Tangkijvanich, P., Tresukosol, D., Sampatanukul, P., Sakdikul, S., Voravud, N., Mahachai, V. et al. Telomerase assay for differentiating between malignancy-related and nonmalignant ascites. Clin Cancer Res 1999; 5(9): 2470–5.

34. Toshima, S., Arai, T., Yasuda, Y., Takaya, T., Ito, Y., Hayakawa, K. et al. Cytological diagnosis and telomerase activity of cells in effusions of body cavities. Oncol Rep 1999; 6(1): 199–203.

35. Tseng, C. J., Jain, S., Hou, H. C., Liu, W., Pao, C. C., Lin, C. T. et al. Applications of the telomerase assay in peritoneal washing fluids. Gynecol Oncol 2001; 81(3): 420–3.

36. Dejmek, A., Yahata, N., Ohyashiki, K., Ebihara, Y., Kakihana, M., Hirano, T. et al. In situ telomerase activity in pleural effusions: a promising marker for malignancy. Diagn Cytopathol 2001; 24(1): 11–15.

37. Hiroi, S., Nakanishi, K. and Kawai, T. Expressions of human telomerase mRNA component (hTERC) and telomerase reverse transcriptase (hTERT) mRNA in effusion cytology. Diagn Cytopathol 2003; 29(4): 212–16.

38. Nagel, H., Schlott, T., Schulz, G. M. and Droese, M. Gene expression analysis of the catalytic subunit of human telomerase (hEST2) in the differential

diagnosis of serous effusions. Diagn Mol Pathol 2001; 10(1): 60–5.

39. Braunschweig, R., Guilleret, I., Delacrétaz, F., Bosman, F. T., Mihaescu, A. and Benhattar, J. Pitfalls in TRAP assay in routine detection of malignancy in effusions. Diagn Cytopathol 2001; 25(4): 225–30.

40. Yamashita, K., Kuba, T., Shinoda, H., Takahashi, E. and Okayasu, I. Detection of K-ras point mutations in the supernatants of peritoneal and pleural effusions for diagnosis complementary to cytologic examination. Am J Clin Pathol 1998; 109(6): 704–11.

41. Yu, C. J., Shew, J. Y., Liaw, Y. S., Kuo, S. H., Luh, K. T., Yang, P. C. et al. Application of mucin quantitative competitive reverse transcription polymerase chain reaction in assisting the diagnosis of malignant pleural effusion. Am J Respir Crit Care Med 2001; 164(7): 1312–18.

42. Sakaguchi, M., Virmani, A. K., Ashfaq, R., Rogers, T. E., Rathi, A., Liu, Y. et al. Development of a sensitive, specific reverse transcriptase polymerase chain reaction-based assay for epithelial tumour cells in effusions. Br J Cancer 1999; 79(3–4): 416–22.

43. Sang, M., Lian, Y., Zhou, X. and Shan, B. MAGE-A family: attractive targets for cancer immunotherapy. Vaccine 2011; 29(47): 8496–500.

44. Hofmann, M. and Ruschenburg, I. mRNA detection of tumor-rejection genes BAGE, GAGE, and MAGE in peritoneal fluid from patients with ovarian carcinoma as a potential diagnostic tool. Cancer 2002; 96(3): 187–93.

45. Saito, T., Kobayashi, M., Harada, R., Uemura, Y. and Taguchi, H. Sensitive detection of small cell lung carcinoma cells by reverse transcriptase-polymerase chain reaction for

prepro-gastrin-releasing peptide mRNA. *Cancer* 2003; 97(10): 2504–11.

46. Fiegl, M., Haun, M., Massoner, A., Krugmann, J., Müller-Holzner, E., Hack, R. *et al.* Combination of cytology, fluorescence in situ hybridization for aneuploidy, and reverse-transcriptase polymerase chain reaction for human mammaglobin/mammaglobin B expression improves diagnosis of malignant effusions. *J Clin Oncol* 2004; 22(3): 474–83.

47. Salani, R., Davidson, B., Fiegl, M., Marth, C., Müller-Holzner, E., Gastl, G. *et al.* Measurement of cyclin E genomic copy number and strand length in cell-free DNA distinguish malignant versus benign effusions. *Clin Cancer Res* 2007; 13(19): 5805–9.

48. Wang, T., Qian, X., Wang, Z., Yu, L., Ding, Y. and Liu, B. Detection of cell-free BIRC5 mRNA in effusions and its potential diagnostic value for differentiating malignant and benign effusions. *Int J Cancer* 2009; 125(8): 1921–5.

49. Mohamed, F., Vincent, N., Cottier, M., Peoc'h, M., Merrouche, Y., Patouillard, B. *et al.* Improvement of malignant serous effusions diagnosis by quantitative analysis of molecular claudin 4 expression. *Biomarkers* 2010; 15(4): 315–24.

50. Ellison, G., Zhu, G., Moulis, A., Dearden, S., Speake, G. and McCormack, R. EGFR mutation testing in lung cancer: a review of available methods and their use for analysis of tumour tissue and cytology samples. *J Clin Pathol* 2013; 66(2): 79–89.

51. Tsai, T. H., Wu, S. G., Chang, Y. L., Wu, C. T., Tsai, M. F., Wei, P. F. *et al.* Effusion immunocytochemistry as an alternative approach for the selection of first-line targeted therapy in advanced lung adenocarcinoma. *J Thorac Oncol* 2012; 7(6): 993–1000.

52. Goto, K., Satouchi, M., Ishii, G., Nishio, K., Hagiwara, K., Mitsudomi, T. *et al.* An evaluation study of EGFR mutation tests utilized for non-small-cell lung cancer in the diagnostic setting. *Ann Oncol* 2012; 23(11): 2914–19.

53. Soda, M., Isobe, K., Inoue, A., Maemondo, M., Oizumi, S., Fujita, Y. *et al.* A prospective PCR-based screening for the EML4-ALK oncogene in non-small cell lung cancer. *Clin Cancer Res* 2012; 18(20): 5682–9.

54. Wu, S. G., Kuo, Y. W., Chang, Y. L., Shih, J. Y., Chen, Y. H., Tsai, M. F. *et al.* EML4-ALK translocation predicts better outcome in lung adenocarcinoma patients with wild-type EGFR. *J Thorac Oncol* 2012; 7: 98–104.

55. Zaidi, S. K., Van Wijnen, A. J., Lian, J. B., Stein, J. L. and Stein, G. S. Targeting deregulated epigenetic control in cancer. *J Cell Physiol* 2013; 228(11): 2103–8.

56. Benlloch, S., Galbis-Caravajal, J. M., Martín, C., Sanchez-Paya, J., Rodríguez-Paniagua, J. M., Romero, S. *et al.* Potential diagnostic value of methylation profile in pleural fluid and serum from cancer patients with pleural effusion. *Cancer* 2006; 107(8): 1859–65.

57. Katayama, H., Hiraki, A., Aoe, K., Fujiwara, K., Matsuo, K., Maeda, T. *et al.* Aberrant promoter methylation in pleural fluid DNA for diagnosis of malignant pleural effusion. *Int J Cancer* 2007; 120(10): 2191–5.

58. Fujii, M., Fujimoto, N., Hiraki, A., Gemba, K., Aoe, K., Umemura, S. *et al.* Aberrant DNA methylation profile in pleural fluid for differential diagnosis of malignant pleural mesothelioma. *Cancer Sci* 2012; 103(3): 510–14.

59. Yang, T. M., Leu, S. W., Li, J. M., Hung, M. S., Lin, C. H., Lin, Y. C. *et al.* WIF-1 promoter region hypermethylation as an adjuvant diagnostic marker for non-small cell lung cancer-related malignant pleural effusions. *J Cancer Res Clin Oncol* 2009; 135(7): 919–24.

60. Hiraki, M., Kitajima, Y., Sato, S., Nakamura, J., Hashiguchi, K., Noshiro, H. *et al.* Aberrant gene methylation in the peritoneal fluid is a risk factor predicting peritoneal recurrence in gastric cancer. *World J Gastroenterol* 2010; 16(3): 330–8.

61. de Matos Granja, N., Soares, R., Rocha, S., Paredes, J., Longatto Filho, A., Alves, V. A. *et al.* Evaluation of breast cancer metastases in pleural effusions by molecular biology techniques. *Diagn Cytopathol* 2002; 27(4): 210–13.

62. Granja Nde, M., Ricardo, S. A., Longatto Filho, A., Alves, V. A., Bedrossian, C. W., Wiley, E. L. *et al.* Potential use of loss of heterozygosity in pleural effusions of breast cancer metastases using the microsatellite marker of the 16q22.1 region of the CDH1 gene. *Anal Quant Cytol Histol* 2005; 27(2): 61–6.

63. Lee, J. H., Hong, Y. S., Ryu, J. S. and Chang, J. H. p53 and FHIT mutations and microsatellite alterations in malignancy-associated pleural effusion. *Lung Cancer* 2004; 44(1): 33–42.

64. Woenckhaus, M., Grepmeier, U., Werner, B., Schulz, C., Rockmann, F., Wild, P. J. *et al.* Microsatellite analysis of pleural supernatants could increase sensitivity of pleural fluid cytology. *J Mol Diagn* 2005; 7(4): 517–24.

65. Economidou, F., Tzortzaki, E. G., Schiza, S., Antoniou, K. M., Neofytou, E., Zervou, M. *et al.* Microsatellite DNA analysis does not distinguish malignant from benign pleural effusions. *Oncol Rep* 2007; 18(6): 1507–12.

66. Nagel, H., Schulten, H. J., Gunawan, B., Brinck, U. and Füzesi, L. The potential value of comparative genomic

hybridization analysis in effusion-
and fine needle aspiration
cytology. *Mod Pathol* 2002; 15(8):
818–25.

67. Pirker, C., Holzmann, K., Spiegl-
Kreinecker, S., Elbling, L.,
Thallinger, C., Pehamberger, H.
*et al.* Chromosomal imbalances in
primary and metastatic
melanomas: over-representation
of essential telomerase genes.
*Melanoma Res* 2003; 13(5):
483–92.

68. Yen, C. C., Liang, S. C., Jong, Y. J.,
Chen, Y. J., Lin, C. H., Chen, Y.
M. *et al.* Chromosomal
aberrations of malignant pleural
effusions of lung adenocarcinoma:
different cytogenetic changes are
correlated with genders and
smoking habits. *Lung Cancer*
2007; 57(3): 292–301.

69. Davidson, B., Zhang, Z.,
Kleinberg, L., Li, M., Flørenes, V.
A., Wang, T. L. *et al.* Gene
expression signatures differentiate
ovarian/peritoneal serous
carcinoma from diffuse malignant
peritoneal mesothelioma. *Clin
Cancer Res* 2006; 12(20 Pt. 1):
5944–50.

70. Davidson, B., Tuft Stavnes, H.,
Holth, A., Chen, X., Yang, Y.,
Shih, le-M. *et al.* Gene expression
signatures differentiate ovarian/
peritoneal serous carcinoma from
breast carcinoma in effusions.
*J Cell Mol Med* 2011; 15(3):
535–44.

71. Davidson, B., Stavnes, H. T.,
Risberg, B., Nesland, J. M.,
Wohlschlaeger, J., Yang, Y. *et al.*
Gene expression signatures
differentiate adenocarcinoma of
lung and breast origin in
effusions. *Hum Pathol* 2012;
43(5): 684–94.

72. Yuan, Y., Nymoen, D. A., Dong,
H. P., Bjørang, O., Shih, le-M.,
Low, P. S. et al. Expression of the
folate receptor genes FOLR1 and
FOLR3 differentiates ovarian
carcinoma from breast carcinoma
and malignant mesothelioma in

serous effusions. *Hum Pathol*
2009; 40(10): 1453–60.

73. Brenne, K., Nymoen, D. A., Reich,
R., Davidson, B. PRAME
(Preferentially Expressed Antigen
of Melanoma) is a novel marker
for differentiating serous
carcinoma from malignant
mesothelioma. *Am J Clin Pathol*
2012; 137(2): 240–7.

74. Brenne, K., Nymoen, D. A.,
Hetland, T. E., Trope, C. G. and
Davidson, B. Expression of the Ets
transcription factor EHF in serous
ovarian carcinoma effusions is a
marker of poor survival. *Hum
Pathol* 2012; 43(4): 496–505.

75. Brusegard, K., Stavnes, H. T.,
Nymoen, D. A., Flatmark, K.,
Trope, C. G., Davidson, B. Rab25
is overexpressed in Müllerian
serous carcinoma compared to
malignant mesothelioma.
*Virchows Arch* 2012; 460(2):
193–202.

76. Bock, A. J., Nymoen, D. A.,
Brenne, K., Kaern, J. and
Davidson, B. SCARA3 mRNA is
overexpressed in ovarian
carcinoma compared to breast
carcinoma effusions. *Hum Pathol*
2012; 43(5): 669–74.

77. Stavnes, H. T., Nymoen, D. A.,
Langerød, A., Hetland Falkenthal,
T. E., Kærn, J., Tropé, C. G. *et al.*
AZGP1 and SPDEF mRNA
expression differentiates breast
carcinoma from ovarian serous
carcinoma. *Virchows Arch* 2013;
462(2): 163–73.

78. Yuan, Y., Nymoen, D. A., Tuft
Stavnes, H., Rosnes, A. K.,
Bjørang, O., Wu, C. *et al.*
Tenascin-X is a novel diagnostic
marker of malignant
mesothelioma. *Am J Surg Pathol*
2009; 33(11): 1673–82.

79. Stancel, G. A., Coffey, D., Alvarez,
K., Halks-Miller, M., Lal, A.,
Mody, D. *et al.* Identification of
tissue of origin in body fluid
specimens using a gene expression
microarray assay. *Cancer
Cytopathol* 2012; 120(1): 62–70.

80. Holloway, A. J., Diyagama, D. S.,
Opeskin, K., Creaney, J.,
Robinson, B. W., Lake, R. A.
*et al.* A molecular diagnostic
test for distinguishing lung
adenocarcinoma from malignant
mesothelioma using cells
collected from pleural effusions.
*Clin Cancer Res* 2006; 12(17):
5129–35.

81. Gueugnon, F., Leclercq, S.,
Blanquart, C., Sagan, C., Cellerin,
L., Padieu, M. *et al.* Identification
of novel markers for the diagnosis
of malignant pleural
mesothelioma. *Am J Pathol* 2011;
178(3): 1033–42.

82. Weber, J. A., Baxter, D. H., Zhang,
S., Huang, D. Y., Huang, K. H.,
Lee, M. J. *et al.* The microRNA
spectrum in 12 body fluids. *Clin
Chem* 2010; 56(11): 1733–41.

83. Wittmann, J. and Jack, H. M.
Serum microRNAs as powerful
cancer biomarkers. *Biochim
Biophys Acta* 2010; 1806(2):
200–7.

84. Xie, L., Chen, X., Wang, L., Qian,
X., Wang, T., Wei, J. *et al.* Cell-
free miRNAs may indicate
diagnosis and docetaxel sensitivity
of tumor cells in malignant
effusions. *BMC Cancer* 2010; 10:
591.

85. Han, H. S., Yun, J., Lim, S. N.,
Han, J. H., Lee, K. H., Kim, S. T.
*et al.* Downregulation of cell-free
miR-198 as a diagnostic
biomarker for lung
adenocarcinoma-associated
malignant pleural effusion. *Int
J Cancer* 2013; 133(3): 645–52.

86. Vaksman, V., Tropé, C.,
Davidson, B. and Reich, R.
Exosome-derived miRNAs and
ovarian carcinoma progression.
*Carcinogenesis* 2014; 35(9):
2113–20.

87. Tyan, Y. C., Wu, H. Y., Lai, W.
W., Su, W. C., Liao, P. C. *et al.*
Proteomic profiling of human
pleural effusion using two-
dimensional nano liquid
chromatography tandem mass

spectrometry. *J Proteome Res* 2005; 4(4): 1274–86.

88. Hsieh, W. Y., Chen, M. W., Ho, H. T., You, T. M. and Lu, Y. T. Identification of differentially expressed proteins in human malignant pleural effusions. *Eur Respir J* 2006; 28(6): 1178–85.

89. Elschenbroich, S., Ignatchenko, V., Clarke, B., Kalloger, S. E., Boutros, P. C. *et al.* In-depth proteomics of ovarian cancer ascites: combining shotgun proteomics and selected reaction monitoring mass spectrometry. *J Proteome Res* 2011; 10(5): 2286–99.

90. Yu, C. J., Wang, C. L., Wang, C. I., Chen, C. D., Dan, Y. M., Wu, C. C. *et al.* Comprehensive proteome analysis of malignant pleural effusion for lung cancer biomarker discovery by using multidimensional protein

identification technology. *J Proteome Res* 2011; 10(10): 4671–82.

91. Davidson, B., Espina, V., Steinberg, S. M. Flørenes, V. A., Liotta, L. A., Kristensen, G. B. *et al.* Proteomic profiling of malignant ovarian cancer effusions: survival and injury pathways discriminate clinical outcome. *Clin Cancer Res* 2006; 12(3 Pt. 1): 791–9.

92. Kim, G., Davidson, B., Henning, R., Wang, J., Yu, M., Annunziata, C. *et al.* Adhesion molecule protein signature in ovarian cancer effusions is prognostic of patient outcome. *Cancer* 2012; 118(6): 1543–53.

93. Bala, L., Sharma, A., Yellapa, R. K., Roy, R., Choudhuri, G. and Khetrapal, C. L.. (1)H NMR

spectroscopy of ascitic fluid: discrimination between malignant and benign ascites and comparison of the results with conventional methods. *NMR Biomed* 2008; 21(6): 606–14.

94. Vettukattil, R., Hetland, T. E., Flørenes, V. A., Kærn, J., Davidson, B. and Bathen, T. F. Proton magnetic resonance metabolomic characterization of ovarian serous carcinoma effusions: chemotherapy-related effects and comparison with malignant mesothelioma and breast carcinoma. *Hum Pathol* 2013; 44(9): 1859–66.

95. Castellarin, M., Milne, K., Zeng, T., Tse, K., Mayo, M., Zhao, Y. *et al.* Clonal evolution of high-grade serous ovarian carcinoma from primary to recurrent disease. *J Pathol* 2013; 229(4): 515–24.

# Academic applications and the future of molecular pathology

Manuel Salto-Tellez and Benedict Yan

## Introduction

In its inception, the purpose of pathology was to understand the nature of diseases, either by the post-mortem examination as in the work of Morgagni (1682 to 1771) or the description of diseases at the microscope, championed by Virchow (1821 to 1902), among others (1). However, towards the latter part of the last century, pathology began to establish itself as a clinical/diagnostic discipline. Indeed, a pathology diagnostic opinion became a *conditio sine qua non* to start any therapeutic intervention, placing pathology at the heart of therapeutic decision making. Pathologists in this new role would not be so interested in the description of a biological process, but in the accurate taxonomy of diseases that would allow a degree of homogeneity in their treatment. This process, together with the importance of high-impact, basic science in the university arena and the wish to separate research and diagnostic administration, polarized the world of pathology, with relatively few pathologists able to keep a significant presence at both ends of this diagnostic-research dichotomy.

Several factors are changing this paradigm, calling for another turn of the pendulum and bringing diagnostics and research closer once again. In our opinion, this process is driven by the following:

1. The increasing importance of translational research – it is an accepted premise that the basic discovery of new biological mechanisms is as important as the description of the clinical/diagnostic significance of such discovery. Figure 21.1 depicts the process of translation of basic science discoveries into clinically relevant uses. The interface between research and diagnostics/therapeutics has been recognized as

the "weakest link" of this process. Needless to say, this area is best attended to by those who understand the diagnostic and therapeutic aspects of the disease; those who are in daily contact with the clinical samples that are the backbone of translational research; those who are populating some of the most important aspects of the clinical databases; those who are traditionally trained to describe pathological processes, classically in tissues and cells, and more recently at a molecular level; in essence, it is the realm of pathology.

2. Biobanking – the clinical relevance of basic science discoveries will only be as robust as the quality of the samples and the background clinico-pathological information that is supporting it. The creation of such high-quality collections of samples and information is one of the most relevant tasks that academic hospitals can undertake (2). By doing so, hospitals will not only be taking care of the patients of today, but also the patients of tomorrow.

3. Clinical databases – finding ways of capturing in a systematic and user-friendly manner the plethora of clinico-pathological information generated in hospitals, and making it available to researchers in a fully anonymized and confidential manner, within the relevant ethical frameworks, is one of the most important challenges of academic medical bioinformatics. Again, the quality of the curation of this information will dictate the clinical utility of scientific discoveries.

4. Technology and laboratory know-how – there are occasions in which certain laboratory equipment can be purchased under broad academic grants, but it is not affordable within current constraints

*Molecular Pathology: A Practical Guide for the Surgical Pathologist and Cytopathologist*, ed. John M. S. Bartlett, Abeer Shaaban and Fernando Schmitt. Published by Cambridge University Press. © Cambridge University Press, 2016.

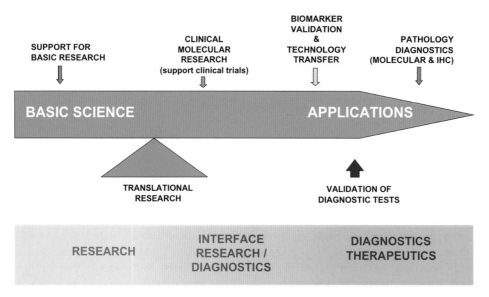

Figure 21.1 Translation of basic science discoveries into clinically relevant uses.

of hospital budgets. On the other hand, sometimes the technical ability to perform certain molecular tests exists in the hospital arena. Hence, the flow of expertise and equipment availability between molecular diagnostics and academia should be encouraged, as it is likely to have a strong synergistic effect in the output of both diagnostics and science. The end result should lead to a more cost-effective paradigm for research development and diagnostic provision.

5. Quality – if we agree with the premise that translational research will generate results directly applicable to diagnostics or therapeutics, and we agree that some of the activities currently accepted within translational research such as clinical trials or biomarker validation will generate results that, in the right ethical context, can be used in diagnosing/treating patients, then it is conceivable that the quality of the laboratory work should be closer to the strict diagnostic standards than the basic discovery ones. The central idea that wherever translational research is carried out, such research should be performed to high standards incorporating GLP, GCP and other robust regulatory frameworks, is understood by the diagnostic industry, and it is slowly percolating through to academic laboratories.

## Understanding molecular diagnostics as an academic discipline

### Biomarkers

The National Institute of Health's definition of biomarker is: "a characteristic that is objectively measured and evaluated as an indicator of normal biologic processes, pathogenic processes, or pharmacologic responses to a therapeutic intervention" (3). Most biomarkers can be measured in biological samples, and can be divided in biomarkers of disease risk, diagnostic markers of disease, biomarkers of prognosis, biomarkers predictive of therapeutic response or pharmacogenomics biomarkers, among others (4). In a world were novel biomarkers can only be defined in full in relation to existing ones, it is essential that molecular diagnostic results are placed in the right context so that they can be related to novel biomarkers detected in these very same cases. Thus, one could say that future biomarker discovery can only take place on the basis of strong molecular diagnostics.

### Areas of molecular diagnostics

Molecular diagnostics involves several key areas, namely:

1. molecular genetics (inherited diseases);
2. molecular infectious diseases;

3. molecular diagnosis of solid tumors (including lymphomas);
4. molecular hemato-oncology; and
5. molecular diagnostics of immunology/ immunodeficiency and transplantation.

In the context of this textbook, molecular pathology/ molecular diagnostics makes reference to "molecular diagnosis of solid tumors" or "molecular diagnostic histopathology or cytopathology" (5). It involves the analysis of all of the biomarker categories stated above. In practical terms, the tests could be described as diagnostic (for instance, sarcoma translocation detection for the diagnosis of sarcoma subtypes), (pre-)genetic (as in the case of MSI and MMR IHC analysis in colorectal cancer prior to genetic analysis) or therapeutic (such as EGFR mutation detection in lung cancer). Interestingly, technologies previously associated to "traditional" pathology, such as immunohistochemistry, are revisited from the point of view of molecular diagnostics, such as HER-2 or Ki-67 IHC in breast cancer. Indeed, one could argue that "therapeutic immunohistochemistry" is therapeutic molecular diagnostics (6).

In view of this, it is not unreasonable to think that the premise once held by many pathologists in the twentieth century that "all diagnostic samples should be treated as potential research samples" is very pertinent these days, and that much needs to be done to populate clinical databases with the results of as many established biomarkers, in a way that is accessible to translational researchers, as is feasible. The measures of quality for this exercise are not different from those which are used in the routine diagnostic setting: relevant laboratory accreditation (CPA, CAP, NATA), strong external quality assurance and internal quality control schemes, turn-around time, a degree of "technical sophistication beyond off-the-shelf kits, etc. Indeed, the foundations of many of these guidelines are found in basic research approaches. Some of these aspects are analyzed in some detail in the next section.

## Molecular pathology – translation research

## Components of a molecular pathology academic programme

The main components of a molecular pathology academic programme, in relation to tissue and cellular

pathology, are shown in Figure 21.2. From looking at these areas and their possible interactions, one could understand the following:

### The need for a synergy between research and diagnostics
#### Clinical trials, biomarker validation and technology transfer

These are areas that clearly sit in the interface between pure diagnostics and research. Although still part of the research endeavor, they are better carried out in laboratory environments adhering to high standards, which ensures that the end product (a diagnosis, a new biomarker or a new diagnostic kit) is fit to be used for patient stratification and therapeutic decision making. As such, one could argue that most of the late stages of research should take place in a laboratory environment that, while investigational in nature, operates as close to accredited standards as possible.

#### Technology availability

The rapid development of technology in molecular diagnostics, together with the move to cost-efficiency and cost-containment in healthcare, suggest that hospitals may not be able to afford the high turnover of technology necessary to detect biomarkers in the best possible manner. Also, the technical know-how to make the most of new technological advances may reside within academia in the first instance. Hence, it would appear that molecular diagnostic laboratories require academic development to maintain their relevance in relation to new technology.

In general, these points explain why many of the leading molecular diagnostic laboratories are within

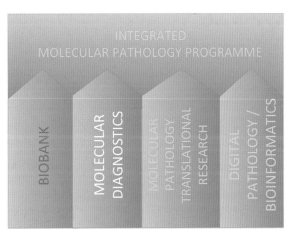

**Figure 21.2** Main components of a molecular pathology academic programme, in relation to tissue and cellular pathology.

academic hospitals, or are run by people with a strong exposure to academic medicine. It also highlights that those who are able to establish that integration in the best possible way will have, as a result, a seamless transition from research to diagnostics, and a cost-efficient diagnostic development.

## Molecular pathology – biobanking

There is no translational research/academic medicine in pathology without high-quality materials and high-quality information (2). As such, the quality of an academic medical center is measured, among other things, by the quality of its biobanking. The collection of tissue, cells, blood or any other human compartment of high quality for research interrogation is necessary, but not sufficient for high-quality research. This material needs to be accompanied by a solid, regularly updated clinicopathological database and, increasingly so, with a record of the research results on those cases kept in biobanks so that, when other users apply for the same materials, they can access the results of those who researched those samples beforehand. This concept transforms the full relevance of biobanks, moving from a "repository of biological samples" to a "repository of science." Again, molecular diagnostics, with good genomic information and excellent left-over DNA and/or RNA materials, are a strong contributor to this holistic view of biobanks.

## Molecular pathology – tissue-based research (FFPE material)

While molecular diagnostic laboratories are generating research materials and research information that is essential for high-quality translational research, the largest and most comprehensive biological collection in pathology departments is the formalin-fixed paraffin-embedded tissue archives (7). These collections should be available for the advancement of molecular pathology (diagnostics and research). There are several ways in which this can be done, which need to take into account the primary interest of the patient, the interest of the diagnostic pathologist with an interest in a particular organ/system, the needs for the diagnostic pathologists of good materials for diagnostic validation and the sample needs for academic research. In our experience, allowing the biobank of the institution to take care of the administration of

these FFPE pathology legacy collections allows the right ethical, scientific and operational framework to make the most of them.

## Academic and diagnostic pathology linked through protocols and technology

These are some of the specific areas where a more coordinated approach between molecular diagnostics in healthcare institutions and academic research would have a synergistic approach in the quality and output of both.

### Morphology

This is the substrate of traditional pathology, but it is also essential for molecular diagnostics and translational research:

1. The histopathological analysis, tissue annotation and macrodissection are, in many cases, absolutely necessary to ensure the best possible quality in tissue-based molecular diagnostics. The morphological analysis prior to molecular testing ensures that: (a) the right sample is analyzed; (b) the area of macrodissection is representative of the lesion, and has a tumor-to-non-neoplastic cellular ratio that is consistent with the sensitivity of the test; (c) areas that may confuse the result of the test are removed from the test itself (such as low-grade adenomas in colorectal cancer KRAS testing or concomitant benign nevi in malignant melanoma BRAF testing); (d) in cases where the final diagnosis is a synthesis of morphological, immunochemistry and molecular analysis, the full integration takes place adequately, as it is the case in lymphoma integrate testing and reporting (8).

2. The interpretation of the molecular research result may be different in the morphological context. For instance, a strong "immunological" signature in gene expression array studies of a certain cancer may mean different things if there is a strong inflammatory response associated to it, or if such response is minimal or absent.

Therefore, it would appear that a morphological analysis is a determinant of molecular diagnostic and research quality. Diagnostic and academic pathology should share such expertise, as a conduit for integration.

## Digital pathology

Quantitation of immunohistochemistry (IHC) or *in situ* hybridization (ISH) is in many ways necessary in the research setting to understand the biological and clinical relevance of a novel biomarker. Similarly, there is already FDA-approved software, related to scanning technology, able to quantitate key biomarkers such as ER, PR and cerbB2/HER2 in breast cancer (9). In general, IHC and ISH in both research and diagnostics should be based on rigorous digitalization and automatic quantitation to allow a process as objective as possible. Digital pathology can be one of those areas where academia and diagnostics can synergize, using the same equipment and similar process for their purpose.

## Tissue microarrays (TMA)

The use of TMA in the process of biomarker discovery and validation is well known in the pathology community (10). There is, however, a diagnostic use of TMA, driven by: (1) the preparation of affordable and manageable controls that can be incorporated to the individual slide, allowing modest savings, but, more importantly, homogeneity in the analytical conditions of both controls and target materials; (2) its use in external quality control programmes (11); (3) TMA can be an excellent framework for specimen exchange, particularly in the context of EQA; and (4) immunophenotyping of a large number of cases (12), where savings are substantial. Again, having a combined service that can provide research and diagnostic TMA services is operationally sound.

## DNA and RNA extractions

Adequate nucleic acid extractions from FFPE material is paramount for both molecular diagnostics and research (7). To date, molecular diagnostics is dominated by single-biomarker PCR testing. In the course of time, the diagnostic community has developed robust protocols for reliable DNA and RNA extraction from FFPE material, incorporating at the same time a series of pre-analytical protocols aiming to have the best tissue sample quality to start with (avoidance of *in vivo* and *ex vivo* ischemia time, consistent time fixation, consistent fixative preparation/purchase, adequate storage of paraffin blocks, etc.). In general, these protocols have also served well the analysis of single biomarkers in the research setting. However, the advent of new technologies, primarily in the research arena at this point, such as high-throughput gene expression or next generation sequencing (NGS), require protocols for RNA/DNA extractions, and protocols to measure the quality of the product, which are much more stringent. Molecular diagnostic operations should adopt these protocols because: (1) they would make better quality nucleic acid available for academic purposes at a shorter turnaround time; and (2) these technologies (particularly NGS) are likely to become the standard of practice in molecular diagnostics in the near future (13, 14).

## High-throughput testing

The application of high-throughput technologies for research and diagnostics follows two differentiated approaches. While in research it is predominantly used for discovery purposes, and thus significant single-biomarker confirmation work goes on after the initial broad discovery exercise, in diagnostics the results need to be ready for diagnostic or therapeutic decision making, with little (if any) need for subsequent confirmation and in a workable turnaround time. The validation of high-throughput testing for diagnostics is a very complex affair, where the usual parameters of the validation are more complex (sensitivity, specificity, accuracy, precision) and others, which are less relevant in single-biomarker testing, can be more determinant (sample source, equipment and operator variability). While there is no question that the molecular diagnostics of the future will have to rely on technologies that are able to interrogate many biomarkers at once, the process of making this technology widely available and affordable will require, yet again, the collaboration between academics and diagnosticians to do so in the shortest possible interval.

## Bioinformatics

Bioinformatics in molecular pathology is paramount at many levels:

1. Digital pathology – the development of diagnostic algorithms that are able to score tissue-based IHC or ISH results in a reliable manner is in the realm of bioinformaticians. More and more often, biomarkers that are IHC/ISH based and the results of which need to be as quantitative as possible to guide therapeutic intervention will need to be analyzed in a bioinformatics-led, digital manner (15). Digital pathologists,

bioinformaticians and diagnostic pathologists will need to work closely so that the final algorithm and the pathway to use it take into account all of the provisos related to the complexity of tissues.

2. Clinicopathological databases – the natural repository of these databases are the biobanks (16), directly associated to pathology departments. Simple databases can be managed by biostatisticians. However, the collection of high-throughput analyses and the correlation with single biomarkers and complex clinicopathological data require the design of bioinfomaticians.

3. High-throughput tests – the product of high-throughput diagnostics, as defined in gene expression signatures (17) and more recently in NGS diagnostic validations (18), requires bioinformatics curation that appears as decisive to the final result and its quality as any other aspect of the diagnostic process.

4. In essence, it is envisaged that bioinformaticians will have a strong presence in the future of "genomic diagnostics," and there are already attempts to define how they should be integrated in healthcare institutions.

## Molecular diagnostics and the future of pathology

## How is molecular testing transforming the practice of pathology?

Most disciplines within the specialty of pathology and laboratory medicine have embraced molecular medicine. Virologists are primarily molecular virologists; hematologists have integrated molecular testing as an integral part of their disease taxonomy and, on many occasions, run molecular diagnostic laboratories within their operations; we do not understand clinical genetics without molecular genetics; blood-banking and immunology is increasingly incorporating molecular techniques. These practitioners are not only aware of the importance of molecular testing in the overall diagnostic or therapeutic opinion, but they also get actively involved in the technical generation of the molecular diagnostic results and, more importantly, in the molecular interpretation of these results.

It is fair to say that, with a few notable exceptions, tissue and cellular pathologists have not risen to this challenge. Histo and cytopathologists are beginning to understand when a sample needs to be submitted for molecular testing and the added value of the molecular result in the overall diagnostic opinion. However, they detach themselves from the whole "molecular diagnostic process." The reasons are many and may be linked to the very epistemological nature of the information-acquisition process in morpho-pathology (1). Regardless of the cause of this detachment, we witness the development of an increasing layer of molecular diagnostic complexity between the original histological and immunohistochemical diagnostic opinion and therapeutic decision making (19), much of which has been illustrated in this book. The result of this process does not negate the value of morphological assessment in the present and the future of medicine. However, while necessary, it is simply not sufficient, and as molecular diagnostics becomes more prominent, morphologists may play a more peripheral role in the process of therapeutic decisions unless they focus on the connection between their current skills and the need to adapt to a new molecular era.

Histopathologists have been for almost a century the key "taxonomists" of disease, and indeed disease classifications involved large morphological detail. This role is now being challenged. The epitome of this change is adenocarcinoma of the lung. The WHO classification of this disease is predominantly morphology-based (20), with numerous subgroups with little (if any) unequivocal clinical/therapeutic significance. This can be compared with the current therapeutic classifications where we are able to define more than half of lung adenocarcinomas with single molecular biomarkers that are actionable or potentially actionable (21). Are we therefore suggesting that the value of morphology is gone? Far from it. In the characterization of lung adenocarcinomas, histo- and cytopathologists need to: (1) establish the diagnosis of adenocarcinoma; (2) assess the suitability of the resection in the surgical specimen; and (3) establish the TNM staging of the disease. These are all absolute requirements before molecular testing kicks in and the whole morpho-molecular picture is completed. Thus, it would appear that the importance of morphology has not diminished: it is just changing.

# Expanding the horizons: non-tissue-based platforms of cancer diagnostics

There are an emerging number of technologies and platforms which seemingly fall outside the domain of conventional tissue-based diagnostics. These include the detection of circulating tumor cells (CTCs) in the blood and *in vitro* drug sensitivity testing akin to that performed in the microbiological setting. A discussion of these subjects follows.

The clinical utility of detecting CTCs lies in their value as prognostic and therapeutic predictive biomarkers. Currently, the only FDA-approved platform for the detection of CTCs is the CELLSEARCH® system, which relies on immunomagnetic isolation of cells in the blood using epithelial-specific antibodies. Immunofluorescence for cytokeratins, CD45 and DNA is performed, following which an operator verifies these cells as CTCs if they express keratin, do not express CD45 and have a nucleus. Other emerging platforms generally also rely on some form of morphological assessment (22). It is our belief that the interests of cancer patients are better served if this platform is managed by a tissue-based diagnostician, since the conceptual framework underpinning CTCs is complex, and requires expertise in both disease mechanisms and morphology.

*In vitro* drug sensitivity testing involves the testing of therapeutic agents using primary cell lines isolated from the tumor, the results of which are used to guide therapy selection for the patient. Although several technical hurdles exist at present, many studies have shown a correlation with *in vitro* and *in vivo* sensitivity in an oncological context (23). We feel that this platform will become increasingly pertinent as high-throughput diagnostic platforms become more established, since the inevitable deluge of actionable targets

as well as targeted therapeutics in the future necessarily complicates therapy selection. Again, because such an assay requires a deep knowledge of tumor biology as well as therapeutics, the tissue-based molecular diagnostician is eminently placed to lead this endeavor.

## The need for a change in training

To maintain a key role in the patient care, morpho-pathology will need to actively embrace molecular diagnostics (24). Failure to do so would have rather detrimental consequences: (1) others will carry out molecular diagnostics in tissue samples, moving a significant component of tissue-based pathology away from anatomic pathologists; (2) the ideal interface to link the clinical practice of medicine and the academic, scientific understanding of diseases will disappear; and (3) we will lose out on the revenue generation that molecular medicine (the fastest growing area of medicine) is generating. To embrace molecular diagnostics: (1) morpho-molecular integration needs to happen where it really matters, namely at the daily clinical practice at sign out; and (2) molecular diagnostics needs to be an integral component of tissue pathology teaching in our residency programs.

## The reward

Eventually, he/she who delivers the morpho-molecular integration in the diagnostic opinion will have the most interesting and most relevant job in laboratory medicine. Incorporating and delivering the molecular testing component of tissue diagnosis will make the overall diagnosis more meaningful for the patient, and will make us better histopathologists and cytopatholgists.

# References

1. Chan, J. Y. and Salto-Tellez, M. Opinion: molecular gestalt and modern pathology. *Adv Anat Pathol* 2012; 19(6): 425–6.

2. Simeon-Dubach, D., Burt, A. D. and Hall, P. A. Quality really matters: the need to improve specimen quality in biomedical research. *Histopathology* 2012; 61(6): 1003–5.

3. Biomarkers Definitions Working, Group. Biomarkers and surrogate endpoints: preferred definitions and conceptual framework. *Clin Pharmacol Ther* 2001; 69(3): 89–95.

4. Kennedy, R. D., Salto-Tellez, M., Harkin, D. P. and Johnston, P. G. Biomarker identification and clinical validation, Chapter 11 in Cassidy, J., Bissett, D., Spence, R. and Payne, M. (eds.), *Oxford Textbook of Oncology,*

4th edn (Oxford University Press, 2015, in press).

5. Siok-Bian, N., Lee, V., Das, K. and Salto-Tellez, M. The relevance of molecular diagnostics in the practice of surgical pathology. *Expert Opin Med Diagn* 2008; 2(12): 1401–14.

6. McCourt, C. M., Boyle, D., James, J. and Salto-Tellez, M. Immunohistochemistry in the era

of personalised medicine. *J Clin Pathol* 2013; 66(1): 58–61.

7. Das, K., Mohd Omar, M. F., Ong, C. W., Bin Abdul Rashid, S., Peh, B. K., Putti, T. C. *et al.* TRARESA: a tissue microarray-based hospital system for biomarker validation and discovery. *Pathology* 2008; 40(5): 441–9.

8. Ireland, R. Haematological malignancies: the rationale for integrated haematopathology services, key elements of organization and wider contribution to patient care. *Histopathology* 2011; 58(1): 145–54.

9. Bloom, K. and Harrington, D. Enhanced accuracy and reliability of HER-2/neu immunohistochemical scoring using digital microscopy. *Am J Clin Pathol* 2004; 121(5): 620–30.

10. Ilyas, M., Grabsch, H., Ellis, I. O., Womack, C., Brown, R., Berney, D. *et al.* Guidelines and considerations for conducting experiments using tissue microarrays. *Histopathology* 2013; 62(6): 827–39.

11. Packeisen, J., Buerger, H., Krech, R. and Boecker, W. Tissue microarrays: a new approach for quality control in immunohistochemistry. *J Clin Pathol* 2002; 55(8): 613–15.

12. Farmer, P. L., Bailey, D. J., Burns, B. F., Day, A. and LeBrun, D. P. The reliability of lymphoma diagnosis in small tissue samples is heavily influenced by lymphoma subtype. *Am J Clin Pathol* 2007; 128(3): 474–80.

13. Mardis, E. R. Next-generation sequencing platforms. *Annu Rev Anal Chem (Palo Alto Calif)* 2013; 6(1): 287–303.

14. Mahoney, D. W., Therneau, T. M., Anderson, S. K., Jen, J., Kocher, J. P., Reinholz, M. M. *et al.* Quality assessment metrics for whole genome gene expression profiling of paraffin embedded samples. *BMC Res Notes* 2013; 6: 33.

15. Minot, D. M., Kipp, B. R., Root, R. M., Meyer, R. G., Reynolds, C. A., Nassar, A. *et al.* Automated cellular imaging system III for assessing HER2 status in breast cancer specimens: development of a standardized scoring method that correlates with FISH. *Am J Clin Pathol* 2009; 132(1): 133–8.

16. Hewitt, R. E. Biobanking: the foundation of personalized medicine. *Curr Opin Oncol* 2011; 23(1): 112–19.

17. Kennedy, R. D., Bylesjo, M., Kerr, P., Davison, T., Black, J. M., Kay, E. W. *et al.* Development and independent validation of a prognostic assay for stage II colon cancer using formalin-fixed paraffin-embedded tissue. *J Clin Oncol* 2011; 29(35): 4620–6.

18. McCourt, C. M., McArt, D. G., Mills, K., Catherwood, M. A., Maxwell, P., Waugh, D. J. *et al.* Validation of next generation sequencing technologies in comparison to current diagnostic gold standards for BRAF, EGFR and KRAS mutational Aanalysis. *PLoS ONE* 2013; 8(7): e69604, doi:10.1371/journal.pone.0069604.

19. Salto-Tellez M. A case for integrated morphomolecular diagnostic pathologists. *Clin Chem* 2007; 53(7): 1188–90.

20. Travis, W. D., Brambilla, E., Noguchi, M., Nicholson, A. G., Geisinger, K. R., Yatabe, Y. *et al.* International Association for the Study of Lung Cancer/American Thoracic Society/European Respiratory Society international multidisciplinary classification of lung adenocarcinoma. *J Thorac Oncol* 2011; 6(2): 244–85.

21. Pao, W. and Hutchinson, K. E. Chipping away at the lung cancer genome. *Nat Med* 2012; 18(3): 349–51.

22. Fischer, A. H. Circulating tumor cells: seeing is believing. *Arch Pathol Lab Med* 2009; 133(9): 1367–9.

23. Yamamoto, Y., Hiasa, Y., Hirooka, M., Koizumi, Y., Takeji, S., Tokumoto, Y. *et al.* Complete response of a patient with advanced primary splenic histiocytic sarcoma by treatment with chemotherapeutic drugs selected using the collagen gel droplet-embedded culture drug sensitivity test. *Intern Med* 2012; 51(20): 2893–7.

24. Lauwers, G. Y., Black-Schaffer, S. and Salto-Tellez, M. Molecular pathology in contemporary diagnostic pathology laboratory: an opinion for the active role of surgical pathologists. *Am J Surg Pathol* 2010; 34(1): 115–17.

# Index

Note: page numbers in *italics* refer to figures and tables, those in **bold** refer to boxes.

MET gene mutations
  lung cancer 267
  renal cell carcinoma 197
metabolomics, serous effusions 367
methylation
  breast cancer 158–60
    blood circulation 158
    blood-based screening 159–60
    nipple fluid 158–9
  CpG islands 120, 158
    blood-based 159–60
    breast cancer 158–60
  promoter hypermethylation
    breast cancer 160
    in carcinogenesis 158
  see also DNA methylation
5'-methylcytosine 109
MGMT gene methylation, serous
    effusions 364
Microarray Quality Control (MAQC)
    project 79–81
microarrays 71–83
  accuracy of analysis 79–81
  analysis 76–7
  applications 72–4
  biochips 74–5
  cancer diagnostics use 83
  classifiers 80–1
  controls 77
  copy-number 73
  data normalization 76–7
  detection 75–6
  development 71–2
  diagnostic use 77–9
  DNA 78
    diagnostic profiling 84
  DNA methylation profiling 73
  evidence levels for use 83
  evolution of technology 72–3
  expression-based 72–3
  fabrication 74–5
  gene signatures 81
    clinical value 81–2
  guidelines 82
  hybridization 74–5
  image processing 75–6
  normalization 75–6
  precision of analysis 79–81
  principles of technology 74–7
  probes 74
  profiling 25
  prognostic indicators 81–2
  protein arrays 73–4
  regulations 82
  RNA 77, 78
    diagnostic profiling 82–4
  sequence polymorphisms 73
  sequence recognition 74
  serous effusions 365–6

single channel analysis 75, 76
status in clinic 82–4
substrates 74
supervised analyses 77
target labeling 75
transformation 75–6
two-channel platforms 75, 76
types in current use 82
validation for clinical use 81
variablity in analyses 80
microdissection 23
  tumor cell enrichment 25
microRNA (miRNA) 16, 16, 66–7
  aberrations 66
  adrenal cortical adenoma 283
  bile duct neoplasia 219
  biogenesis 67
  biomarkers 160–1
  breast cancer 160–2
    disease progression monitoring
      161
    early detection/diagnosis 161
    male 164
    therapeutic agents/targets 161–2
    treatment response prediction
      161
    tumor sensitization 161–2
  circulating 160–1
  functions 160
  gene expression profiling 72–3
  malignancy association 66
  pancreatic neoplasia 219
  profiling 66–7
  serous effusions 366
  in situ hybridization 43
microsatellite instability (MSI)
  colorectal cancer 119–24
    clinical applications 121–2
    detection methods 122–4
    distal sporadic 121
    5-FU response 208
    high phenotype 119–22
    immunohistochemistry of
      mismatch repair proteins 123
    low phenotype 121–2
    mutator phenotype 119
    prognostic/predictive marker 121
  gastrointestinal tract 212
  Lynch syndrome 122, 203, 203
  PCR for markers 122–3
  serous effusions 364–5
microsatellite stability (MSS),
    colorectal cancer 119–21
microscopy, relevance of 2–4
minor groove binding probes (MGB) 61
mismatch repair system (MMR)
  defects
    colorectal cancer 119
    Lynch syndrome 122, 203

immunohistochemistry in colorectal
    cancer 123
MLH1 promoter methylation 123–4
MLK3 gene mutations, colorectal
    cancer 121
molecular beacon probe 61
molecular diagnostic cytopathology,
    gastrointestinal tract 211–13
molecular diagnostics 374–5
  see also diagnostic molecular
    pathology
molecular pathology
  academic programme 375–8
  diagnostic assays 2
  morphology 376
  protocols 376–8
  synergy between research/
    diagnostics 375–6
  technology 376–8
  training 379
  translational research 375–8
  see also diagnostic molecular
    pathology
molecular profiling programs 140–2
  clinical 140–2, 141
  genotype matched treatment 140–2
  sequencing technologies 140
  tumor samples 140
molecular targeted agents 137
  tumors 130–1
molecular testing 378
monoclonal gammopathy of
    undetermined significance
    (MGUS) 317
morphology 376
mRNA alterations
  fine-needle aspiration samples 24–5
  gene expression profiling 72–3
  in situ hybridization 43
  technical aspects of molecular
    studies 26
mRNA decay 16
mRNA expression profiling, breast
    cancer 154
mRNA extraction 23
mTOR pathway, pancreatic
    neuroendocrine tumors 288
MUC gene mutations, serous effusions
    361
mucinous cystic neoplasm (MCN)
    215–16
mucosa-associated lymphoid tissue
    (MALT) lymphoma 316
multi-color FISH 41–2
  variation 42
multiple endocrine neoplasia (MEN)
    syndromes 276
  adrenal cortical adenoma 283
  adrenal cortical carcinoma 283–4